Veterinary Nursing Strategy

Veterinary Nursing Strategy

Crystal Schaeffer
Director of Technician Development
Noah's Animal Hospitals
Indianapolis, IN, USA

Myranda Jennings
Manager of Clinical Development
Noah's Westside Animal Hospital
Indianapolis, IN, USA

WILEY

Published by John Wiley & Sons, Inc., Hoboken, New Jersey.

Library of Congress Cataloging-in-Publication Data applied for:

Paperback ISBN: 9781394330850

Cover Design: Wiley
Cover Image: Crystal Schaeffer

Set in 9.5/12.5pt STIXTwoText by Straive, Pondicherry, India

Printed and bound by CPI Group (UK) Ltd, Croydon, CR0 4YY

C9781394330850_060726

Dedication

"I solemnly dedicate myself to aiding animals and society by providing excellent care and services for animals, by alleviating animal suffering, and by promoting public health. I accept my obligations to practice my profession conscientiously and with sensitivity, adhering to the profession's Code of Ethics, and furthering my knowledge and competence through a commitment to lifelong learning."

Contents

Part I

Foundations of Veterinary Nursing in the Dog and Cat

1

Introduction to Veterinary Nursing

Veterinary nursing is a unique and evolving profession that sits at the intersection of science and compassion. As an essential branch of veterinary medicine, it combines clinical skills with a profound understanding of animal welfare, offering patients both lifesaving care and supportive comfort. Throughout history, veterinary nursing has grown from informal caregiving roles to a specialized, highly respected field with a solid foundation in medical knowledge and technical expertise. This evolution reflects broader shifts in the veterinary profession and society's understanding of the bond between humans and animals.

This introductory chapter delves into the evolution of veterinary nursing, defining it as both an art and a science. In doing so, it highlights the roles that veterinary technicians play, how the profession has developed over the years, and the skills required to support veterinarians in the comprehensive care of animal patients. In exploring veterinary nursing as an art, we examine the critical soft skills—empathy, communication, intuition—that enable technicians to address the nuanced needs of both animal patients and their owners. As a science, veterinary nursing is rooted in evidence-based practices, rigorous technical knowledge, and a commitment to clinical excellence. Together, these dual aspects form a holistic view of veterinary nursing that prioritizes both medical care and humane compassion.

Defining Veterinary Nursing as an Art

The "art" of veterinary nursing is rooted in the human–animal bond, where understanding and empathy play central roles. Veterinary technicians often work with animals that cannot communicate their pain, discomfort, or fear in conventional ways. Therefore, they must develop the skills to interpret nonverbal cues, recognize subtle behavioral changes, and understand the unique personalities and needs of each patient. This empathetic care is essential, as it reduces stress for animals, strengthens patient outcomes, and enhances the caregiver–patient relationship.

Moreover, veterinary technicians must navigate difficult conversations and emotional situations, offering guidance and reassurance to clients who may be distressed about their pets' health. This requires a compassionate and emotionally resilient approach, underscoring the importance of interpersonal skills and sensitivity. Beyond technical expertise, veterinary technicians are expected to cultivate soft skills such as communication, empathy, emotional intelligence, adaptability, teamwork, and conflict resolution. These competencies allow them to collaborate effectively with colleagues, foster trust with clients, and maintain composure in high-stress or emotionally charged situations.

The art of veterinary nursing also involves adapting care practices to each animal's unique context, whether they are working animals, beloved family pets, or exotic species with specialized needs. By integrating technical proficiency with these vital soft skills, veterinary technicians provide holistic care that addresses not only the medical but also the emotional and relational dimensions of veterinary practice.

The Evolution of Veterinary Nursing: Shifts in the Profession and Society's Perception of the Human–Animal Bond

The profession of veterinary nursing has evolved considerably, influenced by advancements in veterinary medicine and shifting societal values around animal welfare. Veterinary nursing was initially perceived as a support role with limited recognition and minimal formal training. However, as the importance of animals in human lives became more prominent, veterinary nursing evolved into a specialized field with structured education, certification, and well-defined roles. This progression reflects not only internal shifts within the veterinary profession but also societal changes in our collective understanding of animals as sentient beings deserving compassionate, individualized care (Figure 1.1).

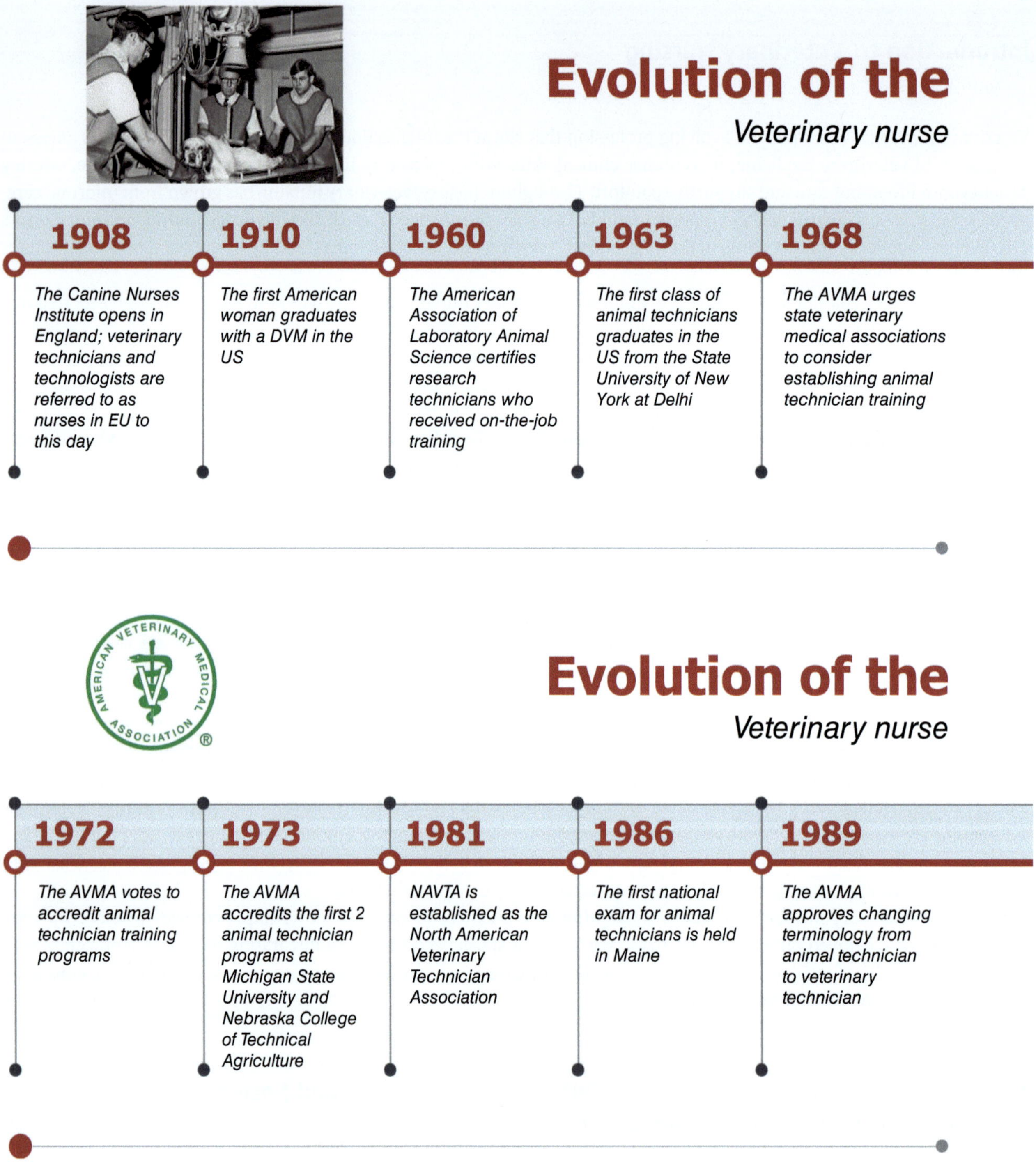

Figure 1.1 Evolution of the veterinary nurse (1908–2018). *Source:* AVMA (2018a, 2024), NAVTA (2024d), AALAS (2024), Purdue University (2018), RCVS (2024a), SUNY Delhi (2024).

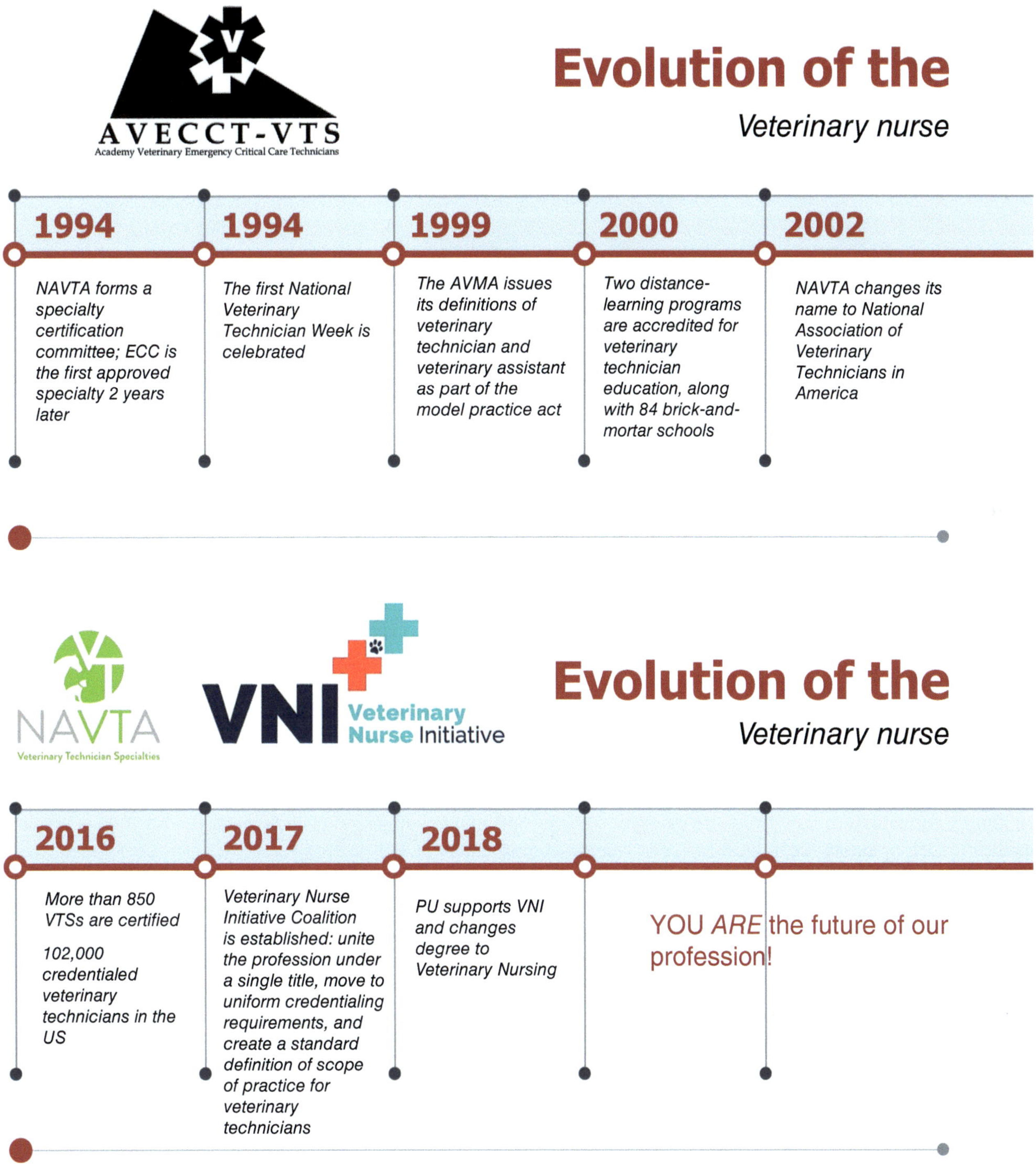

Figure 1.1 (Continued)

The Human–Animal Bond: A Driving Force in Veterinary Nursing's Development

One of the most significant influences on the development of veterinary nursing is the evolving concept of the human-animal bond. Historically, animals served functional roles as sources of labor, protection, and sustenance. However, beginning in the 20th century, animals increasingly assumed companion roles in human lives (AVMA 2018a; Serpell 1996). This shift has resulted in a corresponding expectation for high-quality medical and nursing care for animals, akin to that

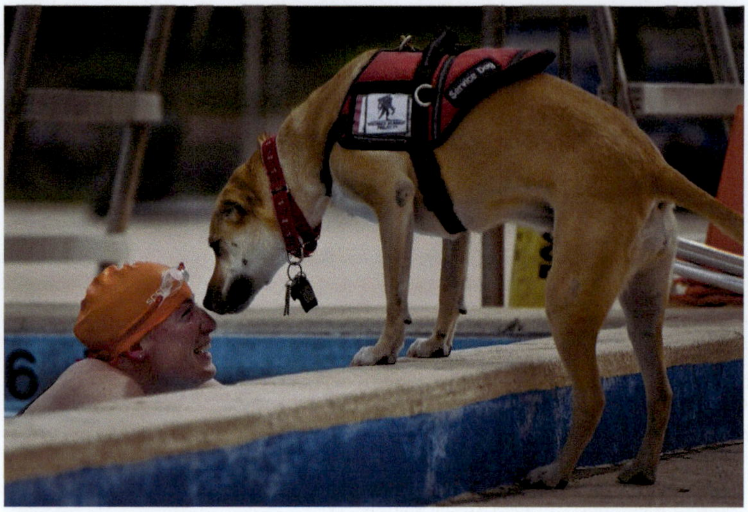

Figure 1.2 A swimmer with a service dog, illustrating the bond and assistance role of service animals. *Source:* US Air Force / Flickr.

provided in human healthcare. Veterinary nursing has thus adapted to meet the needs of animals who are viewed not only as functional beings but as members of families and even as extensions of personal identity.

Research into the human–animal bond has further highlighted the psychological and physiological benefits of animal companionship, influencing the perceived value of veterinary care. Animals are now recognized for their role in reducing human stress, enhancing emotional well-being, and even assisting in medical and psychological therapies (Beck and Katcher 2003; Fine 2019). This understanding has deepened the empathy and dedication within the veterinary nursing profession, as technicians and veterinarians alike strive to honor the emotional connection that humans share with their animals (Figure 1.2).

To meet these evolving expectations, veterinary nursing has transitioned from an auxiliary role to a highly specialized discipline with comprehensive educational pathways. Early veterinary nursing education primarily consisted of on-the-job training, where technical skills were developed through apprenticeship-like models. However, as the profession gained legitimacy, formalized training programs emerged, covering both general nursing care and specific fields within veterinary medicine, such as anesthesia, critical care, and emergency medicine.

Veterinary nursing education now includes rigorous coursework in clinical sciences, such as pharmacology, diagnostic imaging, anesthesia management, and pathology. This academic foundation is complemented by practical training, enabling veterinary technicians to bridge the gap between scientific knowledge and hands-on care. Such specialization allows veterinary technicians to play critical roles in patient assessment, treatment planning, and procedural support, elevating the standard of care for animal patients.

Specialization within veterinary nursing has also expanded in response to the diversification of veterinary medicine itself. For instance, the demand for expertise in oncology, physical therapy, and rehabilitation has grown as animal patients now routinely receive treatment options once reserved for humans. Veterinary technicians with advanced certifications in these areas provide crucial support to veterinarians by conducting assessments, administering specialized treatments, and providing continuity of care across complex medical cases (Table 1.1).

Integration of Ethical Considerations and Patient Advocacy

The evolution of veterinary nursing is also marked by a heightened focus on ethical considerations and patient advocacy. Veterinary technicians serve as advocates for their patients, striving to ensure that animals receive compassionate, humane care. Unlike DVMs, whose advocacy often takes the form of medical decision-making, diagnostics, and treatment planning, veterinary technicians advocate at the bedside level. They are the patient's constant presence, monitoring comfort, observing subtle changes, and ensuring that the animal's voice is represented in every clinical discussion. This close proximity

Table 1.1 Veterinary nursing pathway: education → certification → specialization.

Stage	Description	Examples
Education	Formal veterinary nursing/technology degree programs (associate, bachelor's, or diploma). Coursework includes anatomy, physiology, pharmacology, anesthesia, and clinical practice.	SUNY Delhi, Purdue University, RCVS-accredited programs
Certification	Credentialing via national or state licensing exams (e.g., VTNE in the US). Ensures competency in core nursing knowledge and clinical skills.	VTNE (US), RCVS Veterinary Nurse Registration (UK), provincial licensing exams
Specialization	Advanced Veterinary Technician Specialties (VTS) provide credentialed technicians with opportunities to expand their scope of practice in specific disciplines.	VTS (Anesthesia and Analgesia); VTS (Behavior); VTS (Clinical Pathology); VTS (Clinical Practice [Canine/Feline, Exotic Companion Animal, Production Animal]); VTS (Dentistry); VTS (Dermatology); VTS (Diagnostic Imaging); VTS (Emergency & Critical Care [ECC]); VTS (Equine Veterinary Nursing); VTS (Internal Medicine [Small Animal, Large Animal, Oncology, Neurology, Cardiology]); VTS (Laboratory Animal Medicine); VTS (Nutrition); VTS (Oncology); VTS (Ophthalmology); VTS (Physical Rehabilitation); VTS (Surgery); VTS (Zoological Medicine)

Source: Author's own (2025).

allows technicians to interpret behaviors and nonverbal cues that may otherwise go unnoticed, providing an essential layer of advocacy grounded in the daily lived experience of the patient.

The advocacy of veterinary technicians does not stand in contrast to that of the veterinarian but rather complements it. Where the DVM brings advanced diagnostic acumen and authority in medical decision-making, the veterinary technician contributes a nuanced understanding of the patient's comfort, emotional state, and response to treatment. Together, they form a dual advocacy model—one that unites medical judgment with patient-centered nursing insight. In this collaborative framework, technicians elevate the veterinarian's capacity to make informed decisions, while veterinarians empower technicians to ensure that their observations and recommendations directly shape the patient's care. This synergy strengthens the veterinary team's collective ability to uphold the welfare of the animal while supporting the client's understanding and trust in the process.

Euthanasia, pain management, and quality-of-life decisions exemplify the art of veterinary nursing because they demand a fusion of clinical knowledge, ethical reasoning, and profound empathy. In end-of-life situations, veterinary technicians often provide a quiet, stabilizing presence that reassures both patient and client. They advocate for dignity in the animal's final moments, ensuring comfort through gentle handling, analgesia, and an atmosphere of compassion. In pain management, technicians act as both monitors and interpreters of subtle behavioral cues, pushing for interventions when they recognize signs of discomfort that may not be immediately evident in diagnostic findings. Similarly, in discussions surrounding quality of life, technicians frequently serve as mediators—helping clients voice their concerns, translating clinical data into compassionate terms, and emphasizing the animal's lived experience.

These domains highlight why veterinary nursing is both a science and an art. They showcase not only the technician's technical proficiency in administering analgesics or supporting euthanasia protocols but also the artistry of empathy, presence, and advocacy that transforms medical care into humane care. In this way, veterinary technicians embody the moral and emotional core of veterinary medicine, ensuring that patient welfare remains at the forefront, even in the most ethically complex circumstances.

Euthanasia is one of the most emotionally and ethically challenging aspects of veterinary medicine, requiring veterinary technicians to make decisions that impact the quality and dignity of an animal's final moments. Euthanasia is typically considered when an animal's suffering outweighs its quality of life, often due to terminal illness, severe injury, or chronic, unmanageable pain. In these situations, veterinary technicians play a vital role in advocating for the animal's best interests, sometimes needing to gently guide pet owners toward accepting the difficult decision to say goodbye. Veterinary technicians are trained to assess signs of suffering that may not be immediately obvious to pet owners, such as changes in behavior, decreased appetite, or signs of distress that indicate chronic pain or discomfort. By sharing these insights, technicians can help owners understand when euthanasia may be the most compassionate option, fostering a decision-making process rooted in empathy and a commitment to minimizing suffering. During the euthanasia process itself, veterinary technicians provide support not only to the animal but also to the grieving family, ensuring the procedure is conducted with dignity and respect. Veterinary technicians may offer guidance on how to comfort the pet, explaining each step to reassure the owners and maintain a calm environment. This compassionate involvement supports both the animal and the family through a painful experience, providing solace in the knowledge that their pet's final moments were marked by peace and dignity.

Pain management is a crucial aspect of veterinary nursing, representing one of the purest expressions of the art of care. To alleviate suffering is not only a clinical duty but also an ethical calling that defines the veterinary technician's role as both healer and advocate. Animals entrusted to our care cannot describe their pain in words; instead, their discomfort is written in posture, movement, expression, and the subtle changes only a skilled and attentive eye can perceive. Here lies the artistry of nursing—the ability to interpret these silent languages and transform them into action that restores comfort and dignity.

In practice, pain management requires more than pharmacological precision. It is an act of presence, empathy, and intuition. A technician kneeling by a recovering surgical patient, softly adjusting a blanket, or gently encouraging an arthritic dog to rise after analgesia, embodies the quiet artistry of nursing. These moments go beyond technical administration of opioids, NSAIDs, or adjunctive therapies; they reflect an attunement to the animal's individual experience of pain and healing. Nonpharmacological strategies such as gentle massage, laser therapy, physical rehabilitation, or acupuncture are not merely adjuncts—they are extensions of a holistic, patient-centered philosophy that seeks not only to treat but to comfort.

Collaboration with the veterinarian transforms this artistry into a complete medical and nursing symphony. The DVM designs the pharmacological plan, while the technician ensures it is experienced by the patient as relief, not simply as a prescription. The technician's continuous monitoring, advocacy for adjustments, and intimate knowledge of the animal's demeanor allow the medical plan to evolve into something responsive and humane.

Ultimately, pain management showcases the art of veterinary nursing because it reveals the delicate balance between science and compassion. It requires pharmacology, physiology, and diagnostic insight, but it also demands gentleness, empathy, and an unwavering commitment to comfort. In every tail wag restored, every eased breath, and every softened gaze, the technician's artistry is evident—a testament to the profound responsibility of alleviating suffering and preserving the quality of life that animals so deeply deserve (Table 1.2).

Veterinary technicians are also instrumental in educating pet owners about recognizing signs of pain at home and administering prescribed pain relief safely. This is particularly important in managing chronic pain conditions, such as arthritis in older animals, where ongoing assessment and adjustment of treatment are necessary. By empowering owners with knowledge and support, veterinary technicians extend the reach of pain management beyond the clinic, ensuring that animals experience as little discomfort as possible in their daily lives.

Yet this role demands more than instruction—it calls for perceptive sensitivity to the emotional landscape that often shapes how owners receive and process information. Pain in a beloved pet is rarely understood in purely clinical terms; it is filtered through emotions such as denial, anger, grief, bargaining, and fear. A technician's ability to recognize these emotional responses and gently navigate them is a profound aspect of the art of veterinary nursing. When an owner resists acknowledging their pet's pain out of denial, the technician may lean into subtle observations—demonstrating how the

Table 1.2 Examples of acute vs. chronic pain in dogs and cats.

Category	Dogs	Cats
Acute pain	• Postoperative pain (spay/neuter, orthopedic surgery) • Acute trauma (fractures, lacerations) • Otitis externa (sudden severe ear pain) • Pancreatitis (acute onset abdominal pain) • Dental extraction pain	• Postsurgical pain (OHE, mass removal) • Acute trauma (HBC, bite wounds) • Urethral obstruction (painful straining) • Acute pancreatitis • Dental extraction pain
Chronic pain	• Osteoarthritis and degenerative joint disease • Chronic intervertebral disc disease (IVDD) • Chronic otitis • Chronic pancreatitis • Cancer-associated pain (osteosarcoma, soft tissue tumors)	• Osteoarthritis (often subtle, decreased mobility) • Stomatitis and chronic gingivostomatitis • Chronic kidney disease (musculoskeletal pain, oral ulcers) • Cancer-associated pain • Chronic cystitis (FIC-related pain)

Source: Author's own (2025).

animal hesitates to climb stairs or avoids certain movements. When anger or grief emerges, the technician's calm presence and empathetic listening create a safe space for owners to express their distress while still receiving critical education.

This perceptive advocacy ensures that the animal's suffering is not masked by human emotion. By combining clinical expertise with emotional intelligence, veterinary technicians bridge the gap between what the animal experiences and what the owner can accept. In doing so, they honor both the patient's silent needs and the client's very human vulnerability, fostering trust, clarity, and ultimately, better patient outcomes.

Quality of life encompasses more than just the absence of pain; it also includes mobility, appetite, social interactions, and the intangible joys that give an animal's life meaning. The art of veterinary nursing emerges in this space, where clinical observation blends with compassion and empathy. Veterinary technicians, often spending the most time with patients, are uniquely positioned to notice subtle changes that reflect well-being—the dog that no longer greets with a wagging tail, the cat that retreats from family interactions, or the aging pet whose eyes no longer brighten at the sight of a favorite toy. These observations go beyond medical data; they are windows into the lived experience of the patient.

As advocates, veterinary technicians champion the preservation and enhancement of these moments of joy, comfort, and connection. In cases of chronic or degenerative disease, their artistry lies in balancing science with sensitivity: interpreting laboratory results and clinical findings while also weighing how mobility, appetite, rest, and emotional engagement contribute to an animal's daily life. This holistic view of care acknowledges that animals, like humans, exist within an emotional and physical continuum, where suffering is not always measurable by diagnostic values but can be deeply felt through changes in spirit and behavior.

The art of veterinary nursing in quality-of-life care is also reflected in the technician's role as communicator and mediator. They help clients see beyond fear and grief, guiding them with compassion through difficult choices while ensuring that the animal's perspective remains at the center. Through their presence, empathy, and perceptive advocacy, veterinary technicians transform quality-of-life assessment from a checklist into a profoundly human–animal experience—one that honors dignity, nurtures comfort, and cherishes the bond that defines why veterinary nursing is both a science and an art.

In palliative and hospice care, veterinary technicians often serve as the primary caregivers guided by indirect supervision of veterinarians, providing comfort measures that focus on quality rather than cure. This may involve adjustments to diet, environmental modifications to ease mobility, and the use of pain relief or appetite stimulants. These interventions are designed to help the animal enjoy its remaining time, even if a complete recovery is not possible. By advocating for these quality-of-life measures, veterinary technicians ensure that animals receive compassionate care tailored to their individual needs and circumstances.

The artistry of this role rests heavily on communication, critical thinking, and in-the-moment understanding. Communication is essential not only with the veterinarian but also with the client, who may be navigating anticipatory grief, denial, or fear. Veterinary technicians must convey complex medical concepts with clarity and empathy, ensuring that clients feel supported while decisions remain centered on the animal's well-being. Critical thinking allows technicians to interpret subtle clinical signs in real time—recognizing, for example, when decreased mobility signals worsening discomfort, or when an intervention is no longer providing benefit.

Equally important is the technician's capacity for in-the-moment understanding, the ability to balance medical judgment with compassion in dynamic, emotionally charged situations. A patient may suddenly refuse food, collapse, or exhibit new behaviors, requiring immediate adaptation of the care plan. In these moments, the technician draws upon their knowledge, intuition, and emotional intelligence to provide both clinical guidance and comfort, bridging science with humane care. Through this integration of communication, critical reasoning, and presence, veterinary technicians elevate palliative and hospice care into an art form—one that honors life, eases suffering, and preserves dignity during an animal's final chapter.

The Role of Ethical Standards and Professional Guidelines

The ethical framework of veterinary nursing provides both structure and support in navigating the complexity of clinical decision-making. Regulatory bodies and professional associations establish ethical standards that define the responsibilities of veterinary technicians, emphasizing principles of animal welfare and patient-centered care. These codes of ethics provide scientific and professional scaffolding—the rules, standards, and boundaries—that guide technicians in advocating for their patients even in the most difficult of circumstances.

Yet within this framework, the art of veterinary nursing flourishes. Ethical codes outline what should be done, but it is the technician's perception, empathy, and ability to interpret each unique situation that breathes humanity into these standards. A technician may rely on their scientific training to recognize indicators of suffering, but it is their artistry—listening to the unspoken cues of an animal or recognizing the grief and denial in an owner's voice—that allows them to translate ethical principles into compassionate action.

This balance of art and science allows veterinary technicians to serve as patient advocates with both credibility and compassion. Science provides the framework: evidence-based guidelines, professional standards, and regulatory expectations. The art provides the interpretation: understanding when to push for stronger pain management, how to support a client through the stages of grief, and how to ensure the patient's silent needs are honored amid conflicting viewpoints. Together, art and science transform ethical codes from abstract doctrine into lived practice, ensuring that the welfare of animals remains at the very center of veterinary nursing.

These ethical guidelines are essential for navigating end-of-life care, pain management, and quality-of-life decisions, as they provide a foundation upon which veterinary technicians can base their actions. By adhering to these standards, veterinary technicians uphold the integrity of their profession and foster trust with both clients and the veterinary team.

Ethical standards in veterinary nursing are influenced by both regulatory guidelines and societal expectations. Veterinary technician associations and regulatory bodies have established codes of ethics that outline the responsibilities of veterinary technicians, including principles of animal welfare, client communication, and professional conduct. Adhering to these ethical standards is essential not only for the well-being of animal patients but also for maintaining public trust in the veterinary profession. This trust is vital, as clients increasingly expect veterinary professionals to provide compassionate and ethical care that respects the dignity of their animals.

Technological Advancements and Their Impact on Veterinary Nursing

Technology has played a transformative role in veterinary nursing, enabling more accurate diagnostics, advanced treatments, and improved patient monitoring. The integration of technology into veterinary practices has expanded the capabilities of veterinary technicians, allowing them to perform complex procedures and manage sophisticated medical equipment.

For example, advancements in diagnostic imaging, such as digital radiography, ultrasound, and magnetic resonance imaging (MRI), have revolutionized the way diseases are diagnosed and treated in animals. Veterinary technicians are often responsible for operating these machines, as well as interpreting diagnostic quality and ensuring patient comfort during imaging procedures. Additionally, anesthesia management has become increasingly sophisticated, with veterinary technicians administering and monitoring anesthesia levels using computerized systems that ensure greater precision and safety for patients.

The emergence of telemedicine in veterinary practice represents another significant technological shift, broadening access to veterinary care and allowing veterinary technicians to support remote patient monitoring and consultations. Telemedicine platforms enable veterinary technicians to engage with clients in real time, providing advice on postoperative care, medication administration, and routine health assessments (Volk et al. 2021). This immediacy demands both real-time decision-making and critical thinking, as technicians must quickly assess clinical information presented virtually, interpret patient status through owner descriptions and visual cues, and provide guidance that is both safe and effective.

Here, the art and science of veterinary nursing intersect seamlessly. Science lies in evidence-based recommendations, pharmacological accuracy, and adherence to clinical protocols. The art emerges in the technician's ability to listen perceptively, interpret nonverbal cues from both the patient and the client, and tailor communication with empathy and clarity. A dog reluctant to eat after surgery, or a cat displaying subtle signs of discomfort, may not be easily quantified over a screen; yet through careful questioning, observation, and intuition, technicians can identify underlying issues and advise the owner with confidence.

Telemedicine also reflects the holistic evolution of veterinary care, where the goal extends beyond the clinic walls to encompass the well-being of both patient and owner. By guiding owners through postoperative challenges, chronic disease management, or medication protocols in the comfort of their home, veterinary technicians reduce stress for the animal while empowering the client. This integrative approach not only enhances continuity of care but also deepens trust, reinforcing the human–animal bond and the technician's role as both clinical professional and compassionate advocate.

Ultimately, telemedicine exemplifies how veterinary nursing continues to evolve—leveraging advancements in technology to provide broader access, more responsive care, and stronger partnerships with owners. It is in this balance of rapid clinical reasoning, scientific rigor, and the artistry of empathy that veterinary technicians ensure that patients and their families receive the highest standard of care, no matter where they are.

Equally transformative has been the role of social media and digital learning platforms. Veterinary technology and technician influencers have created widely accessible educational content, making continuing education and skill development possible far beyond the walls of traditional conferences or urban veterinary hubs. Through podcasts, video demonstrations, case discussions, and interactive forums, technicians in rural or resource-limited areas can now learn advanced anesthesia protocols, emergency triage strategies, or patient handling techniques without the barrier of travel. This digital democratization of knowledge has not only expanded professional growth opportunities but has also strengthened a sense of community among technicians, connecting individuals across geographic and cultural divides. In this way, technology does more than enhance diagnostics and patient care—it also amplifies the reach of veterinary nursing education itself. By combining sophisticated medical tools with the immediacy of social media–driven learning, veterinary technicians can continually refine their skills, ensuring that patients everywhere, regardless of location, benefit from high-quality, modern veterinary nursing (Table 1.3).

Table 1.3 Veterinary technician social media and digital learning platforms.

Platform/Resource	Type	Accessibility/ Audience	Access Model	References
Veterinary Support Personnel Network (VSPN)	Online community and CE	Credentialed and noncredentialed veterinary staff	Free (membership required for full access)	VSPN (2025)
Vetfolio	Subscription CE and resources	Veterinary technicians, assistants, DVMs	Paid subscription (with some free trials)	Vetfolio (2025)
NAVTA online CE portal	Professional association CE hub	Members of NAVTA	Paid (NAVTA membership benefit)	NAVTA (2024a)
IVC Journal/IVC Journal Online Learning	Digital learning and articles	Veterinary professionals worldwide	Mixed—free articles, paid CE	IVC Journal (2025)
Veterinary Anesthesia Nerds (Facebook Group)	Peer-to-peer education and case sharing	Technicians with interest in anesthesia/ analgesia	Free (Facebook community)	Veterinary Anesthesia Nerds (2025)
VetTechLife (Instagram and TikTok)	Influencer-led microlearning and skills demos	Technicians, students, broader public	Free (social media content)	VetTechLife (2025)
Veterinary Technician Podcasts (e.g., Radio Vet Nurse, Internal Medicine for Vet Techs)	Audio-based learning and case discussions	Technicians and students seeking ongoing education	Mixed—free episodes, some paid CE credit	Radio Vet Nurse Podcast (2025), Internal Medicine for Vet Techs Podcast (2025)
YouTube Channels (e.g., VIN Foundation, VetTechPrep)	Video demonstrations and tutorials	Students, early-career professionals, rural learners	Mixed—free content, paid advanced modules	VIN Foundation (2025)
Coursera/EdX Veterinary Courses	General MOOC platform	Technicians, students, interdisciplinary learners	Free/low-cost (depending on course)	Coursera (2025)

Source: Compiled by author from NAVTA (2024a), Vetfolio (2025), VSPN (2025), IVC Journal (2025), Veterinary Anesthesia Nerds (2025), VetTechLife (2025), Radio Vet Nurse Podcast (2025), Internal Medicine for Vet Techs Podcast (2025), VIN Foundation (2025), Coursera (2025), LinkedIn Learning (2025).

Challenges and Future Directions in Veterinary Nursing

Despite the significant advancements in veterinary nursing, the profession faces ongoing challenges, including high levels of occupational stress, compassion fatigue, and issues related to professional recognition and compensation (Hatch 2021; Moses et al. 2018). As veterinary technicians are frequently involved in emotionally demanding situations, such as end-of-life care and intensive patient monitoring, managing compassion fatigue has become a priority within the profession. Support systems, mental health resources, and professional resilience training are increasingly recognized as essential for sustaining the well-being of veterinary technicians.

Professional recognition and fair compensation remain pivotal issues within veterinary nursing, despite the critical role veterinary technicians play in patient care. Data from NAVTA's 2024 Demographic Survey shows that the average annual income for technicians is approximately $53,759—yet 39% identify low salary as their biggest concern, and a majority see compensation as the greatest challenge overall (NAVTA 2024a). Many technicians also report feeling underutilized, with nearly half noting little distinction between their responsibilities and those of support staff, and only about a third feel fully valued in clinical roles (NAVTA 2024a; Portland Veterinary Medical Association 2023).

To address this, professional associations like NAVTA and the AVMA have undertaken concerted advocacy efforts. NAVTA's Government Relations Committee has engaged in legislative action across 25 states to establish title protection, standardized credentialing, and a clearly defined scope of practice (NAVTA 2023). In a landmark move, the Colorado legislature enacted House Bill 24-1047, which formally recognizes the expertise of RVTs and VTSs, authorizes appropriate delegation of duties, and clarifies supervision structures—reflecting an urgent need for both recognition and systemic evolution (Colorado Veterinary Medical Association 2024). At the regulatory level, the AAVSB has developed a Practice Act Model to support greater uniformity in credentialing and regulation across jurisdictions, enhancing professional mobility and reinforcing technician roles within veterinary teams (Figure 1.3) (AAVSB 2025).

Where ethical and regulatory frameworks provide the science, this evolving landscape demands the artistry of advocacy, empathy, and professional integrity. Veterinary technicians must navigate not only clinical responsibilities but also the emotional labor of asserting their professional worth, negotiating for recognition, and contributing to the welfare of both patients and the profession.

Looking to the future, veterinary nursing is poised for further evolution, driven by advances in medical knowledge, technology, and societal values. Continued advocacy for the professionalization of veterinary nursing, combined with an emphasis on ethical, compassionate care, will shape the trajectory of the profession. As veterinary technicians expand their roles and expertise, they will continue to enhance the quality of care available to animal patients, honoring the human–animal bond that lies at the heart of their work.

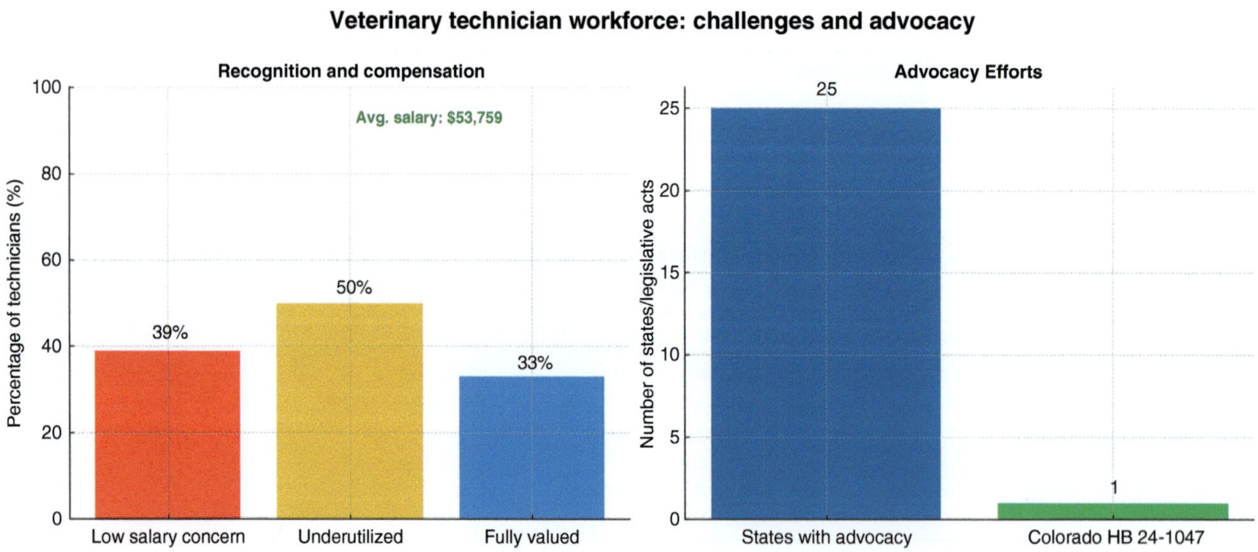

Figure 1.3 NAVTA Demographic Survey 2024. *Source:* Portland Veterinary Medical Association (2023), NAVTA (2023), Colorado HB 24-1047.

Veterinary nursing has evolved from a role of simple assistance to a multifaceted profession that embodies both art and science. This evolution mirrors broader changes within the veterinary field and society's recognition of the value of animals as sentient beings. Veterinary technicians are not only caregivers but also advocates, educators, and essential members of the veterinary healthcare team.

As the field continues to grow, veterinary nursing will remain grounded in its commitment to evidence-based practice, ethical standards, and compassionate care. This dual commitment to scientific rigor and empathetic service defines veterinary nursing as a unique and vital profession. The journey of veterinary nursing reflects our shared responsibility to provide animals with the highest quality of care and to honor the deep, intrinsic connection that humans share with the animal world.

Veterinary Nursing as a Science

On the other hand, veterinary nursing is a scientific discipline that requires a strong foundation in anatomy, physiology, pharmacology, and pathology. Veterinary technicians perform a wide range of clinical tasks, from administering medications and managing anesthesia to assisting in surgeries and providing critical care. These tasks demand precise technical knowledge, as well as an understanding of diagnostic and therapeutic procedures. For detailed application of these clinical skills, readers may refer to Chapters 3 and 7, which explore the integration of theory with hands-on practice in greater depth (Figure 1.4).

Evidence-based practice is the basis of veterinary nursing as a science. Technicians must remain up to date with current research and best practices, ensuring that the care they provide is both safe and effective. Additionally, the scientific aspect of veterinary nursing involves a commitment to continuous learning and professional development, as advances in veterinary medicine and technology create new treatment options and protocols.

The Role of Veterinary Technicians in Modern Veterinary Medicine

In contemporary veterinary practice, veterinary technicians are indispensable members of the healthcare team, embodying both the science and the art of veterinary nursing. Scientifically, they bring technical expertise grounded in anatomy, physiology, pharmacology, and evidence-based practice. This allows them to administer treatments, monitor anesthetic depth, interpret diagnostic results, and adjust care plans with clinical precision. Artistically, they blend empathy, perception, and intuition, providing comfort, reassurance, and individualized care that acknowledges each animal's unique needs and personality.

Veterinary technicians often serve as the primary caregivers for hospitalized animals in both emergency and general practice settings. In emergency and critical care, this role may include rapid triage, round-the-clock monitoring, and dynamic

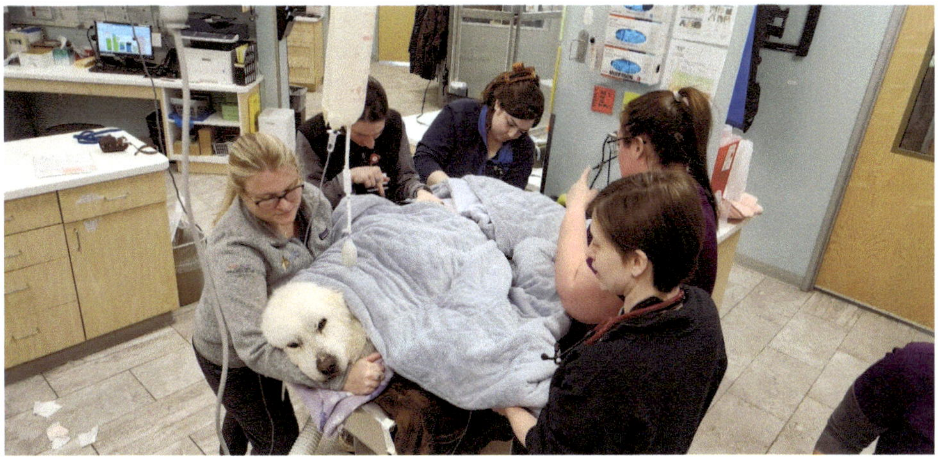

Figure 1.4 Schaeffer, Crystal. (2025). Veterinary nurse monitoring critical patient. *Source:* Photo by Crystal Schaeffer.

adjustment of therapeutic interventions—requiring quick decision-making that merges science with in-the-moment judgment. In general practice, however, the technician's role may take on a more preventive and longitudinal dimension: monitoring chronic conditions such as diabetes or osteoarthritis, assisting with wellness visits, and supporting surgical patients through routine anesthesia and recovery. In both settings, technicians act as the consistent presence that supports the patient's journey, from the critical moment of crisis to the quieter rhythms of preventive care.

Beyond direct patient care, veterinary technicians also play a vital role in client education and support. Scientifically, they translate diagnostic findings and treatment protocols into clear, actionable instructions for owners. Artistically, they draw on communication skills, empathy, and emotional intelligence to help clients navigate the fear, grief, or uncertainty that may accompany a pet's illness. This client-centered approach is particularly impactful in managing chronic disease in general practice—such as guiding owners through insulin administration or arthritis management—as well as in emergency settings where timely education can save a life.

Veterinary technicians are also unwavering advocates for animal welfare, both within the clinic and in the broader community. They apply ethical frameworks and evidence-based standards to ensure humane and respectful treatment, but they also rely on their perceptive artistry to speak for the patient when owners or clinicians are conflicted. By blending science with compassion and by adapting their advocacy to the context—whether in the fast pace of an ER or the continuity of care in a GP setting—veterinary technicians advance a culture of respect, dignity, and patient-centered practice across the full spectrum of veterinary medicine.

The Future of Veterinary Nursing

Looking to the future, veterinary nursing is poised for continued growth and development. As public awareness of animal welfare increases, there is likely to be greater demand for skilled veterinary technicians who can provide high-quality care and support. Additionally, the integration of veterinary nursing into research and public health initiatives could open new career paths and opportunities for professional advancement.

The future of veterinary nursing will also be shaped by ongoing efforts to standardize education and certification requirements worldwide. These efforts aim to establish a global standard of care, ensuring that veterinary technicians everywhere are equipped to meet the demands of modern veterinary medicine. By strengthening the profession's foundation, these initiatives will help veterinary technicians continue to make meaningful contributions to animal health and welfare.

Conclusion

Veterinary nursing is a multifaceted profession that requires a balance of scientific knowledge and compassionate care. As both an art and a science, it demands not only technical skills but also the ability to connect with and advocate for patients and clients. The evolution of veterinary nursing reflects the broader advancements in veterinary medicine and the growing recognition of animals as sentient beings deserving of compassionate and ethical care.

As this textbook explores the principles and practices of veterinary nursing, it is guided by the understanding that veterinary nursing is more than a collection of tasks; it is a calling that requires dedication, empathy, and a lifelong commitment to learning. Through this journey, we will examine the science behind nursing interventions, as well as the art of building trust, communicating effectively, and providing comfort to patients and their owners. This dual perspective on veterinary nursing will provide a foundation for excellence in practice and set the stage for future contributions to the field.

References

AAVSB (2025). Practice act model. American Association of Veterinary State Boards. https://www.aavsb.org/wp-content/uploads/2025/05/PracticeActModel.pdf (accessed 11 March 2025).

American Association for Laboratory Animal Science (AALAS) (2024). History of AALAS. (Online). www.aalas.org (accessed 8 March 2025).

American Veterinary Medical Association (AVMA) (2024). Veterinary technology programs. (Online). https://www.avma.org/education/accreditation/programs/veterinary-technology (accessed 1 July 2025).

Beck, A.M. and Katcher, A.H. (2003). Future directions in human-animal bond research. *American Behavioral Scientist* 47 (1): 79–93. https://doi.org/10.1177/0002764203255206.

Colorado Veterinary Medical Association (2024). New legislation expands roles for veterinary technicians in Colorado. https://colovma.org/new-legislation-expands-roles-for-veterinary-technicians-in-colorado (accessed 2 January 2025).

Coursera (2025). Veterinary courses on Coursera. www.coursera.org (accessed 11 March 2025).

Fine, A.H. (ed.) (2019). *Handbook on Animal-Assisted Therapy: Foundations and Guidelines for Animal-Assisted Interventions*, 5e. Cambridge, MA: Academic Press.

GetArchive (n.d.). Swimmer handicapped service dog, emotions. Public domain stock photo. https://itoldya420.getarchive.net/amp/media/swimmer-handicapped-service-dog-emotions-66611b (accessed 19 August 2025).

Hatch, P.H. (2021). *The Veterinary Nurse's Survival Guide*, 88–102. London: CRC Press.

Internal Medicine for Vet Techs Podcast (2025). Internal Medicine for Vet Techs. https://imfppodcast.podbean.com (accessed 11 March 2025).

IVC Journal (2025). IVC Journal online learning. https://ivcjournal.com (accessed 10 March 2025).

Moses, L., Malowney, M.J., and Wesley Boyd, J. (2018). Ethical conflict and moral distress in veterinary practice: a survey of north American veterinarians. *Journal of Veterinary Internal Medicine* 32 (6): 2115–2122. https://doi.org/10.1111/jvim.15315.

NAVTA (2023). NAVTA response to AVMA statement on scope of practice. National Association of Veterinary Technicians in America. https://navta.net/news/navta-response-to-avma-statement-on-scope-of-practice (accessed 8 March 2025).

Portland Veterinary Medical Association (2023). Credentialed veterinary technician underutilization: How do we move forward? https://www.portlandvma.org/ovtaa/credentialed-veterinary-technician-underutilization-how-do-we-move-forward (accessed 11 March 2025).

Purdue University College of Veterinary Medicine (2018). Purdue veterinary nursing degree name change. (Online). https://vet.purdue.edu (accessed 11 March 2025).

Radio Vet Nurse Podcast (2025). Radio vet nurse. https://radiovetnurse.libsyn.com (accessed 10 April 2025).

Serpell, J. (1996). *In the Company of Animals: A Study of Human-Animal Relationships*. Cambridge: Cambridge University Press.

SUNY Delhi (2024). Veterinary science technology program history. (Online). https://www.delhi.edu/academics/programs/vet-science (accessed 27 January 2025).

Veterinary Anesthesia Nerds (2025). Veterinary anesthesia nerds—Facebook group. https://www.facebook.com/groups/472601212799491 (accessed 25 March 2025).

Veterinary Support Personnel Network (VSPN) (2025). Veterinary support personnel network. https://www.vin.com/vspn (accessed 8 April 2025).

Vetfolio (2025). Vetfolio—veterinary continuing education. www.vetfolio.com (accessed 9 April 2025).

VIN Foundation (2025). VIN foundation YouTube channel. https://www.youtube.com/@VINFoundation (accessed 28 March 2025).

Volk, J.O., Felsted, K.E., Thomas, J.G., and Siren, C.W. (2021). The impact of COVID-19 on the veterinary profession: telemedicine and beyond. Schaumburg, IL: American Veterinary Medical Association. www.avma.org (accessed 1 July 2025).

2

History of Veterinary Nursing

Veterinary nursing is a multifaceted profession that combines the art of compassionate care with the science of clinical expertise. Over centuries, the role has transformed from an informal, auxiliary function to a specialized and essential discipline within veterinary medicine. This chapter explores the rich history of veterinary nursing, tracing its roots from early animal caregivers to modern-day veterinary nurses and technicians. By examining key milestones, the contributions of early pioneers, and recent advancements, we uncover the evolution of the profession and its growing recognition as a vital component of animal healthcare.

Early Pioneers and Foundations

Premodern Animal Care

The origins of veterinary nursing are deeply rooted in the foundational relationship between humans and animals. Throughout history, this bond has transcended utilitarian needs, reflecting a profound respect for animals as vital to human survival and companionship. The earliest evidence of human–animal interactions reveals that care for animals emerged as a natural extension of this bond, with responsibilities often falling to those closest to the animals, such as farmers, herders, and household caregivers. Among Indigenous peoples of North America, this relationship was especially evident in their deep spiritual and practical connections to horses and bison. Horses, introduced to the continent in the 16th century, became integral to Indigenous lifeways, not only transforming mobility, hunting practices, and warfare but also symbolizing strength, freedom, and kinship. Likewise, the bison served as both a physical and spiritual cornerstone, providing food, clothing, shelter, and tools, while also representing sacred interdependence between humans, animals, and the land. In both cases, care and respect for these animals were woven into cultural traditions, oral histories, and communal practices, underscoring that the earliest forms of animal care were not purely functional but reflected a worldview in which animals were recognized as partners in survival and identity (Figure 2.1).

Early Animal Care in Ancient Civilizations

The ancient Egyptians are among the first recorded societies to demonstrate organized animal care (Salisbury and Van Valkenburgh 2007). Renowned for their deep spiritual and practical connection to animals, they considered many species sacred. Hieroglyphs and papyrus texts reveal that Egyptians not only revered animals like cats, which were associated with the goddess Bastet, but also placed significant importance on livestock such as cattle and donkeys. Tomb art depicts scenes of wound cleaning and splinting, suggesting a rudimentary understanding of medical intervention. Archaeological evidence of healed fractures in animal remains points to intentional efforts to nurse animals back to health, a precursor to veterinary nursing principles (Figure 2.2) (Salisbury and Van Valkenburgh 2007).

Similarly, the ancient Greeks held animals in high regard, particularly those linked to agriculture and mythology. Their literature and philosophy often underscored the ethical treatment of animals. Figures like Aristotle documented observations on animal anatomy and behavior, indirectly influencing caregiving practices. Hippocrates, often hailed as the "Father of Medicine," profoundly influenced the development of medical thought, and his work also holds significant implications for veterinary care (Smith 2005). His writings and philosophy revolved around the concept of health as a balance of natural forces, emphasizing the interconnectivity of all living beings. While his primary focus was on human health, Hippocrates frequently drew comparisons between humans and animals, laying the groundwork for a holistic approach that later influenced both human and veterinary medicine (Figure 2.3).

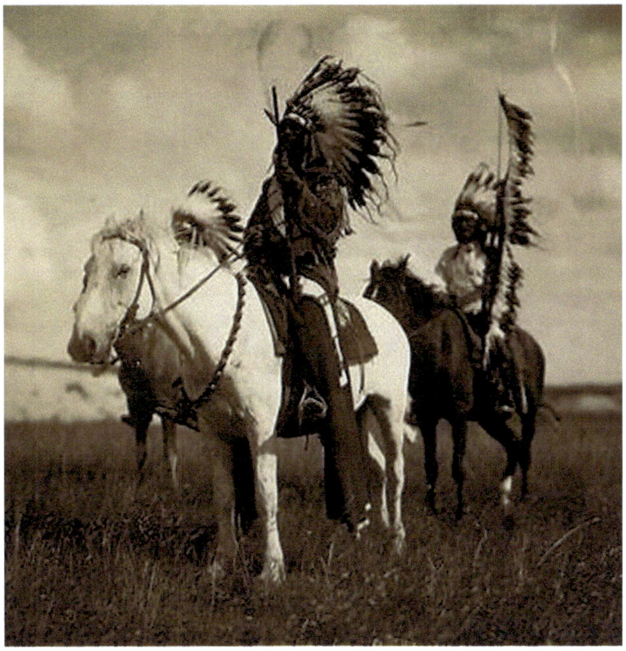

Figure 2.1 Indigenous riders on horseback. *Source:* ArtsyBee / Pixabay / CC0.

Hippocrates recognized that the principles governing health and disease in humans often paralleled those in animals. For example, his observations on diet, environment, and physical activity as critical factors in maintaining health applied universally. In his seminal work *On Airs, Waters, and Places*, Hippocrates discussed how environmental factors—such as climate, geography, and seasonal changes—could influence the health of living organisms (Hippocrates, trans. Jones 1923). This acknowledgment extended implicitly to animals, particularly those living alongside humans in shared environments. His insights reflected an early understanding of what is now referred to as One Health: the interdependence of human, animal, and environmental health.

Hippocrates also noted the physiological similarities between humans and animals, particularly in the context of disease processes. In his anatomical and physiological studies, he used animal models to extrapolate knowledge about human health. For example, his dissections and observations of animal anatomy provided foundational knowledge that informed early surgical practices and disease treatment in both humans and animals (Ghosh 2015). These practices implicitly acknowledged that health was a shared state across species, driven by common biological principles.

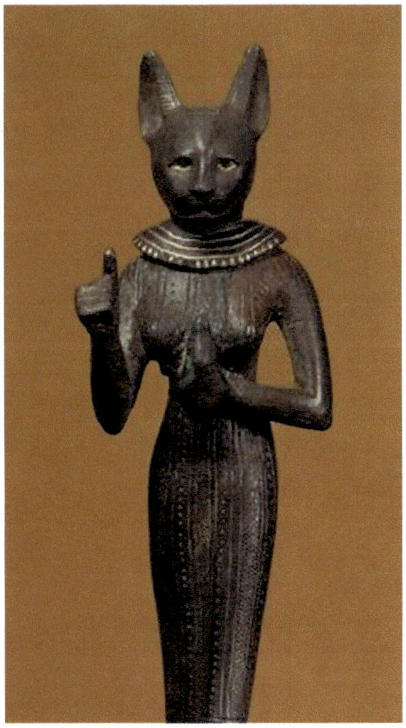

Figure 2.2 Bronze statuette of Bastet, the cat-headed goddess, late Ptolemaic period to Ptolemaic period. *Source:* Henry Walters / The Walters Art Museum / CC0.

One of Hippocrates' most enduring contributions to medicine was his emphasis on treating the patient, not just the disease (Hippocrates, trans. Jones 1923). He advocated for a holistic approach that considered the physical, emotional, and environmental factors influencing health. This philosophy naturally extended to animals under human care, as caretakers began to see the value in addressing not only an animal's immediate physical ailments but also its overall well-being. For example, a sick horse or livestock animal would not only be examined for physical injuries or disease but also assessed in terms of its diet, workload, and living conditions—a concept clearly inspired by Hippocratic thought.

In ancient Rome, the structured documentation of animal care marked a significant advancement in veterinary practices. This systematic approach to livestock management and healthcare is particularly evident in the works of Columella, a Roman agriculturalist and writer whose contributions remain invaluable to understanding early veterinary methods. His comprehensive treatise, *De Re Rustica* (*On Agriculture*), offers a meticulous account of animal husbandry, encompassing the care, maintenance, and treatment of livestock, which were essential to the Roman economy and society (Columella, trans. Ash 1941). Columella's work is a cornerstone of Roman agricultural literature, reflecting a practical yet detailed understanding of animal health. His insights into livestock management were shaped by the central role of animals in Roman life, particularly in agriculture, transportation, and military contexts. Livestock such as cattle, horses, sheep, and goats were not only sources of food and labor but also symbols of wealth and status. Consequently, their health and productivity were of paramount importance (Figure 2.4).

Columella's text provides specific instructions for addressing injuries and ailments in animals, emphasizing both prevention and treatment. For example, he describes the importance of cleaning and dressing wounds to prevent infection—a

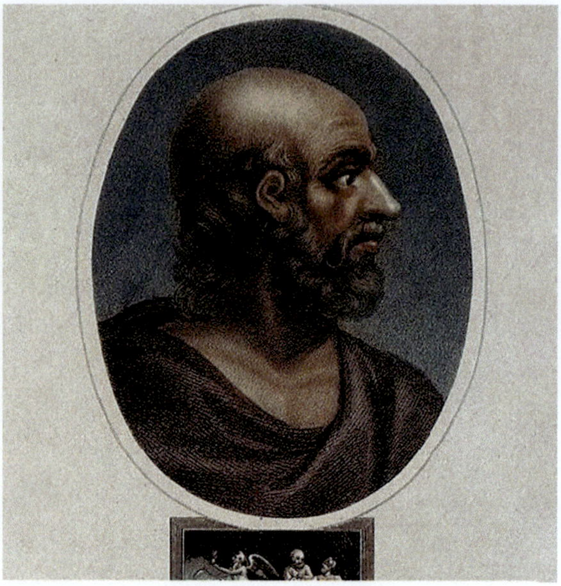

Figure 2.3 Portrait of Hippocrates, colored stipple engraving by J. Chapman, 1809. *Source:* Wellcome Collection / Public domain.

practice that aligns with modern antiseptic techniques. He also details methods for immobilizing animals during treatment, ensuring both the safety of the handler and the welfare of the animal (Columella, trans. Ash 1941). These techniques highlight an early understanding of animal restraint and stress reduction, concepts that remain integral to veterinary nursing today (Figure 2.5).

In cases of fractures or lameness, Columella recommended setting broken bones using splints made from readily available materials, such as wood or leather, bound with cloth or rope (Columella, trans. Ash 1941). This practice demonstrates an early application of biomechanical principles and the use of improvised but effective medical tools. His emphasis on gentle handling and the proper immobilization of injured limbs underscores the compassionate aspect of caregiving, a hallmark of veterinary nursing.

Beyond treating individual injuries, Columella stressed the importance of herd health as a collective concept. He recognized that the overall well-being of a herd was critical for sustained productivity. His recommendations included maintaining clean and dry living quarters for animals, rotating grazing pastures to

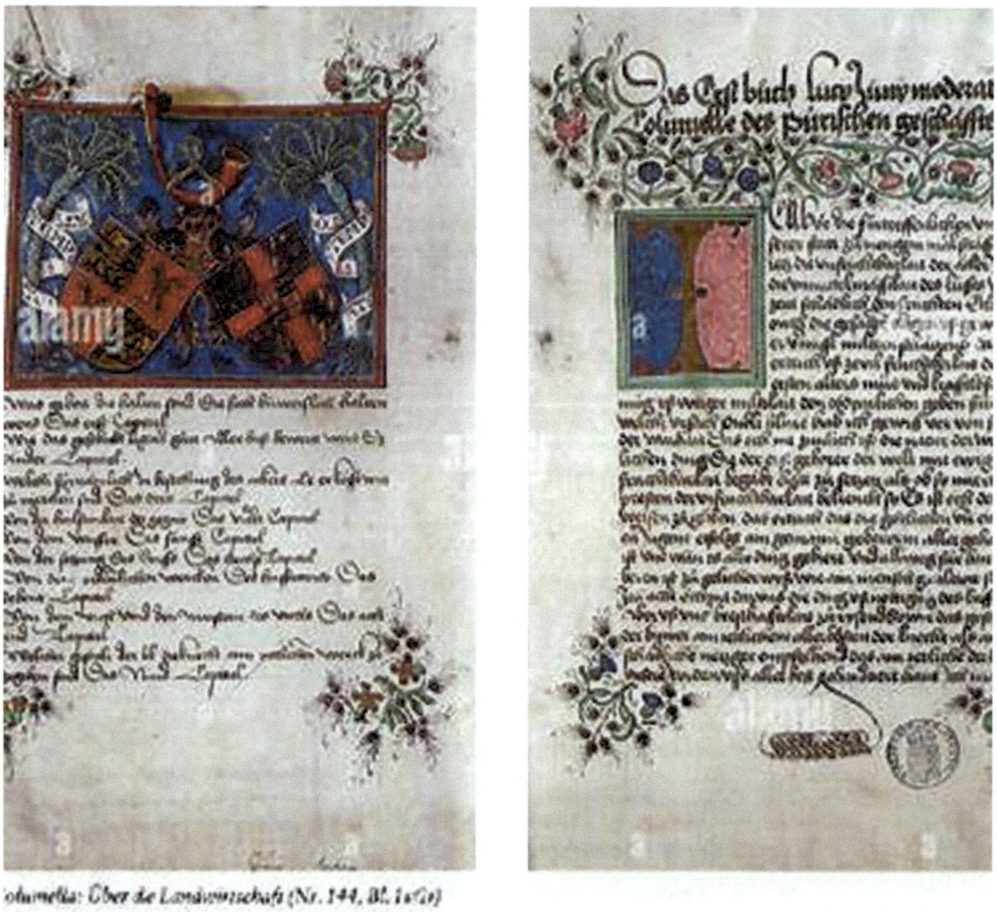

Figure 2.4 Portrait of Columella, artistic depiction by Jean de Tournes (1559). *Source:* Heinrich Österreicher / Wikimedia Commons / Public Domain / https://commons.wikimedia.org/wiki/File:Columella_stuttgart.jpg / last accessed on 27 Oct, 2025.

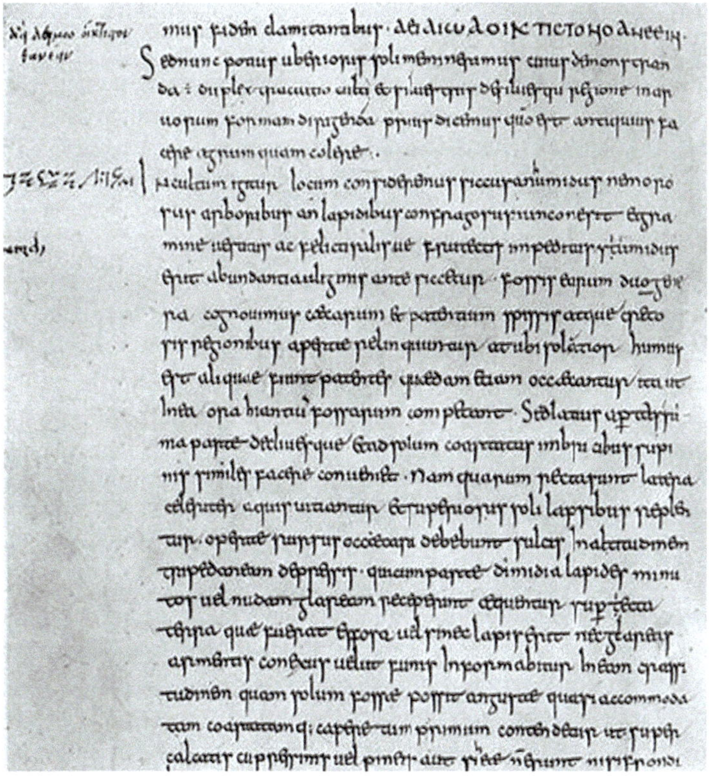

Figure 2.5 Excerpt from a 9th-century manuscript of De Re Rustica by Columella. *Source:* Lucius Junius Moderatus Columella / Wikimedia Common / Public Domain / https://commons.wikimedia.org/wiki/File:Columella,_De_re_rustica,_Milano,_L_85_sup.jpg / last accessed on 27 Oct, 2025.

prevent overuse and contamination, and providing a balanced diet tailored to the needs of each species (Columella, trans. Ash 1941). These practices reflect an early understanding of environmental and nutritional factors in disease prevention.

Columella also advocated for regular health inspections of animals to detect early signs of disease or injury. By promoting a proactive approach to health management, he anticipated modern preventive veterinary medicine, which prioritizes regular wellness checks and vaccinations. His writings highlight the role of observation and early intervention, principles that form the foundation of contemporary veterinary nursing.

In Roman society, the economic value of animals was closely tied to their health and productivity (Columella, trans. Ash 1941). Columella recognized this connection and provided guidelines to maximize efficiency while ensuring humane treatment. For example, he emphasized the importance of rest and recovery for working animals, such as oxen and horses, to prevent overexertion and chronic injuries. He also recommended breeding practices that prioritized the health and vitality of offspring, reflecting an understanding of genetics and selective breeding. Additionally, Columella detailed methods for addressing common ailments that could impair productivity, such as hoof diseases in horses and parasitic infections in sheep. His focus on early detection and treatment highlights a pragmatic approach to preserving the utility and longevity of animals, which was vital to sustaining the agricultural economy.

Columella's *De Re Rustica* stands as a testament to the advanced agricultural and veterinary knowledge of ancient Rome. His systematic and practical approach to animal care laid the groundwork for more formalized veterinary practices in later centuries. The emphasis on observation, preventive care, and the humane treatment of animals in his writings resonates with the core principles of modern veterinary technicians. Roman mosaics and inscriptions also depict veterinarians (referred to as *medicus pecuarius*) tending to animals, indicating a nascent professional class involved in animal health (Totelin 2017). However, much of the day-to-day caregiving remained in the hands of laypersons, such as farmers and slaves, who were tasked with the immediate care of sick or injured animals.

The Role of Lay Caregivers

In these ancient societies, the individuals responsible for animal care were typically those who worked closest to the animals. Farmers and herders, often motivated by economic necessity, became adept at performing basic tasks like cleaning wounds, setting broken bones, and applying rudimentary treatments (Clutton-Brock 1992). These practices, while unscientific by modern standards, were innovative for their time and underscored the intuitive understanding of animal needs.

Ancient herders were among the earliest practitioners of animal care, relying on keen observation, practical experience, and collective community knowledge to address the health needs of their livestock. Their intimate relationship with their animals—born out of necessity and daily interaction—allowed them to recognize subtle signs of illness or injury that might otherwise go unnoticed. These early caregiving practices laid a critical foundation for the development of veterinary medicine and nursing as we know it today.

Recognizing Signs of Illness or Injury

Herders often observed their animals closely as part of their daily routines, looking for deviations in behavior or physical condition that might indicate underlying health issues. For instance, lameness in a working animal like an ox or horse might suggest an injury to the hoof or leg, while a lack of appetite or lethargy could point to systemic illness. Behavioral changes, such as a normally docile animal becoming irritable or restless, were also important indicators. This observational skill—essentially a form of early diagnostic ability—was honed through experience and a deep familiarity with the animals under their care. These herders understood that timely intervention could mean the difference between recovery and loss, especially in societies where animals were indispensable for agriculture, transportation, and sustenance. Their ability to identify and address health issues quickly was therefore not only a matter of animal welfare but also of economic survival.

Once a problem was identified, ancient herders turned to the resources available in their environment to treat their animals. They frequently used natural remedies derived from local plants, minerals, and other organic materials. Herders might apply crushed leaves, bark, or resin with antibacterial properties to open wounds to prevent infection. Plants like *Aloe vera*, known for their soothing and healing properties, were likely used in such treatments. Similarly, honey—a natural antibiotic—may have been employed to treat and dress wounds. Herbal poultices and teas made from plants with analgesic properties, such as willow bark (a precursor to modern aspirin), could have been used to alleviate pain in injured animals. Certain herbs, such as wormwood or garlic, were believed to have antiparasitic effects and may have been included in feed or used topically to combat infestations. Aromatic herbs like thyme or eucalyptus could have been burned to produce soothing vapors, helping animals with respiratory distress (Scarborough 1991; Touwaide and Appetiti 2013). These remedies were often discovered through trial and error, with successful treatments becoming part of the community's collective knowledge. Over time, these practices evolved into more sophisticated forms of herbal and holistic medicine, which continue to influence modern veterinary and human healthcare.

Oral Tradition and Community Knowledge

The reliance on practical, experience-based knowledge fostered a rich oral tradition of animal caregiving. Techniques and remedies were passed down from one generation to the next, often shared within families, villages, or nomadic tribes. This transmission of knowledge ensured that each successive generation of herders was equipped with the skills necessary to care for their animals. Oral tradition also encouraged collaboration and innovation. Communities would gather to share stories of successful treatments, compare practices, and exchange insights about the health challenges faced by their livestock. In this way, herders collectively refined their understanding of animal health, creating a dynamic repository of veterinary knowledge. This reliance on shared knowledge also served to standardize certain practices within regions, giving rise to early forms of localized veterinary customs. For example, a particular plant known for its efficacy in treating wounds might become a staple in one region's animal care practices, while another community might develop expertise in managing respiratory ailments using local herbs (Landsberg 2002; Touwaide and Appetiti 2013).

The Evolution of Holistic Practices

The integration of observation, natural remedies, and oral tradition reflects the holistic nature of ancient animal caregiving. Herders recognized that an animal's health was influenced not only by injuries or diseases but also by factors such as diet, workload, and environmental conditions. This early holistic perspective aligns closely with current veterinary nursing's emphasis on treating the whole patient rather than focusing solely on isolated symptoms (Figure 2.6).

Over centuries, these early practices evolved and were refined as societies advanced. The herbal remedies and caregiving techniques of ancient herders formed the basis for more formalized systems of medicine, including traditional Chinese veterinary medicine and Ayurvedic practices, both of which continue to influence contemporary veterinary care (Dhama et al. 2005; Xie and Preast 2010). The practices of ancient herders highlight the origins of veterinary nursing as an art and science grounded in empathy, observation, and innovation. By addressing the immediate needs of their animals through natural

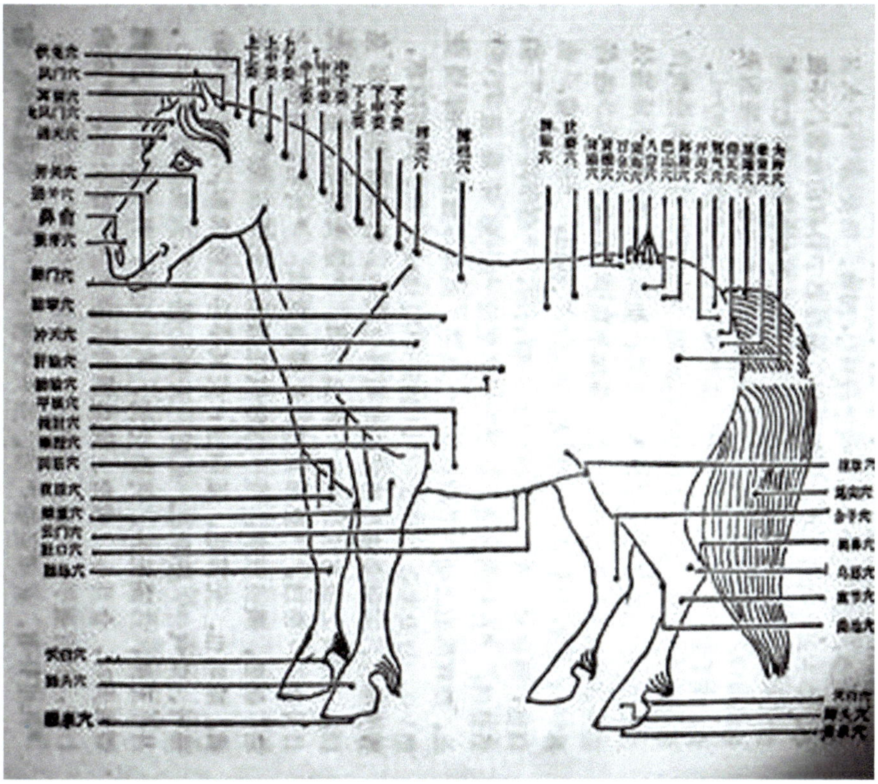

Figure 2.6 Traditional Chinese veterinary illustration of equine acupuncture points—riginating from the Bo Le Ming Tang Lun chapter—highlighting the historical foundation of TCVM. *Source:* Unknown illustrator (Han–Song period).

remedies and collaborative knowledge, they laid the groundwork for the development of systematic veterinary care. Their approach underscores the timeless importance of practical experience and holistic thinking in animal health, principles that remain central to the field today. Moreover, the act of nourishing and nurturing sick animals reflected an intrinsic empathy that would later define the art of nursing. These lay caregivers often developed close relationships with their animals, understanding their individual temperaments and behaviors. This deep connection fostered a caregiving ethic that went beyond mere survival, emphasizing the welfare of the animal as a being with intrinsic value. In many ways, this mirrors the ethos of modern veterinary nursing, where patient-centered care remains central to the profession. Veterinary technicians today employ not only technical expertise in anesthesia, pharmacology, and diagnostic procedures, but also draw upon the same attentiveness to individual behaviors, comfort, and emotional well-being that early caregivers embodied. The continuity lies in the recognition that effective veterinary care is not solely about curing disease or prolonging life, but also about alleviating suffering, preserving dignity, and strengthening the human–animal bond. Thus, while the science of veterinary nursing has advanced considerably, the underlying philosophy of compassionate advocacy for animals remains remarkably consistent across time.

Foundations of Animal Caregiving

Although these early efforts lacked the formalized training and scientific framework that define today's veterinary nursing, they laid the groundwork for the profession. The ability to recognize illness, administer basic treatments, and provide comfort reflected a core set of skills that would eventually become codified in veterinary nursing education. Furthermore, these practices highlighted the dual nature of caregiving—one that requires both practical skill and a compassionate understanding of the patient.

In summary, the roots of veterinary nursing are entwined with the history of human–animal relationships. Ancient civilizations, through their documented practices and enduring traditions, established a baseline for caregiving that reflected both necessity and empathy. These early caregivers, often unsung and informal in their roles, created a legacy of animal care that would evolve into the structured and recognized field of veterinary nursing. The practices they developed, from wound treatment to nourishment, continue to resonate in the modern principles of veterinary care, blending the art of empathy with the science of medicine.

The Birth of Veterinary Medicine

The formalization of veterinary medicine in the 18th century marked a pivotal moment in the history of animal healthcare. The establishment of dedicated veterinary schools, beginning with the École Nationale Vétérinaire de Lyon in 1761, represented the first structured effort to professionalize the field (Pugh 2002). These institutions emerged in response to significant agricultural and economic challenges, particularly the devastating impact of livestock diseases on human societies.

The Context of Veterinary Medicine's Emergence

The 18th century was a period of rapid agricultural and industrial transformation in Europe. Livestock played a critical role in sustaining economies, providing food, labor, and materials like wool and leather. However, recurring outbreaks of devastating diseases such as rinderpest, anthrax, and foot-and-mouth disease threatened the stability of these systems. These epidemics not only caused widespread animal mortality but also disrupted trade, diminished food supplies, and undermined public health by exacerbating zoonotic disease risks (Smith 2012; Wilkinson 1992). Governments and scientific communities began to recognize the need for specialized expertise to combat these challenges. This recognition catalyzed the founding of veterinary schools to formalize the study of animal health and disease (Figure 2.7).

Establishment of the École Nationale Vétérinaire de Lyon

In 1761, French veterinarian Claude Bourgelat founded the École Nationale Vétérinaire de Lyon, widely regarded as the world's first veterinary school (Pugh 2002). Bourgelat's vision was to create a rigorous academic institution dedicated to the study of animal health, modeled after medical schools for human physicians. The curriculum focused on anatomy, pathology, pharmacology, and disease prevention, with an emphasis on addressing the agricultural crises of the time.

Bourgelat's school quickly gained prominence and set the standard for veterinary education. Students were trained in diagnostic techniques, disease management, and surgical procedures, enabling them to serve as experts in controlling livestock epidemics. The school's success inspired the establishment of similar institutions across Europe, including the École Nationale Vétérinaire d'Alfort in France in 1765, and the Tierarzneischule in Vienna, Austria, in 1776 (Pugh 2002; Dunlop and Williams 1996) (Figure 2.8).

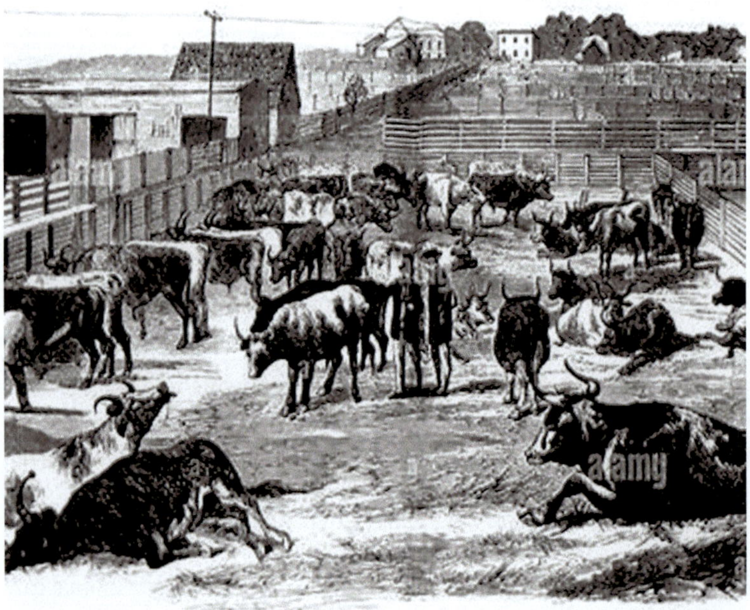

Figure 2.7 Engraving depicting cattle afflicted with rinderpest (cattle plague) during a 19th-century outbreak—illustrative of the devastation caused by recurrent livestock diseases. *Source:* Science History Images / Alamy Stock Photo.

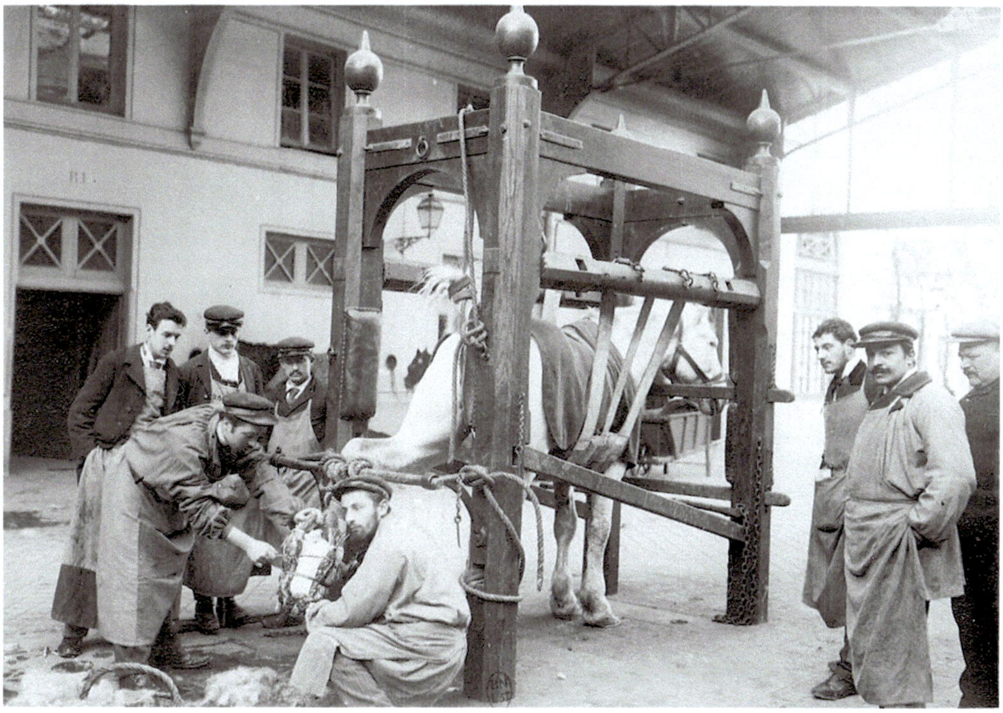

Figure 2.8 Historic view of the École Nationale Vétérinaire d'Alfort, founded in 1765 and modeled after Bourgelat's Lyon school. *Source:* Joseph Jules Beau / Wikimedia Commons / Public Domain / https://commons.wikimedia.org/wiki/File:%C3%89cole_nationale_v%C3%A9t%C3%A9rinaire_d%27Alfort_(1899).jpg / last accessed on 27 Oct, 2025.

The early veterinary schools were primarily concerned with livestock diseases, reflecting the priorities of the agricultural economies they served. The goal was not only to protect individual animals but also to safeguard entire herds and flocks, thereby ensuring a stable food supply and supporting economic growth. Veterinary students were trained to identify, contain, and eradicate infectious diseases, often collaborating with governmental authorities to implement public health measures. Veterinarians were also involved in early zoonotic disease management, studying conditions that could be transmitted between animals and humans. This focus laid the groundwork for the One Health concept, emphasizing the connection between human, animal, and environmental health.

While the establishment of veterinary schools professionalized the role of the veterinarian, the need for trained assistants was largely overlooked during this period. Animal care outside the purview of veterinarians continued to rely heavily on laypersons, apprentices, and laborers who worked alongside trained professionals or independently in rural areas. These informal caregivers often performed essential tasks such as wound care, birthing assistance, and the administration of basic treatments, much as they had for centuries. They relied on practical knowledge and traditional remedies, filling gaps in veterinary care, particularly in regions where trained veterinarians were unavailable. Apprenticeships remained a common pathway for those interested in animal care. Aspiring practitioners would learn directly from veterinarians or experienced caregivers, gaining hands-on experience rather than formal education. While effective in transferring skills, this system lacked the standardization and theoretical grounding provided by veterinary schools (Figure 2.9).

Early Contributions and Limitations

Although the veterinary schools of the 18th century represented a major advancement, their narrow focus on veterinarians as sole practitioners of animal health created limitations. By neglecting to train a broader spectrum of animal healthcare providers, these institutions perpetuated a gap between theory and practice in day-to-day animal care. Tasks that could have been delegated to trained assistants were instead left to individuals with varying levels of experience and expertise. Furthermore, the emphasis on livestock meant that companion animals, such as dogs and cats, received little attention in these early veterinary programs. These animals were typically cared for by their owners or informal caregivers, with veterinarians intervening only in cases of severe illness or injury.

By the mid-19th century in Victorian England, however, the role of dogs began to shift significantly, moving from primarily working animals to beloved household companions. This period saw the emergence of the "pet-keeping culture," where

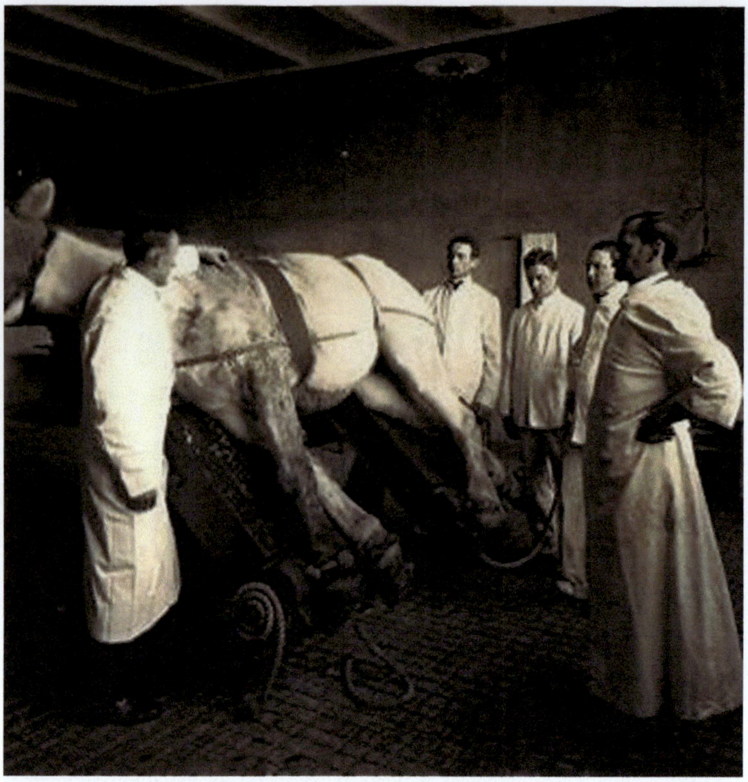

Figure 2.9 Veterinary school interior, showing assistants and students working with a horse in a treatment area. *Source:* Unknown photographer (1908).

middle- and upper-class families increasingly valued dogs for companionship, emotional support, and as symbols of social refinement. The rise of urban living and the influence of Queen Victoria, an avid dog owner, further elevated the cultural status of dogs. Breed societies and kennel clubs were established, reflecting a growing interest in canine care and breeding standards. Despite this cultural transformation, veterinary education still lagged behind, with little formal training available in the care of companion animals. As a result, much of the responsibility for canine welfare during this period continued to rest with owners and informal caregivers rather than trained veterinary professionals (Howell 2015; Ritvo 1987).

Despite these limitations, the 18th-century veterinary schools laid the foundation for the modern veterinary profession. They established veterinary medicine as a legitimate field of study and created a framework for addressing animal health systematically and scientifically. The success of these schools demonstrated the value of specialized training and set a precedent for expanding the scope of animal care. In later centuries, the growing recognition of the need for veterinary support roles would lead to the emergence of veterinary nursing and technology. These professions evolved to address the practical and logistical challenges of animal care, complementing the work of veterinarians and enhancing the overall quality of care.

The formalization of veterinary medicine in the 18th century was a transformative period that brought structure, legitimacy, and scientific rigor to animal healthcare. While the focus on veterinarians as primary practitioners left gaps in the broader caregiving ecosystem, the establishment of veterinary schools like the École Nationale Vétérinaire de Lyon marked a critical step forward. This era not only addressed urgent agricultural and public health needs but also set the stage for the eventual development of complementary roles, such as veterinary nursing, that would enrich and expand the profession.

The Emergence of Veterinary Nursing

Formalizing the Role

The mid-20th century represents a critical juncture in the evolution of veterinary nursing, characterized by the formalization of the profession and the establishment of structured training programs. This period was marked by a growing awareness of the need for skilled support staff to assist veterinarians, particularly in increasingly complex clinical and surgical settings. The Royal College of Veterinary Surgeons (RCVS) in the United Kingdom emerged as a pioneer in this effort,

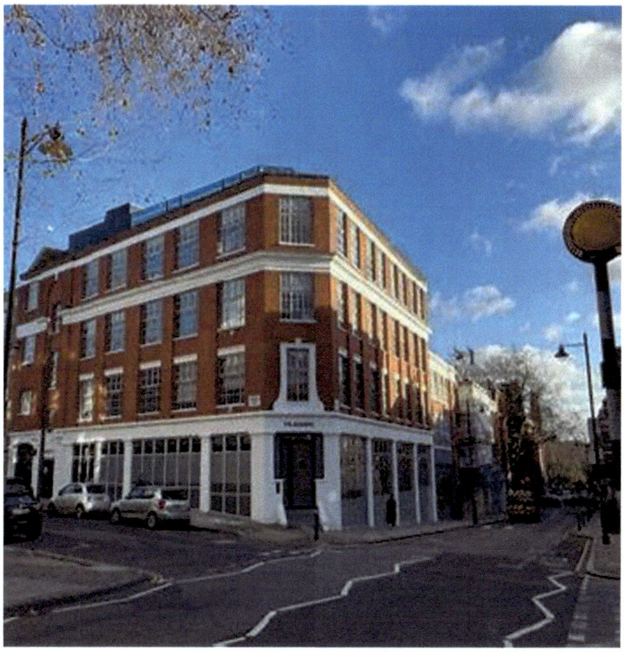

Figure 2.10 The current headquarters of the Royal College of Veterinary Surgeons, representing the modern institutional face of the profession. *Source:* with permission of Royal College of Veterinary Surgeons.

launching the first formal veterinary nursing program in 1961 (RCVS 2011). This initiative not only addressed practical needs in veterinary medicine but also transformed veterinary nursing into a recognized and professionalized field (Figure 2.10).

By the mid-20th century, veterinary medicine had undergone significant advancements. The development of new diagnostic tools, surgical techniques, and therapeutic modalities had increased the complexity of veterinary care. Veterinarians faced growing demands in both general practice and specialized settings, requiring additional support to manage patient care efficiently. Simultaneously, societal changes, including the increasing prominence of companion animals in households, heightened expectations for veterinary services. Pet owners began seeking higher-quality care for their animals, paralleling trends in human healthcare. This shift emphasized the need for skilled professionals who could provide hands-on care, monitor patients, and facilitate communication between veterinarians and clients.

Alongside these developments, broader societal pressures began shaping how animals were perceived, particularly in relation to sentience and welfare. Upton Sinclair's *The Jungle* (1906), while primarily exposing the exploitation of human workers in the Chicago meatpacking industry, also drew public attention to the brutal conditions in which animals were slaughtered. Although Sinclair's intent was to advocate for labor reform, the graphic depictions of animal suffering resonated with readers and provoked a wider conversation about the ethical treatment of animals in industrial systems. This cultural moment contributed to a gradual shift in societal attitudes, where animals were increasingly recognized not merely as commodities but as sentient beings capable of experiencing pain and distress (Ritvo 1987; Sinclair 1906). This growing awareness paralleled the heightened expectations for veterinary care and reinforced the profession's evolving responsibility to address both the medical and ethical dimensions of animal treatment (Figure 2.11).

Despite these growing demands, the role of veterinary technicians remained informal and largely unregulated. Tasks such as patient monitoring, anesthesia management, and postoperative care were often delegated to untrained assistants or learned through informal apprenticeships. This lack of standardization created inconsistencies in care quality and highlighted the need for formal education and credentialing in veterinary nursing.

The RCVS took a groundbreaking step in 1961 by introducing the first structured veterinary nursing program. This initiative represented a deliberate effort to address the need for a professional, well-trained workforce to support veterinarians. The program was designed to equip veterinary nurses with the theoretical knowledge and practical skills required to deliver high-quality care in clinical settings. The RCVS veterinary nursing program combined classroom instruction with hands-on clinical training. Topics ranged from animal anatomy and physiology to pharmacology, surgical nursing, and client communication (RCVS 2011). This comprehensive approach ensured that graduates were prepared for the multifaceted demands of the role. A significant portion of the program was dedicated to supervised clinical experience. Students worked

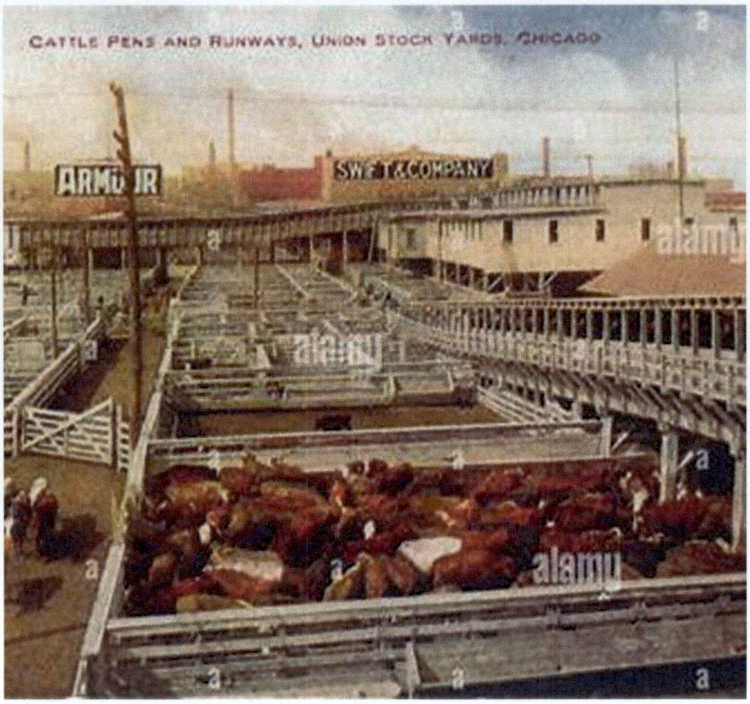

Figure 2.11 "The Great Union Stock Yards of Chicago" lithograph (c. 1878) by Charles Rascher—depicting the industrial scale of meatpacking and setting the stage for Upton Sinclair's revelations about animal suffering. *Source:* Zip Lexing / Alamy Stock Photo.

alongside veterinarians in practices, gaining firsthand experience in patient care, anesthesia, radiography, and laboratory procedures. This emphasis on practical training bridged the gap between theoretical knowledge and real-world application. RCVS introduced standardized examinations to assess students' knowledge and competence. Upon successful completion, graduates receive professional qualifications, marking the first instance of veterinary nursing being recognized as a distinct and legitimate profession (RCVS 2011).

The introduction of professional qualifications for veterinary technicians was a transformative milestone. It legitimized the role by establishing clear educational and ethical standards, distinguishing veterinary nursing from informal or auxiliary roles. Veterinary nurses gained professional status, earning respect within the veterinary community and among the public. Their specialized training and qualifications underscored their value as integral members of the healthcare team. Standardized training ensured that veterinary nurses possessed the skills and knowledge necessary to perform critical tasks, such as monitoring anesthesia, administering medications, and providing postoperative care. This improvement in care quality enhanced patient outcomes and allowed veterinarians to focus on diagnostic and surgical procedures. The formalization of veterinary nursing created pathways for career advancement, including opportunities for specialization in areas such as emergency and critical care, anesthesia, and behavior. These advancements not only enriched the profession but also attracted individuals seeking a fulfilling career in animal healthcare.

Role of Professional Associations in Advancing Veterinary Nursing

The establishment of professional associations was a pivotal step in the evolution of veterinary nursing, providing advocacy, community, and a framework for professional standards. These organizations not only advanced the interests of veterinary technicians but also played a crucial role in shaping the identity and recognition of the profession. The formation of the British Veterinary Nursing Association (BVNA) in 1965 marked a significant milestone in this journey, with similar movements gaining momentum globally, particularly in the United States in the 1970s (Burns 2006; BVNA 2015).

The BVNA was founded in 1965 as the first professional organization dedicated exclusively to veterinary nurses. Its establishment was driven by the growing need for a unified voice to represent the interests of veterinary nurses and to provide a platform for collaboration, education, and advocacy. The BVNA served as a powerful advocate for veterinary nurses, lobbying for improved recognition, fair working conditions, and opportunities for career advancement. One of its primary goals was to promote the professional identity of veterinary nurses, ensuring they were seen as skilled practitioners rather than mere auxiliary staff. This advocacy extended to legislative efforts, pushing for regulations that defined the scope of practice and protected the title of "veterinary nurse" (BVNA 2015; Lord et al. 2018).

The BVNA worked closely with the RCVS to develop and refine professional standards for veterinary nursing. By contributing to the design of training programs, certification requirements, and codes of conduct, the BVNA helped ensure that veterinary nurses were equipped with the skills and knowledge necessary to excel in their roles. These standards not only elevated the quality of care but also fostered public trust in the profession. Beyond advocacy and standard setting, the BVNA provided a vital sense of community for veterinary nurses. Through conferences, workshops, and networking events, the association created opportunities for professional development and peer support. These gatherings fostered a culture of continuous learning and collaboration, encouraging members to share best practices and innovations. Inspired by developments in the United Kingdom, similar efforts to formalize veterinary nursing began to take shape in the United States during the 1970s. Here, the role was referred to as "veterinary technician" to distinguish it from human nursing and to reflect the technical skills required for the job.

The Role of NAVTA

The National Association of Veterinary Technicians in America (NAVTA) was established in 1981 as the primary professional association for veterinary technicians in the United States (NAVTA 2020). Like the BVNA, NAVTA focused on advocacy, education, and community building. Its efforts included:

- Advocating for state licensure and certification to standardize the profession across the country.
- Developing the Veterinary Technician National Examination (VTNE), which became a critical step in credentialing veterinary technicians.
- Establishing specialty certifications in areas such as, but not limited to, anesthesia, emergency and critical care, and dentistry, allowing technicians to pursue advanced roles within the field.

NAVTA's work paralleled that of the BVNA, emphasizing the importance of professional identity and recognition while addressing the unique challenges of the American veterinary landscape. In the United States during the early 1980s, veterinary technicians faced a fragmented regulatory environment, with credentialing and scope of practice varying widely from state to state. This lack of uniformity created barriers to professional identity and complicated efforts to standardize education and practice. Furthermore, public awareness of the role of veterinary technicians remained limited, with many clients perceiving them as "assistants" rather than trained professionals. These challenges were compounded by relatively low wages and limited career advancement opportunities, which threatened retention and professional sustainability. NAVTA sought to address these issues by advocating for standardized credentialing, clearer role definitions, and greater recognition of veterinary technicians as essential members of the healthcare team (NAVTA 2011; Smith 2019; Volk et al. 1984).

Global Influence and Parallel Developments

The formation of professional associations for veterinary nurses and technicians was not limited to the United Kingdom and the United States. Similar movements emerged worldwide, reflecting the universal need for skilled animal caregivers. In Australia and New Zealand, veterinary nursing gained formal recognition in the 1970s and 1980s, with the establishment of professional associations and training programs (ANZCVS 2010; AVA 2013). These organizations worked to standardize the profession and advocate for the unique needs of veterinary nurses in their regions. Countries such as Germany, Sweden, and the Netherlands followed the UK's lead, creating national associations and educational pathways for veterinary nurses. These efforts were often supported by broader European initiatives to harmonize veterinary standards across the continent. The establishment of international organizations, such as the International Veterinary Nurses and Technicians Association (IVNTA), fostered global collaboration and knowledge exchange (FVE, 2012; IVNTA, 2014). These organizations provided a platform for discussing shared challenges, such as workforce shortages and mental health, and for promoting best practices.

Professional associations played a central role in advocating for legislative and regulatory changes that enhanced the profession. In both the United Kingdom and the United States, associations worked to secure title protection, ensuring that only qualified individuals could use the titles of "veterinary nurse" or "veterinary technician." This was a critical step in elevating the status of the profession and safeguarding its integrity. Additionally, these associations prioritized education as the basis for professional development. By offering continuing education opportunities, such as seminars, certifications, and online courses, they ensured that veterinary nurses and technicians could keep pace with advancements in veterinary medicine. This commitment to lifelong learning helped the profession evolve in tandem with the broader field of veterinary science.

Equally important was the role of state-level veterinary technician associations, particularly in the United States. These organizations provided a vital sense of community and solidarity for technicians, many of whom worked in professional environments where their roles were poorly understood or undervalued. State associations offered platforms for technicians to network, share knowledge, and build collective identity, while also serving as advocacy bodies that amplified their members' voices in local legislative and regulatory debates. Through newsletters, regional conferences, and mentorship programs, these associations cultivated professional pride and fostered leadership among technicians at the grassroots level. By bridging the gap between national initiatives and local realities, state associations played a pivotal role in strengthening the visibility, cohesion, and influence of the profession across diverse geographic and regulatory landscapes (Fox 2014; NAVTA 2011; Smith 2019).

Development of Educational Programs

The Shift to Formal Education in Veterinary Nursing

The transition from on-the-job training to formalized education in veterinary nursing represented a transformative moment in the profession. This shift, which gained momentum in the 1960s and 1970s, marked the beginning of a standardized approach to veterinary nursing education (Burns 2006; Orpet and Welsh 2011). Veterinary technology programs accredited by the American Veterinary Medical Association (AVMA) became a cornerstone of this change, establishing structured curricula and degree pathways. These programs elevated the profession by ensuring that veterinary technicians were equipped with both theoretical knowledge and practical skills to meet the growing complexities of veterinary medicine.

Prior to the establishment of formal education programs, veterinary nurses and technicians typically learned through on-the-job training. While this method provided hands-on experience, it lacked consistency and often depended on the availability and expertise of the supervising veterinarian. Training varied widely between practices, leading to discrepancies in knowledge and skill levels across individuals. On-the-job training often emphasizes immediate clinical needs, with little attention to broader theoretical concepts such as anatomy, physiology, or pharmacology. The absence of structured educational pathways restricted opportunities for career growth and recognition within the profession.

The Emergence of Accredited Veterinary Technology Programs

In response to the need for standardization and professionalization, the AVMA began accrediting veterinary technology programs in the 1960s and 1970s. These programs were developed in collaboration with veterinary professionals, educators, and industry leaders to ensure they met the demands of modern veterinary practice (AVMA 2011). The AVMA-accredited programs introduced a comprehensive curriculum that combined theoretical and practical components. Core areas of study included anatomy and physiology, pharmacology, diagnostic procedures, surgical nursing, anesthesia management, and client communication. This structured approach ensured that all graduates met a uniform standard of competence, regardless of the institution they attended. In addition to classroom instruction, accredited programs emphasized practical experience through clinical rotations and internships. These placements allowed students to apply their knowledge in real-world settings, working under the supervision of experienced veterinarians and technicians. This hands-on training was integral to bridging the gap between theory and practice. These programs typically culminated in an Associate of Science (AS) or Associate of Applied Science (AAS) degree in Veterinary Technology. The curricula were designed to provide a comprehensive foundation in veterinary nursing, encompassing both theoretical knowledge and practical skills.

Associate Degree Programs

Courses covered essential topics such as animal anatomy and physiology, pharmacology, surgical nursing, diagnostic imaging, laboratory procedures, and client communication. This comprehensive approach ensured that graduates were well-prepared for the diverse responsibilities of veterinary nursing. Integral to these programs was hands-on training through clinical rotations in veterinary hospitals, research facilities, or animal shelters. This practical experience allowed students to apply classroom knowledge in real-world settings, fostering competence and confidence in their skills (AVMA 2011; Orpet and Welsh 2011). Graduates became eligible to sit for the VTNE, a standardized test assessing proficiency in veterinary technology. Successful completion of the VTNE led to credentialing as a Licensed Veterinary Technician (LVT), Certified Veterinary Technician (CVT), Registered Veterinary Technician (RVT), or Licensed Veterinary Medical Technician (LVMT), depending on state regulations. In addition to associate degrees, some institutions offered Bachelor of Science

(BS) programs in Veterinary Technology. These programs provided advanced training and opportunities for specialization, catering to individuals seeking to deepen their expertise or pursue leadership roles within the field.

Advanced Degree Programs

Building upon the associate degree foundation, Bachelor of Applied Science in veterinary technology (BAS) programs delved into specialized areas such as advanced anesthesia techniques, exotic animal care, veterinary practice management, and research methodologies. This advanced coursework prepared graduates for more complex clinical roles and supervisory positions. Students could focus on specific areas of interest, such as emergency and critical care, dentistry, or behavior, allowing for career advancement and the pursuit of specialty certifications. The bachelor's curriculum often included components on leadership, ethics, and communication, equipping graduates with the skills necessary for effective team management and client relations. The establishment of these degree pathways marked a significant shift in veterinary nursing education, promoting standardization and elevating the profession's status. Formal education ensured that veterinary technicians possessed a consistent and comprehensive skill set, enhancing the quality of animal care and fostering greater professional recognition.

In recent years, the field has continued to evolve with the introduction of advanced degree programs, such as the Master of Veterinary Clinical Care (MVCC) offered by Lincoln Memorial University (LMU). Launched in August 2022, the MVCC program is the first of its kind in the United States, designed specifically for credentialed veterinary technicians seeking to build upon the knowledge and skills acquired in AVMA-accredited programs (LMU 2022). The curriculum focuses on patient case management, evidence-based medicine, critical thinking, practice management, and both clinical and professional skills. Courses are co-instructed by Doctors of Veterinary Medicine (DVMs) and Veterinary Technician Specialists (VTS), providing advanced critical thinking and clinical reasoning training. The program aims to prepare graduates to work with diverse populations, providing exceptional veterinary care with sensitivity to various cultural contexts and experiences of patient owners.

The introduction of the MVCC program represents a significant advancement in veterinary nursing education, providing a pathway for veterinary technicians to attain master's-level expertise and assume greater responsibilities within the veterinary healthcare team. This progression reflects the ongoing commitment to elevating the profession through advanced education and specialized training.

In summary, the transition from on-the-job training to formal education, encompassing associate, bachelor's, and now master's degree programs, has profoundly transformed veterinary nursing. These educational advancements have standardized training, expanded the scope of practice, and enhanced the professional standing of veterinary nurses and technicians, ultimately contributing to improved animal healthcare outcomes.

Equally significant, the establishment of formal degree programs provided veterinary technicians not only with clinical knowledge but also with a professional trajectory. Associate degree programs created a foundational entry point into the field, while the introduction of bachelor's and master's degrees offered opportunities for academic advancement, specialization, and leadership. These programs reinforced the idea that veterinary technology and nursing were not static auxiliary roles, but dynamic professions with the capacity to evolve alongside veterinary medicine. Higher education also encouraged the integration of research, pedagogy, and evidence-based practice into veterinary nursing, fostering a culture of scholarship that positioned technicians to contribute to advancing the discipline itself.

In parallel, the development of VTS credentialing provided an advanced professional track that complemented academic degree programs. Technicians who pursued specialization in areas such as emergency and critical care, anesthesia, dentistry, internal medicine, and nutrition demonstrated not only technical mastery but also a commitment to lifelong learning and professional excellence. The VTS pathway, overseen by NAVTA and its Academy system, provided external validation of advanced competency and created new opportunities for technicians to engage in teaching, research, leadership, and policy development. Together, formal higher education and the VTS framework expanded both the credibility and visibility of veterinary technicians, demonstrating their capacity to contribute to clinical outcomes, academic advancement, and the strategic evolution of veterinary medicine as a whole (Bissett et al. 2021; NAVTA 2011).

The Role of Formal Credentials in Protecting the Title of Veterinary Technician

The establishment of formal credentials for veterinary technicians marked a turning point in defining the role and scope of practice for these professionals. By instituting standardized education, examinations, and licensure, credentialing systems ensured that veterinary technicians were recognized as skilled professionals, distinct from individuals whose training had previously been acquired solely through informal, on-the-job experience without the benefit of a structured educational framework. Title protection laws, largely dictated at the state level in the United States, provided a legal framework to safeguard the title of "veterinary technician" and specify the tasks that credentialed individuals could perform. However, these laws vary significantly between states, reflecting differing levels of professional recognition and scope of practice. Unlike many professions with federally standardized licensure, the regulation of veterinary technicians in the United States falls to individual states. Title protection laws define who may legally use the title "veterinary technician" and outline their authorized scope of practice. These regulations vary widely, leading to differing levels of professional recognition and responsibilities across states. Title protection ensures that only individuals who meet specific educational and credentialing requirements can use the title "veterinary technician." This distinction prevents untrained individuals from performing technical tasks that require specialized knowledge, thus protecting both animal welfare and public safety.

Defining Scope of Practice

State laws also establish the scope of practice for veterinary technicians, delineating which tasks they can perform under veterinary supervision. Common responsibilities include administering medications, anesthesia management, diagnostic procedures, and client communication/education. However, the extent of these responsibilities varies depending on the state.

Comparative Examples of State Regulations

State with Comprehensive Title Protection: New York

New York provides robust title protection and a well-defined scope of practice for veterinary technicians (New York State Education Department 2021):

- **Title Protection:** In New York, only individuals who have graduated from an accredited veterinary technology program, passed the VTNE, and obtained state licensure can use the title "Licensed Veterinary Technician" (LVT).
- **Scope of Practice:** LVTs in New York are authorized to perform a wide range of tasks under the direct or indirect supervision of a licensed veterinarian, including:
  - Administering anesthesia and monitoring surgical patients.
  - Conducting laboratory diagnostics and radiographic imaging.
  - Assisting in dental procedures.
  - Handling emergency situations, such as administering CPR or stabilizing critical patients.

New York's regulations clearly define the roles and responsibilities of veterinary technicians, fostering professional recognition and ensuring high standards of care.

A State with Limited Title Protection: Alabama

In contrast, Alabama provides limited title protection and scope of practice regulation for veterinary technicians (Alabama State Board of Veterinary Medical Examiners 2021):

- **Title Protection:** Alabama does not have comprehensive title protection laws. This allows individuals who have not completed accredited education or passed the VTNE to perform many of the same tasks as credentialed technicians, leading to potential inconsistencies in care quality.
- **Scope of Practice:** The state's laws offer minimal guidance on the scope of practice, leaving significant discretion to individual veterinary practices. While credentialed technicians may perform technical tasks such as assisting in surgeries or administering medications, there is less regulatory oversight to ensure uniform standards.

This lack of regulation creates challenges in distinguishing credentialed technicians from untrained staff, potentially undermining the professional identity of veterinary technicians in the state (Tables 2.1 and 2.2).

Table 2.1 Veterinary technician credentialing and title protection by state in the United States.

State/Territory	Credential Type (LVT/RVT/CVT/ Registration/License/Certification)	Protected Titles (If Any)	Title Protection Status
Alabama	LVT (state license)	Licensed Veterinary Technician (LVT)	General title protection (NAVTA snapshot)
Alaska	LVT (state license)	Licensed Veterinary Technician (LVT)	Regulated, but no explicit title protection (NAVTA snapshot)
Arizona	CVT (state certification or private/ association)	Certified Veterinary Technician (CVT)	Regulated, but no explicit title protection (NAVTA snapshot)
Arkansas	CVT (state certification or private/ association)	Certified Veterinary Technician (CVT)	General title protection (NAVTA snapshot)
California	RVT (state registration)	Registered Veterinary Technician (RVT)	General title protection (NAVTA snapshot)
Colorado	CVT (state certification or private/ association)	Certified Veterinary Technician (CVT)	No title protection (NAVTA snapshot)
Connecticut	No state credential (verify local/ association options)	None (no state credential)	No title protection (NAVTA snapshot)
Delaware	LVT (state license)	Licensed Veterinary Technician (LVT)	General title protection (NAVTA snapshot)
District of Columbia	CVT (state certification)	Certified Veterinary Technician (CVT)	Regulated, but no explicit title protection (NAVTA snapshot)
Florida	CVT (state certification or private/ association)	Certified Veterinary Technician (CVT)—voluntary via FVMA, not statutory	No title protection (NAVTA snapshot)
Georgia	RVT (state registration)	Registered Veterinary Technician (RVT) [statute uses term "RVT"]	General title protection (NAVTA snapshot)
Hawaii	RVT (state registration)	Registered Veterinary Technician (RVT)	General title protection (NAVTA snapshot)
Idaho	CVT (state certification or private/ association)	Certified Veterinary Technician (CVT)	Regulated, but no explicit title protection (NAVTA snapshot)
Illinois	CVT (state certification or private/ association)	Certified Veterinary Technician (CVT)	Limited title protection (NAVTA snapshot)
Indiana	RVT (state registration)	Registered Veterinary Technician (RVT)	General title protection (NAVTA snapshot)
Iowa	RVT (state registration)	Registered Veterinary Technician (RVT)	Regulated, but no explicit title protection (NAVTA snapshot)
Kansas	RVT (state registration)	Registered Veterinary Technician (RVT)	Regulated, but no explicit title protection (NAVTA snapshot)
Kentucky	LVT (state license)	Licensed Veterinary Technician (LVT)	Regulated, but no explicit title protection (NAVTA snapshot)
Louisiana	RVT (state registration)	Registered Veterinary Technician (RVT)	Limited title protection (NAVTA snapshot)
Maine	LVT (state license)	Licensed Veterinary Technician (LVT)	Regulated, but no explicit title protection (NAVTA snapshot)
Maryland	RVT (state registration)	Registered Veterinary Technician (RVT)	Limited title protection (NAVTA snapshot)
Massachusetts	CVT (state certification or private/ association)	Certified Veterinary Technician (CVT)—association only	No title protection (NAVTA snapshot)
Michigan	LVT (state license)	Licensed Veterinary Technician (LVT)	Limited title protection (NAVTA snapshot)
Minnesota			

(*Continued*)

Table 2.1 (Continued)

State/Territory	Credential Type (LVT/RVT/CVT/ Registration/License/Certification)	Protected Titles (If Any)	Title Protection Status
	CVT (state certification or private/ association)	Certified Veterinary Technician (CVT)—association only	No title protection (NAVTA snapshot)
Mississippi	CVT (state certification or private/ association)	Certified Veterinary Technician (CVT)	Regulated, but no explicit title protection (NAVTA snapshot)
Missouri	RVT (state registration)	Registered Veterinary Technician (RVT)	Limited title protection (NAVTA snapshot)
Montana	CVT (state certification or private/ association)	Certified Veterinary Technician (CVT)—association only	No title protection (NAVTA snapshot)
Nebraska	LVT (state license)	Licensed Veterinary Technician (LVT)	Limited title protection (NAVTA snapshot)
Nevada	LVT (state license)	Licensed Veterinary Technician (LVT)	General title protection (NAVTA snapshot)
New Hampshire	CVT (state certification or private/ association)	Certified Veterinary Technician (CVT)	No title protection (NAVTA snapshot)
New Jersey	CVT (state certification or private/ association)	Certified Veterinary Technician (CVT)—association only	No title protection (NAVTA snapshot)
New Mexico	RVT (state registration)	Registered Veterinary Technician (RVT)	Regulated, but no explicit title protection (NAVTA snapshot)
New York	LVT (state license)	Licensed Veterinary Technician (LVT)	General title protection (NAVTA snapshot)
North Carolina	RVT (state registration)	Registered Veterinary Technician (RVT)	Regulated, but no explicit title protection (NAVTA snapshot)
North Dakota	LVT (state license)	Licensed Veterinary Technician (LVT)	Regulated, but no explicit title protection (NAVTA snapshot)
Ohio	RVT (state registration)	Registered Veterinary Technician (RVT)	Regulated, but no explicit title protection (NAVTA snapshot)
Oklahoma	RVT (state registration)	Registered Veterinary Technician (RVT)	General title protection (NAVTA snapshot)
Oregon	CVT (state certification or private/ association)	Certified Veterinary Technician (CVT)	Regulated, but no explicit title protection (NAVTA snapshot)
Pennsylvania	CVT (state certification or private/ association)	Certified Veterinary Technician (CVT)	Limited title protection (NAVTA snapshot)
Rhode Island	CVT (state certification or private/ association)	Certified Veterinary Technician (CVT)—association only	No title protection (NAVTA snapshot)
South Carolina	LVT (state license)	Licensed Veterinary Technician (LVT)	Regulated, but no explicit title protection (NAVTA snapshot)
South Dakota	RVT (state registration)	Registered Veterinary Technician (RVT)	Regulated, but no explicit title protection (NAVTA snapshot)
Tennessee	LVMT (state license)	Licensed Veterinary Medical Technician (LVMT)	General title protection (NAVTA snapshot)
Texas	LVT (state license)	Licensed Veterinary Technician (LVT)	Limited title protection (NAVTA snapshot)
Utah	No state credential (verify local/ association options)	None (no state credential)	Limited title protection (NAVTA snapshot)
Vermont	CVT (state certification or private/ association)	Certified Veterinary Technician (CVT)—association only	No title protection (NAVTA snapshot)
Virginia	LVT (state license)	Licensed Veterinary Technician (LVT)	Regulated, but no explicit title protection (NAVTA snapshot)

Table 2.1 (Continued)

State/Territory	Credential Type (LVT/RVT/CVT/ Registration/License/Certification)	Protected Titles (If Any)	Title Protection Status
Washington	LVT (state license)	Licensed Veterinary Technician (LVT)	Regulated, but no explicit title protection (NAVTA snapshot)
West Virginia	RVT (state registration)	Registered Veterinary Technician (RVT)	Limited title protection (NAVTA snapshot)
Wisconsin	CVT (state certification or private/ association)	Certified Veterinary Technician (CVT)	Regulated, but no explicit title protection (NAVTA snapshot)
Wyoming	CVT (state certification or private/ association)	Certified Veterinary Technician (CVT)—association only	No title protection (NAVTA snapshot)
Puerto Rico	Unclear/verify (no consistent statewide credential info)	Unclear/verify (no consistent statewide credential info)	No title protection (NAVTA snapshot)

This condensed table lists each state/territory with credential type, protected titles, and NAVTA title-protection status for quick reference.
Source: Adapted from NAVTA (2022), AAVSB (2023), and AVMA (2025).

Table 2.2 Comparison of veterinary technician/nurse credentialing in the United States and the United Kingdom.

Category	United States	United Kingdom
Credential title(s)	United States: Licensed Veterinary Technician (LVT), Registered Veterinary Technician (RVT), Certified Veterinary Technician (CVT), Licensed Veterinary Medical Technician (LVMT)—varies by state.	United Kingdom: Veterinary Nurse (VN), regulated nationally by the Royal College of Veterinary Surgeons (RCVS).
Credentialing authority	State veterinary boards; requirements differ across all 50 states plus DC and PR. Some states have no statutory credentials.	Royal College of Veterinary Surgeons (RCVS)—single national authority.
Educational pathway	Associate's degree (two years) is most common. Increasing number of bachelor's (four years) and some master's programs. State licensure/certification/registration required in most but not all jurisdictions.	RCVS-approved Level 3 Diploma in Veterinary Nursing (further education) or bachelor's degree in Veterinary Nursing (higher education).
Title protection	Fragmented. Some states offer general title protection, some limited, some none. In nonregulated states, titles may be used without credentials.	Protected nationally. Only individuals listed on the RCVS Register may legally use the title "Veterinary Nurse."
Scope of practice	Defined state-by-state. Commonly includes anesthesia induction/monitoring, dental prophylaxis, radiography, lab work, and patient nursing care. Diagnosis, prescribing, and surgery reserved for veterinarians. Some states allow limited dental extractions.	Defined nationally by RCVS Day-One Competences. Includes anesthesia monitoring, radiography, dentistry, medical nursing, and surgical nursing. Diagnosis, prescribing, and surgery reserved for veterinarians.
Continuing education (CE/CPD)	Mandatory in most states with varying hours per renewal cycle (e.g., 10–20 CE hours biennially). Some states still have no CE requirement.	Mandatory CPD: 15 hours/year for registered veterinary nurses (RCVS requirement).
Professional associations	NAVTA (National Association of Veterinary Technicians in America) advocates nationally; state associations provide community and local voice.	British Veterinary Nursing Association (BVNA) provides advocacy, professional development, and community.
Professional identity challenges	Ongoing debate around fragmented credentialing, title protection, underutilization, and pursuit of a unified title ("Veterinary Nurse").	Greater consistency due to national regulation; challenges focus more on professional recognition, pay equity, and utilization.

This chart provides a high-level comparison between the credentialing, title protection, and professional identity frameworks in the United States and the United Kingdom.
Source: Adapted from NAVTA (2022), RCVS (2023), and BVNA (2023).

The Impact of Title Protection and Scope of Practice Variations

In states with robust title protection, credentialed veterinary technicians enjoy greater professional recognition and respect. Their defined roles and responsibilities underscore their value within the veterinary team, fostering trust among clients and colleagues. Comprehensive regulations help ensure consistency in the quality of care, as credentialed technicians are held to standardized educational and ethical standards. Conversely, states with limited regulation risk variability in care quality, which can affect patient outcomes.

States with limited title protection may face challenges in attracting and retaining credentialed technicians, as the lack of professional distinction diminishes incentives for pursuing formal education and credentialing. Professional organizations, such as NAVTA, advocate for national title protection and a standardized scope of practice. Initiatives like the Veterinary Nurse Initiative (VNI) aim to unify state regulations and elevate the profession by transitioning the title "veterinary technician" to "veterinary nurse," aligning with international terminology and fostering broader recognition.

The Veterinary Nurse Initiative (VNI): Elevating and Unifying the Veterinary Nursing Profession

The VNI is a groundbreaking effort spearheaded by NAVTA aimed at standardizing the title and scope of practice for veterinary technicians across the United States (NAVTA 2018). By transitioning the title "veterinary technician" to "veterinary nurse," the initiative seeks to align the profession with international standards, enhance public understanding, and foster greater professional recognition. The VNI represents a comprehensive approach to addressing inconsistencies in state regulations and elevating the role of veterinary technicians within the veterinary healthcare system. The VNI is driven by the recognition that the current designation of "veterinary technician" lacks consistency and fails to convey the full scope of expertise and responsibilities inherent in the role (NAVTA 2018). The term "nurse" is widely understood and respected across medical professions, making it a more accurate and recognizable title for the work performed by veterinary technicians.

Goals of the VNI

The initiative aims to (VNI 2024):

- **Standardize Title and Scope:** Establish a unified title ("veterinary nurse") and consistent scope of practice across all states.
- **Align with International Standards:** Bring the US profession in line with countries like the United Kingdom, Australia, and New Zealand, where "veterinary nurse" is the standard title.
- **Enhance Public Understanding:** Improve client awareness and appreciation of the role by adopting terminology familiar to human healthcare.
- **Elevate Professional Recognition:** Foster respect for veterinary technicians as skilled, essential members of the veterinary healthcare team.

One of the primary motivations behind the VNI is the inconsistency in state-level regulations governing veterinary technicians. Variability in title protection, credentialing requirements, and scope of practice has led to disparities in professional recognition and utilization.

The VNI has also encountered significant opposition. Critics argue that the initiative places undue emphasis on changing the professional title rather than addressing deeper issues such as compensation, utilization, and inconsistent state regulation. Some veterinarians and technicians have expressed concern that adopting the title "nurse" may create legal and professional conflicts with human nursing boards, several of which have formally opposed the use of the term in veterinary medicine (National Council of State Boards of Nursing 2018). Opponents also contend that the initiative risks diverting resources and attention away from more urgent priorities, such as securing stronger state-level title protection and expanding technician scope of practice (Bassert and Thomas 2021). In addition, certain state associations have resisted implementation, citing fears of legislative setbacks, confusion among clients, and resistance from nursing organizations that view the title change as an encroachment on their protected professional identity (Miller and Kogan 2019). These tensions illustrate why the VNI, despite its aspirational goals, has faced a sustained push to dismantle or reframe the process in favor of strategies that directly improve workplace conditions and retention.

Conclusion

The history of veterinary nursing is a testament to its remarkable journey of evolution, resilience, and innovation. From its roots as an informal caregiving role grounded in instinct and necessity, the profession has transformed into a highly specialized, indispensable discipline that embodies both the art of compassionate care and the science of clinical expertise. Veterinary nursing has consistently adapted to meet the challenges of advancing medicine, evolving animal healthcare needs, and the growing recognition of its critical role within the veterinary team. By honoring the pioneering efforts that laid its foundation, embracing the current advancements that define its excellence, and proactively shaping its future through education, advocacy, and innovation, veterinary nursing is poised to not only thrive but also lead in shaping the future of veterinary medicine. In doing so, it will continue to make profound and meaningful contributions to animal welfare, public health, and the interconnected well-being of human and animal communities worldwide.

References

Alabama State Board of Veterinary Medical Examiners, 2021. *Administrative Code and Practice Act*. Montgomery, AL: ASBVME. https://www.asbvme.alabama.gov (accessed 1 July 2025).

American Veterinary Medical Association (AVMA), 2011. *50 Years of Veterinary Technology Education*. Schaumburg, IL: AVMA. www.avma.org (accessed 1 July 2025).

Australian and New Zealand College of Veterinary Scientists (ANZCVS) (2010). *Veterinary Nursing in Australia and New Zealand: A Historical Overview*. Brisbane: ANZCVS Publications.

Australian Veterinary Association (AVA) (2013). *The Role of Veterinary Nurses in Australia: Position Statement*. www.ava.com.au (accessed 1 July 2025).

Bassert, J.M. and Thomas, J.A. (2021). *McCurnin's Clinical Textbook for Veterinary Technicians and Nurses*, 10e. St. Louis: Elsevier.

Bissett, S., Robertson, I., and McKeegan, D. (2021). Veterinary nursing education: Building professional identity through degree pathways. *Veterinary Record* 188 (4): 145–148.

British Veterinary Nursing Association (BVNA) (2015) *History of the British Veterinary Nursing Association*. [online] London: BVNA. Available at: https://www.bvna.org.uk/about-us/our-history/ (accessed: 1 July 2025).

Burns, K. (2006). Veterinary technology and nursing: the evolving profession. *Journal of the American Veterinary Medical Association* 229 (3): 357–359. https://doi.org/10.2460/javma.229.3.357.

Caré, X. (2013) École nationale vétérinaire de Lyon (former school building at Clos des Deux-Amants). [online image]. CC BY-SA 4.0. Wikimedia Commons (accessed 24 August 2025).

Clutton-Brock, J. (1992). *The Walking Larder: Patterns of Domestication, Pastoralism, and Predation*, 88–92. London: Unwin Hyman.

Columella, L.J.M. (1941). *On Agriculture (De Re Rustica)*. Translated by H.B. Ash. Cambridge, MA: Harvard University Press.

Dhama, K., Chauhan, R.S., Singhal, L., and Saini, U. (2005). Ayurvedic and herbal remedies in veterinary medicine: An overview. *International Journal of Cow Science* 1 (2): 26–29.

Dunlop, R.H. and Williams, D.J. (1996). *Veterinary Medicine: An Illustrated History*, 82–85. St. Louis: Mosby.

Federation of Veterinarians of Europe (FVE), 2012. *Veterinary Nursing and Paraprofessionals in Europe: Survey Report*. Brussels: FVE. https://www.fve.org/publications (accessed 1 July 2025).

Fox, M.W. (2014). The evolving role of veterinary technicians: Local and state perspectives. *Journal of Veterinary Medical Education* 41 (3): 293–300.

Ghosh, S. (2015). *A History of Medicine: From Prehistory to the Year 2020*, 45–48. Lanham, MD: University Press of America.

Hippocrates, 400 BCE(1923). On airs, waters, and places. In: *Hippocrates*, vol. I (ed. W.H.S. Jones), trans. Cambridge, MA: Harvard University Press.

Howell, P. (2015). *At Home and Astray: The Domestic Dog in Victorian Britain*. Charlottesville: University of Virginia Press.

International Veterinary Nurses and Technicians Association (IVNTA) (2014). Mission and history. www.ivnta.org (accessed 1 July 2025).

Jean de Tournes (1559). Portrait of Lucius Junius Moderatus Columella, in *Insignium aliquot virorum icones*. [online image]. Public domain. Available via Picryl (accessed 24 August 2025).

Landsberg, G. (2002). Traditional veterinary medicine: Regional knowledge and ethnoveterinary practices. In: *Health, Disease and Healing in Animal History* (ed. P. Mathias and G. McNeill), 61–74. London: Routledge.

Landseer, E. (1837) Her Majesty's Favourite Pets. [online image]. Public domain. https://commons.wikimedia.org/wiki/File:Her_Majesty%27s_Favourite_Pets_by_Sir_Edwin_Henry_Landseer.jpg

Lincoln Memorial University (LMU) (2022). *Master of Veterinary Clinical Care (MVCC) program launch*. Harrogate, TN: Lincoln Memorial University College of Veterinary Medicine Available at: https://www.lmunet.edu/college-of-veterinary-medicine/mvcc/index.php (accessed: 1 July 2025).

Lord, L.K., Wittum, T.E., Neer, T.M. et al. (2018). Scope-of-practice issues for veterinary technicians: A national survey and policy analysis. *Journal of the American Veterinary Medical Association* 252 (5): 531–539. https://doi.org/10.2460/javma.252.5.531.

The Met (n.d.) *Bastet statuette (cat-headed goddess), Late Period–Ptolemaic Period, Egypt*. [online image]. Public domain. The Metropolitan Museum of Art Open Access (accessed 24 August 2025).

Miller, H. and Kogan, L.R. (2019). Perceptions of the Veterinary Nurse Initiative among veterinary professionals in the United States. *Journal of the American Veterinary Medical Association* 255 (12): 1420–1426.

National Council of State Boards of Nursing (NCSBN) (2018). *Policy statement on the use of the title "nurse" in veterinary medicine*. NCSBN www.ncsbn.org.

NAVTA (2011). *History of the National Association of Veterinary Technicians in America*. National Association of Veterinary Technicians in America www.navta.net.

National Association of Veterinary Technicians in America (NAVTA), 2018. *Veterinary Nurse Initiative (VNI) Overview*. https://www.navta.net/page/vni (accessed 1 July 2025).

National Association of Veterinary Technicians in America (NAVTA) (2020) NAVTA history and professional advocacy. [online] NAVTA. Available at: https://www.navta.net/page/AboutNAVTA (accessed: 1 July 2025).

New York State Education Department, 2021. *Veterinary Technology: License Requirements*. Albany, NY: Office of the Professions. https://www.op.nysed.gov/professions/veterinary-technology (accessed 1 July 2025).

Orpet, H. and Welsh, P. (2011). *Handbook of Veterinary Nursing*, 2e, 1–4. Oxford: Wiley-Blackwell.

PickPik (n.d.) *Native Americans on horseback*. [online image]. https://www.pickpik.com/native-americans-horse-green-grass-grass-field-photo-historical-52406

Pugh, L.F. (2002). *From Farriery to Veterinary Medicine 1785–1795*, 12–15. Cambridge: Royal College of Veterinary Surgeons.

Ritvo, H. (1987). *The Animal Estate: The English and Other Creatures in the Victorian Age*. Cambridge, MA: Harvard University Press.

Royal College of Veterinary Surgeons (RCVS) (2011). *A short history of veterinary nursing*. London: RCVS Available at: (Accessed: 1 July 2025).

Salisbury, R.B. and Van Valkenburgh, B. (2007). The archaeology and history of veterinary medicine. In: *Veterinary Medicine: Origins and Historical Foundations* (ed. P.J. Pastoret), 15–28. Paris: World Organisation for Animal Health (OIE).

Scarborough, J. (1991). Roman medicine and the regulation of animal health. In: *Veterinary Medicine and Human Health in the Ancient World* (ed. B. Boddington), 37–49. Oxford: Oxford University Press.

Sinclair, U. (1906). *The Jungle*. New York: Doubleday, Page & Company.

Smith, C. (2019). The evolution of the veterinary technician profession in the United States. *Journal of the American Veterinary Medical Association* 254 (5): 562–568.

Smith, C.F. (2005). *A Historical Perspective on Veterinary Medicine*, 22–28. Oxford: Blackwell Publishing.

Smith, F. (2012). *Animals and Disease: An Introduction to the History of Comparative Medicine*, 45–52. London: Equine Veterinary Journal/UK Veterinary History Society.

Totelin, L.M.V. (2017). *Ancient Botany*, 112–115. London: Routledge.

Touwaide, A. and Appetiti, E. (2013). Food and medicines in the Mediterranean tradition: A systematic analysis of the earliest extant body of textual evidence. *Journal of Ethnopharmacology* 148 (2): 321–336. https://doi.org/10.1016/j.jep.2012.09.037.

Unknown photographer (1908). *Interior scene at a veterinary school: attendants assisting with equine treatment*. [online image]. Public domain. Wikimedia Commons (accessed 24 August 2025).

Unknown photographer (1899) *École nationale vétérinaire d'Alfort, Maisons-Alfort, France*. [online image]. Public domain. https://commons.wikimedia.org/wiki/File:École_nationale_vétérinaire_d%27Alfort_en_1899.jpg

Veterinary Nurse Initiative (VNI) (2024). *Unifying the Title of Veterinary Nurse.* [online] NAVTA. https://www.navta.net/page/vni (accessed 1 July 2025).

Volk, J.O., Felsted, K., Thomas, J.G., and Siren, C.W. (1984). *The Status and Future of Veterinary Technicians in the United States.* Schaumburg, IL: American Veterinary Medical Association.

Wellcome Collection (n.d.) *Hippocrates.* Coloured stipple engraving by J. Chapman, 1809. [online image]. Public Domain (CC0). Wellcome Collection (accessed 24 August 2025).

Wilkinson, L. (1992). *Animals and Disease: An Introduction to the History of Comparative Medicine*, 33–40. Cambridge: Cambridge University Press.

Xie, H. and Preast, V. (2010). *Traditional Chinese Veterinary Medicine: Fundamental Principles.* Coral Springs, FL: Chi Institute Press.

3

Nursing Basics

Introduction

Veterinary nursing is dynamic and multifaceted, demanding technical competence, clinical reasoning, and compassionate care in equal measure. Many technicians already perform the "basics" daily—handling and restraint, venipuncture, medication administration, anesthesia monitoring, surgical assistance, laboratory sampling and interpretation, radiography, accurate documentation, and clear client communication. This chapter affirms those foundations while inviting you to sharpen them: not as a checklist of tasks to complete, but as a craft to refine.

Our goal is to move beyond how to perform a procedure and explore why each step matters—physiologically, behaviorally, ethically, and in terms of patient welfare and team safety. We will examine decision points, common pitfalls, and failure-prevention strategies; connect small technique choices to patient outcomes; and highlight microskills. You will see how subtle adjustments—reading early stress signals, selecting the least-restrictive effective restraint, calibrating analgesia, confirming drug calculations, or structuring a client explanation—compound into better medicine and smoother workflows.

By approaching familiar skills with a deeper lens, technicians strengthen judgment, adaptability, and advocacy. The result is greater confidence in detecting early changes, responding to complications, communicating clearly with clients and colleagues, and aligning care with best practices. In short, this chapter is a springboard from competence to mastery—grounding everyday techniques in their underlying principles so holistic, proactive, and specialized care can take shape with intention and consistency (Table 3.1).

Section 1: Animal Handling and Restraint

Effective animal handling and restraint are essential competencies for veterinary technicians, ensuring the safety of both the patient and the handler while facilitating optimal patient care. Proper handling techniques minimize stress, prevent injury, and enhance the overall veterinary experience (Overall 2013). Restraint should be approached with a balance of control and compassion, as excessive force or improper techniques can exacerbate fear and defensive behaviors, leading to increased risk of injury (Becker and Bain 2020).

Principles of Low-stress Handling

The use of low-stress handling is central to reducing anxiety and promoting cooperation in veterinary patients. Effective restraint begins with an understanding of species-specific behavior and the ability to read early signs of fear or arousal so techniques can be adjusted before stress escalates. Subtle indicators—such as lip licking, panting, tail flicking, ear flattening, pupil dilation, and avoidance—should prompt a pause, a softer touch, or a change in approach to preserve the patient's sense of control (Stella et al. 2013). Creating a calm environment further supports this goal: minimize sudden noise, harsh lighting, rushing, and direct staring; use nonslip surfaces and familiar scents; and consider pheromone diffusers (e.g., Feliway for cats, Adaptil for dogs) which have shown benefit for some patients (Frank et al. 2010). Throughout the interaction, pair handling with positive reinforcement—food, gentle praise, or a brief break—so that cooperation is reinforced and handling aversion diminishes over time.

Restraint tools should be selected and applied judiciously to provide security without unnecessary force. Towels, well-fitted muzzles, and slip leads can offer controlled, predictable contact while maintaining comfort when used with

Table 3.1 Core nursing skills.

Chapter Section	Skill Area	Key Topics Included
1	Animal handling and restraint	Low-stress techniques, species-specific restraint, FAS scoring
2	Venipuncture and IV access	Site selection, catheter types, aseptic technique, troubleshooting
3	Medication administration	Oral, topical, injectable, ophthalmic, complication prevention
4	Anesthesia monitoring	HR, BP, SpO_2, $ETCO_2$, anesthetic depth, hypotension management
5	Surgical assisting	Sterile prep, instrument handling, intraoperative support, specialty procedure tips
6	Laboratory skills	CBC, chemistry, urinalysis, cytology, error prevention
7	Imaging and radiology	Positioning, digital systems, ultrasound, artifact correction
8	Dentistry	Dental charting, cleaning, radiographs, assisting with extractions
9	Patient nursing and monitoring	Pain scoring, nutritional support, neonatal/geriatric care, record keeping
10	Client communication	History taking, client education, grief support, conflict resolution
11	Professional soft skills	Time management, adaptability, emotional resilience, teamwork

steady hands and clear contingencies for release. When behavioral history or real-time responses indicate that physical restraint alone will likely provoke defensive behavior or compromise welfare, previsit pharmaceuticals or in-clinic chemical restraint may be the kindest, safest option for the patient and team (Stewart et al. 2019). The guiding principle is progressive, least-restrictive handling: start with the lightest effective method, monitor continuously for stress signals, and scale up or down as the patient shows you what they can tolerate.

Handling should be tailored to species and temperament, as well as to the procedure. For dogs, commonly used positions—standing restraint, sternal recumbency, and lateral recumbency—offer graduated control and should be selected to match the task while allowing frequent microreleases as the patient succeeds. A properly fitted muzzle is appropriate for dogs with a history of fearful or defensive behavior, or when a procedure is likely to be painful; basket styles that permit panting and treat delivery are ideal for longer tasks, while fabric muzzles are reserved for brief moments. After procedures, an e-collar may help prevent self-trauma, but it should be fitted and introduced calmly with reinforcement to minimize confusion or distress.

Cats require a "less is more" philosophy that emphasizes guided movement over gripping and preserves the cat's choice to hide, perch, or settle. Begin with environmental adjustments—quiet room, dimmer light, carrier base or familiar towel as the handling surface—and slow, predictable touch, pausing early if arousal rises. Towel techniques are often the next step when a bit more containment is needed: a simple burrito for general security, a half-wrap to steady the thorax for auscultation, or a targeted limb-exposure wrap for venipuncture. Each should be applied smoothly, with the cat's body fully supported, and released as soon as the task is complete. Feline muzzles that cover the eyes may be used briefly to reduce visual stimuli during short procedures when calmer methods are insufficient. Scruffing, once routine, should not be a first-line method; many cats cope better with towel-based support and gentle head control, and scruffing can heighten fear or defensive responses (ISFM 2016). If scruffing is used at all, it should be limited to urgent, time-critical situations when immediate safety is at risk and other options have failed, performed with full body support, the lightest effective pressure, and the shortest duration possible before transitioning back to low-stress methods.

Across species, the technician's role is to plan for success—anticipating triggers, staging equipment, arranging pharmacologic support when indicated, and setting clear stop-points if the patient's welfare is trending the wrong way. When restraint is framed as cooperative, minimally aversive, and paired with reinforcement, patients learn that clinical handling is predictable and safe, which reduces anxiety and promotes smoother care over time (Frank et al., 2010; ISFM 2016; Stella et al. 2013; Stewart et al. 2019).

Put It Into Practice: Handling and Restraint for Dogs and Cats

Begin by staging the environment before the patient arrives. Prepare a quiet space with minimal foot traffic, have nonslip mats on the table and floor, and lay out the least-restrictive tools you expect to use first—high-value treats, a familiar towel or the cat's carrier base, a well-fitting basket muzzle, and a clean slip lead. Decide on a progressive plan with your team: a

Green plan (calm handling only), an Amber plan (add towel support, light head control, basket muzzle for dogs, or a brief eye covering feline muzzle), and a Red plan (abort, regroup, and consider previsit pharmaceuticals or in-clinic sedation per protocol). Assign roles so one person leads handling while another watches for early stress signals and verbalizes "green/amber/red" status in real time.

For dogs, approach in an arc rather than head-on, soften your body posture, and let the dog choose proximity. Pair initial touch with a steady stream of tiny food rewards to create a cooperative frame. Start with the lightest effective position that fits the task—standing for vaccines or quick auscultation, sternal recumbency for blood draws from a cephalic vein, or lateral recumbency for wound care—while offering microreleases as the dog succeeds. If defensive signals appear or the procedure is likely to be uncomfortable, fit a basket muzzle before escalation; choose a size that permits panting and treat delivery, introduce it with food, and keep your hands quiet once it is on. Fabric muzzles are reserved for very brief moments because they limit panting. Throughout, keep one hand for guidance and one for support rather than gripping; adjust pressure with the same sensitivity you would use to steady a glass of water, and return to neutral as soon as control is no longer needed.

For cats, let the carrier be your starting surface and avoid pouring the cat onto a cold table. Open the door, remove the top if possible, and allow the cat to remain on or in familiar bedding. Use slow hands and predictable contact, pausing at the first sign of rising arousal. When more containment is needed, move up one step at a time: a simple towel "burrito" to provide whole-body security; a half-wrap to steady the thorax for auscultation; or a targeted limb-exposure wrap for venipuncture. Apply each wrap smoothly while fully supporting the cat's weight, and release immediately after the task. Brief use of a feline muzzle that covers the eyes can reduce visual input for short procedures, but it should follow failed low-intensity attempts, not precede them. Scruffing is not a first-line method; if used at all, it is reserved for urgent, time-critical safety moments when other options have failed, and it must be as light and brief as possible with full body support before transitioning back to low-stress techniques.

Build in explicit "stop points" before you begin. Agree that two unsuccessful attempts at any task trigger a pause to lower arousal, change the plan, or reschedule with previsit medication. Use simple, shared language to keep the team aligned: "Pausing—ears are pinning and tail is tucked; moving from Green to Amber," or "Switching to burrito wrap for one venipuncture attempt; if no go, we'll stop and plan PVP." The goal is not to "get it done at all costs," but to complete necessary care without teaching the patient that handling is unpredictable or aversive. Reinforcement should be woven throughout, not saved for the end. For food-motivated dogs, maintain a gentle, continuous "chip-rate" of pea-sized treats during touch and needle placement; for cats, use lickable treats, a warm towel, or short breaks in a covered carrier. When a patient refuses food, treat the absence of eating as data about stress and lighten your approach accordingly. Keep your voice low and neutral, minimize direct staring, and coordinate hands so only one person changes pressure at a time.

Close the loop with documentation that helps the next visit go better. Record the handling plan that worked, the patient's stress signals, the point at which you escalated, the tools that helped, and whether previsit medication is recommended. Offer owners a brief debrief: what their pet handled well, what signs of stress you saw, and how you plan to make future visits smoother. Repeatable notes like "carrier top removed; half-wrap tolerated; eye-covering muzzle for 30 seconds; recommend gabapentin three hours pre-visit" turn a one-time success into a durable protocol.

Finally, practice these skills when the stakes are low. Run five-minute team drills—basket-muzzle fitting with treat delivery on a stuffed dog, towel wraps on a cat mannequin, or "green/amber/red" call-outs during mock venipuncture positioning—so the mechanics are automatic when you need them. The combination of prepared environment, progressive planning, crisp microskills, and honest stop rules is what keeps handling both kind and effective.

Recognizing and Managing Aggression

Aggression in veterinary patients is often a result of fear, pain, or previous negative experiences. Veterinary technicians must be able to differentiate between offensive aggression, where an animal is actively attempting to control a situation, and defensive aggression, which occurs when an animal perceives no means of escape. The use of Fear, Anxiety, and Stress (FAS) scoring provides a structured approach to assessing a patient's emotional state and modifying handling strategies accordingly (Landsberg et al. 2012).

Fear, Anxiety, and Stress (FAS) Scoring

FAS scoring is based on observable behaviors and provides an objective way to evaluate a patient's level of stress. The scale ranges from FAS 1 (relaxed, minimal fear) to FAS 5 (extreme fear and aggression) (Table 3.2) (Landsberg et al. 2012).

Table 3.2 Fear, anxiety, and stress (FAS) scoring with behavioral signs and handling considerations.

FAS Score	Behavioral Signs	Handling Considerations
1 (Relaxed)	Normal body posture, soft eyes, calm demeanor	Minimal restraint needed
2 (Mild anxiety)	Slight panting, lip licking, hesitant approach	Use treats, speak softly
3 (Moderate anxiety)	Tense posture, pinned ears, scanning environment	Proceed slowly, use towel wraps if needed
4 (Severe fear)	Attempts to flee, growling, hissing, rigid body	Minimize handling, consider chemical restraint
5 (Extreme fear/aggression)	Snapping, lunging, dilated pupils, defensive biting	Sedation or full chemical restraint recommended

Adapted from Fear Free FAS Spectrum handouts and the AAFP/ISFM Cat Friendly Veterinary Interaction Guidelines.
Source: Fear Free (n.d.), Rodan et al. (2022).

When handling patients with FAS levels 4 or 5, modifications to the standard approach are necessary. Allowing a fearful patient time to acclimate to the environment before restraint, reducing visual stimulation, and using previsit pharmaceuticals or injectable sedatives can significantly reduce handling stress (Stewart et al. 2019). Protective equipment such as bite gloves, muzzles, and restraint poles should only be used as a last resort and in a manner that prioritizes patient welfare. For extremely reactive animals, preemptive chemical restraint is often the safest option. Sedation or anxiolytic medications should be considered in aggressive or highly fearful patients to minimize stress and ensure the safety of veterinary staff (Becker and Bain 2020).

Mastering animal handling and restraint is a fundamental skill for veterinary technicians. Utilizing low-stress handling techniques, recognizing species-specific behavioral cues, and assessing patients using structured FAS scoring allows for safer, more effective patient care. By applying these principles, veterinary professionals can enhance patient welfare, improve clinical efficiency, and reduce the risk of injury to both animals and staff.

Handling, Restraint, and the Role of Chemical Sedation

Mastery of animal handling and restraint is a fundamental competency in veterinary nursing, serving as the foundation for safe, effective, and compassionate patient care. While physical restraint techniques are essential, they must always be guided by a low-stress philosophy, incorporating species-specific behavioral assessment and structured fear, anxiety, and stress (FAS) scoring. By recognizing subtle behavioral cues and adjusting approach in real time, veterinary technicians can mitigate patient distress and prevent escalation. The ultimate goal is to safeguard both patient welfare and staff safety while maintaining the integrity of the patient–practitioner bond (Becker and Bain 2020).

Chemical restraint is not a last resort but a proactive and humane component of care, particularly in patients exhibiting aggression, fear, or extreme reactivity. Previsit pharmaceuticals such as acepromazine, gabapentin, and trazodone—colloquially termed "Happy Dog" or "Happy Cat" packs—reduce stress, enhance compliance, and improve overall safety. Acepromazine, a phenothiazine derivative, provides tranquilization via dopamine antagonism but lacks true anxiolytic effects and carries risk in cardiovascularly compromised patients. Gabapentin modulates calcium channels, providing anxiolysis and mild analgesia, particularly useful in feline practice. Trazodone, a serotonin antagonist and reuptake inhibitor (SARI), offers anxiolytic and sedative benefits in dogs, supporting low-stress handling during examinations and procedures.

In-hospital injectable sedation protocols frequently incorporate dexmedetomidine, ketamine, and butorphanol, either alone or in combination. Dexmedetomidine, an alpha-2 agonist, produces sedation, analgesia, and muscle relaxation but requires vigilant monitoring due to biphasic cardiovascular effects. Ketamine, an NMDA receptor antagonist, provides dissociative anesthesia with preserved airway reflexes and is often paired with other agents to minimize excitatory effects. Butorphanol, a kappa-opioid agonist and mu-antagonist, provides mild sedation and analgesia with minimal respiratory depression, making it a frequent choice in multimodal protocols. Full mu-opioid agonists (e.g., hydromorphone, morphine, methadone, fentanyl) may be integrated for greater analgesia, reducing sympathetic arousal and facilitating handling in highly anxious or dysphoric patients.

Importantly, unmanaged stress elevates endogenous cortisol levels, potentiating cardiovascular instability, arrhythmias, and impaired recovery. Proactive sedation not only facilitates restraint but also prevents the physiologic sequelae of sympathetic overactivation. Veterinary technicians must therefore advocate for chemical restraint when arousal surpasses safe thresholds, pausing or terminating sessions when necessary. This is not failure but patient advocacy.

Client education is integral to compliance with previsit medication protocols. Framing pharmaceuticals as "emotional support tools" emphasizes their role in reducing trauma, protecting staff, and improving the patient's long-term perception of veterinary care. Providing written dosing instructions, transparent communication, and follow-up support strengthens owner trust and ensures successful outcomes.

Ultimately, restraint in veterinary nursing is an art informed by science. Through the judicious integration of behavioral observation, low-stress physical handling, and evidence-based pharmacologic support, veterinary technicians serve as patient advocates, enhancing welfare, improving safety, and transforming veterinary visits into more positive experiences for all involved.

Section 2: Venipuncture and IV Catheter Placement

Venipuncture and intravenous (IV) catheter placement are fundamental skills in veterinary nursing, allowing for blood collection, medication administration, and fluid therapy. Mastery of these techniques requires a thorough understanding of anatomy, patient handling, and catheter maintenance. While cephalic, saphenous, and jugular veins are commonly used, advanced knowledge of alternative venous access sites is crucial for challenging cases, such as patients with poor perfusion, coagulopathies, or extensive trauma (Bateman 2021).

Fundamentals of Venipuncture

Venipuncture involves inserting a needle into a vein to obtain a blood sample or administer fluids. Proper technique minimizes patient discomfort and prevents complications such as hematoma formation, thrombosis, or vessel damage. The choice of venipuncture site depends on the patient's species, size, temperament, and the procedure being performed (Hopper and Silverstein 2020).

The cephalic vein, located on the cranial aspect of the forelimb, is commonly used for both venipuncture and catheter placement due to its accessibility. The lateral saphenous vein, found on the lateral aspect of the hind limb, is frequently utilized in dogs, particularly in fractious patients where restraining the forelimb is challenging. In contrast, the medial saphenous vein, located on the inner thigh, is preferred for feline venipuncture due to ease of control and reduced risk of hematoma (Hall et al. 2020). The jugular vein is the preferred site for large volume blood collection and central venous pressure monitoring, but requires precise technique to minimize the risk of arterial puncture (Mathews et al. 2017).

Intravenous Catheter Placement

Intravenous (IV) catheterization underpins safe anesthesia, fluid therapy, and timely delivery of critical medications. The technical steps are familiar to most technicians, yet outcomes improve markedly when placement is framed as a patient-centered, least-restrictive procedure that anticipates stress, pain, and physiologic goals. In other words, technique choices—site, gauge, securement, and maintenance—should be justified by the patient's needs and the intended therapy, not habit alone (Table 3.3) (AAHA 2020; Silverstein and Hopper 2020).

Plan for cooperation before touching the vein. Stage a quiet space with a nonslip surface, dim lighting, and species-appropriate reinforcement (lickables for cats, pea-sized treats for dogs). Handle with the lightest effective restraint: guide rather than grip, support the limb rather than stretch it. Warm the distal limb or use a warm pack to promote vasodilation, and apply a tourniquet only as long as needed. For awake patients, consider dermal/local analgesia—topical anesthetic per protocol or a tiny intradermal lidocaine bleb at the entry site—to reduce needle aversion and improve first-pass success. These microinvestments decrease struggling, preserve venous integrity, and make future visits smoother (AAHA 2020; Grimm et al. 2015). Choose the largest practical gauge and the shortest effective length the patient will comfortably tolerate: by Poiseuille's law, larger radius and shorter length sharply increase flow—crucial for resuscitation, anesthetic induction, and rapid drug delivery. Start distal to preserve proximal options: common sites include the cephalic or lateral/medial saphenous in dogs and the cephalic or medial saphenous/femoral in cats. Reserve jugular access for central venous lines or when repeated peripheral attempts fail, and do not hesitate to use previsit anxiolytics or in-clinic sedation when the welfare calculus favors pharmacologic cooperation over force (Silverstein and Hopper 2020). Clip widely enough to keep

Table 3.3 IV access devices commonly used in small-animal practice.

Device	Also Called	Typical Use	Common Sites	Typical Duration[a]	Advantages	Limitations
Over-the-needle peripheral catheter (OTN)	Peripheral IV	Most frequent everyday IV access: fluids, CRIs, peri-op meds	Cephalic, lateral/ medial saphenous	Hours to a few days (24–72 hours per hospital policy)	Quick to place, inexpensive, wide gauge range (24–18 G)	Can kink if over a joint; not ideal for frequent blood sampling
Through-the-needle catheter	Legacy jugular/ central placement (often replaced by Seldinger CVC kits)	Central access for longer therapy, hyperosmolar/ irritant infusions, CVP sampling	Jugular vein	Days (protocol-dependent)	Allows central infusions and blood sampling from line	Larger introducer needle; bleeding risk; requires strict asepsis and securement
Winged infusion set	"Butterfly"	Short procedures: single-dose injections, brief infusions, blood draws	Cephalic, saphenous	Minutes to short sessions	Low profile; helpful for small/ fragile veins; excellent for venipuncture	Not suited for unattended/ continuous fluids; easily dislodged

Author's summary of common intravenous access devices for dogs and cats, with typical clinical uses, sites, and limitations.
[a] Always follow your hospital's dwell-time and site-rotation policy.
Source: Table 3.3: AAHA, 2020; Silverstein & Hopper, 2015; Grimm et al., 2015

adhesive and gloves off hair, then perform a target-style skin prep using chlorhexidine with adequate contact time followed by alcohol for defatting. Use firm friction in concentric passes from clean to cleaner, and avoid repalpating the site after final prep unless using a sterile glove. Replace any item that becomes contaminated rather than "working around it." Contamination at insertion is a leading predictor of phlebitis and catheter-associated bloodstream infection (AAHA 2020). Stabilize the vessel with gentle counter-tension, advance the catheter smoothly once flashback appears, and avoid pistoning the stylet within the vein. After confirming placement and flushing easily, secure the catheter so it cannot lever at the hub. Create adhesive "stirrups," anchor with a chevron or U-loop of tape, and attach an extension set or T-port to keep connections off the hub. Choose a breathable, transparent dressing so the insertion site remains visible; bulky wraps hide early inflammation and can impair perfusion. Check distal circulation after bandaging and again after the patient walks or flexes the joint (Silverstein and Hopper 2020). Label the dressing with date/time, gauge/length, site, and initials. Disinfect injection caps before each access, flush with the minimum volume needed to clear dead space before and after medications, and inspect at least once per shift for pain, swelling, heat, discharge, wet dressings, or migration. Many services achieve lower complication rates by replacing peripheral catheters "for cause" (e.g., signs of phlebitis, occlusion, contamination) rather than by rigid time alone, while still observing typical dwell times of 24–72 hours depending on patient and policy. Document the maintenance plan so the next shift continues the same bundle without drift (AAHA 2020; Silverstein and Hopper 2020). Record site, gauge/length, number of attempts, securement method, flushes and medications delivered, maintenance checks, and any complications with the team's response.

Ultrasound guidance improves first-pass success in dehydrated, edematous, or critically ill patients and reduces iatrogenic hematomas by visualizing vessel depth and needle tip location (McMichael and Powell 2021). If rapid access is lifesaving and peripheral attempts have failed, intraosseous catheterization provides central-like flow for fluids, hypertonic solutions, and many emergency drugs until IV access is secured. For prolonged therapy, frequent blood sampling, or infusion of irritant/vesicant solutions, a jugular central venous catheter placed under full sterile technique with a central-line care bundle is often the kindest and safest choice (Silverstein and Hopper 2020). See Chapter 7 for more information on alternative access points when common catheterization techniques fail or advanced techniques are required.

Section 3: Medication Administration

Administering medications is one of the most routine, and most critical, tasks performed by veterinary technicians. It is far more than a mechanical act; it is a responsibility that directly impacts patient safety, treatment success, and client trust. Every dose given carries the potential for healing or harm, making accuracy, knowledge, and clinical judgment essential.

Veterinary technicians must approach medication administration with both technical skill and a clear understanding of why a drug is being used, how it works, and what the potential risks are. This requires a foundational knowledge of pharmacokinetics, including how a drug is absorbed, distributed, metabolized, and excreted by the patient. Recognizing how different administration routes influence the onset, intensity, and duration of drug action is essential for ensuring therapeutic effectiveness and minimizing adverse effects.

The route of administration, whether oral, topical, injectable, or ophthalmic, should never be chosen or carried out blindly. The technician must first consider the patient's condition, the drug's formulation and intended effect, and any contraindications based on current health status. For example, administering an oral NSAID to a vomiting patient or giving a nephrotoxic drug to a dehydrated animal may cause serious complications if done without proper assessment.

Moreover, technicians must take ownership of the medications they administer. This means reviewing drug labels, confirming correct dosage and timing, understanding potential side effects, and communicating clearly with both the veterinary team and the pet owner. When a technician gives medication, they are not simply following instructions; they are acting as a medical professional entrusted with the well-being of a nonverbal patient.

Oral Medication Administration

Oral (PO) administration is one of the most frequently used routes in veterinary medicine, offering a convenient and noninvasive option for many patients. However, ease of administration does not diminish the importance of clinical oversight. Veterinary technicians must verify that oral medications are appropriate for the patient's current condition and can be safely absorbed by the gastrointestinal system.

Before administration, technicians should confirm whether the drug requires an empty stomach, should be given with food, or may interact with other medications or supplements. For example, certain antibiotics and thyroid medications lose effectiveness when given with calcium-containing foods, while some analgesics may cause GI upset without a meal buffer. Understanding the pharmacological profile of the drug is essential to ensure compliance and avoid adverse effects. Additionally, technicians are responsible for confirming proper formulation, liquid, tablet, capsule, or compounded, based on the patient's species, size, and temperament. For fractious or inappetent patients, technicians must advocate for alternatives such as transdermal, injectable, or compounded formulations to ensure safe and stress-free dosing. By viewing oral medication administration as a clinical responsibility rather than a task, veterinary technicians uphold safety, efficacy, and patient comfort with every dose.

Advanced Tip: Avoiding Esophageal Stricture

Doxycycline tablets in cats can cause esophageal ulcers, leading to esophageal strictures if not followed by water. Always administer a minimum of 5 mL of water or use compounded liquid formulations to reduce the risk (Padrid 2021).

Topical Medication Administration

Topical medications, whether transdermal gels, ear drops, or dermal treatments, may seem straightforward but require diligent handling and a strong understanding of drug absorption and patient behavior. Unlike other routes, topicals may remain on the patient's body for extended periods, posing risks of ingestion, cross-contamination, or environmental degradation.

Technicians must be aware of the exact location, absorption rate, and potential systemic effects of topical drugs. Transdermal methimazole, for instance, can be inadvertently ingested during grooming if applied improperly or without protective measures. Otic medications must be verified as safe for use with a ruptured tympanic membrane; applying ototoxic agents to a ruptured eardrum could cause permanent hearing loss or vestibular damage.

Part of a technician's responsibility includes counseling owners on post-application precautions, such as preventing pets from licking treated areas, using e-collars, or keeping treated animals separate from housemates or children. Technicians must also confirm that topicals are compatible with the pet's lifestyle and environment. Properly administered, topical medications are effective and minimally invasive. Improperly handled, they can result in toxicity, treatment failure, or even human exposure. Recognizing this responsibility ensures safer outcomes for both patients and their caregivers.

Clinical Insight: Otic Medication Penetration

Ceruminous debris can prevent otic medication absorption. Applying ear cleaners 15–30 minutes before medicated drops increases penetration and efficacy, particularly for Pseudomonas otitis cases (Rosychuk 2019).

Injectable Medication Administration

Injectable medications are a cornerstone of veterinary care, offering rapid absorption and precise control over dosage and effect. Because these drugs bypass the gastrointestinal system, they often take effect more quickly, but they also carry an increased risk if given incorrectly. Veterinary technicians must understand both the mechanics of injection technique and the pharmacodynamics of what they are administering.

Whether the route is subcutaneous (SQ), intramuscular (IM), intravenous (IV), or intraosseous (IO), technicians must confirm the correct dosage, dilution, and injection site. Certain medications, such as chemotherapeutics, hypertonic solutions, or some NSAIDs, can cause severe tissue damage if extravasated or given via the wrong route. For example, injecting dexamethasone acetate IV can result in embolism or necrosis, while lidocaine administered IV too quickly may cause cardiovascular collapse. Preadministration checks, such as verifying drug compatibility, reviewing expiration dates, confirming patient ID, and ensuring no contraindications, are not optional steps. They are part of the technician's duty of care.

In addition, technicians must be prepared to monitor for immediate adverse reactions, particularly with vaccines, sedatives, and newly initiated therapies. Administering injectable medications demands vigilance, respect for pharmacology, and a deep understanding of patient status before, during, and after the injection (Table 3.4).

Expert Tip: Preventing Necrosis with IM Injections

Injecting NSAIDs or corticosteroids IM can lead to muscle necrosis. Always verify formulation instructions. For example, dexamethasone SP can be given IV or IM, but dexamethasone acetate should never be given IV (Mathews et al. 2017).

Ophthalmic Medication Administration

Ophthalmic medications require precision, restraint skill, and a keen awareness of the sensitivity of the eye. Unlike systemic treatments, topical ocular drugs must be administered directly to a delicate and highly reactive surface. Misapplication, whether due to poor technique, expired drugs, or failure to identify corneal damage, can lead to permanent vision impairment or pain.

Table 3.4 Injectable medication administration sites.

Injection Type	Common Abbreviation	Description/Notes	Tips and Tricks
Subcutaneous	SQ or SC	Administered under the skin, often over the scruff or flank.	Tent the skin to form a pocket; avoid injecting too deeply or into muscle.
Intramuscular	IM	Delivered into a muscle such as the epaxial or quadriceps. **Cats and small dogs:** $\leq$ **2 mL IM per site.** **Medium–large dogs:** up to **5 mL IM per site.**	Use a swift motion; aspirate to avoid blood vessels; massage the site after.
Intravenous	IV	Delivered directly into the vein, usually via catheter; it allows rapid absorption.	Always check patency; inject slowly to monitor for adverse reactions.
Intradermal	ID	Given just under the dermis; used for allergy or TB testing.	Create a small bleb; use a very small gauge needle; do not massage the site.
Intraosseous	IO	Administered into medullary cavity when IV access isn't possible; rapid absorption.	Requires sterile technique; use a specialized IO needle and secure well.

Source: M. Jennings (2025). Author's own compilation.

Technicians must confirm that the chosen product is appropriate for the eye's condition. For example, steroid-containing ointments are contraindicated in patients with corneal ulcers, where they may delay healing and worsen tissue damage. Before administering any medication, technicians should assess for signs of discharge, cloudiness, or pain and communicate concerns to the veterinarian before proceeding. Technique is equally critical. Contact with the corneal surface must be avoided to prevent trauma or contamination of the medication container. In multidrug regimens, technicians should ensure the correct order of application and spacing between doses, applying solutions before ointments and waiting 5–10 minutes between them to allow absorption. Finally, education is key. Technicians must coach owners on safe restraint, correct dosing intervals, and when to discontinue or adjust treatment. Mastery of ophthalmic administration reflects a technician's blend of technical skill, pharmacological knowledge, and empathetic patient handling.

Pro Tip: Preventing Cross-Contamination

When treating infectious keratoconjunctivitis, use separate applicators for each affected eye to prevent spreading pathogens like *Chlamydophila felis*.

Complications and Best Practices

Veterinary technicians are not just administrators of medication; they are responsible stewards of pharmacologic care. With every dose comes the duty to ensure that the right drug is given to the right patient, in the right way, for the right reason. That level of responsibility demands not only technical precision but a deep awareness of potential complications and proactive prevention strategies.

Each route of administration carries its own risks:

- Oral medications can lead to aspiration pneumonia if given to patients with dysphagia, sedation, too quickly without voluntary swallowing, or neurologic compromise.
- Intramuscular injections may cause tissue necrosis if given improperly, especially with irritating drugs like corticosteroids or certain antibiotics.
- Intravenous medications must be administered with vigilance to avoid phlebitis, extravasation, or embolism.
- Medication incompatibilities, such as mixing incompatible drugs in the same syringe or line, can lead to precipitation, inactivation, or toxicity.
- Hypersensitivity reactions, including anaphylaxis, can occur unexpectedly and require immediate recognition and intervention.

Best practices begin with knowledge. Technicians must understand the pharmacology of the drug being administered, including its expected effects, contraindications, and interactions with other medications or conditions. This knowledge base allows technicians to question an unfamiliar dose, advocate for route changes in compromised patients, or pause administration until clarification is obtained. Technicians also play a vital role in client education. Owners must be taught not only *how* to administer medications at home, but also *why* adherence matters. Strategies such as using pill pockets, demonstrating techniques, providing clear written instructions, and recommending compounding options can significantly improve compliance and reduce treatment failure (Plumb 2020). Ultimately, the safest and most effective medication administration occurs when technicians act as both technical experts and critical thinkers, anticipating risks, adapting for each patient, and embracing full ownership of the medications they deliver. This proactive approach reduces adverse effects, builds client trust, and elevates the quality of care across every aspect of veterinary nursing.

Section 4: Anesthesia Monitoring—Basic

Anesthesia Monitoring

Anesthesia monitoring is far more than a checklist of vital signs; it is a moment-by-moment responsibility that can mean the difference between a safe procedure and a life-threatening emergency. Veterinary technicians serve as the eyes and ears of the anesthetized patient, acting with intention, vigilance, and deep understanding to ensure every patient under anesthesia receives the highest standard of care.

To monitor anesthesia effectively, technicians must go beyond rote measurements. They must interpret what each change in heart rate, respiratory effort, or blood pressure means in the context of the anesthetic plan, the patient's condition, and the surgical stimulus. This level of care demands a solid grasp of anesthetic pharmacology, physiology, and the way different monitoring parameters reflect perfusion, ventilation, and oxygenation status.

Each phase of anesthesia, premedication, induction, maintenance, and recovery presents its own challenges and risks. Technicians must adapt their monitoring strategies in each phase to anticipate complications such as hypotension, hypoventilation, hypoxemia, arrhythmias, airway obstruction, and thermal loss. Monitoring is not passive observation; it is active problem prevention.

This section explores the technician's role in anesthesia from preparation to full recovery. With each patient, the goal is not just survival, it is stability, comfort, and a smooth anesthetic experience with minimal complications. Through vigilance, knowledge, and critical thinking, veterinary technicians become powerful advocates for anesthetized patients.

Premedication Monitoring

The premedication phase is the first opportunity for the technician to shape a safe and predictable anesthetic experience. Administering sedatives and analgesics is not merely preparatory, it is a calculated effort to reduce patient stress, ease induction, and stabilize physiologic parameters before anesthetic agents are introduced.

Before giving any premedication, the technician should obtain and record baseline vital signs, including temperature, heart rate (HR), respiratory rate (RR), and, when possible, blood pressure (BP) and SpO_2. These values serve as a critical point of comparison throughout the anesthetic event, helping the technician recognize abnormal trends and differentiate drug effects from pathology.

Each premedication protocol must be tailored to the individual patient's signalment, temperament, health status, and planned procedure. For instance, acepromazine may be inappropriate in hypotensive or geriatric patients due to its vasodilatory effects, while dexmedetomidine may cause profound bradycardia in small dogs or patients with cardiac disease. Understanding why a particular drug is chosen and how it may impact perfusion, thermoregulation, or airway reflexes is essential to anticipating and mitigating risk.

During this phase, the technician monitors for early signs of over-sedation, paradoxical excitement, or adverse reactions such as vomiting or allergic response. A quiet environment, gentle handling, and close observation of the patient's response help guide next steps and alert the team to potential complications before they escalate.

Technicians must also ensure that emergency drugs, intubation supplies, and monitoring equipment are prepared and functional before proceeding. Premedication is not just a sedative, it is the first moment where preparation, foresight, and clinical insight protect the patient from harm.

Induction Monitoring

Induction is the most physiologically unstable phase of anesthesia. During this transition from consciousness to unconsciousness, rapid changes in heart rate, blood pressure, respiratory drive, and muscle tone occur, often in the span of seconds. The technician's role is to manage this transition safely and skillfully, maintaining control while minimizing stress and complications.

Before induction begins, technicians should confirm that all necessary equipment is ready: an appropriately sized endotracheal tube, laryngoscope, oxygen flow, anesthetic machine, and suction. The patient's IV catheter should be secured and flushed, and induction agents must be double-checked for dose accuracy and compatibility.

Understanding the mechanism of action and side effects of each induction drug is essential. For example, propofol can cause apnea if administered too quickly, while ketamine may increase heart rate and blood pressure but cause muscle rigidity and poor intubation conditions if not paired with a muscle relaxant. Technicians must adjust the rate of administration based on patient response, titrating to effect rather than administering a full dose by default.

Airway management is a top priority. Loss of protective reflexes occurs quickly, and the technician must be prepared to intubate without delay while ensuring proper tube placement and securing the airway. Pulse oximetry, heart rate, and respiratory rate should be monitored continuously, even in the brief moments before full machine monitoring is initiated.

Importantly, the technician must anticipate complications such as vomiting, regurgitation, laryngospasm, or apnea. Early interventions such as suctioning, providing supplemental oxygen, or beginning manual ventilation can prevent a manageable issue from becoming a crisis.

Induction is a moment of heightened responsibility. With full attention and clinical awareness, the technician ensures that the patient passes safely from consciousness into anesthesia, without injury, oxygen deprivation, or unnecessary stress.

Pro Tip: Preoxygenation Before Induction
Providing 3–5 minutes of 100% oxygen before induction prevents perianesthetic hypoxia, particularly in brachycephalic breeds and critical patients (Grimm et al. 2021).

Maintenance Phase Monitoring

Once the patient is anesthetized and the procedure is underway, the technician's role shifts from induction support to continuous, dynamic monitoring. The maintenance phase is often assumed to be the most stable portion of anesthesia, but this assumption can lead to complacency. In reality, patients under maintenance are at constant risk for physiological compromise. Vigilance during this stage is critical.

The goal of the maintenance phase is to sustain a safe and appropriate depth of anesthesia; deep enough to prevent pain and movement, but light enough to avoid cardiovascular or respiratory depression. Every patient responds differently to anesthetic agents, and even minor surgical stimuli can trigger abrupt shifts in vital signs. The technician must anticipate, detect, and respond to these changes in real time.

Monitoring during maintenance is not about collecting numbers, it is about interpreting trends, correlating data, and making informed decisions. A rising ETCO, a sudden drop in MAP, or an irregular heart rhythm may indicate underlying issues such as inadequate ventilation, hypoperfusion, or excessive anesthetic depth. Understanding *why* these changes occur enables the technician to take timely corrective action or alert the veterinarian before complications escalate.

It is during this phase that the technician becomes the patient's primary advocate. Machines can alarm, but only a well-trained technician can recognize patterns, connect physiology to pharmacology, and apply appropriate interventions.

Advanced Insight: Minimum Alveolar Concentration (MAC) Adjustments
The MAC of inhalants (e.g., isoflurane, sevoflurane) can be influenced by hypothermia, age, and concurrent drugs. Opioids and sedatives lower MAC requirements, reducing the needed vaporizer setting and improving hemodynamic stability (Steffey et al. 2020).

Anesthetic monitoring is a dynamic, interpretive process that extends far beyond recording vital signs; it is the synthesis of physiologic assessment, pharmacologic knowledge, and clinical judgment. Veterinary technicians occupy a pivotal role in this continuum, safeguarding patients by anticipating complications, recognizing subtle deviations from normal physiology, and initiating timely interventions. Each anesthetic stage—from premedication through induction, maintenance, and recovery—presents unique challenges that demand vigilance, adaptability, and technical proficiency.

Ultimately, the technician's responsibility is not solely to ensure survival but to preserve patient stability, comfort, and welfare throughout the perianesthetic period. The ability to interpret physiologic trends in the context of anesthetic depth, surgical stimulation, and the individual patient's health status elevates monitoring from a passive duty to an active form of patient advocacy. This standard of care requires continuous development of critical thinking, communication with the veterinary team, and mastery of both manual and electronic monitoring modalities.

For a more comprehensive discussion of specific monitoring parameters—including electrocardiography, blood pressure measurement, pulse oximetry, capnography, and temperature regulation—readers are directed to Chapter 7, which provides an in-depth analysis of physiologic monitoring techniques and their clinical applications.

Section 5: Surgical Assisting: Preparation, Sterility, and Intraoperative Support

Surgical assisting is more than a technical task, it is an active role in patient safety, surgical success, and overall case efficiency. Veterinary technicians are essential members of the surgical team, not only because of their ability to maintain asepsis and handle instruments, but because of the clinical judgment, foresight, and intention they bring to the operating room.

Every action during a surgical procedure carries consequences: a poorly prepared site can lead to infection; a break in sterility can compromise healing; a delayed instrument handoff can extend anesthesia time and increase risk. When veterinary technicians understand the *why* behind each protocol, they move from reactive assistants to proactive surgical partners, anticipating needs, minimizing complications, and advocating for the patient at every step.

Pre-Surgical Preparation and Asepsis

A successful surgery begins long before the first incision. Technicians are responsible for ensuring that all preoperative requirements are met, including confirming correct patient identity, verifying surgical consent, ensuring appropriate fasting, and reviewing diagnostics such as CBC, chemistry panels, coagulation tests, and blood typing for transfusion-prone cases.

Understanding the *why* behind these tasks is crucial. For example, skipping a coagulation panel in a liver patient could result in intraoperative hemorrhage, and failing to fast a patient could increase the risk of aspiration during the perianesthesia periods. These details are not administrative; they are clinical safeguards (Table 3.5).

In the high-stakes environment of surgery, missed steps can compromise patient safety. A pre-surgical checklist is not about bureaucracy, it's about protecting the patient through structured, intentional preparation. Technicians are the front-line defenders against preventable mistakes.

Using a checklist reinforces critical thinking, reduces cognitive overload during busy shifts, and fosters consistent habits that benefit every patient. Most importantly, it allows the technician to pause, review, and ask, *"Have we done everything possible to ensure this patient enters surgery safely?"*

Surgical Site Preparation

Sterile technique is the technician's first defense against surgical site infections (SSIs), which can prolong healing, increase patient suffering, and lead to costly complications. A thorough and intentional approach to site preparation ensures that bacteria are minimized before the surgical field is established.

The three-step site prep process includes:

1) **Clipping**: Extending the clip 5–10 cm beyond the intended incision site not only provides room for draping but helps prevent hair and debris from entering the field.
2) **Scrubbing**: Using antiseptic (typically chlorhexidine) with alcohol helps disrupt biofilms and mechanically remove dirt and microorganisms.
3) **Final Paint**: A final antiseptic layer creates a long-lasting bactericidal barrier just before the patient is draped.

Table 3.5 Pre-surgical checklist for veterinary technicians.

Task	Why It Matters
Confirm patient identity and procedure	Prevents wrong-patient or wrong-site errors; aligns team on expectations
Verify informed consent is documented	Ensures legal and ethical compliance; confirms owner understands risks
Review pre-surgical diagnostics	Identifies anesthetic or surgical risks (e.g., anemia, coagulopathy, organ disease)
Confirm NPO status	Reduces risk of aspiration from passive regurgitation.
Assess temperament and FAS score	Helps select appropriate premedication and handling techniques
Prepare and label all pre-meds/induction drugs	Prevents dosing errors and ensures readiness during time-sensitive events
Check and flush IV catheter	Confirms patency and avoids delays in emergency drug delivery
Gather and test monitoring equipment	Early detection of anesthetic complications depends on functional equipment
Clip and clean surgical site	Reduces bacterial contamination; ensures clean surgical field
Set up sterile packs and instruments	Ensures aseptic technique; avoids surgical delays
Verify surgical team roles	Improves coordination and communication during procedure
Check emergency crash cart and oxygen	Readiness to respond to anesthetic emergencies improves survival odds

Source: M. Jennings (2025). Author's owner illustration.

Advanced Insight: Chlorhexidine vs. Povidone-Iodine

Chlorhexidine provides persistent bactericidal action for up to six hours and is less affected by organic matter than povidone-iodine, making it superior for surgical site preparation (Weese et al. 2021).

Maintaining Sterility in the OR

Once the patient is prepped and draped, sterility must be actively protected throughout the procedure. The technician plays a critical role in enforcing aseptic boundaries, understanding that even a minor breach in protocol could have major consequences.

The sterile field includes:

- The draped area around the patient
- The surgical table and sterile instrument packs
- The surgeon's gown and gloves (above waist level only)

Pro Tip: "Sterile Bubble" Awareness

If an item dips below the sterile field (e.g., below the waist or table edge), it is no longer sterile. Always inform the surgeon and replace contaminated items (Fossum 2019).

Instrument Handling and Intraoperative Techniques

A well-trained surgical technician must anticipate the surgeon's needs and handle instruments with precision and efficiency. Passing instruments correctly is essential to maintaining the flow of the procedure. Forceps and scissors should always be held by the box lock and passed in a firm, ready-to-use position, ensuring the surgeon can grasp and use them without repositioning. Keeping instruments organized throughout the surgery is equally important, as a logical layout allows for quick and accurate retrieval. Grouping instruments by function, such as retractors, clamps, and suturing tools, reduces the risk of delays and enhances procedural efficiency.

Additionally, the surgical assistant must be proficient in using suction and hemostasis devices. Understanding the appropriate application of suction tips, such as the Poole tip for abdominal procedures and the Yankauer tip for general use, ensures optimal fluid removal. Familiarity with hemostatic agents, including bone wax and gel foam, allows for better intraoperative bleeding control, ultimately improving surgical outcomes (Table 3.6).

Expert Tip: Avoiding Instrument Damage

Never use tissue scissors (e.g., Metzenbaum) to cut sutures, as this dulls the cutting edge, making fine dissection less precise (Weese et al. 2021).

Table 3.6 Common surgical instruments and their uses.

Instrument Type	Example	Primary Function
Clamps	Kelly, Mosquito, Rochester-Carmalt	Hemostasis, tissue grasping
Scissors	Metzenbaum, Mayo, Iris	Cutting tissue, sutures
Needle holders	Mayo-Hegar, Olsen-Hegar	Holding suture needles
Retractors	Gelpi, Army-Navy, Balfour	Exposure of the surgical site

Source: M. Jennings (2025). Author's own illustration.

Section 6: Laboratory Testing

Laboratory diagnostics form the cornerstone of veterinary clinical decision-making, providing essential insights into homeostatic balance, organ function, and infectious or neoplastic disease processes. As such, the veterinary technician must exhibit a high degree of proficiency in specimen collection, preparation, and preliminary interpretation. A failure in any stage—particularly during the preanalytical phase—can profoundly affect diagnostic accuracy, delay treatment, or result in misdiagnosis.

Venipuncture should be performed with both anatomical precision and procedural awareness. The jugular vein remains the preferred site for large volume blood collection in dogs and cats due to its caliber and consistent flow. Smaller veins—such as the cephalic, lateral saphenous, or medial saphenous (in cats)—may be utilized when a smaller sample is needed or jugular access is contraindicated. In certain cases, dorsal pedal, auricular, or femoral veins may be appropriate, provided proper restraint and post-collection hemostasis are maintained.

An appropriate needle gauge must be chosen to prevent hemolysis while achieving rapid blood flow. Typically, a 22-gauge needle is sufficient for most dogs and cats. Larger breeds may accommodate a 20- or 18-gauge, while fragile or anemic patients may require a 25-gauge, recognizing the increased risk for red cell trauma and sample compromise.

The proper order of filling blood tubes is critical to avoid cross-contamination of additives, which may significantly interfere with laboratory values. The following order is recommended in veterinary practice, adapted from human medicine protocols:

1) **Citrate Tube (Blue Top)**: Used for coagulation testing; drawn first to prevent contamination with procoagulant or anticoagulant agents.
2) **Plain Red Top**: Contains no additives; ideal for serum collection.
3) **Serum Separator Tube (SST or Tiger Top)**: Contains clot activator and gel for serum separation.
4) **Heparin Tube (Green Top)**: Used for plasma chemistry; must be filled properly to ensure accurate electrolyte values.
5) **EDTA Tube (Purple or Lavender Top)**: Used for hematology; EDTA can chelate calcium and interfere with coagulation tests if drawn prematurely.

Failure to adhere to this sequence may result in erroneous results. For example, EDTA contamination of a serum sample can cause pseudohyperkalemia, hypocalcemia, and prolonged clotting times—compromising clinical interpretation and potentially leading to inappropriate therapy.

Each tube has a calibrated vacuum to collect a predetermined volume of blood, necessary for appropriate blood-to-additive ratios. Underfilling or overfilling a tube may dilute or concentrate the additive, leading to invalid results. Minimum volume recommendations are as follows:

- **EDTA Tube**: ~1 mL for CBC; underfilling can lead to cellular distortion and platelet clumping.
- **Heparin Tube**: ~0.5–1 mL minimum for chemistry; especially important for electrolytes and critical care analytes.
- **Citrate Tube**: Must be filled precisely (9:1 blood to anticoagulant); underfilling leads to falsely prolonged PT/aPTT.
- **Serum Tubes**: Ideally 2–3 mL to allow for repeat testing or add-ons; allow full clotting before centrifugation.

When limited by patient size or clinical condition, prioritization of tests must be made in conjunction with the attending clinician to ensure critical diagnostics are preserved.

In addition to proper site selection, tube order, and sample handling, veterinary technicians must also calculate the total volume of blood that can be safely removed from a patient at one time. This is especially critical in small or critically ill animals where excessive blood loss—even from diagnostic sampling—can induce iatrogenic anemia, hypovolemia, or compromise tissue perfusion. The volume of blood drawn should always be guided by species-specific total blood volume (TBV) estimations and the physiological status of the patient.

For healthy, normovolemic patients, total blood volume can be approximated using standard values: approximately 80–90 mL/kg in dogs and 60–70 mL/kg in cats. For conservative and consistent clinical calculations, 80 mL/kg is commonly used for dogs and 65 mL/kg for cats. No more than 10% of this total blood volume should be removed at one time for diagnostic purposes. In stable, normovolemic canine donors, up to 15–20% may be collected for transfusion purposes when appropriate post-collection fluid support is provided and the patient is monitored closely.

To apply these calculations clinically, consider the following example. A 25-kg mixed-breed dog presents for routine bloodwork. The estimated total blood volume is calculated as 25 kg multiplied by 80 mL/kg, resulting in 2,000 mL. Ten percent of this volume is 200 mL, which is the maximum safe amount of blood that may be drawn in a single event without inducing clinical compromise. If the requested diagnostics require only 7.2 mL of blood—for example, 1.5 mL for a complete blood count in an EDTA tube, 2 mL for serum chemistry, 2.7 mL for coagulation testing, and 1 mL for blood typing—then the volume to be collected is well within the safe limit. Nonetheless, care must still be taken to use the appropriate gauge needle and adhere to the designated fill lines on each blood tube to ensure blood-to-additive ratios are preserved.

In contrast, a 4-kg adult cat undergoing similar diagnostics would have a total blood volume of 260 mL, using 65 mL/kg as the estimated TBV. Ten percent of this total is only 26 mL. Although the diagnostics may still require less than this threshold, this example underscores the importance of scaling blood collection volumes to patient size. In small or debilitated patients, it is prudent to limit collection to 5–7% of the total blood volume. Additionally, fluid support and clinical monitoring should be considered when volumes approach these limits. In all patients, especially those with reduced circulatory reserve, using microcollection tubes can preserve diagnostic integrity while minimizing iatrogenic harm.

The veterinary technician must remain vigilant to signs of volume depletion, such as tachycardia, prolonged capillary refill time, pale mucous membranes, hypotension, and altered mentation following large volume collection. When in doubt, diagnostic needs should be prioritized, and sampling should be deferred or spaced over time to support patient safety.

Understanding the physiological basis of safe blood volume removal and performing accurate calculations based on patient weight ensures that diagnostic sampling remains both clinically effective and medically responsible. It is the responsibility of the veterinary technician to advocate for patient welfare by aligning technical skill with evidence-based limits for blood collection.

Serum Biochemistry: Assessing Organ Function and Metabolic Health

Serum biochemistry profiles analyze a wide range of physiological parameters, including liver, kidney, pancreatic, muscle, and endocrine function, as well as electrolyte and protein balance. Proper sample handling is essential for accurate results, as hemolysis, lipemia, and prolonged clotting times can alter readings. Technicians must ensure that serum or plasma is separated promptly and that patients are properly prepared for testing, for example, fasting is necessary for lipid and glucose evaluations to prevent artificially elevated values (Weiss et al. 2021).

Liver function is commonly assessed using markers such as alanine aminotransferase (ALT) and alkaline phosphatase (ALP), which indicate hepatocellular damage or cholestasis. Increased gamma-glutamyl transferase (GGT) and bilirubin levels provide additional information about liver function and bile duct obstruction. Renal function is evaluated by measuring blood urea nitrogen (BUN), creatinine, and symmetric dimethylarginine (SDMA), all of which reflect glomerular filtration rate (GFR) and help diagnose kidney disease or dehydration status. The pancreas is assessed using lipase, amylase, canine pancreatic lipase immunoreactivity (cPLI), and feline pancreatic lipase immunoreactivity (fPLI), which aid in diagnosing pancreatitis and exocrine pancreatic insufficiency. Electrolyte levels, including sodium, potassium, chloride, calcium, and phosphorus, help identify fluid imbalances, endocrine disorders such as Addison's disease and diabetes, and neuromuscular dysfunction. Protein levels, including albumin, globulin, and total protein, provide information about hydration status, liver function, and potential chronic disease processes (Thrall et al. 2022).

Veterinary technicians must be vigilant in identifying abnormal biochemical trends and communicating findings to the veterinary team. Detecting hypoglycemia in a neonate prompts immediate intervention with dextrose supplementation, while elevated creatinine and SDMA in a geriatric patient may indicate chronic kidney disease requiring fluid therapy adjustments. Recognizing hyperkalemia in a blocked cat ensures rapid medical intervention, preventing potentially fatal arrhythmias.

Complete Blood Count (CBC): Evaluating Hematologic and Immune Function

A complete blood count (CBC) provides vital information on red blood cells (RBCs), white blood cells (WBCs), and platelets (PLTs), offering insight into oxygen transport, immune response, and clotting ability. Abnormalities in CBC results can indicate infection, anemia, inflammation, or bone marrow disorders.

Red blood cell parameters such as hematocrit, hemoglobin concentration, and mean corpuscular volume (MCV) assess the blood's oxygen-carrying capacity. Changes in these values help differentiate between anemia types, such as regenerative anemia caused by hemorrhage or hemolysis and nonregenerative anemia linked to bone marrow suppression or chronic disease. The white blood cell differential, which includes neutrophils, lymphocytes, monocytes, eosinophils, and basophils, aids in diagnosing infection, inflammation, stress responses, and immune-mediated diseases. An elevated neutrophil count may indicate an active bacterial infection or inflammatory response, while an increased eosinophil count suggests a parasitic infection or allergic reaction. Platelet count and morphology are essential for assessing coagulation status, as low platelet counts may suggest immune-mediated thrombocytopenia (ITP) or disseminated intravascular coagulation (DIC) (Weiss et al. 2021).

Beyond automated hematology analyzers, veterinary technicians must be proficient in performing manual hemograms when automated equipment is unavailable, yields questionable results, or when specific cellular abnormalities require morphological evaluation. A manual hemogram allows for the evaluation of red blood cells, white blood cells, and platelets using both quantitative and qualitative methods. Accurate performance of a hemogram requires appropriate sample preparation, microscope technique, and mathematical calculation. The analysis is typically conducted from a well-prepared, well-stained blood smear obtained from an EDTA-anticoagulated sample.

To perform a hemogram, the veterinary technician begins by preparing a blood smear using the push-slide technique, allowing the smear to air dry completely before staining with a Romanowsky-type stain such as Diff-Quik or Wright-Giemsa. The slide should be examined under low power to evaluate smear quality and distribution, and then under oil immersion (100× objective) to assess cell morphology and perform differential counts.

The white blood cell (WBC) differential is conducted by counting a total of 100 leukocytes in the monolayer region of the smear and classifying each as a neutrophil (segmented or band), lymphocyte, monocyte, eosinophil, or basophil. The relative percentage of each leukocyte type is then converted into absolute numbers by using the total WBC count, which may be obtained from an automated counter or estimated manually using a hemocytometer. The formula for absolute count is:

$$\text{Absolute leukocyte count} = (\%\text{ of cell type}) \times (\text{Total WBC count}) \div 100$$

For example, if the WBC count is 12,000/μL and 78% of the cells are segmented neutrophils:

$$\text{Absolute neutrophil count} = 78 \times 12{,}000 \div 100 = 9{,}360\ \text{neutrophils}/\mu\text{L}$$

Similarly, if 10% are lymphocytes:

$$\text{Absolute lymphocyte count} = 10 \times 12{,}000 \div 100 = 1{,}200\ \text{lymphocytes}/\mu\text{L}$$

This quantitative approach is essential for detecting leukocytosis, leukopenia, or shifts in leukocyte populations that may indicate inflammation, infection, neoplasia, or immunologic processes.

The packed cell volume (PCV) is obtained via microhematocrit centrifugation and visually measured using a hematocrit reader card. When PCV is known, the red blood cell indices can be manually calculated if a total red cell count and hemoglobin concentration are available. These include:

- **Mean Corpuscular Volume (MCV)**: Reflects average size of RBCs

$$\text{MCV (fL)} = (\text{PCV} \times 10) \div \text{RBC count (in millions}/\mu\text{L)}$$

- **Mean Corpuscular Hemoglobin (MCH)**: Average hemoglobin per RBC

$$\text{MCH (pg)} = (\text{Hb} \times 10) \div \text{RBC count (in millions}/\mu\text{L)}$$

- **Mean Corpuscular Hemoglobin Concentration (MCHC)**: Average hemoglobin concentration in RBCs

$$\text{MCHC (g/dL)} = (\text{Hb} \times 100) \div \text{PCV}$$

For instance, if a patient has a PCV of 45%, hemoglobin of 15 g/dL, and RBC count of 5.5 million/μL:

- MCV = (45 × 10) ÷ 5.5 = 81.8 fL
- MCH = (15 × 10) ÷ 5.5 = 27.3 pg
- MCHC = (15 × 100) ÷ 45 = 33.3 g/dL

These indices assist in classifying anemias as microcytic, normocytic, or macrocytic, and as hypochromic or normochromic.

While automated hematology analyzers have become increasingly accurate and efficient in veterinary practice, they are not without limitations. One of the most clinically significant drawbacks is the potential for inaccurate platelet counts, particularly in feline patients. As such, every in-house automated complete blood count (CBC) should be supplemented with a manual platelet estimation, regardless of the species, and especially in cats (Harvey 2012).

Automated analyzers often misidentify small platelets as erythrocytes or cellular debris or fail to count clumped platelets altogether. Feline platelets are not only smaller and more variable in size compared to their canine counterparts, but they are also prone to spontaneous aggregation during or shortly after sample collection. This aggregation is frequently artifactually interpreted by the analyzer as thrombocytopenia, leading to a falsely low platelet count and potentially unnecessary concern for bleeding disorders such as immune-mediated thrombocytopenia or bone marrow suppression.

To mitigate this diagnostic error, a manual platelet estimate should be performed on every blood smear. Using the 100× oil immersion objective, the technician should evaluate the monolayer and count the number of platelets in at least 10 fields, then calculate the average number of platelets per field. This average is multiplied by a standard factor—typically 15,000 to 20,000—to generate an estimated platelet count per microliter.

For example, if an average of 10 platelets per high-power field is observed:

$$\text{Estimated platelet count} = 10 \times 15{,}000 = 150{,}000/\mu\text{L}$$

This manual estimation serves two purposes: it confirms or corrects the automated count, and it allows for the detection of platelet clumping or morphological abnormalities. If large clumps are seen, particularly at the feathered edge or near the smear origin, it is essential to note that the actual platelet count may be substantially higher than reported. In such cases, the result should be interpreted as artifactually low due to aggregation, and clinical decisions should be made accordingly.

In feline patients, where platelet clumping is almost expected during sample handling, the reliance on an automated count without visual confirmation risks misdiagnosis, inappropriate further testing, or unnecessary intervention. Furthermore, certain disease states—including FeLV-related marrow disorders, DIC, or infectious thrombocytopenias—require platelet assessments that include morphology, size variation (macroplatelets), and the presence or absence of clumps, which can only be evaluated microscopically.

In summary, the integration of manual platelet estimation into routine CBC review is not optional—it is essential, particularly when using in-house hematology platforms. Veterinary technicians are uniquely positioned to perform this function accurately and must be trained to recognize the limitations of automated counts and apply microscopic verification as part of comprehensive diagnostic laboratory practice.

A manual hemogram also allows for qualitative assessment of cellular morphology, including anisocytosis, polychromasia, spherocytosis, Heinz bodies, toxic neutrophil changes, and reactive lymphocyte morphology—findings which may be overlooked by automated analyzers but are diagnostically significant in many disease states.

By mastering the performance of manual hemograms and accompanying calculations, the veterinary technician not only ensures diagnostic accuracy in resource-limited settings but also enhances their role as a diagnostic partner within the medical team. Manual hematology skills require practice, attention to detail, and critical thinking, and remain a cornerstone of competent laboratory nursing practice.

Error Recognition and Quality Control

Preanalytical errors—such as hemolysis, lipemia, sample dilution from IV fluids, incorrect tube usage, or improper filling—are the most common and preventable source of diagnostic error. Analytical errors stem from machine calibration issues, operator inexperience, or sample contamination. Postanalytical mistakes include transcription errors, misinterpretation, or failure to correlate lab data with clinical signs.

Veterinary nurses must adopt a quality control mindset. This includes:

- Double-checking patient identifiers and sample labels.
- Using proper collection techniques and adhering to tube order.
- Documenting collection times and storage methods.
- Recognizing when lab results do not match clinical findings and advocating for repeat testing or alternative diagnostics.

Expert Tip: Hemolysis and Lipemia Artifacts

Hemolysis falsely elevates potassium and phosphorus, while lipemia can falsely increase triglycerides and glucose. Always assess sample quality before interpreting results (Thrall et al. 2022).

Cytology

Cytologic examination represents a minimally invasive and cost-effective diagnostic modality that is widely utilized in small animal medicine. When performed correctly, it offers rapid, in-clinic evaluation of cellular morphology and can provide essential diagnostic insight into neoplastic, inflammatory, infectious, or degenerative processes. However, the diagnostic value of cytology is heavily dependent on meticulous sample collection, appropriate slide preparation, and careful staining technique to preserve cellular architecture and minimize artifacts.

Fine needle aspiration (FNA) is one of the most common sampling techniques in veterinary cytology and can be employed to evaluate cutaneous and subcutaneous masses, lymph nodes, internal organs, and fluid accumulations. To perform an FNA, a 22- to 25-gauge needle is typically attached to a 6–12 mL syringe. The site is clipped and aseptically prepared. Two methods may be employed: aspiration and non-aspiration (capillary) technique. In the aspiration method, negative pressure is generated by retracting the plunger while moving the needle back and forth within the lesion. In contrast, the non-aspiration technique omits the syringe; the needle alone is rapidly redirected within the target tissue, relying on capillary action to draw cells into the hub. The latter method is often preferred for highly vascular or fragile tissues to reduce hemodilution or mechanical distortion of cells.

Once the sample is collected, the contents of the needle are expelled onto a clean glass microscope slide by reattaching the needle to an air-filled syringe and gently depressing the plunger. The manner in which the sample is spread is contingent upon its viscosity and cellularity. Three commonly used smear techniques include:

1) **Compression or "Squash" Technique**: This method is ideal for solid mass aspirates. A second slide is placed perpendicularly over the slide containing the sample, and gentle, even pressure is applied to spread the material without crushing the cells. The top slide is then slid off in one smooth motion to produce a uniform monolayer.
2) **Starfish Technique**: Useful for highly viscous or particulate samples, such as those from mucosal surfaces, abscesses, or joint fluid. Using the tip of a needle or applicator stick, the sample is teased outwards in multiple directions from a central drop, creating a radial "starfish" pattern. This technique minimizes cell disruption while allowing visualization of large particles or mucus strands.
3) **Feathered-Edge or Blood-Smear Technique**: This technique is preferred for fluid samples or aspirates with low cellularity. A second slide is angled at approximately 30–45° and drawn backward into the fluid sample, then pushed forward smoothly to create a thin film with a feathered edge. This gradient allows for optimal distribution of cells and enhances the identification of cell populations under varying densities.

Prepared slides should be air-dried rapidly to preserve cellular detail and prevent artifacts from water-induced lysis. Once dry, the slides must be fixed in 100% methanol for a minimum of two to three minutes prior to staining. In the clinical setting, Romanowsky-type stains such as Diff-Quik or Wright-Giemsa are commonly used. It is imperative to adhere strictly to the manufacturer's protocols, including immersion times and reagent freshness, as overstaining or understaining can obscure nuclear and cytoplasmic features. Reagents should be replaced regularly to prevent contamination or precipitation artifacts.

When submitting cytologic samples to an external laboratory, it is recommended to prepare and submit multiple slides—ideally three to five—to improve diagnostic yield. Slides should be clearly labeled with patient identifiers and site of collection. A thorough clinical history should accompany the submission, including the anatomic location and gross appearance of the lesion, duration and progression, relevant laboratory findings, and any tentative differential diagnoses. This contextual information significantly enhances the pathologist's ability to render an accurate and clinically relevant interpretation.

Maximizing Diagnostic Value

Veterinary technicians contribute significantly to the accuracy of cytological results by recognizing common pitfalls that could lead to inconclusive or misleading diagnoses. Poor sample quality due to excessive hemodilution, thick smears, or delayed staining can obscure key cytological findings. Ensuring that multiple slides are prepared from a single sample increases the likelihood of obtaining a representative cellular population. Additionally, communicating any relevant patient history, such as prior infections, systemic illness, or suspected neoplasia, provides essential context for interpretation.

Urinalysis: Methodology and Clinical Interpretation

Urinalysis is one of the most accessible and informative diagnostic tools available in veterinary medicine, offering vital insight into renal concentrating ability, urinary tract health, and systemic metabolic disturbances. In-house urinalysis should consist of three components: physical examination, chemical analysis via dipstick, and microscopic sediment evaluation, which allows direct observation of cellular and noncellular elements within the urine.

Urine Collection Techniques in Small Animal Veterinary Practice

The method by which urine is collected can profoundly influence the reliability of results, the risk of contamination, and patient safety. The four primary techniques used in small animal patients include free catch, manual bladder expression, cystocentesis, and urinary catheterization. Selection of an appropriate collection method should be guided by the diagnostic objective, patient temperament, clinical condition, and the need for sterility.

Free catch, also referred to as voided sample collection, is a noninvasive technique in which urine is collected midstream during spontaneous micturition. This method is useful for initial screening urinalysis, particularly in cooperative patients or those in which invasive techniques are contraindicated. The veterinary technician should wait until the animal begins to urinate and then slide a clean or sterile container into the urine stream, ideally collecting the midstream portion to reduce contamination from external genitalia. The perineal area should be wiped clean beforehand using sterile saline or dilute chlorhexidine to reduce skin or hair contamination. While this method is minimally stressful and easily performed, it carries a higher risk of contamination from the distal urethra, genital tract, or skin, limiting its utility for culture and sensitivity testing.

Manual bladder expression involves the application of gentle, steady pressure to the caudal abdomen to initiate micturition and evacuate the bladder. It is best employed in patients with normal bladder tone and unobstructed outflow tracts, such as anesthetized animals or those with neurologic compromise requiring voiding assistance. The veterinary technician should place both hands on either side of the caudal abdomen and apply gradual bilateral pressure until urine flows. Proper technique requires sensitivity to bladder distension and resistance; excessive force can cause discomfort, rupture the bladder in compromised patients, or retrograde urine flow into the ureters, increasing the risk of pyelonephritis. This technique should never be used in patients suspected of urinary obstruction or with recent abdominal surgery. Due to the high risk of contamination, samples obtained by bladder expression are unsuitable for urine culture.

Cystocentesis is the preferred method for obtaining a sterile urine sample suitable for urinalysis and bacterial culture, as it bypasses the distal urethra and external genitalia, minimizing contamination. While generally safe, the procedure requires anatomical precision and situational awareness, as improper technique may result in significant iatrogenic complications. Veterinary technicians play a central role in patient positioning, restraint, aseptic preparation, and postprocedural monitoring, and must remain vigilant to detect early signs of adverse events.

The procedure is performed with the patient in lateral or dorsal recumbency. The urinary bladder is identified via abdominal palpation or ultrasonography, and the ventral abdomen is aseptically prepared using alcohol. A 22-gauge needle attached to a 6–12 mL syringe is advanced into the bladder wall, typically at a caudodorsal angle or perpendicular to the abdominal wall, depending on bladder positioning and operator preference. Aspiration is performed using gentle negative pressure. Once urine is collected, the needle is withdrawn, and pressure is applied briefly to the puncture site.

One important complication of cystocentesis is a vagal response, triggered by abrupt stimulation of the parasympathetic nervous system via excessive abdominal pressure, rapid bladder decompression, or mechanical stimulation of visceral afferent fibers during needle penetration (Ettinger et al. 2017). This response may lead to bradycardia, hypotension, pale mucous membranes, hypersalivation, lethargy, or syncope. Veterinary technicians must monitor patients carefully during and immediately after the procedure, particularly in brachycephalic breeds, geriatric patients, or those with preexisting vagal tone. If signs of vagal stimulation occur, the procedure should be aborted, and supportive care—including oxygen supplementation and anticholinergic administration, if indicated—should be initiated under veterinary supervision.

A second and potentially serious complication is the development of hemoperitoneum secondary to inadvertent vascular puncture. While rare, improper angling of the needle or excessive advancement may result in perforation of major abdominal vessels, including branches of the caudal abdominal, deep circumflex iliac, or epigastric arteries. This may result in intraperitoneal hemorrhage, particularly in hypocoagulable patients or those with neoplastic abdominal masses. Clinical signs that warrant concern include abdominal distension, hypovolemia (e.g., prolonged capillary refill time, weak pulses), sudden tachycardia, or signs of discomfort such as vocalization or guarding. Serial abdominal girth measurements, ultrasound evaluation for free abdominal fluid, and monitoring of packed cell volume (PCV) may be indicated following a traumatic attempt.

Another critical concern is iatrogenic renal puncture, particularly when using ultrasound guidance in small patients, or when bladder volume is minimal and the adjacent kidneys become inadvertently included within the imaging field. In such cases, the kidney may be mistaken for a partially filled bladder or be unintentionally contacted if the needle is advanced too cranially. Penetration of the renal cortex may result in localized pain, gross hematuria, or transient azotemia, and may induce acute hypertension or renal capsule irritation, both of which require prompt recognition. Veterinary technicians should be trained to confirm bladder identity using sonographic landmarks (i.e., thin-walled, anechoic, spherical organ without corticomedullary definition) and never advance the needle without full visualization of the target structure. If a renal puncture is suspected, the patient should be monitored for lumbar discomfort, hematuria, or signs of systemic inflammatory response, and the incident should be immediately reported to the attending veterinarian.

Ultimately, successful cystocentesis requires an understanding not only of anatomy but of the subtle physiological responses that may occur during the procedure. Veterinary technicians must approach each collection with precision, patience, and preparation to safeguard patient welfare and uphold sample integrity.

Urinary catheterization allows for the collection of urine from patients who cannot voluntarily void, who are undergoing anesthesia, or who require continuous urine output monitoring. Catheterization is the preferred method for obtaining a sterile sample in male dogs when cystocentesis is contraindicated. However, the procedure carries risks including urethral trauma, infection, and discomfort, and requires strict aseptic technique. Samples collected immediately after catheter placement are most representative; however, repeated sampling or prolonged indwelling catheterization may increase the risk of bacterial contamination.

In summary, the selection of a urine collection technique must balance the need for sterility, patient safety, and diagnostic utility. Veterinary technicians play a pivotal role in assessing patient condition, preparing for and performing or assisting with collection, maintaining aseptic technique, and recognizing signs of patient discomfort or procedural complications. Proper technique and informed decision-making not only preserve sample integrity but also ensure the safety and welfare of the patient.

Sample Technique

Following centrifugation of 3–5 mL of well-mixed urine at 1,500–2,000 rpm for five minutes, the supernatant is gently decanted, leaving approximately 0.5 mL of urine with the sediment. This remaining volume is gently resuspended by flicking or gentle agitation. From this, a single drop is applied to a microscope slide for evaluation. There are two primary methods of preparing a slide for sediment analysis: the line mount technique and the conventional drop mount, both of which may be assessed either unstained or with a stain such as Sedi-Stain or Sternheimer-Malbin.

In the line mount technique, a drop of resuspended urine sediment is placed near one end of a clean glass slide. A second slide is used to spread the drop in a linear fashion, similar to the preparation of a blood smear. This technique offers a concentrated distribution of formed elements and improves visibility of rare structures such as casts or crystals, which may be missed with traditional drop mounting. However, this method may physically distort fragile cells and requires a practiced hand to maintain a monolayer distribution.

In contrast, the standard drop mount technique involves simply placing one drop of urine sediment on the slide and applying a coverslip. This method preserves cellular architecture more effectively and allows for a more consistent field during low- and high-power examination. It is generally preferred for routine microscopic evaluation.

Urine sediment may be evaluated unstained, which preserves the native appearance and refractivity of cellular and crystalline elements. However, the use of stains such as Sedi-Stain or Sternheimer-Malbin can enhance the visualization of nuclear detail, aiding in the differentiation of leukocytes, epithelial cells, and granular casts. While staining may improve diagnostic yield, it also introduces artifacts such as crystal dissolution and background debris. Therefore, both stained and unstained preparations should ideally be examined, especially in cases of suspected pathology.

Regardless of preparation, the slide should be examined under low power (10×) to identify casts, crystals, and large aggregates, and under high power (40×) to assess red and white blood cells, epithelial cells, bacteria, and other fine elements. Oil immersion is not used for urine sediment.

Each constituent of the urine sediment provides diagnostic insight:

- **Red Blood Cells (RBCs)**: Normally absent or present in low numbers (<5/HPF). Increased numbers may indicate hemorrhage, trauma, inflammation, or iatrogenic collection (e.g., catheterization).

- **White Blood Cells (WBCs)**: Normally <5/HPF. Elevated counts suggest inflammation or infection.
- **Epithelial Cells**: Squamous cells (from distal urethra or genital tract) are common in voided samples; transitional and renal tubular epithelial cells in high numbers may suggest pathology, including neoplasia or tubular injury.
- **Casts**: Cylindrical proteinaceous structures formed in the renal tubules. Hyaline casts may be seen in health or proteinuria; granular casts suggest tubular degeneration; waxy casts are indicative of chronic renal disease; cellular casts reflect acute inflammation or injury.
- **Crystals**: Struvite and calcium oxalate are common; significance depends on patient context. Ammonium biurate, cystine, or calcium oxalate monohydrate crystals can indicate metabolic disease or toxicity.
- **Bacteria and Yeast**: Their presence in sediment from cystocentesis-obtained samples is clinically relevant and should prompt culture. Yeast is rare and may reflect contamination or systemic infection.
- **Artifacts**: Contaminants such as pollen, fibers, or starch granules may mimic pathological elements and must be distinguished through experience and careful observation.

Urine specific gravity (USG) is another critical component of urinalysis, reflecting the kidney's ability to concentrate or dilute urine in response to hydration and homeostatic demands. It is measured using a refractometer, which quantifies the refractive index of urine. Veterinary refractometers are calibrated specifically for canine and feline urine and must not be substituted with human medical instruments.

To measure USG, a drop of well-mixed urine is placed on the refractometer prism and the cover plate is closed. The instrument is held up to a light source, and the scale is read at the meniscus of the urine line. The refractometer must be calibrated regularly with distilled water (which should read 1.000) to ensure accuracy.

USG interpretation must be performed in the context of hydration status and concurrent laboratory values. In general:

- **Canine USG:**
  - 1.030 indicates adequate concentration
  - 1.013–1.030 is equivocal
  - <1.013 suggests hyposthenuria or isosthenuria in the face of azotemia
- **Feline USG:**
  - 1.035 is considered adequate
  - 1.015–1.035 is borderline
  - <1.015 may indicate impaired concentrating ability

Hyposthenuria (actively diluted urine) implies preserved tubular function but is inappropriate in dehydrated patients and may indicate disorders such as hyperadrenocorticism, pyometra, or psychogenic polydipsia. Isosthenuria (urine SG of ~1.008–1.012) suggests that the kidneys are neither concentrating nor diluting and is often seen in renal insufficiency or failure.

The combination of physical, chemical, and microscopic assessment—performed with methodical precision—makes urinalysis a cornerstone of laboratory diagnostics. Mastery of slide preparation, microscope technique, and accurate interpretation of findings empowers the veterinary technician to identify disease processes early and with confidence, thereby playing a pivotal role in patient care.

Fecal Diagnostics: Techniques and Sensitivity

Fecal diagnostics remain a cornerstone of gastrointestinal health evaluation, particularly in young animals, those with incomplete deworming histories, immunocompromised patients, shelter populations, and individuals presenting with gastrointestinal signs such as diarrhea, vomiting, weight loss, tenesmus, hematochezia, or failure to thrive. Routine fecal examinations are also critical for wellness screening, boarding facility intake, and pre-treatment assessments in patients scheduled for immunosuppressive therapy or group housing.

Fecal analysis is designed to identify parasitic ova, protozoan cysts, motile trophozoites, occult blood, and occasionally bacterial or fungal elements. Fecal samples should be fresh (ideally <12 hours old), stored in an airtight, clean plastic container, and kept refrigerated if not analyzed immediately. Room temperature degradation of protozoal forms and desiccation of ova can lead to false negatives. Veterinary technicians must also use personal protective equipment when handling feces to mitigate zoonotic transmission of pathogens such as *Toxocara* spp., *Ancylostoma* spp., *Giardia*, and *Cryptosporidium*.

There are several methods of fecal testing, each with distinct diagnostic objectives:

Direct Smear (Saline Wet Mount)

The direct smear is used to evaluate motile protozoa such as *Giardia lamblia* trophozoites, *Tritrichomonas foetus* (in cats), or flagellated commensals. Although sensitivity is low due to the small sample size, this technique is rapid and useful for identifying active swimming organisms in diarrheic feces.

To prepare a direct smear:

1) Place a drop of isotonic saline (0.9% NaCl) onto a clean microscope slide.
2) Using an applicator stick, collect a small amount of feces (about the size of a match head) and emulsify it into the saline to form a homogenous suspension.
3) Cover with a coverslip and examine under 10× and 40× objectives immediately, as trophozoite motility diminishes quickly with time or temperature changes.

Trophozoites appear as teardrop-shaped, flagellated organisms with a jerky or "falling leaf" motion, most easily appreciated under high-power magnification.

Wet Mount with Lugol's Iodine

When structural detail of cysts and ova is preferred over motility evaluation, a second wet mount may be prepared using Lugol's iodine solution. This enhances nuclear detail of protozoal cysts and highlights morphological features of helminth ova, though it kills motile forms. The procedure is identical to a saline wet mount, except the saline is replaced with a drop of dilute iodine solution, and the slide is examined for structural features rather than movement.

Centrifugal Fecal Flotation

Centrifugation is the gold standard technique for detecting helminth ova (e.g., *Toxocara*, *Ancylostoma*, *Trichuris*, *Taenia*) and protozoal cysts (e.g., *Giardia*, *Isospora*). Passive flotation (gravity-based) techniques are still used in some practices but have inferior sensitivity, particularly for light infections or intermittent shedders.

To perform a centrifugal fecal flotation:

1) Combine approximately 1–2 g of feces (roughly a pea-sized amount) with 10 mL of a flotation solution, such as zinc sulfate (1.18–1.20 specific gravity) or Sheather's sugar solution (1.27 specific gravity).
2) Mix thoroughly to homogenize the feces and break up debris.
3) Strain the suspension through gauze or a sieve into a clean centrifuge tube to remove particulate matter.
4) Fill the tube to the brim with the same flotation solution, creating a slight meniscus at the top.
5) Place a coverslip gently on top of the meniscus.
6) Centrifuge at 1,200–1,500 rpm for 5–10 minutes.
7) Following centrifugation, remove the coverslip vertically and place it on a clean slide for microscopic examination.

Examination is performed under 10× for scanning and 40× for detailed morphology. The flotation solution's specific gravity is critical: it must be high enough to cause ova and cysts to float, while not so high as to distort or collapse delicate protozoal forms.

Antigen Detection (Fecal ELISA)

Enzyme-linked immunosorbent assays (ELISAs) are available in-clinic and through reference laboratories for the detection of *Giardia*, hookworm, and roundworm antigens. These tests detect soluble parasite antigens, increasing sensitivity over flotation alone and reducing false negatives in patients shedding low numbers of ova or cysts.

ELISAs are particularly valuable for detecting *Giardia* spp., which often shed cysts intermittently and in low numbers. These tests may be used as stand-alone diagnostics or as part of composite testing protocols that include flotation and smear techniques.

Molecular Diagnostics (PCR)

Fecal PCR panels are increasingly used for the identification of enteropathogens in patients with chronic diarrhea or unresponsive gastrointestinal disease. These panels can detect genetic material from a variety of pathogens, including

Salmonella, *Clostridium perfringens*, *Campylobacter* spp., *Giardia*, *Tritrichomonas*, and others. While PCR provides excellent specificity, it detects both viable and nonviable organisms, and results must always be interpreted in light of clinical signs.

Gross Examination of Feces

Veterinary technicians should begin every fecal evaluation with a gross assessment. Important observations include:

- **Color**: Black (melena), red (hematochezia), pale or clay-colored (biliary obstruction)
- **Consistency**: Diarrheic, formed, or constipated
- **Mucus**: Often associated with large bowel disease
- **Blood**: Indicates mucosal irritation or bleeding
- **Parasites**: Proglottids or adult worms may be visible externally

A detailed and methodical fecal diagnostic approach maximizes the detection of gastrointestinal parasitism and infectious disease while minimizing false negatives. By understanding the principles and procedures of each technique and combining microscopic skill with clinical context, the veterinary technician enhances both the diagnostic process and patient care outcomes.

Section 7: Radiology and Imaging: Seeing Beyond the Surface

Radiology and imaging are more than technical tasks, they are acts of interpretation, preparation, and precision that directly influence the diagnostic journey of every patient. Veterinary technicians are not just image takers; they are diagnostic facilitators, responsible for the clarity, safety, and usefulness of every image acquired.

A poorly positioned radiograph can obscure a fracture. An overexposed film can hide a mass. A technician who understands *why* each element of imaging matters becomes an essential part of the diagnostic process, ensuring every image has clinical value and every patient is handled with care.

The Technician's Diagnostic Role

Imaging begins long before the machine is turned on. Technicians must consider the patient's history, presenting complaints, and anatomy to plan the most informative views. This includes choosing appropriate positioning aids, adjusting exposure settings based on tissue density, and selecting restraint methods that are both effective and low-stress.

Every step requires intention: *Why are we taking this view? Is it the most appropriate projection for the clinical question? What can I do to reduce stress and motion?* The answers to these questions distinguish a technician who performs imaging from one who practices imaging.

This role becomes even more critical in emergency situations. Patients in respiratory distress, for example, may not tolerate traditional restraint or positioning. In these moments, the technician must think creatively and advocate clearly. Standing lateral or DV thoracic radiographs, oxygen supplementation during positioning, and minimizing handling time can all make the difference between stabilizing and decompensating a patient.

When imaging a dyspneic cat or a trauma patient, the technician must balance the need for diagnostic quality with the patient's current ability to cope. That may mean:

- Asking the veterinarian if radiographs can wait until oxygenation improves.
- Offering oxygen supplementation in the radiology room to the patient.
- Adjusting technique to capture quick, informative images with minimal movement.
- Staging views captured to offer the patient a break between series.
- Being prepared to pause or abort imaging if patient distress worsens.

In cases of pain, such as fractures or abdominal emergencies, the technician's advocacy might involve recommending sedation, adjusting padding to reduce discomfort during positioning, or ensuring premedication is administered before imaging. These moments aren't just about comfort, they're about making the imaging process safe, humane, and diagnostically valuable. The best imaging comes from a technician who is attuned to both the patient's physiology and emotional state. It's not only about getting the picture, but also about getting it safely, compassionately, and intentionally (Table 3.7).

Table 3.7 Quick reference: imaging considerations for emergency patients.

Clinical Situation	Recommended Adjustments	Why It Matters
Respiratory distress	• Minimize handling time • Use oxygen support (flow-by or oxygen cage) • Prefer DV or standing lateral views • Avoid lateral recumbency when possible • Capture critical view first • Minimize respiratory anxiety with butorphanol	Reduces stress, prevents decompensation, and allows for rapid stabilization
Severe pain or trauma	• Provide analgesia or sedation when feasible • Use extra padding and gentle handling • Limit limb manipulation • Consider chemical restraint early	Prevents worsening of injuries and improves image quality while protecting staff
Unstable or critical patients	• Communicate clearly with the veterinarian about urgency vs. patient stability • Prepare all equipment and settings before touching the patient • Assign specific roles to the team to streamline the process	Ensures safety and speed; avoids unnecessary delays that can harm the patient

Source: M. Jennings (2025). Author's own illustration.

Positioning with Purpose

Correct positioning is fundamental to diagnostic imaging and demands far more than physical manipulation of the patient. Veterinary technicians must be able to obtain orthogonal views, typically lateral and ventrodorsal or dorsoventral, to provide complete spatial understanding of internal structures. This process requires careful attention to detail to minimize distortion and magnification, center the anatomical region of interest, and reduce stress that could cause motion artifacts. Positioning tools such as sandbags, foam wedges, and troughs are not simply aids for convenience; they are instruments of diagnostic accuracy and patient comfort. When dealing with painful or fractious patients, the use of chemical restraint should not be considered a last resort, but rather a proactive welfare-based decision that benefits both image quality and the patient's experience.

Exposure Settings: Understanding the Variables

The diagnostic value of a radiograph hinges on proper exposure settings, and veterinary technicians must understand how kilovoltage (kV), milliamperage (mA), and exposure time interact. These variables must be adjusted thoughtfully based on the patient's size and the density of the tissues being imaged. Inadequate settings can lead to overexposure, which can obscure subtle lesions, or underexposure, which diminishes clarity and interpretability. Motion artifacts caused by long exposure times or poor patient handling can also render nondiagnostic images. Technicians who understand and anticipate these factors are able to suggest or implement adjustments confidently, contributing to a more effective and efficient diagnostic process.

Digital Radiography: The Modern Standard

With the advent of digital radiography, veterinary imaging has become faster, more adaptable, and better suited to clinical decision-making. However, the speed and convenience of these systems do not lessen the technician's responsibility to capture high-quality images on the first attempt. Digital radiography includes two main types: computed radiography (CR), which uses a phosphor plate that must be scanned into a digital reader, and direct digital radiography (DDR), which uses a flat-panel detector that transmits images instantly to a computer. Although digital platforms allow for manipulation of image brightness and contrast after exposure, they cannot compensate for improper positioning, poor timing, or technical errors. Recognizing common artifacts such as motion blur, grid cutoff, or image saturation is essential to prevent diagnostic delays, avoid retakes, and maintain clinical accuracy.

Radiation Safety: Protecting Ourselves and Others

Radiation safety is both a professional obligation and an ethical responsibility. Every veterinary technician must understand and implement safety protocols to protect themselves, their colleagues, and their patients. Following the ALARA principle, keeping radiation exposure As Low As Reasonably Achievable, requires minimizing exposure time, maximizing distance from the beam, and using appropriate shielding such as lead aprons, gloves, and thyroid protectors. However, shielding is not a substitute for smart planning. Technicians must develop workflows that reduce retakes and avoid unnecessary exposure. Furthermore, technicians are often in a leadership position when it comes to modeling proper safety practices and educating newer team members about responsible radiographic procedures.

Advanced Imaging: Ultrasound and CT

Ultrasound and computed tomography (CT) represent advanced diagnostic tools that require more than just familiarity with the equipment, they demand a technician's ability to think critically and execute procedures with precision. In many cases, veterinary technicians are responsible for setting up imaging protocols, sedating or restraining the patient, and acquiring usable images under veterinary supervision. Understanding probe orientation, recognizing common artifacts, and adjusting depth, gain, and frequency settings are critical for producing diagnostic-quality images. A technician trained in these skills will be able to identify when an image is nondiagnostic, troubleshoot issues such as poor resolution or acoustic shadowing, and ensure that each scan is labeled and saved correctly. Advanced imaging requires intention, clarity of purpose, and a deep understanding of what the image is meant to reveal. It is not about pushing buttons, it is about seeing with insight and capturing the internal story of the patient.

Expert Tip: Thinking Like the Diagnostician

Before capturing an image, ask yourself:
What am I trying to show? What could go wrong with this image? Will this answer the clinical question?
When veterinary technicians approach imaging with diagnostic curiosity and clinical accountability, they transform from technicians into essential diagnostic collaborators.

Ultrasound Imaging: Principles and Technician Role

Ultrasound is a real-time, noninvasive imaging modality used to evaluate soft tissues, fluid-filled structures, and vascular flow. Unlike radiography, ultrasound does not use ionizing radiation but relies on high-frequency sound waves that interact with tissues to produce an image. Veterinary technicians play a critical role in probe positioning, image optimization, and patient restraint for ultrasound examinations (Table 3.8).

Clinical Pearl: Optimizing Image Clarity

Using an acoustic gel layer between the probe and skin eliminates air interference, ensuring better sound wave transmission and image resolution (Nyland and Mattoon 2015).

Table 3.8 Ultrasound probes and their uses.

Probe Type	Frequency	Use
Linear probe	High-frequency (7–15 MHz)	superficial structures like tendons, thyroid glands, and small abdominal organs
Curvilinear probe	Mid-frequency (3–8 MHz)	abdominal imaging and general organ assessment
Phased array probe	Low-frequency (2–5 MHz)	cardiac imaging due to its small footprint and deep penetration

Source: M. Jennings (2025). Author's own illustration.

Proper probe positioning is essential for acquiring accurate and diagnostic ultrasound images. Technicians must consistently align the probe marker according to established anatomical conventions to ensure proper orientation. When scanning in the sagittal plane, the probe marker should be directed toward the patient's head, providing a longitudinal view of internal structures. In the transverse plane, the probe marker should point toward the patient's right side, allowing for cross-sectional visualization. Maintaining correct orientation throughout the procedure ensures consistency in image interpretation and supports effective communication among the veterinary team.

Choosing the Right Modality: Radiography vs. Ultrasound

Veterinary technicians play a vital role in selecting and executing imaging techniques based on the clinical question at hand. Radiography and ultrasound are not interchangeable tools, they provide complementary information that, when used thoughtfully, guide diagnostic clarity and patient care.

Radiographs offer unmatched visualization of bones, gas-filled spaces, and high-density structures. For example, thoracic radiographs are essential for assessing pulmonary patterns, cardiac silhouette, and evidence of pleural effusion. Abdominal radiographs help identify gastrointestinal obstructions, urinary tract calculi, or abnormal organ shapes. Skeletal radiographs remain the gold standard for diagnosing fractures, arthritis, and osseous tumors. However, obtaining useful images requires more than pushing a button; technicians must understand how positioning, timing, and patient condition influence what the image reveals, and what it might miss.

Ultrasound, by contrast, excels at evaluating soft tissue and fluid-filled structures. It allows real-time assessment of organ architecture, vascular flow, and subtle lesions that may be invisible on radiographs. In abdominal imaging, ultrasound offers detailed insight into hepatic or splenic masses, bowel motility, and free fluid. Echocardiography provides dynamic assessment of cardiac function, helping to identify valve insufficiencies, chamber enlargement, or pericardial effusion. In emergency settings, the FAST (Focused Assessment with Sonography for Trauma) protocol empowers technicians and clinicians to rapidly detect free abdominal or thoracic fluid, often guiding life-saving decisions within minutes.

Understanding the capabilities and limitations of each modality allows technicians to advocate for the most appropriate diagnostic approach. It also enables them to anticipate the veterinarian's next steps, prepare the patient accordingly, and recognize when a repeat image or alternative view may be necessary. Diagnostic imaging is not passive, it is an extension of clinical thinking, and the technician's grasp of modality selection plays a key role in accurate, timely diagnosis.

Avoiding Common Imaging Pitfalls

Veterinary technicians must be proficient in recognizing and correcting technical errors to ensure diagnostic accuracy (Table 3.9).

> **Expert Tip: i3Using Radiographic Contrast Studies**
>
> If standard radiographs do not provide enough detail, contrast agents (e.g., barium sulfate for GI studies, iodinated contrast for urinary studies) enhance visualization of soft tissue structures.

Table 3.9 Imagining pitfalls with common causes and corrections.

Imaging Pitfall	Common Cause	Correction
Motion artifact	Patient movement during exposure	Use sedation or shorten exposure time
Poor contrast	Incorrect kV setting	Adjust kV for better differentiation between tissues
Ultrasound shadowing	Bone or gas interference	Adjust probe angle or use alternative imaging plane

Source: M. Jennings (2025). Author's own illustration.

Section 8: Dentistry

Veterinary dentistry is far more than a cosmetic or elective procedure; it is a foundational component of patient health. With over 80% of dogs and cats affected by periodontal disease by the age of three, veterinary technicians must approach dental care with purpose, precision, and a clear understanding of their role in preventing pain and improving quality of life. From charting and cleaning to radiographic imaging and surgical assistance, each task has a direct impact on a patient's comfort, systemic health, and long-term well-being.

Oral Anatomy and Dental Charting

A strong foundation in oral anatomy is essential for every technician involved in dental procedures. The Triadan system provides a standardized method of numbering teeth, improving accuracy in dental records and communication between staff. Each quadrant of the mouth has a corresponding numerical series: the right maxilla begins with the 100s, the left maxilla with the 200s, the left mandible with the 300s, and the right mandible with the 400s. For example, the upper right canine is designated as 104, while the lower left first molar is labeled 309.

Technicians must not only understand this system but also apply it with confidence during dental procedures. Charting includes documentation of missing teeth, enamel defects, fractures, resorptive lesions, and periodontal disease grading. Recognizing the stages of periodontal disease, from gingivitis with no attachment loss to advanced periodontitis with significant bone loss, guides treatment planning and client communication. Dental charts are legal records, but they also serve as a map to improve future outcomes.

Professional Dental Cleaning (COHAT)

A Complete Oral Health Assessment and Treatment (COHAT) is not simply a "cleaning," it is a comprehensive medical procedure that addresses the visible and invisible threats to oral health. The veterinary technician must conduct each component with both thoroughness and purpose. Supragingival scaling removes plaque and tartar above the gumline, but it is the subgingival scaling that truly prevents periodontal disease by disrupting the bacterial colonies hidden beneath the surface. Polishing smooths the enamel to delay plaque reattachment, and fluoride or sealant applications strengthen enamel and reduce bacterial adhesion.

Full-mouth intraoral radiographs are a standard part of a COHAT; guidelines strongly recommend them for every dental patient because much of the dentoalveolar pathology is invisible on oral exam. Approximately two-thirds of each tooth lies below the gingiva, and studies show that radiographs uncover clinically important disease in 28% of dogs and 42% of cats whose teeth appeared grossly normal (AAHA 2019; AVDC position) (Table 3.10).

Radiography in Dentistry

Veterinary dental radiographs are indispensable for diagnosing diseases not visible on oral exam. Fractured roots, resorptive lesions, endodontic disease, and retained deciduous teeth often evade detection without radiographic imaging. Technicians must be proficient in positioning, technique, and troubleshooting to obtain high-quality films.

The bisecting angle technique is commonly used in veterinary dentistry to prevent distortion of the tooth image. This requires aligning the X-ray beam perpendicular to the imaginary line that bisects the angle between the tooth axis and the sensor. Misalignment can lead to common errors, such as elongation, foreshortening, or overlapping roots, each of which reduces diagnostic value. A technician who understands and adjusts technique accordingly enhances the accuracy of diagnosis and reduces the need for repeat exposure (Table 3.11).

Common Dental Disorders and Recognition

Gingivitis and periodontitis represent a progressive spectrum of disease triggered by bacterial plaque and the immune system's response. Technicians must understand this continuum to better advocate for treatment, whether that be routine cleaning, root planing, or extraction of unsalvageable teeth. Fractured teeth are another common finding, particularly in dogs with inappropriate chew toys or trauma. If pulp exposure is confirmed radiographically, the technician should anticipate discussion of extraction or referral for endodontic therapy.

Table 3.10 COHAT procedural checklist for veterinary technicians.

Step	Purpose
1. Review history and diagnostics	Confirm anesthesia clearance, recent bloodwork, and any oral health notes
2. Pre-anesthetic assessment	Check TPR, hydration, oral discomfort, and inform vet of any new findings
3. Pre-op imaging (optional)	If indicated, obtain pre-cleaning radiographs (e.g., fractured tooth)
4. Supragingival scaling	Remove visible plaque and tartar from the crown with ultrasonic scaler
5. Subgingival scaling	Use curette or ultrasonic tip beneath the gumline to remove hidden plaque
6. Full-mouth radiographs	Identify pathology under the gumline, root resorption, bone loss, abscesses
7. Chart findings thoroughly	Use Triadan system, periodontal grading, note lesions or abnormalities
8. Polishing	Smooth enamel to reduce plaque adherence postscaling
9. Fluoride or sealant application	Strengthen enamel and provide a protective barrier
10. Vet evaluation and extractions	Assist during oral exam and extractions if needed; take post-op radiographs
11. Postprocedural monitoring	Monitor for bleeding, pain, or complications as patient recovers
12. Client education	Discuss findings, home care strategies, and next steps

Source: M. Jennings (2025). Author's own illustration.

Table 3.11 Quick-reference table: common dental radiograph errors and corrections.

Error Type	Cause	How to Correct
Elongation	X-ray beam too perpendicular to the tooth	Adjust the beam to follow the *bisecting angle* between the tooth and sensor
Foreshortening	X-ray beam too perpendicular to the sensor	Reposition the beam more parallel to the tooth's long axis
Overlapping roots	Inadequate horizontal angulation of the beam	Shift the X-ray tube head slightly mesially or distally for better separation
Cone cut	Sensor not fully covered by the X-ray beam	Reposition the cone to fully center over the sensor
Motion blur	Patient movement during exposure	Use sedation when appropriate and ensure rapid, confident image capture
Poor detail/ contrast	Incorrect exposure settings or outdated sensor plates	Verify proper kV/mA/time, use fresh sensors, and adjust for patient size

Source: M. Jennings (2025). Author's own illustration.

Malocclusions may be congenital or acquired, and while mild cases can be monitored, others require intervention to prevent trauma to soft tissue or abnormal wear patterns. Technicians are often the first to recognize these conditions during a routine exam and must be prepared to discuss concerns with the veterinarian and owner.

Discoloration of a tooth, often pink, gray, or purple, indicates pulp necrosis. These teeth are frequently painful and may become chronically infected. Their identification, even in asymptomatic patients, is a key example of how veterinary technicians serve as patient advocates in silent pain scenarios.

Client Education and Home Care

A technician's responsibility does not end with the procedure. Educating clients on daily home care is essential to long-term oral health. The gold standard remains daily brushing with veterinary-approved enzymatic toothpaste. However, in pets that resist brushing, alternatives such as dental wipes, chlorhexidine rinses, prescription dental diets, or VOHC-approved dental chews can be used to support oral hygiene.

Technicians should tailor recommendations to the client's lifestyle and the pet's temperament. Simply handing the owner a toothbrush is rarely effective. Demonstration, coaching, and follow-up conversations are key to building long-term compliance. The technician's credibility and trust with the client can directly influence whether that pet receives meaningful preventive care at home.

Expert Tip: Avoiding Harmful Dental Chews
Hard chews like antlers and bones can cause tooth fractures. The "thumbnail test" is a simple way to assess safety, if you can't dent it with your fingernail, it's too hard for a pet's teeth (Gorrel 2021).

Section 9: Veterinary Patient Care and Nursing

Veterinary patient care is a dynamic, hands-on discipline that bridges science, compassion, and critical thinking. At the heart of this work are veterinary technicians, whose daily actions directly influence patient recovery, comfort, and long-term outcomes. Through pain management, nutritional support, specialized nursing for vulnerable populations, and diligent documentation, technicians uphold the standards that define high-quality veterinary care.

The Intangible Art of Veterinary Nursing

Not every aspect of nursing care can be measured, charted, or taught through a textbook. As veterinary technicians gain experience, they develop a deeper, often intuitive sense of what their patients need. This internal compass, sometimes referred to as "spidey senses" by seasoned technicians, is not guesswork. It is the result of a thousand small observations: the subtle change in a dog's posture, the hesitation in a cat's breathing, the flick of an ear that signals discomfort before vital signs ever change.

This intuitive awareness is a hallmark of excellent nursing care. Technicians often become the first to notice that something isn't right, even when objective data is still within normal limits. A patient who "just doesn't look like himself" or seems "off" may be developing hypoglycemia, pain, or early shock. Trusting those instincts and voicing them confidently is not just valuable, it can be lifesaving.

Beyond physiology, veterinary technicians often connect with patients in ways that transcend clinical routines. There is a quiet, profound language spoken through gentle touch, presence, and empathy. Sitting on the floor with a trembling dog or letting a hospitalized cat crawl into their lap during treatments is more than comfort, it's communication. These moments of stillness and emotional connection foster trust, reduce stress, and support healing in ways that are just as critical as medications and procedures.

Veterinary nursing is not only about what we *do* for our patients, but how we *listen* to them, through behavior, body language, and energy. When technicians embrace this deeper level of communication, they become powerful advocates and caregivers, ensuring that patients are not only treated, but truly understood.

Developing Intuition Through Intentional Practice

For technicians who haven't yet experienced this intuitive connection, or who are still learning to trust their instincts, know that this is a skill that grows with time, reflection, and presence. It begins with slowing down, even in a fast-paced environment, and choosing to truly observe your patients beyond the checklist. Pay attention to how they move when no one is near them. Notice how their demeanor shifts around different people or in different spaces. Start to ask yourself not just *what* a patient is doing, but *why*.

Practice sitting with patients without rushing, hold space for them without needing to fix something right away. Learn their language. Let discomfort guide curiosity, not fear. Talk through your observations with trusted mentors and ask for their insight. Over time, patterns will emerge, and what once felt subtle, or abstract will become your most reliable internal alarm.

Intuition is not a mysterious gift given only to a few; it is a form of clinical perception built on experience, empathy, and engagement. If you are seeking to deepen this skill, be patient with yourself. The act of showing up with genuine intention and attention is the first step toward developing the kind of technician presence that patients feel safe around, and that colleagues trust without hesitation.

Cultivating Intuition as a Veterinary Technician

Not every technician feels an immediate connection to their patients, and that's okay. Intuition isn't magic. It's a skill that grows from deep observation, clinical experience, and genuine presence. Start by slowing down, watching your patients closely, and asking why, not just what.

Trust builds as you reflect on subtle signs: the shift in a patient's eyes, the tension in their body, the way they respond to your presence. Talk through your gut feelings with mentors. Over time, these instincts become a vital part of your nursing care.

You don't have to be born with intuition. You can build it.

Pain Management: Recognizing and Responding with Intention

Pain compromises healing, alters physiology, and diminishes quality of life. Because animals cannot self-report discomfort, veterinary technicians must become experts at recognizing the subtle and overt signs of pain. Posture, vocalization, facial expression, and behavior shifts all serve as cues that something isn't right. Tools like the Glasgow Composite Pain Scale for dogs and the Feline Grimace Scale for cats offer structured ways to assess discomfort, but it is often the technician's daily interaction that reveals a change before a scale confirms it.

When pain is suspected, immediate action is warranted. Multimodal analgesia, using a combination of drug classes like NSAIDs, opioids, local anesthetics, and adjuncts, provides comprehensive relief while minimizing side effects. Technicians administer medications, monitor for efficacy, and advocate for adjustments when a patient remains restless, guarded, or withdrawn. Sedation may also be needed to manage opioid-induced dysphoria in sensitive patients, improving recovery without compromising analgesia.

Beyond pharmacology, nursing interventions like soft bedding, heat therapy, and passive range-of-motion exercises support musculoskeletal comfort and prevent secondary complications. Pain management is not a single task; it is an ongoing process requiring critical observation and clinical judgment.

Clinical Insight: Subtle Signs of Pain in Cats

Cats often hide signs of pain, displaying behaviors such as hunched posture, reluctance to jump, sudden change in behavior, and decreased grooming. These changes should prompt pain management interventions.

Multimodal Analgesia and Pain Control

Effective pain management in veterinary patients requires more than just a single drug or protocol, it demands a strategic, multimodal approach tailored to the patient's condition, procedure, and overall health. By combining different classes of analgesics that target pain at various points along the nociceptive pathway, veterinary teams can achieve more complete pain control while minimizing the risk of side effects. Veterinary technicians play a central role in implementing these strategies, assessing patient responses, and advocating for necessary adjustments in analgesia plans.

Multimodal pain control typically involves four primary categories: nonsteroidal anti-inflammatory drugs (NSAIDs), opioids, local anesthetics, and adjunctive medications. Each has unique properties, benefits, and limitations, which technicians must understand to monitor effectiveness and identify adverse reactions.

NSAIDs such as carprofen, meloxicam, and robenacoxib are cornerstones of inflammatory pain management. These drugs work by inhibiting cyclooxygenase enzymes (COX-1 and COX-2), reducing prostaglandin synthesis, and thereby decreasing inflammation and peripheral sensitization. While highly effective, NSAIDs must be used judiciously, patients with renal disease, GI ulcers, or coagulopathies may not be appropriate candidates. Veterinary technicians must closely monitor hydration status, appetite, vomiting, diarrhea, and bloodwork trends in patients receiving NSAIDs.

Opioids remain essential for managing moderate to severe pain, especially in surgical and trauma patients. Drugs like buprenorphine, hydromorphone, and methadone act on the central nervous system, dampening the perception of pain and improving patient comfort. Opioids may be administered as intermittent boluses or as continuous rate infusions (CRIs), with technician monitoring vitals observing sedation level, respiratory rate, and signs of dysphoria or bradycardia.

Technicians must also understand breed-specific sensitivities, for example, sighthounds and cats may react differently to opioid administration and require adjusted protocols.

Local anesthetics, such as lidocaine and bupivacaine, offer the benefit of regional analgesia without systemic effects. When used in nerve blocks, line blocks, or splash blocks, these agents can desensitize a specific area and significantly reduce the need for systemic analgesics. Bupivacaine provides a longer duration of action, making it ideal for surgical wound infiltration. Technicians trained in local block techniques contribute to smoother recoveries and reduced postoperative pain.

Adjunctive medications expand the toolkit for managing complex or chronic pain cases. Gabapentin and amantadine are commonly used for neuropathic pain or long-term osteoarthritis management. Gabapentin works by modulating calcium channels in the nervous system, while amantadine targets NMDA receptors to reduce central sensitization. These medications are often introduced during recovery or in outpatient settings, and veterinary technicians must guide owners through proper administration, potential side effects (e.g., sedation), and expected timelines for improvement.

By applying a multimodal strategy, veterinary technicians help create individualized analgesic plans that are both effective and sustainable. Their hands-on role in preparation for medication, patient monitoring, documentation, and owner education makes them essential contributors to comprehensive pain management, improving patient outcomes, recovery quality, and long-term welfare (Table 3.12).

Expert Tip: Preventing Opioid-Induced Dysphoria

post-surgical patients, especially cats and sighthounds, may exhibit opioid dysphoria (restlessness, vocalization). A low dose dexmedetomidine or acepromazine can provide sedation and improve recovery quality (Mathews et al. 2017).

Clinical Example: Advocating for Multimodal Pain Management in a Geriatric Orthopedic Case

Sadie, a 12-year-old, FS, Labrador Retriever, presented for a tibial plateau leveling osteotomy (TPLO) after rupturing her cranial cruciate ligament. As the assigned surgical technician, Emily noted Sadie's age, history of mild kidney compromise, and signs of preexisting osteoarthritis in her contralateral limb. Recognizing that a single analgesic approach might not be sufficient, and could even be contraindicated, Emily initiated a discussion with the attending veterinarian before the procedure.

Drawing on her knowledge of pharmacodynamics and current pain management protocols, Emily proposed a multimodal plan: a preoperative epidural, perioperative fentanyl and lidocaine CRI, and postoperative NSAIDs (pending renal monitoring) paired with adjunctive gabapentin for long-term comfort. She also recommended laser therapy and passive range-of-motion exercises to aid recovery and reduce stiffness.

Table 3.12 Overview of multimodal analgesia drug classes.

Drug Class	Examples	Mechanism of Action	Clinical Considerations
NSAIDs	Carprofen, Meloxicam, Robenacoxib	Inhibit COX enzymes to reduce prostaglandin production and inflammation	Monitor GI, renal, and hepatic function. Avoid in dehydrated or coagulopathic patients.
Opioids	Buprenorphine, Hydromorphone, Methadone	Bind to opioid receptors in the CNS to block pain perception	Watch for respiratory depression, dysphoria, bradycardia. Consider CRI or titration based on patient response.
Local anesthetics	Lidocaine, Bupivacaine	Block sodium channels to prevent nerve depolarization and pain signal transmission	Used for nerve blocks and wound infiltration. Bupivacaine offers prolonged duration.
Adjunctive medications	Gabapentin, Amantadine, Ketamine	Gabapentin modulates calcium channels; amantadine inhibits NMDA receptors	Often used for chronic or neuropathic pain. Monitor for sedation or ataxia.

Source: M. Jennings (2025). Author's own illustration.

The veterinarian adjusted the treatment plan to include Emily's suggestions. Postoperatively, Sadie showed improved comfort, required fewer breakthrough pain interventions, and ambulated earlier than expected. Bloodwork remained stable, and the owners reported a smoother recovery compared to her last orthopedic procedure. Emily documented all pain scores in the medical record using the Glasgow Composite Pain Scale and adjusted nursing interventions accordingly.

Outcome: Emily's proactive advocacy and clinical reasoning helped deliver tailored, layered analgesia that reduced adverse effects, improved Sadie's quality of recovery, and built client trust. Her involvement showcased the critical role of the technician in ensuring evidence-based, compassionate pain control.

Nutritional Support: Diet, Tube Feeding, and Obesity Management

Nutrition as a Therapeutic Tool

Malnutrition silently undermines healing. It impairs immune function, delays tissue repair, and lowers resilience to stress. Yet it often goes unnoticed until weight loss or muscle wasting becomes obvious. Veterinary technicians are uniquely positioned to detect early signs of nutritional compromise, from poor appetite to changes in body condition.

A structured Body Condition Score (BCS) system helps guide evaluation, but technicians must also consider medical status, caloric demands, and patient preferences. For patients unable to meet their needs orally, enteral feeding through nasogastric, esophagostomy, or gastrostomy tubes ensures continued support. Monitoring tube placement, preventing clogging, and calculating daily caloric intake are essential nursing tasks.

Assessing Nutritional Status

A Body Condition Score (BCS) is a standardized method for evaluating a patient's fat and muscle stores. The nine-point scale is commonly used (Table 3.13):

Enteral Feeding and Feeding Tube Management

When patients are unwilling or unable to eat on their own, the veterinary technician plays a pivotal role in initiating and managing enteral support. From selecting the most appropriate tube to maintaining cleanliness and monitoring tolerance, technicians are central to the success of nutritional interventions.

Technicians are often the first to recognize signs of inadequate intake, such as weight loss, muscle wasting, or prolonged anorexia. Their advocacy may prompt early nutritional intervention, improve patient outcomes, and shorten recovery time. Enteral feeding options vary depending on the duration of support needed and the patient's underlying condition.

Nasogastric (NG) tubes are typically chosen for short-term support, especially in hospitalized patients with mild anorexia or gastrointestinal motility disorders. Technicians are responsible for measuring and placing NG tubes under veterinary supervision, confirming placement via radiography, and securing the tube with minimal discomfort to the patient. Regular flushing, documentation of intake, and monitoring for regurgitation or dislodgement are all within the technician's purview.

For longer-term support, esophagostomy tubes (E-tubes) are often selected, particularly in cats or dogs with oral trauma, neoplasia, or chronic disease. Once placed by a veterinarian, technicians manage all aspects of care: preparing and administering meals, monitoring for tube site infection, and teaching owners how to continue care at home. Clear communication and compassionate coaching are essential when helping clients feel confident in providing at-home tube feedings.

In cases where even longer nutritional support is needed, or when bypassing the upper GI tract is necessary, gastrostomy tubes (G-tubes) are utilized. These tubes require advanced nursing care, especially in patients with neurologic conditions, severe trauma, or cancer. Technicians must be vigilant in monitoring the tube site, securing the port correctly, and

Table 3.13 Quick reference nine-point body condition score.

BCS	Description
1–3 (underweight)	Prominent ribs, spine, pelvic bones
4–5 (ideal)	Ribs palpable with slight fat covering
6–9 (overweight/obese)	Ribs difficult to palpate, abdominal fat deposits

Source: M. Jennings (2025). Author's own illustration.

recognizing early signs of complications such as peritonitis, clogging, or vomiting. Thorough documentation and timely communication with the veterinarian allow for prompt adjustments in care if complications arise.

Across all feeding tube types, the technician's role extends beyond the mechanical aspects. Monitoring stool quality, body condition, appetite return, and patient demeanor provide important feedback on nutritional response. When technicians observe subtle changes, like signs of nausea during feeding or a drop in energy, they become the voice for the patient who cannot speak, helping to fine-tune the care plan accordingly.

Enteral feeding management is not just about delivering calories, it's about restoring strength, protecting dignity, and supporting recovery with the same attentiveness as any other critical intervention. The veterinary technician's knowledge, consistency, and intuition can make the difference between a patient who simply survives and one who thrives.

Environmental Enrichment and Nursing Considerations

Veterinary patient care extends beyond medication and monitoring; it also includes the emotional and cognitive well-being of animals in unfamiliar or stressful environments. Environmental enrichment is often overlooked but plays a key role in improving patient outcomes, particularly in long-term hospitalization or boarding settings. Enrichment strategies should be tailored to the species and individual temperament. For dogs, this may include short walks, scent-based games, or stuffed food toys. Cats often benefit from vertical spaces, hiding boxes, and visual stimulation. Calm lighting, soft bedding, noise reduction, and minimizing unnecessary handling are critical elements of a healing-focused environment. In ICU or isolation settings, even small comforts, like familiar blankets, pheromone diffusers, or gentle music, can ease anxiety and promote recovery. Veterinary technicians act as advocates for hospitalized patients, ensuring their physical needs are met alongside their emotional well-being. Documenting enrichment interventions and behavioral responses allows technicians to refine care plans and inform the broader team of what works best for each patient.

Infection Control: A Foundational Responsibility in Nursing Care

Infection prevention is one of the most fundamental responsibilities of a veterinary technician. Every patient interaction, surface cleaned, or protocol followed contributes to maintaining a safe, healing-centered environment for animals and staff alike. In a hospital setting, pathogens spread easily through hands, equipment, and aerosols. Veterinary technicians must remain vigilant, recognizing that infection control is not limited to isolation wards, it is a daily, hospital-wide discipline.

Standard precautions begin with proper hand hygiene before and after each patient contact, using either soap and water or alcohol-based hand rubs depending on visible soiling. Personal protective equipment (PPE), such as gloves, gowns, and masks, must be worn consistently in designated areas, and disinfectants should be selected based on efficacy against targeted organisms (e.g., parvovirus, MRSP). Equipment such as stethoscopes, thermometers, and clippers must be disinfected between uses to prevent cross-contamination.

Technicians also play a pivotal role in managing patients under isolation. This includes enforcing barrier protocols, maintaining designated supplies, and ensuring correct waste disposal. Properly labeled signage, color-coded garments, and clear communication help reduce the risk of transmission. By modeling adherence to infection control protocols, veterinary technicians protect vulnerable patients, limit hospital-acquired infections, and uphold the integrity of the clinical environment.

Mobility Assistance and Nursing Support

Mobility is a key component of recovery and comfort in veterinary patients. Whether due to postoperative pain, neurologic impairment, or orthopedic injury, restricted mobility can contribute to pressure sores, delayed healing, incontinence, and even respiratory compromise. Veterinary technicians must assess each patient's mobility status and apply appropriate assistance strategies to promote safety and dignity.

Nursing interventions begin with proper bedding and patient positioning. Soft, absorbent materials help distribute weight evenly and prevent skin breakdown, especially in recumbent or geriatric patients. Technicians should reposition nonambulatory patients every four to six hours and monitor for early signs of decubital ulcers or limb stiffness. For patients capable of limited movement, assisted ambulation using slings, harnesses, or towel support encourages circulation, maintains muscle tone, and improves morale. Early mobility, when appropriate, also helps reduce complications such as ileus or atelectasis. Documenting changes in gait, reluctance to move, or signs of pain allows technicians to advocate for pain management, physical therapy, or environmental modifications. In cases of chronic immobility, veterinary technicians also collaborate in bladder expression, hygiene care, and mobility device fitting. Thoughtful, attentive mobility support demonstrates a commitment to whole-patient care.

Documentation: The Language of Patient Advocacy

Accurate recordkeeping is the foundation of safe and consistent patient care. Every medication given, every change observed, and every decision made must be documented clearly and objectively. Trends in temperature, pulse, respiration, blood pressure, and oxygenation help identify improvement or decline, especially when care is shared across multiple shifts.

More than a legal safeguard, documentation is a communication tool. Behavior notes, appetite logs, urination patterns, and responses to medications give the broader medical team insight into how the patient is progressing. Veterinary technicians carry the responsibility of being their patient's voice on the record, ensuring that nothing is missed and every concern is communicated.

Patient Handoffs and IPASS Rounding: Enhancing Continuity of Care

Effective communication during patient handoffs is critical for reducing medical errors and ensuring consistent, high-quality care (Mathews et al., 2017). The IPASS system is a structured approach originally developed in human medicine and now adapted in many veterinary settings to improve clarity during shift changes, rounds, and case transfers.

IPASS stands for:

- **I**: *Illness Severity*: Brief description of the patient's condition (e.g., stable, critical).
- **P**: *Patient Summary*: A concise summary of the reason for hospitalization, diagnostics performed, and current treatment plan.
- **A**: *Action List*: What needs to be done next, pending diagnostics, medication times, or specific monitoring tasks.
- **S**: *Situational Awareness and Contingency Planning*: What to watch for (e.g., "If vomiting continues, alert DVM") and any anticipated complications.
- **S**: *Synthesis by Receiver*: The receiving technician or team member repeats the key points to confirm understanding and clarify next steps.

Clinical Example

A veterinary technician ending a shift might say: "Bella is a four-year-old spayed female Labrador. Illness severity is stable but guarded, she's recovering from exploratory laparotomy. Summary: surgery revealed a linear foreign body, and a resection-anastomosis was performed. She's NPO, on IV fluids and fentanyl CRI. Action list: Monitor for pain, check abdominal incision at 3 p.m., and recheck vitals in 1 hour. Situational awareness: Watch for signs of dehiscence or increased abdominal pain. If present, notify the surgeon immediately. Synthesis?" IPASS helps prevent missed treatments, duplicated efforts, or overlooked symptoms by creating a culture of clear, accountable handoff communication. It reinforces technician's responsibility not just in performing tasks, but in ensuring information continuity.

Section 10: Client Communication and Education

Effective communication with pet owners is a cornerstone of veterinary nursing, forming the bridge between medical expertise and real-world outcomes. Veterinary technicians, as the primary point of contact for many clients, serve as educators, translators of clinical information, and compassionate supporters. Through clear communication, active listening, and strategic education, technicians help ensure that owners are informed, empowered, and able to actively participate in their pet's care. This relationship not only strengthens compliance but also enhances the emotional experience of veterinary care for both the client and patient (Shaw et al. 2020).

The Clinical Relevance of Patient Signalment

Among the many tools available to veterinary professionals in the diagnostic process, few are as essential, encompassing, and profoundly informative as signalment. Defined as the compilation of a patient's age, species, breed, sex, and reproductive status, signalment provides the clinician and veterinary technician with the foundational framework upon which differential diagnoses are built. It is often referred to as the "holy grail" of patient history for good reason—it anchors every diagnostic consideration, shapes the interpretation of clinical signs, and guides therapeutic decision-making with precision and context.

Signalment is not a superficial descriptor; it is a biologically and behaviorally predictive profile. Age informs the clinician of developmental or degenerative processes. Species and breed signal predispositions to congenital anomalies, metabolic patterns, or inherited conditions. Sex and reproductive status determine hormonal influences, potential for reproductive disease, and relevant behavioral factors. Taken collectively, signalment contextualizes every physical finding and laboratory abnormality, providing a lens through which data becomes meaning.

The utility of signalment cannot be overstated. In an emergency setting, it may be the most important piece of information available prior to diagnostic imaging or laboratory testing. In general practice, it tailors wellness recommendations and preventive strategies. For the veterinary technician, understanding and recalling the signalment should be second nature—used to assess risk, anticipate complications, and customize nursing care plans.

Consider the following clinical example: A four-year-old, male, castrated Doberman Pinscher presents with a history of exercise intolerance and recent collapse. On presentation, the patient is alert but tachycardic, with weak femoral pulses and pale mucous membranes. Without even ausculting the heart, the signalment immediately points to a high index of suspicion for dilated cardiomyopathy (DCM). Doberman Pinschers are genetically predisposed to this condition, and the age and sex align with the demographic most commonly affected. While the clinical signs could be indicative of several disorders—including hypovolemia, hemorrhage, or metabolic collapse—the breed-specific context provided by signalment rapidly narrows the field and prioritizes cardiac assessment, such as electrocardiography and echocardiography. Treatment protocols and triage urgency likewise shift, with the veterinary technician anticipating the need for oxygen therapy, arrhythmia monitoring, and rapid intervention.

In another instance, the presentation of an intact female cat with lethargy and purulent vaginal discharge vs. a sexually altered female cat with purulent vaginal discharge, alters the diagnostic and therapeutic path drastically. In the first case, observation and the patient's signalment bring concern for pyometra—a life-threatening uterine infection—which guides immediate diagnostics and potential surgical intervention. Again, it is signalment that frames the approach before diagnostics confirm the pathology.

In teaching settings, one of the most valuable exercises in clinical rounds is the formulation of differentials based on signalment alone. Such exercises cultivate clinical reasoning and reinforce the vital importance of this patient descriptor (Fossum 2019). The absence of this data, or its inaccuracy in a medical record, can delay diagnosis and compromise patient care. As such, the veterinary technician must be a steward of accurate, complete, and readily accessible signalment information.

As we move forward in this text, signalment will continue to serve as the silent yet powerful informant in every case study, nursing plan, and procedural discussion. Mastering its use is not optional—it is essential to competent, evidence-informed veterinary nursing practice.

History Taking: Gathering the Full Picture

Patient History and the Veterinary Technician's Role

Accurate and thorough patient history is the cornerstone of effective veterinary diagnostics and nursing care. This process is not simply about asking questions but about crafting a structured, investigative dialogue that encourages clarity, honesty, and clinical depth from the pet owner. Veterinary technicians, who are often the first and most consistent point of contact, must balance empathy, medical awareness, and critical thinking to elicit information that directly shapes diagnostic reasoning and treatment planning.

The framework of a successful history can be visualized as an inverted triangle. At the broad base, open-ended questions such as "Can you tell me more about what you've been noticing?" or "Walk me through what you've seen over the past few days," allow owners to narrate their observations freely. This unstructured format often reveals subtle clinical cues. As the interview progresses, questions narrow in scope, becoming more specific and targeted to refine differential diagnoses and symptom progression. For example, closed-ended questions such as "Has there been any vomiting?" or "How many times per day is the patient defecating?" provide measurable, diagnostic detail.

The technician's role is not limited to following a checklist. Low medical literacy in the general population means many clients may struggle to articulate symptoms or may misattribute clinical signs. A client who reports "excessive drinking because it has been hot" may, in fact, be describing polyuria and polydipsia associated with endocrine or renal disease. In such cases, the technician's medical knowledge directs follow-up questions, such as, "Have you noticed changes in appetite or energy levels?" or "Are you seeing larger puddles of urine than usual?" This combination of guided inquiry and medical reasoning elevates the history into an active diagnostic tool.

Concrete examples illustrate this process. For a patient presenting with vomiting and diarrhea, the technician may begin broadly: "Tell me what made you decide to bring [patient name] in today?" As the client responds, the technician guides the conversation into more precise inquiries: "When did the vomiting start?," "What does it look like—food, bile, foam, blood?," "Is the patient still eating or drinking?," and "Has there been diarrhea as well, and what is its consistency and color?" These details help assess hydration status, potential dietary indiscretion, or more severe gastrointestinal pathology (Illustration 3.1).

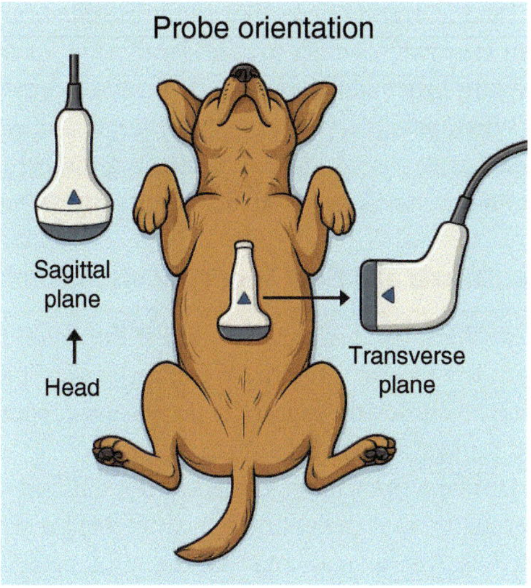

Illustration 3.1 Ultrasound probe orientation. *Source:* M. Jennings (2025). Author's own illustration.

For a coughing patient, the dialogue may begin with, "When did you first notice your pet coughing?" followed by "What does the cough sound like—dry, honking, moist?" and "Does it occur at rest, after activity, or at night?" Here, vaccination history, exposure to other dogs, or cardiac history become critical components of history-taking, guiding differentiation between infectious, structural, or cardiopulmonary etiologies.

Similarly, in dermatologic concerns, a technician might start with, "What made you concerned about the skin or coat today?" before progressing into detailed questions about duration, distribution, self-trauma behaviors, diet, and parasite prevention. Recognizing the potential for misattribution, such as blaming itching on "new bedding" rather than ectoparasites or allergic disease, the technician uses medical awareness to refine the inquiry.

The history-taking process also incorporates observational data. While collecting vitals or visually inspecting the patient, technicians may notice distended abdomens, poor body condition, or ectoparasite evidence. These findings can redirect or expand the owner interview. Noticing a patient's muscle wasting, for example, might prompt further exploration into appetite, activity level, or chronic disease processes. Observing flea dirt could lead to questions about preventive compliance and exposure risk.

Additional clinical examples reinforce the value of structured inquiry. For anal sac concerns, the dialogue may begin with, "What behaviors have you noticed that made you think something might be wrong?" before exploring scooting, licking, discharge, or bowel movement changes. In hyporexia, the conversation might start with, "How has your pet's appetite changed recently?" followed by targeted questions about selective feeding, treat interest, and concurrent systemic signs. For ocular issues, questions such as "What changes have you noticed with your pet's eyes?" and "Has vision or navigation been affected?" help differentiate between superficial irritation, infection, or deeper pathology. In orthopedic cases, asking when lameness was first noticed, whether it is constant or intermittent, and whether it worsens after activity, helps contextualize musculoskeletal disease.

Adaptability in communication style is also essential. Instead of asking, "Have you noticed polyuria or polydipsia?" technicians may reframe to, "Have you noticed your pet drinking more water or needing to urinate more often?" This ensures clarity while building client trust. When clients appear overwhelmed, visual aids or rephrased explanations provide support without sacrificing accuracy.

Ultimately, patient history is both art and science. It is an investigative process where veterinary technicians integrate structured dialogue, medical knowledge, observation, and client education. By combining broad, open-ended questions with specific, diagnostic follow-ups, technicians capture critical clinical data while simultaneously strengthening client relationships. This approach transforms history-taking into a dynamic diagnostic tool, reinforcing the technician's role as patient advocate and integral member of the veterinary healthcare team.

Delivering Instructions That Stick

Once a diagnosis has been made or a treatment plan outlined, it is often the technician's responsibility to ensure the client understands what comes next. This role involves more than handing over discharge paperwork, demands empathy, adaptability, and a strong grasp of the material being explained. Veterinary technicians must use accessible language that avoids jargon, tailoring their explanation based on the client's level of comfort and understanding. Instead of telling an owner that "NSAIDs are contraindicated due to hepatopathy," a technician might say, "Because of liver changes, this medication isn't safe right now, but we have other ways to manage your pet's pain."

Demonstrating tasks like administering oral medications to a cat, cleaning an ear, or administering subcutaneous fluids can empower owners to confidently care for their pet at home. Encouraging clients to ask questions and inviting them to explain instructions back in their own words can reveal misunderstandings before they lead to complications.

When possible, providing both verbal and written instructions reinforces retention. A calm, unrushed explanation, combined with visual aids or physical demonstrations, allows owners to feel capable and engaged. The technician, in this moment, serves as an advocate not only for medical accuracy but for owner success.

Euthanasia and Grief Support: Compassion in the Hardest Moments

Veterinary technicians are often at the emotional heart of the euthanasia process. They set the tone in the room, prepare both the patient and client, and serve as a compassionate anchor during an overwhelmingly difficult moment. However, many technicians, especially newer ones, report discomfort with what to say, how to offer support, and how to remain present amid client grief.

Unlike more technical procedures, euthanasia does not come with a fixed checklist. It requires emotional flexibility, vulnerability, and the courage to sit in silence when silence is the most supportive thing we can offer. The discomfort technicians feel is real and normal. But avoiding eye contact, rushing the process, or falling back on purely clinical language can unintentionally leave grieving clients feeling more alone.

Technicians can be trained to recognize that their presence *is* an intervention. Sitting on the floor beside a client, quietly offering a tissue, or simply acknowledging the weight of the moment with phrases like *"Take all the time you need,"* or *"We're here when you're ready"* can create space for grief. Emotional intelligence is just as essential here as any clinical skill.

When a Client Asks, "What Would You Do?"

Perhaps one of the most difficult moments for veterinary technicians is when an owner looks to them and asks, *"What would you do if it were your pet?"* It's a question loaded with emotion, seeking reassurance, clarity, and validation. Many technicians feel frozen by this, afraid of overstepping, unsure how to answer truthfully without imposing personal bias. The key is to reframe rather than deflect. A technician does not need to make the decision for the client, but they can help the client clarify their own values. Consider responses such as:

> *"That's such a hard place to be. Every pet and every family is different, but I can help talk through what we're seeing today."*
>
> *"I always try to focus on what brings quality to their life, whether they're eating, enjoying their time, or still having those "good moments." What are you seeing at home?"*
>
> *"It's never an easy choice, but from a medical perspective, we are starting to see signs that comfort is declining. I can help you think through what Max's day-to-day looks like now."*

These responses don't avoid the question, they guide the client to reflect on their own observations, while gently reinforcing the medical and emotional framework for making end-of-life decisions.

Support After the Goodbye

Once the euthanasia is complete, veterinary technicians often transition from clinical support to emotional caregiving. Clients may cry, collapse into silence, or share stories. The technician's job is not to fix grief, but to honor it. Sitting in silence without trying to cheer them up can be one of the most compassionate acts. Offering small, meaningful support; a paw print, a condolence card, or simply remembering the pet's name at a later visit, reinforces that their loss was acknowledged and respected.

Resolving Conflict Through Empathy and Structure

Not all client interactions are serene. Veterinary teams encounter high-stress conversations daily, ranging from financial frustration to emotional outbursts, and technicians are often the first to respond. The ability to de-escalate situations using structure and empathy is an essential skill. One widely used model is L.E.A.R.N.: Listen, Empathize, Ask, Respond, Navigate. Listening without interruption demonstrates respect. Empathizing acknowledges the client's emotional reality. Asking open-ended questions uncovers the root of the concern. Responding with facts and compassion provides clarity. Finally, navigating to a solution, such as finding a more affordable medication option or offering a payment plan, can restore trust and ensure the patient receives care.

Consider a technician assisting an overwhelmed client whose dog has just been diagnosed with diabetes. Faced with emotional distress and financial concern, the technician listens without judgment, empathizes with the weight of the diagnosis, asks what the client feels comfortable managing, and responds with information about low-cost insulin brands and home glucose monitoring. By doing so, the technician turns a moment of panic into one of clarity, giving the client the tools to care for their pet rather than surrender to fear.

Section 11: Professional and Soft Skills in Veterinary Nursing

Veterinary technicians operate at the intersection of clinical precision and human connection. Success in this role depends not only on technical knowledge but also on mastering the interpersonal, cognitive, and emotional skills that allow a technician to navigate the daily complexities of patient care. Time management, teamwork, adaptability, and resilience are not "extras," they are essential nursing competencies that support both the patients we treat and the professionals we hope to become. These soft skills enable technicians to lead with intention, respond proactively to challenges, and provide consistent, compassionate care under pressure.

Time Management: Clinical Efficiency Without Compromising Care

The pace of veterinary practice is relentless. A technician might find themselves juggling a recovering surgery patient, triaging an emergency, assisting with a radiograph, and preparing for the next outpatient appointment, all within the same hour. Time management in this setting means more than checking boxes; it's about prioritizing care based on patient need, anticipating team flow, and creating systems that reduce chaos rather than contribute to it.

For example, a technician managing multiple inpatients might implement a whiteboard system to track scheduled treatments and rechecks while setting phone reminders for time-sensitive medications. They will also delegate tasks appropriately to keep the team moving in rhythm. The goal is to maximize time *without sacrificing thoroughness*. When a technician approaches each shift with a plan: rounding efficiently, organizing supplies, reviewing the day's surgical cases in advance, they set the tone for the entire team and improve patient outcomes.

A guiding principle in time management is the "one-touch rule": if a task can be completed immediately, do it. Delaying charting, cage card updates, or medical record entries only creates more work later and risks critical information being lost or delayed. In high-functioning hospitals, this kind of foresight makes the difference between controlled urgency and preventable chaos.

Pro Tip: The "One-Touch Rule" for Efficiency

When handling paperwork, medical records, or task assignments, aim to complete them immediately rather than postponing them. Delays lead to backlogs and increased stress (Gantt 2021).

Team Collaboration: Owning Your Role in Patient-Centered Care

Veterinary medicine is inherently collaborative. No technician works in isolation, and every patient's success story is the result of shared responsibility. When veterinary teams function well, it's because each member knows their role, respects the expertise of others, and communicates with purpose. An exceptional technician doesn't just complete their own tasks; they take responsibility for the success of the team. This means actively listening during rounds, clarifying doctor orders, looping in assistants when support is needed, and confirming handoffs to ensure continuity of care. It means offering help when others are drowning and asking for help before falling behind. Mutual respect and shared accountability are what transform a group of coworkers into a cohesive nursing team.

Structured communication models like SBAR (Situation, Background, Assessment, Recommendation) provide technicians with a powerful tool to communicate concerns, propose solutions, and collaborate effectively with veterinarians. When a technician uses SBAR to report a post-op patient's sudden lethargy and hypotension, while simultaneously suggesting diagnostics and supportive care, they demonstrate critical thinking, situational awareness, and team leadership. These are not just soft skills; they are clinical tools in disguise.

Expert Tip: The SBAR Communication Model

Using SBAR ensures clear, concise communication when relaying patient updates to veterinarians (Cobb et al. 2022).

Real-World Example: Using the SBAR Communication Model in Veterinary Practice

The SBAR model is a structured communication framework designed to ensure clear, concise, and effective communication between veterinary team members. This model is particularly useful when relaying patient updates, discussing critical cases, or handing off information during shift changes (Cobb et al. 2022).

Scenario: Post-Surgical Complication in a Canine Patient

A veterinary technician is reporting a concern about a postoperative patient to the veterinarian. The patient, Luna, a six-year-old, F, Labrador Retriever, underwent a spay surgery earlier in the day and is now exhibiting signs of hypotension and lethargy.

S—SITUATION: *"Dr. Smith, I'm concerned about Luna, the Labrador who had her spay this morning. She is significantly more lethargic than expected, and her blood pressure is reading low at 80/50 mmHg."*

B—BACKGROUND: *"Luna was a healthy patient prior to surgery. The procedure went smoothly, and she was given hydromorphone for pain management, followed by carprofen postoperatively. She recovered uneventfully from anesthesia but has remained quiet in her kennel since then. An initial post-op assessment showed normal vitals, but her blood pressure has now dropped, and she is reluctant to get up."*

A—ASSESSMENT: *"Her mucous membranes are pink but slightly tacky, and her heart rate has increased from 90 bpm earlier to 120 bpm now. Her respiratory rate is also slightly elevated. There is no visible bleeding at the incision site, but her abdomen appears slightly distended. Given the combination of hypotension, tachycardia, and her lethargy, I'm concerned about possible internal bleeding or a reaction to her medications."*

R—RECOMMENDATION: *"I suggest we check a PCV/TP and perform an abdominal ultrasound to rule out post-op hemorrhage. We may also want to consider IV fluid boluses to address her hypotension. Would you like me to prepare these diagnostics while you examine her?"*

The SBAR model is effective in this situation because it allows for clear, structured, and efficient communication between the veterinary technician and the veterinarian. By starting with the most urgent concern, the technician immediately alerts the veterinarian to Luna's hypotension and lethargy, ensuring that the critical issue is addressed without delay. Providing relevant background information concisely gives the veterinarian a clear picture of the patient's medical history without unnecessary details, allowing them to quickly understand the context of the case. The technician then presents an objective assessment, highlighting key observations such as changes in vital signs, mucous membrane status, and possible complications like internal bleeding or a reaction to medications. This approach ensures that the veterinarian has a well-rounded view of the patient's condition before making a decision. Finally, by proactively offering a recommendation, the technician demonstrates critical thinking and initiative, suggesting diagnostic and treatment options while allowing the veterinarian to make the final call. This structured communication ensures a timely response, minimizes misunderstandings, and enhances patient care in a fast-paced clinical setting.

Adaptability and Problem-Solving: Staying Grounded When the Plan Falls Apart

No shift ever goes exactly as planned. Machines fail, medications run out, patients crash, and schedules unravel. What distinguishes a skilled veterinary technician is their ability to respond rather than react. Adaptability in this field means staying calm when faced with unexpected challenges, knowing how to pivot efficiently, and using problem-solving skills to protect both patient and team. This starts with a mindset of curiosity and control. Rather than panicking when the blood pressure monitor fails mid-procedure, the technician calmly grabs a Doppler and confirms the reading manually. If an oxygen concentrator stops functioning, they know how to switch to a backup tank. It's not just about having a plan B, it's about trusting your ability to think on your feet.

One strategy that supports adaptability is the "pause and prioritize" approach. In an emergency, it can be tempting to jump into action without a clear direction, but the most experienced technicians know that a brief moment of stillness allows them to triage effectively and act with purpose. In many ways, adaptability is not about being unshakable, it's about knowing where to plant your feet when the ground moves beneath you.

Advanced Insight: The "Pause and Prioritize" Method

In high-stress moments, technicians should pause briefly to assess priorities before acting. This prevents rushed decisions that could compromise patient care (Mills 2020).

Attention to Detail: The Technician as the First Line of Defense

In every hospital, there are stories that begin with, *"It's a good thing the tech caught it."* Whether it's a patient's respiratory rate increasing by two breaths per minute, a tiny shift in mucous membrane color, or a subtle change in behavior, the veterinary technician is often the first to notice when something isn't right. This kind of vigilance isn't instinctual, it's cultivated.

Veterinary technicians develop clinical intuition by staying attuned to patterns. They know not to dismiss a trend in vital signs, even if the current reading appears normal. They're able to detect a decrease in grooming or interaction in a hospitalized cat and recognize that pain or nausea may be developing. They read bloodwork not just for individual values, but for the story they tell together. These observations may seem small, but they often lead to early intervention, preventing decline and improving outcomes. Technicians who approach patient care with consistency, focus, and clinical curiosity become indispensable to their teams and to the lives they care for.

Clinical Insight: The "Trend, Don't Just Read" Method

When monitoring patients, look at patterns over time rather than isolated readings. A gradual decline in blood pressure or rising lactate levels may indicate worsening shock before overt clinical signs appear (Mathews et al. 2017).

Pro Tip: The Power of Debriefing

After emotionally challenging cases, holding a team debriefing provides an outlet for stress, promotes learning, and strengthens team cohesion (Cobb et al. 2022). It is important that a psychologically safe space is provided during the debriefing. By encouraging open and honest feedback, the team is able to identify areas of needed improvement, ultimately improving patient care.

Emotional Resilience: Caring for Others Without Losing Yourself

There's a quiet emotional toll to veterinary nursing, one that builds slowly. It's the heaviness that lingers after euthanasia, the frustration of financial barriers to care, the helplessness during a code, and the pressure of never feeling caught up. Over time, this can wear on even the most passionate technicians. Building emotional resilience is not about "toughing it out," it's about learning how to feel without drowning, how to care deeply without collapsing. Recognizing burnout, compassion fatigue, or emotional exhaustion early is essential. Technicians may notice they're becoming numb to patient stories, easily irritable with clients, or increasingly disconnected from the job they once loved. These are not signs of weakness, they're signs that care has outpaced recovery.

Resilient technicians take proactive steps to recharge. This might mean setting clear boundaries around work-life balance, creating rituals of reflection (such as journaling or debriefing with peers), and seeking support through mentorship or mental health professionals. It also means celebrating small wins, a patient that walks out of the ICU, a thank-you note from a client, or a moment of laughter with a teammate.

While technical proficiency is essential, the ability to process and release the emotional weight of difficult experiences is equally vital. Debriefing, whether formal or informal, offers veterinary technicians a structured way to reflect, gain support, and reset before the next case. By creating space for processing both clinical outcomes and emotional responses, debriefing

Table 3.14 Debriefing outline table.

Debriefing Step	Key Discussion Points	Example Questions
1. Introduction and purpose	Explain the goal of the debriefing: to reflect on the case, improve future responses, and provide emotional support.	*"Let's take a few minutes to discuss what happened, what went well, and what we can improve. This is a learning opportunity, and it's also okay to talk about how we're feeling."*
2. Review of the case	Summarize the case, including patient history, interventions performed, and final outcome.	*"We treated a nine-year-old Golden Retriever for hypovolemic shock due to a ruptured splenic tumor. Despite initiating CPR and emergency interventions, the patient did not survive. Let's go over the events."*
3. Identify what went well	Acknowledge strengths in teamwork, communication, and clinical execution.	*"What do you think we handled effectively? Were there any aspects of teamwork that stood out?"*
4. Identify areas for improvement	Discuss challenges encountered, decision-making processes, and areas where workflow could be improved.	*"Were there any moments where we could have been more efficient or communicated better? Are there any protocol changes we should consider?"*
5. Emotional check-in	Provide space for team members to express how they feel about the case, especially if it involved a loss.	*"How is everyone feeling about the case? Does anyone need additional support or time to process?"*
6. Develop actionable steps	Summarize key takeaways and propose solutions to improve future responses.	*"Going forward, what adjustments can we make to enhance patient care and team coordination? Who will take responsibility for implementing these changes?"*
7. Closing and support resources	Reinforce appreciation for the team's efforts and provide resources for additional support if needed.	*"I want to thank everyone for their hard work today. If anyone wants to discuss this further or needs a break, please don't hesitate to step away or reach out."*

Source: M. Jennings (2025). Author's own illustration.

allows technicians to leave work at work, reducing the risk of compassion fatigue and burnout while fostering long-term resilience and team cohesion (Table 3.14).

Real-World Example: Debriefing After a Critical Emergency Case

Scenario: Post-CPR Debriefing in an Emergency Hospital

A veterinary team has just finished performing CPR on a nine-year-old, Golden Retriever named Bailey, who presented in hypovolemic shock due to a ruptured splenic tumor. Despite the team's best efforts, Bailey did not regain a heartbeat, and the owners elected to discontinue CPR. After the case concludes, the lead emergency veterinarian gathers the team for a debriefing.

VETERINARIAN: *"I know that was a difficult case, and I appreciate everyone's hard work. Let's take a few minutes to go over what happened and discuss how we all feel. First, let's talk about what went well. What do you think we handled effectively during the code?"*

TECHNICIAN 1: *"I think we did a great job initiating CPR quickly. As soon as Bailey coded, we started compressions immediately and rotated every two minutes, just like in RECOVER guidelines."*

TECHNICIAN 2: *"Yes, and I thought communication was clear. When I was drawing up emergency drugs, the doctor confirmed the doses before I administered them, which helped avoid any confusion."*

VETERINARIAN: *"Agreed. We had a strong team effort and followed protocol well. Now, let's consider what we could improve. Were there any challenges you noticed?"*

TECHNICIAN 3: *"I felt like there was some hesitation in deciding whether to continue CPR or stop. The owners were struggling with their decision, and I wasn't sure when we should have guided them toward stopping CPR."*

VETERINARIAN: *"That's a great point. Sometimes, when owners are emotionally overwhelmed, it's hard to balance giving them time while also making the best decision for the patient. In the future, we could have one team member assigned to communicate with the family while the rest of us continue the medical efforts. This might help make the transition to euthanasia smoother."*

TECHNICIAN 1: *"I also think we could have been more prepared with postmortem care. The owners wanted to stay with Bailey for a while, and we were rushing to clean up."*

VETERINARIAN: *"That's good feedback. Maybe we should have a designated person for postmortem preparation so we can focus on both the medical and emotional aspects of the case."*

After discussing workflow improvements, the veterinarian shifts the conversation toward **emotional support** for the team.

VETERINARIAN: *"This was a tough case. How is everyone feeling? Does anyone need to step away for a moment or talk things through?"*

TECHNICIAN 3: *"It's always hard losing a patient, but I feel better knowing we did everything we could."*

VETERINARIAN: *"Absolutely. Cases like these remind us why teamwork is so important. I really appreciate everyone's hard work today. If anyone needs to talk more later, let me know. And don't forget to take a break if you need one."*

This debriefing session allows the team to reflect on their clinical performance, learn from the case, and acknowledge the emotional impact of patient loss. By fostering an open discussion, veterinary teams can continuously improve patient care while supporting one another's well-being in an emotionally demanding profession (Mills 2020).

Section 12: End-of-Chapter Skills Table

This table is designed to help veterinary technicians evaluate their understanding and readiness before progressing to the more advanced material in this book. Each skill listed below corresponds with a major concept covered in the chapter, grouped into clinical and professional domains. As you review each item, use the checkboxes to self-assess your confidence level. If any area feels uncertain, revisit the relevant section or seek mentorship opportunities to strengthen your proficiency. Mastery of these foundational concepts will ensure success as you move into more specialized aspects of veterinary nursing.

Core Veterinary Nursing Skills Checklist

Use this table at the end of the chapter to evaluate your readiness to move into advanced nursing topics. Mark each skill based on your confidence level: 1 = Novice, 2 = Developing, 3 = Proficient. For any items rated 1 or 2, refer back to the relevant section in this chapter for review (Table 3.15).

Conclusion

Veterinary nursing is more than a checklist of technical competencies, it is a deeply human, multifaceted practice that balances clinical precision with empathy, communication, and critical thinking. Veterinary technicians are not simply task-completers; they are advocates, problem-solvers, and collaborators who influence every stage of a patient's journey through the hospital.

This chapter has laid the groundwork for the essential responsibilities of the veterinary technician: managing pain, nutrition, and special-needs populations while ensuring clear and compassionate communication with clients and colleagues alike. From interpreting pain scores to guiding euthanasia discussions, every action a technician takes has the potential to shape outcomes and enhance the quality of life for patients.

Just as important as the hands-on skills are the soft skills that support teamwork, adaptability, time management, and emotional resilience. A technician who can remain composed under pressure, navigate difficult conversations, and recognize their own limits is better equipped to deliver consistent, high-quality care. These foundational skills are not the endpoint of your learning, but the springboard into deeper knowledge, advanced procedures, and specialized roles.

As you move forward into the chapters ahead, revisit these principles often. Mastery in veterinary nursing is not a fixed destination, but a continual process of learning, reflecting, and evolving. By carrying both competence and compassion into your practice, you will not only succeed clinically, but you will also lead, inspire, and transform the standard of care in veterinary medicine.

Table 3.15 Core skills scoring tool.

Skill Area	Skill Description	Confidence Rating (1–3)
Pain assessment	Use of validated pain scales (e.g., GCPS, FGS) and recognition of subtle signs	
Analgesia understanding	Knowledge of multimodal pain management and drug classes	
Monitoring for pain	Tracking post-op patients and recognizing signs of discomfort	
Nutritional assessment	Use of BCS, weight trends, and RER calculation for nutritional planning	
Feeding tube care	Knowledge of NG, E-tube, and G-tube use, placement, and maintenance	
Medical record keeping	Documenting medications, vitals, treatments, and behavioral observations	
Infection control	Adhering to hospital sanitation protocols and using PPE correctly	
Mobility assistance	Providing safe, supported movement and repositioning for comfort and recovery	
Client education	Explaining treatment plans, home care, and medications in clear, layperson terms	
History taking	Gathering thorough patient histories and clarifying inconsistencies	
Team communication (SBAR)	Using structured formats like SBAR to present patient updates and advocate effectively	
Conflict resolution	Using empathy and communication models (e.g., LEARN) to manage difficult situations	
Time management	Prioritizing tasks, avoiding time traps, and using tools like checklists effectively	
Adaptability	Responding to emergencies, equipment failure, or procedural changes with calm clarity	
Attention to detail	Recognizing subtle shifts in behavior or trends in vitals before overt signs appear	
Emotional resilience	Practicing self-care, recognizing burnout, and accessing peer or professional support	
Debriefing participation	Engaging in post-event team debriefs to reflect, learn, and release emotional tension	

Source: M. Jennings (2025). Author's own illustration.

References

American Animal Hospital Association (2019). 2019 AAHA fluid therapy guidelines for dogs and cats. *Journal of the American Animal Hospital Association* 55 (2): 83–99.

American Animal Hospital Association (2020). 2020 AAHA anesthesia and monitoring guidelines for dogs and cats. *Journal of the American Animal Hospital Association* 56 (2): 59–82.

Bateman, S. (2021). Practical fluid therapy in veterinary patients. *Veterinary Clinics of North America: Small Animal Practice* 51 (6): 1235–1249.

Becker, M. and Bain, M.J. (2020). *Fear Free Veterinary Visits: Techniques for Reducing Stress in Veterinary Patients*. AAHA Press.

Ettinger, S.J., Feldman, E.C., and Côté, E. (2017). *Textbook of Veterinary Internal Medicine*, 8e. Elsevier.

Fear Free, LLC. (n.d.). *Fear, anxiety, and stress (FAS) spectrum*.

Fossum, T.W. (2019). *Small Animal Surgery*, 5e. Elsevier.

Frank, D., Beauchamp, G., Palestrini, C., and Shofer, F.S. (2010). Systematic review of the use of pheromones for treating stress-related behaviors in dogs and cats. *Journal of the American Veterinary Medical Association* 236 (12): 1308–1316.

Grimm, K.A., Lamont, L.A., Tranquilli, W.J. et al. (2015). *Lumb & Jones' Veterinary Anesthesia and Analgesia*, 5e. Wiley-Blackwell.

Grimm, K.A., Lamont, L.A., Tranquilli, W.J. et al. (2021). *Veterinary Anesthesia and Analgesia: The Fifth Edition of Lumb & Jones*. Wiley-Blackwell.

Hall, L.W., Clarke, K.W., and Trim, C.M. (2020). *Wright's Veterinary Anaesthesia and Analgesia*, 11e. Elsevier.

Harvey, J.W. (2012). *Veterinary Hematology: A Diagnostic Guide and Color Atlas*. Elsevier.

Hopper, K. and Silverstein, D.C. (2020). *Small Animal Critical Care Medicine*, 3e. Elsevier.

International Society of Feline Medicine (ISFM) (2016). Handling techniques for reducing feline stress. *Journal of Feline Medicine and Surgery* 18 (7): 606–614.

Landsberg, G.M., Hunthausen, W., and Ackerman, L. (2012). *Behavior Problems of the Dog and Cat*, 3e. Saunders Elsevier.

Mathews, K.A., Sinclair, M., and Steele, A.M. (2017). Analgesia and anesthesia for the ill or injured cat. *Journal of Feline Medicine and Surgery* 19 (7): 627–636.

McMichael, M. and Powell, L.L. (2021). *Critical Care Monitoring and Therapy in Small Animals*. Wiley-Blackwell.

Mills, J. (2020). Supporting veterinary team wellbeing through structured debriefing and reflection. *Veterinary Nursing Journal* 35 (6): 192–197.

Nyland, T.G. and Mattoon, J.S. (2015). *Small Animal Diagnostic Ultrasound*, 3e. Elsevier.

Overall, K.L. (2013). *Manual of Clinical Behavioral Medicine for Dogs and Cats*. Elsevier.

Padrid, P.A. (2021). Feline respiratory medicine and doxycycline risks. *Journal of Feline Medicine and Surgery* 23 (4): 299–307.

Plumb, D.C. (2020). *Plumb's Veterinary Drug Handbook*, 9e. Wiley-Blackwell.

Rodan, I., Dowgray, N., Carney, H. C., Carozza, E., Ellis, S. L. H., Heath, S., Niel, L., St Denis, K., & Taylor, S. (2022). 2022 AAFP/ISFM cat friendly veterinary interaction guidelines: Approach and handling techniques. *Journal of Feline Medicine and Surgery*, 24, 1093–1132. doi:10.1177/1098612X221128760.

Rosychuk, R.A. (2019). Otitis externa and otitis media. *Veterinary Clinics of North America: Small Animal Practice* 49 (1): 1–20.

Shaw, J.R., Bonnett, B.N., and Adams, C.L. (2020). *Communication in Veterinary Medicine: Theory and Practice*. Wiley-Blackwell.

Silverstein, D.C. and Hopper, K. (2015). *Small animal critical care medicine*, (2nd ed.)e. Elsevier.

Silverstein, D.C. and Hopper, K. (2020). *Small Animal Critical Care Medicine*, 3e. Elsevier.

Stella, J.L., Croney, C.C., and Buffington, C.A.T. (2013). Effects of stressors on the behavior and physiology of domestic cats. *Journal of the American Veterinary Medical Association* 243 (1 2): 1726–1735.

Steffey, E.P., Mama, K.R., and Brosnan, R.J. (2020). Inhalation anesthetics. In: *Veterinary Anesthesia and Analgesia*, 5e (ed. K.A. Grimm, L.A. Lamont, W.J. Tranquilli, et al.), 297–331. Wiley-Blackwell.

Stewart, M., Taylor, M., and Baldwin, C. (2019). The use of pre-visit pharmaceuticals for veterinary patients. *Veterinary Record* 184 (19): 593–598.

Thrall, M.A., Weiser, G., Allison, R.W., and Campbell, T.W. (2022). *Veterinary Hematology and Clinical Chemistry*, 3e. Wiley-Blackwell.

Weese, J.S., Blondeau, J.M., Boothe, D. et al. (2021). Antimicrobial use guidelines for treatment of urinary tract disease in dogs and cats. *Journal of Veterinary Internal Medicine* 35 (1): 50–77.

Weiss, D.J., Wardrop, K.J., and Schalm, O.W. (2021). *Schalm's Veterinary Hematology*, 7e. Wiley-Blackwell.

4

Ethical Considerations in Veterinary Nursing

Understanding Veterinary Ethics

Veterinary nursing is a profession deeply rooted in ethical responsibility, requiring practitioners to balance medical knowledge, patient advocacy, client relations, and legal considerations. Ethics in veterinary nursing extend beyond mere compliance with laws and regulations; they encompass moral obligations to patients, clients, colleagues, and society as a whole (Rollin 2011). Veterinary technicians frequently encounter situations where they must apply ethical principles to ensure the well-being of animals while respecting the rights and decisions of pet owners.

Historical Context of Veterinary Ethics

The principles of veterinary ethics have evolved significantly over time, paralleling changes in societal attitudes toward animal welfare and human-animal relationships. In the early 20th century, veterinary medicine primarily served agricultural needs, with a focus on maintaining the health of livestock for economic purposes. Ethical considerations were largely utilitarian, prioritizing efficiency and productivity over individual animal welfare.

The mid-20th century marked a shift with the rise of companion animal care. As pets became integral members of families, veterinary medicine expanded to prioritize quality of life, pain management, and humane euthanasia. The development of professional codes of ethics, such as those established by the American Veterinary Medical Association (AVMA), helped formalize ethical standards in the profession.

By the early 21st century, veterinary ethics incorporated broader concerns, including conservation medicine, animal rights advocacy, and the One Health initiative, which recognizes the interconnectedness of human, animal, and environmental health. In 2025, veterinary nursing continues to grapple with emerging ethical challenges, such as addressing antimicrobial resistance, ethical sourcing of pharmaceuticals, and the impact of climate change on animal populations.

Fundamental Ethical Principles

Veterinary ethics is broadly categorized into descriptive, normative, and applied ethics. Descriptive ethics involves observing and analyzing moral behavior within the profession, whereas normative ethics establishes standards for what ought to be done in given situations. Applied ethics involves utilizing these principles in practical, real-world scenarios (Beauchamp and Childress 2019). The foundational ethical principles in veterinary nursing include beneficence, non-maleficence, autonomy, justice, and fidelity.

Beneficence

Beneficence refers to the ethical duty to act in the best interest of the patient. Veterinary technicians must prioritize patient welfare, ensuring that treatments and interventions aim to improve health, reduce suffering, and enhance quality of life. This principle often comes into play in emergency situations where immediate intervention is required to save an animal's life. For example, a veterinary technician may need to provide pain management and stabilize a patient before a veterinarian can fully assess the condition. Beneficence also extends to preventive care, such as administering vaccinations and educating pet owners on proper nutrition and hygiene.

Non-Maleficence

Non-maleficence, or "do no harm," requires veterinary technicians to avoid causing unnecessary suffering or harm to their patients. This principle is particularly relevant in surgical procedures, anesthesia monitoring, and restraint techniques. Veterinary technicians must ensure that handling methods minimize stress and discomfort while performing necessary medical procedures. Ethical conflicts can arise when certain treatments may prolong an animal's life but also increase suffering, leading to difficult decisions regarding palliative care and euthanasia.

Autonomy

Autonomy refers to respecting the informed decisions of pet owners regarding their animal's care. Veterinary technicians must provide clients with comprehensive, unbiased information to facilitate informed decision-making. Challenges occur when an owner's decision contradicts what the veterinary team believes is in the animal's best interest. For instance, if a client refuses life-saving surgery due to financial concerns, the veterinary technician must balance respecting autonomy with advocating for the patient's well-being.

Justice

Justice in veterinary ethics entails ensuring fair and equal treatment of all patients and clients, regardless of socioeconomic status, breed, or species. This principle also applies to resource allocation, such as prioritizing emergency cases in a triage setting. Veterinary technicians must remain impartial, treating each case with professionalism and without bias. Justice also extends to ethical considerations in shelter medicine, where limited resources must be distributed fairly among many animals in need.

Fidelity

Fidelity includes maintaining trust and honesty in professional relationships, including those with clients, veterinarians, and colleagues. Veterinary technicians must uphold confidentiality, accurately document medical records, and provide truthful information to pet owners. Breaking trust by withholding information or misrepresenting a patient's condition can lead to ethical breaches and professional consequences. These principles guide veterinary technicians in decision-making and provide a framework for ethical behavior in clinical practice. However, the complexity of real-life cases often leads to ethical dilemmas that require critical thinking and compassionate negotiation.

Ethical Dilemmas and Decision-making

Veterinary technicians frequently encounter ethical dilemmas where competing interests and responsibilities create conflicts. These situations require a structured approach to ethical decision-making to balance the needs of patients, clients, and veterinary teams.

Ethical Theories Relevant to Veterinary Nursing

Utilitarianism

Utilitarianism emphasizes outcomes, advocating for actions that produce the greatest good for the greatest number. In veterinary practice, this may involve prioritizing treatments that benefit the most animals, such as mass vaccination programs or population control initiatives in shelters (Yeates 2020). However, utilitarian reasoning can be controversial, particularly in decisions involving euthanasia or resource allocation. For example, a shelter may have limited space and funds, leading to difficult choices about which animals receive medical care. A utilitarian approach would prioritize treating the most adoptable or easily rehabilitated animals to maximize overall positive outcomes. However, this can raise ethical concerns about fairness and the intrinsic value of each animal's life.

Deontology

Deontology focuses on duties and rules rather than consequences. Veterinary technicians following deontological ethics adhere strictly to professional guidelines, legal requirements, and institutional policies. For example, even if an owner wishes to forgo pain relief for their pet due to cost concerns, a deontologically minded veterinary technician will insist on providing appropriate analgesia, as it aligns with their ethical duty to prevent suffering. A common deontological dilemma arises when veterinary professionals encounter cases of suspected animal abuse. Even if reporting the case may strain the client-veterinary relationship or lead to financial repercussions, the duty to protect animal welfare outweighs these concerns. Deontologists prioritize adherence to laws and ethical codes, regardless of potential negative consequences (Rollin 2018).

Virtue Ethics

Virtue ethics emphasizes the moral character of individuals making ethical decisions. Veterinary technicians who embody traits such as compassion, integrity, and empathy naturally make ethical choices that prioritize animal welfare and professional integrity. According to Beauchamp and Childress (2019), the cultivation of virtues is essential in guiding moral actions, particularly in healthcare settings where rigid rules or outcomes may not address every ethical nuance.

Virtue ethics also plays a role in professional interactions. A veterinary technician who practices kindness and patience will likely foster stronger relationships with both clients and colleagues, contributing to a positive workplace culture. Unlike utilitarianism or deontology, which focus on external rules and consequences, virtue ethics highlights personal growth and ethical character development over time. By integrating these ethical theories into daily practice, veterinary technicians can develop a more nuanced approach to ethical dilemmas, balancing patient welfare, client needs, and professional obligations.

Common Ethical Dilemmas in Veterinary Nursing

Euthanasia and Quality of Life Decisions: One of the most emotionally taxing ethical dilemmas in veterinary nursing involves euthanasia. While euthanasia is often performed to alleviate suffering, disagreements can arise between veterinary staff and pet owners regarding the appropriate timing and necessity of the procedure (Batchelor and McKeegan 2012). Veterinary technicians must navigate these discussions with empathy, providing clear communication about the doctor's prognosis, pain management, and end-of-life options.

Financial Constraints and Treatment Limitations: Veterinary care is often limited by the financial means of pet owners, which can lead to ethical conflicts. A veterinary technician may recognize an optimal treatment plan but must work within the financial constraints of the client (Moses et al. 2018). Finding a balance between advocating for the best medical care and respecting the owner's financial limitations requires professional judgment and ethical reasoning.

Informed Consent and Client Education: Ensuring informed consent is a critical ethical responsibility. Veterinary technicians must provide clients with accurate and comprehensible information about their pet's condition and available treatment options (Robinson 2020). Ethical conflicts may arise when clients misunderstand or refuse treatment based on misinformation.

Animal Welfare and Neglect: Cases involving suspected animal neglect or abuse place veterinary technicians in difficult ethical positions. They must balance their duty to report neglect with maintaining professional relationships with clients (Yeates and Main 2009). Legal obligations to report suspected cruelty vary by jurisdiction, but the ethical obligation to advocate for animal welfare remains universal.

Ethical Decision-making Models

To systematically navigate ethical dilemmas, veterinary technicians can utilize structured decision-making models. These models provide a framework for analyzing complex ethical situations and ensuring that ethical principles are upheld. The most commonly used models in veterinary nursing include:

The Four Quadrant Approach

The Four Quadrant Approach, originally adapted from human medical ethics, provides a structured method for analyzing complex ethical dilemmas. This model was developed to facilitate ethical reasoning in clinical medicine by systematically organizing relevant factors into four key areas (Beauchamp and Childress 2019). In veterinary nursing, this framework helps practitioners apply core ethical principles while navigating the additional complexity of substituted decision-making

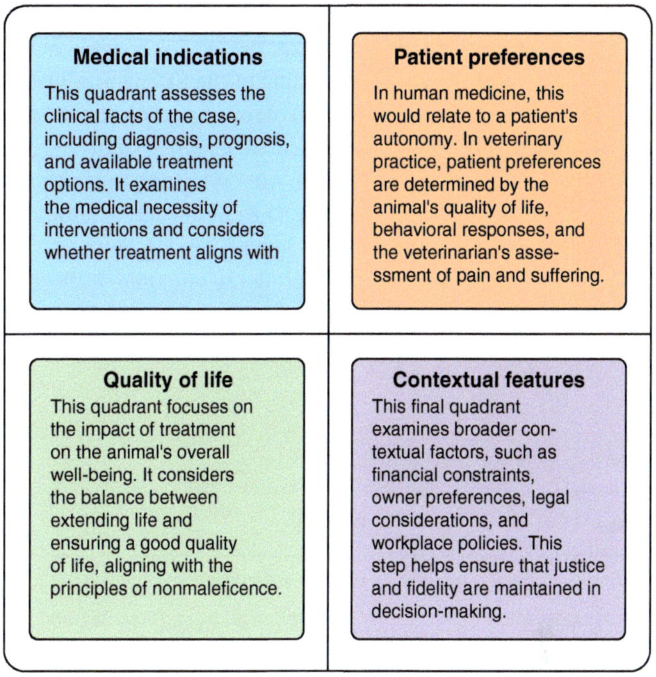

Figure 4.1 The four quadrant approach to ethical decision-making in veterinary nursing. *Source:* M. Jennings (2025).

on behalf of nonverbal patients. By evaluating medical indications, patient preferences, quality of life, and contextual features, veterinary technicians can make ethically sound decisions that respect both animal welfare and client concerns (Figure 4.1).

Case Study 4.1 End-of-life Decision in a Terminally Ill Dog

A 12-year-old Labrador Retriever, Max, presents with late-stage osteosarcoma. The veterinarian outlines three options: aggressive amputation and chemotherapy, palliative pain management, or euthanasia. The veterinary technician uses the Four Quadrant Approach to navigate the ethical dilemma (Table 4.1).

Table 4.1 Four Quadrant framework applied to ethical decision-making in a complex end-of-life case.

Quadrant	Case Assessment
Medical indications	Amputation may prolong life but may not be curative; pain management offers temporary relief.
Patient preferences	Max exhibits moderate discomfort without signs of acute suffering, suggesting quality of life remains acceptable for now.
Quality of life	Max continues to eat and socialize, but his mobility is declining, creating concern about future comfort.
Contextual features	The owner is emotionally hesitant about euthanasia and has limited financial resources, influencing the treatment decision.

Source: M. Jennings (2025).

By systematically evaluating these quadrants, the veterinary team recommends palliative care with a transition to euthanasia when Max's quality of life declines further.

The Five-step Model

The Five-step Model provides a structured yet flexible approach to ethical decision-making in veterinary nursing. It begins by encouraging veterinary professionals to clearly define the ethical concern at hand. This involves identifying conflicts, such as a tension between client wishes and patient welfare, and recognizing the ethical principles in question.

Once the problem is outlined, the next step involves gathering all relevant information. This includes clinical facts, the patient's prognosis, financial constraints, legal requirements, and contextual considerations like institutional policies or team input. A thorough understanding of the full picture lays the foundation for sound decision-making. From there, veterinary technicians explore all available options. This means considering every reasonable course of action, evaluating their benefits, risks, and ethical consequences. Creative solutions or compromises may emerge during this process, particularly when ideal outcomes aren't feasible. After weighing the options, a decision is made based on ethical reasoning, professional standards, and practical limitations. The chosen action should aim to protect patient welfare, honor client communication, and remain aligned with legal and institutional guidelines.

The model concludes with evaluating the outcome. Reflection is a key component—assessing whether the decision met ethical standards and what impact it had on the patient, client, and team. This evaluation helps veterinary professionals grow in confidence and improve future decision-making (Table 4.2).

Table 4.2 The five-step model table.

Phase	Description
Define the ethical concern	Clearly articulate the ethical issue and identify the conflicting principles or responsibilities involved.
Gather relevant information	Collect clinical, legal, financial, and contextual details to fully understand the situation and inform next steps.
Explore possible actions	Consider all viable options, weighing the ethical pros and cons of each. Include both ideal solutions and realistic compromises.
Select an ethical path forward	Decide on the most ethically justifiable course of action, balancing professional responsibilities with practical limitations.
Reflect and learn from the outcome	Review the results and determine whether the action upheld ethical integrity. Use the experience to strengthen future ethical reasoning and decision-making.

Case Study 4.2 Financial Constraints in a Treatable Condition

A client brings in a cat, Luna, suffering from pyometra. The condition is treatable with an emergency ovariohysterectomy surgery, but the owner cannot afford the procedure. The veterinary technician applies the Five-step Model (Table 4.3).

Table 4.3 Case application of the five-step model: Luna the cat.

Phase	Case Details
Define the ethical concern	The cat requires emergency surgery for pyometra, but the owner's financial limitations create a conflict between beneficence and justice.
Gather relevant information	The team reviews the clinic's payment plan policy, available financial resources, and the urgency of the medical condition.
Explore possible actions	Alternatives are considered, including referral to an animal welfare organization that may offer financial assistance.
Select an ethical path forward	A partial payment plan is approved by the clinic, and the client is referred to a local rescue for supplemental support.
Reflect and learn from the outcome the outcome	Luna successfully undergoes surgery, and the clinic creates a formal protocol to guide similar ethically complex cases in the future.

Source: M. Jennings (2025).

Table 4.4 Core factors of the Ethical Matrix used in veterinary nursing decision-making.

Matrix Factor	Explanation
Well-being	The direct impact on the animal's health and quality of life.
Autonomy	The rights and choices of pet owners, including financial, emotional, and personal considerations.
Justice	The broader impact on society, the veterinary profession, and other animals.

The Ethical Matrix

The Ethical Matrix, developed by Mepham (2005), provides a more comprehensive approach that considers multiple perspectives by evaluating the interests of different stakeholders in veterinary decision-making. This model ensures a balanced approach by assessing how different groups, patients, clients, veterinary teams, and society are affected by ethical choices.

The three key factors considered in the Ethical Matrix (Table 4.4).

Case Study 4.3 Contagious Disease in a Shelter

A local shelter detects an outbreak of feline calicivirus, a highly contagious disease. The team must decide whether to quarantine affected cats or euthanize them to prevent further spread.

The Ethical Matrix applied (Table 4.5).

Table 4.5 Ethical Matrix factors considered in decision-making for euthanasia.

Matrix Factor	Explanation
Well-being	Euthanasia prevents suffering but permanently removes any chance of recovery; quarantine may risk further infections.
Autonomy	The shelter must consider its mission to save lives while being responsible with resources.
Justice	Limited funding means prolonged care for sick cats may reduce resources for healthier, adoptable animals.

Source: M. Jennings (2025).

Navigating Ethical Challenges

Applying ethical principles and decision-making frameworks in veterinary practice requires practical skills, emotional intelligence, and resilience. Veterinary technicians must develop strategies to handle ethical challenges effectively while maintaining their well-being.

The Role of Communication in Ethical Challenges

Effective communication is one of the most essential skills for veterinary technicians when navigating ethical challenges. Ethical dilemmas often arise due to miscommunication or misunderstanding between veterinary professionals and clients. Clear, honest, and empathetic communication helps prevent conflicts and fosters mutual understanding.

Active Listening: Veterinary technicians should practice active listening when discussing treatment options with pet owners. This involves giving undivided attention, acknowledging concerns, and asking clarifying questions. For example, when a client is hesitant about euthanasia, a veterinary technician should listen to their fears, provide compassionate responses, and offer educational support.

Delivering Difficult News: Ethical challenges often involve difficult conversations—helping a client process the veterinarian's findings, clarifying the implications for the pet's comfort and quality of life, and navigating financial constraints. While technicians do not deliver a diagnosis or prognosis, they play a central role in creating psychological safety, reinforcing the veterinarian's message, and guiding owners through the next steps. Clear, plain language, a calm pace, and intentional pauses for questions help owners absorb information without feeling rushed. Techniques such as "chunk and check" and brief teach-back (e.g., "Just to be sure I explained that clearly, how would you describe the plan in your own words?") support understanding and shared decision-making.

A light-touch application of the SPIKES framework can structure these moments without duplicating the veterinarian's medical discussion (Baile et al. 2000). In Setting, technicians prepare a private, quiet space, minimize interruptions, and ensure tissues/water are available. During Perception, they assess what the client already understands and what matters most to them, listening for values, constraints, and support systems. With the Invitation, technicians confirm how much detail the client wants from them now and what should be deferred to the veterinarian. In Knowledge, technicians confine themselves to clarifying the veterinarian's information using lay terms, avoiding new interpretations or estimates about outcomes. Empathy involves naming and validating emotions ("I can see how overwhelming this feels") and allowing silence. Finally, Summary/Strategy focuses on immediate, concrete next steps—what will happen today, what to monitor at home, whom to call, and when the veterinarian will rejoin the conversation—so the owner leaves with a clear, written plan.

Financial discussions require the same ethical clarity and empathy. Technicians should present medically appropriate options already endorsed by the veterinarian, outline cost ranges transparently, and connect clients with approved resources such as written estimates, staged care when clinically appropriate, reassessment points, third-party financing, charitable funds, or hospital-specific assistance. Language should remain nonjudgmental and choice-supportive ("Let's look at what's possible within your budget while keeping [pet's name] comfortable"), and technicians must avoid promising outcomes, pressuring decisions, or agreeing to plans outside hospital policy or the veterinarian's recommendations. When questions exceed their scope—particularly about prognosis, likelihood of success, or changes to the medical plan—technicians should promptly loop the veterinarian back in to maintain accuracy, trust, and team integrity (Baile et al. 2000).

Managing Client Expectations: Ethical tension often arises when a client's hopes do not match medical reality. Technicians do not diagnose or predict outcomes, yet they are essential to align expectations by clarifying what the veterinarian has said, exploring the client's goals and constraints, and ensuring that next steps are medically appropriate and clearly understood. Early alignment begins with brief, open questions ("What matters most to you for Milo right now?"), followed by an ask–tell–ask rhythm: elicit the client's understanding, offer concise information in lay language, and then check comprehension with a quick teach-back. Throughout, avoid guarantees or new interpretations; when questions turn to prognosis or likelihood of success, bring the veterinarian back into the conversation to preserve accuracy and team integrity (Adams and Kurtz 2017).

When a client pushes for aggressive treatment in the face of a terminal condition, the technician's role is to validate the client's concern, surface the values behind that request, and translate the veterinarian's guidance into practical choices that minimize suffering. Helpful language is both empathic and boundary-aware: "I can hear how important more time feels. Let's look at what care options the doctor recommends and what they might mean for comfort day-to-day." Where appropriate, frame a time-limited trial that the veterinarian has endorsed, with clear, observable stopping rules (e.g., appetite, mobility, interaction, and distress signals) and a pre-planned pivot to comfort-focused or hospice care if criteria are not met. Quality-of-life tools and written home-care plans support shared decision-making and reduce later conflict, while neutral phrasing avoids judgment ("Here's what this option would involve for pain control, monitoring, and rechecks"). If disagreement persists or the requested plan falls outside medical standards or hospital policy, the technician should pause the discussion and re-engage the veterinarian to set clinical and ethical boundaries. This approach centers the pet's welfare, respects the client's values, and keeps the team aligned, using brief, structured communication techniques that we elaborate later in the book (Baile et al. 2000).

The Influence of Personal Background on Ethical Perceptions

Educational Background

The way a veterinary technician is educated plays a crucial role in how they identify, interpret, and respond to ethical dilemmas in clinical practice. Unlike a standardized pathway, veterinary technicians may receive varying levels of formal education before becoming credentialed, ranging from certificate programs and associate degrees to bachelor's degrees in veterinary technology. These differences in academic preparation can significantly influence a technician's ethical awareness, clinical reasoning, and ability to recognize moral complexity in patient care. Evidence for these links between educational depth and ethical competence appears across accreditation standards and health-professions research (American

Veterinary Medical Association 2023, 2024; Hernandez et al. 2018; Khaghanizadeh et al. 2023; Lincoln Memorial University 2025; Shadi et al. 2024; U.S. Bureau of Labor Statistics 2025).

Technicians who complete more in-depth or academically rigorous programs are often exposed to formal coursework in ethics, communication, and professional standards, helping them develop a structured framework for evaluating ethical challenges. They are more likely to recognize nuanced issues, such as power dynamics in informed consent or conflicts between patient welfare and financial limitations, that may go unnoticed by those with more limited training. These individuals may also be familiar with ethical theories and decision-making models, such as utilitarianism or the Four Quadrant Approach, which can support confident and thoughtful navigation of complex situations.

It's also important to note that some technicians pursue education well beyond entry-level credentials. Increasingly, veterinary technicians are enrolling in bachelor's or even master's degree programs in veterinary nursing, public health, bioethics, or related fields. These advanced degrees provide deeper knowledge not only in clinical practice, but also in areas like leadership, research ethics, and systems-level thinking. As technicians further their education, they gain a broader understanding of the ethical landscape in veterinary medicine, positioning them to serve as ethical leaders and advocates within their teams and the profession at large.

Ultimately, a technician's educational background shapes their ethical lens determining not only what they know, but also how they think, question, and act when faced with moral dilemmas. Continued education, mentorship, and reflective practice remain key to developing the ethical competence necessary for today's complex veterinary environment.

Gender and Ethical Perspectives

Gender may play a meaningful role in how veterinary professionals perceive and respond to ethical dilemmas. According to survey data, there are observable trends in ethical decision-making that correlate with gender, particularly in how individuals prioritize different aspects of patient care (Batchelor and McKeegan 2012). Some studies suggest that female veterinary professionals may be more likely to focus on the emotional and welfare-centered dimensions of care. This includes a heightened sensitivity to patient suffering, a stronger inclination toward preserving quality of life, and a more empathetic approach in client communication. These tendencies often align with relational ethics, which emphasize compassion, communication, and trust in the decision-making process.

In contrast, male veterinary professionals may more frequently approach ethical situations through a procedural or outcome-driven lens, prioritizing clinical protocols, efficiency, and financial sustainability. While this approach is by no means devoid of compassion, it often emphasizes structure, logical sequencing, and practical viability. These differing emphases do not indicate superiority of one approach over the other; rather, they reflect diverse ways of interpreting complex moral scenarios within veterinary practice.

Understanding these gender-influenced perspectives is valuable for improving team dynamics and fostering ethical collaboration. When a veterinary team comprises individuals with a variety of ethical priorities, such as empathy-driven care alongside outcome-oriented reasoning, it creates an opportunity for more balanced and well-rounded decision-making. Encouraging open dialogue among team members about how they view, and approach ethical situations can reduce misunderstandings, promote mutual respect, and ultimately support patient care that is both medically sound and ethically grounded.

It is important to acknowledge that gender is not the sole determinant of ethical perspective. Cultural background, educational experience, and personal values all play a role in shaping how professionals navigate ethical tension. Furthermore, emerging data on gender diversity in the veterinary field suggests a growing need to recognize and support nonbinary professionals. The AVMA's 2024 workforce survey identified 159 veterinarians who identify as nonbinary, reflecting a small but important demographic within the profession. Organizations such as the Pride Veterinary Medical Community (PrideVMC) have taken significant steps to advance inclusion. According to PrideVMC (2021), the Gender Identity Bill of Rights outlines essential protections for transgender, nonbinary, and gender nonconforming individuals, while additional implementation tools continue to be developed to support inclusive practices across veterinary settings (Pride Veterinary Medical Community, n.d.). As the profession becomes more diverse, veterinary teams must remain open to learning from all perspectives—gender-based or otherwise—to build ethical environments rooted in equity, respect, and collaboration.

Cultural and Religious Influences

Cultural and religious beliefs also significantly shape attitudes toward veterinary ethics, influencing both how clients make decisions and how veterinary professionals interpret their responsibilities. For example, in certain religious traditions, euthanasia may be viewed as morally unacceptable under any circumstances, while in others, it may be seen as a compassionate act to relieve suffering. These deeply held values can strongly influence client choices during emotionally charged situations such as end-of-life care, spaying and neutering, or dietary management.

Veterinary technicians must develop a high degree of cultural competence to navigate these conversations respectfully and effectively. This involves not only avoiding assumptions but also seeking to understand the client's perspective without judgment. Culturally informed care allows technicians to better anticipate potential ethical conflicts and tailor communication in a way that promotes trust and mutual understanding. Additionally, veterinary professionals must be prepared to balance cultural sensitivity with their ethical and legal obligations. For instance, if a client's beliefs result in a decision that may cause prolonged suffering to a patient, the technician may face moral distress and need to advocate for alternative options while still honoring the client's values. In multicultural communities, it is particularly important to create space for open dialogue about beliefs and practices that may affect veterinary decision-making.

By remaining culturally aware and ethically grounded, veterinary technicians can foster inclusive care environments that honor client diversity while prioritizing animal welfare. Ongoing training in cultural humility, religious literacy, and inclusive communication can further support this effort, helping teams navigate the intersection of ethics and belief with compassion and professionalism.

Personal Values

Personal values form the internal compass by which veterinary professionals navigate ethical challenges. These values—shaped by upbringing, life experiences, moral philosophy, and even past clinical encounters—can profoundly influence how an individual interprets right and wrong, prioritizes conflicting duties, and responds to morally ambiguous situations. While professional guidelines and legal standards provide a framework, it is often a veterinary technician's personal convictions that drive real-time decisions in complex or emotionally charged scenarios. For example, a technician who strongly values animal autonomy may feel deeply conflicted when asked to assist with a procedure the client insists on, but the technician perceives it as unnecessary or distressing to the patient. Another technician who places a high value on loyalty and teamwork may find it challenging to report a colleague's mistake, even when patient safety is at risk. In each case, the professional's values can either align with or challenge the institutional norms and ethical expectations of the workplace. Due to personal values varying significantly from one individual to another, veterinary teams must recognize that ethical perspectives will not always be uniform. These differences can be a source of strength, offering diverse viewpoints that enrich ethical discussions and decision-making. However, they can also lead to conflict if not managed with respect and open communication.

Veterinary technicians are encouraged to engage in regular self-reflection to understand how their values influence their practice. Participating in ethics rounds, journaling after difficult cases, or discussing dilemmas with mentors can help technicians gain clarity on their personal ethical framework. Institutions can support this process by fostering environments where open dialogue about values is encouraged, not avoided. Ultimately, while personal values should not override established standards of care or professional codes of ethics, acknowledging and integrating them into ethical reasoning helps technicians approach each case with greater authenticity, empathy, and moral clarity.

Building Emotional Resilience

To prevent burnout and compassion fatigue, veterinary technicians must adopt proactive self-care practices that promote both mental and physical well-being. Engaging in mindfulness exercises, such as meditation or deep-breathing techniques, can help professionals manage stress and remain present during difficult ethical discussions. Regular physical activity, including yoga, jogging, or strength training, has been shown to reduce stress hormones and improve overall resilience. Finding hobbies outside of work, whether creative arts, reading, or gardening, can offer an essential mental break from the emotional toll of veterinary practice.

Seeking peer support is another crucial aspect of emotional resilience. Veterinary technicians should foster connections within professional networks, support groups, or mentorship programs to share experiences and receive emotional validation. Having a safe space to discuss ethical challenges can alleviate the burden of moral distress and provide new perspectives on problem-solving. Accessing mental health resources, such as professional counseling or veterinary wellness programs, can further support emotional well-being and provide coping mechanisms for handling ethical dilemmas.

Participating in ethics training and case discussions is an effective way to strengthen confidence when facing ethical dilemmas. Regular engagement in continuing education courses focused on veterinary ethics enables veterinary technicians to refine their decision-making skills and stay informed on emerging ethical issues in the field. Role-playing exercises and simulated case studies within team meetings allow veterinary professionals to practice handling difficult conversations and develop structured approaches to ethical challenges.

Setting healthy emotional boundaries is essential for maintaining long-term resilience in veterinary practice. Recognizing personal limits and knowing when to step away from emotionally taxing cases prevents burnout and ensures sustained professional effectiveness. Veterinary technicians must learn to compartmentalize difficult cases while still providing compassionate care. Taking scheduled breaks, establishing clear work-life boundaries, and avoiding excessive emotional investment in every case are crucial strategies for maintaining psychological well-being. In cases where moral distress becomes overwhelming, seeking guidance from supervisors or ethical review boards can provide additional support and reassurance.

Case Study 4.4 Managing an Ethical Conflict Between a Veterinarian and a Client

A veterinary technician working in an emergency clinic encounters a challenging case in which a veterinarian recommends euthanasia for a severely injured stray dog. However, the client who found the dog is emotionally invested and insists on pursuing extensive treatment, despite the poor prognosis and significant financial limitations. The technician is caught between supporting the veterinarian's clinical judgment and acknowledging the client's strong emotional attachment.

To navigate this ethical dilemma, the technician begins by practicing active listening to better understand the client's motivations and concerns. They provide compassionate education about the dog's prognosis, outlining the treatment options and the potential for continued suffering. Using the Ethical Matrix as a guide, the technician evaluates the interests of all stakeholders—the patient, the client, the veterinary team, and the shelter's broader mission and resources. They then collaborate with the veterinarian to identify feasible alternatives, such as reaching out to an animal rescue organization for additional support. Through this collaborative and empathetic process, the technician helps facilitate a compromise in which the dog receives pain management and a short trial period of treatment, allowing for reassessment before a final decision is made. This solution honors the client's emotional investment while still prioritizing ethical patient care.

Ethical Challenges in a Multidisciplinary Veterinary Team

Veterinary medicine is inherently team-based, requiring collaboration between veterinarians, veterinary technicians, assistants, and administrative staff to provide high-quality patient care. However, with a diverse team comes the potential for ethical challenges, as each role within the hospital brings its own perspectives, values, and professional responsibilities. Veterinary technicians often find themselves navigating ethical dilemmas related to patient care, financial limitations, and communication between clients and veterinary staff. Addressing these challenges requires critical thinking, ethical reasoning, and adherence to professional standards to ensure that patient welfare remains at the forefront of decision-making (Rollin 2018).

Differing Perspectives in Veterinary Ethics

Veterinary teams comprise individuals with varying levels of education, experience, and ethical viewpoints. Veterinarians are primarily responsible for diagnosing conditions, prescribing treatments, and making medical decisions, whereas veterinary technicians focus on patient care, treatment administration, and client communication. Administrative staff, such as practice managers and customer service representatives, often prioritize financial considerations and hospital policies, while veterinary assistants support clinical operations. These differing roles can sometimes lead to conflicting priorities, particularly in cases where medical recommendations, client expectations, and financial constraints are misaligned (Moses et al. 2018). For instance, a veterinary technician may advocate for aggressive treatment of a critically ill patient, while a veterinarian, understanding the client's financial limitations, may opt for a more conservative approach. In such cases, technicians may struggle with moral distress, feeling that financial considerations are preventing optimal patient care. Conversely, administrative staff may emphasize profitability and business sustainability creating further ethical tension between clinical staff who focus on patient advocacy and management personnel who must ensure the financial viability of the hospital (Yeates and Main 2019).

Conflicts Over Treatment Plans and Medical Decisions

Disagreements over treatment plans are among the most common ethical challenges within a veterinary team. Veterinary technicians, who spend the most time with hospitalized patients, may recognize subtle changes in patient condition that influence treatment decisions. However, if a veterinarian disregards or downplays their observations, technicians may feel undervalued or powerless in advocating for their patients. This can lead to frustration and ethical distress, particularly if the technician believes that an alternative treatment approach could yield better outcomes (Rollin 2018).

Conflicts may also arise when multiple veterinarians within the same hospital hold differing opinions on how to proceed with a case. One veterinarian may suggest euthanasia for a terminally ill patient, while another may propose palliative care options. In such scenarios, veterinary technicians may struggle with their own ethical stance, especially if they personally disagree with the recommended course of action. Remaining professional and respectful while balancing personal ethics with hospital protocols is essential in these situations (Yeates and Main 2019).

Financial Considerations and Ethical Dilemmas

Financial limitations present some of the most difficult ethical challenges in veterinary practice. Unlike human medicine, which is often subsidized by insurance or government programs, veterinary care is largely out-of-pocket, leading to situations where clients cannot afford the recommended treatment. Veterinary technicians, who frequently handle cost discussions and client interactions, may feel torn between advocating for the patient and understanding the client's financial constraints. For example, in emergency settings, a technician may triage a patient with a life-threatening condition, knowing that aggressive medical intervention could save its life. However, if the client declines treatment due to financial concerns, the technician must accept the reality that the patient may not receive the necessary care. This moral conflict can lead to compassion fatigue and burnout, particularly when technicians experience repeated cases where economic euthanasia is the only option (Moses et al. 2018).

Finding solutions to these ethical dilemmas often requires creative problem-solving and open communication within the veterinary team. Offering payment plans, discussing alternative treatment options, or referring clients to financial assistance programs can sometimes bridge the gap between affordability and necessary medical care. Encouraging a team-based discussion that includes both medical and administrative perspectives can help veterinary professionals reach ethically sound decisions that prioritize patient welfare while acknowledging financial realities (Rollin 2018).

Navigating Ethical Disagreements and Maintaining Team Cohesion

Addressing ethical conflicts within a veterinary team requires a culture of open communication, respect, and shared ethical principles. Veterinary hospitals should foster an environment where all team members feel heard and valued, recognizing that each role contributes to patient care in different but equally important ways.

One effective approach to resolving ethical dilemmas is the ethical case review, where the team discusses difficult cases, evaluates different viewpoints, and collectively determines the best course of action. This not only strengthens team cohesion but also helps establish consistent hospital policies that align with ethical best practices (Yeates and Main 2019). Additionally, veterinary technicians should be empowered to voice their concerns through structured communication models such as the SBAR (Situation, Background, Assessment, Recommendation) method, which ensures that observations and recommendations are clearly conveyed to veterinarians and hospital leadership. Training in ethical reasoning, conflict resolution, and communication strategies can also help veterinary professionals navigate these challenges with confidence and professionalism (Moses et al. 2018).

Case Study 4.5 Disagreement Over Treatment Approaches

In a general practice setting, a veterinarian recommends aggressive chemotherapy for a cat diagnosed with late-stage cancer, believing that treatment may extend the patient's life. However, a veterinary technician involved in the case strongly feels that palliative care would be a more humane approach, as the cat is already showing significant signs of pain, inappetence, and reduced quality of life. The technician experiences moral distress, feeling torn between their professional duty to support the veterinarian's medical plan and their personal ethical belief that the patient may suffer

Table 4.6 Four quadrant approach applied to chemotherapy decision for a terminally Ill cat.

	Medical Indications	Patient Welfare
Client Preferences	Has the client been fully informed of all options, including palliative care and hospice support?	Does the treatment align with the best interests of the patient? Is pain management adequately addressed?
Contextual Factors	Are financial constraints influencing the recommendation? Does the hospital have a policy on quality-of-life assessments?	What are the expected outcomes of chemotherapy? Will it improve quality of life or prolong suffering?

Source: M. Jennings (2025).

unnecessarily. To navigate this challenge, the technician engages in an open discussion with the veterinarian, using the Four Quadrant Approach to ensure that the decision is evaluated from multiple ethical perspectives. This method considers (Table 4.6).

A team meeting is being held, allowing the veterinarian, technician, and other staff members to discuss ethical concerns openly, ensuring that all perspectives are acknowledged. Ultimately, a compromise is reached in which the veterinarian presents all treatment options to the client, providing transparent information on prognosis, potential side effects, and palliative alternatives. The final decision is left to the client, ensuring an ethically sound, patient-centered approach.

This case study illustrates the ethical tension between medical intervention and humane palliative care. This directly ties into earlier discussions about team collaboration, professional ethics, and the role of veterinary technicians in patient advocacy. The case emphasizes the importance of structured ethical frameworks, such as the Four Quadrant Approach, and how open team discussions can prevent moral distress while ensuring patient-centered care. It also reinforces the role of effective communication and compromise in navigating conflicting viewpoints, reflecting the LEARN and SBAR models commonly used in clinical communication (Robinson 2020).

Case Study 4.6 Financial Constraints and Ethical Tension

An emergency veterinary hospital receives a three-year-old Labrador Retriever in critical condition after being hit by a car. The dog has sustained a severely fractured femur and internal bleeding, requiring immediate stabilization, surgery, and intensive post-operative care. The attending veterinarian recommends emergency surgery, but after receiving an initial estimate, the owners state that they cannot afford the full cost of treatment. They request only pain management and euthanasia, despite the dog having a good prognosis with surgical intervention. The veterinary technician, who has been monitoring the dog's vital signs and providing initial stabilization, feels ethical distress knowing that the patient could survive with proper medical care. The technician struggles with the emotional burden of watching a treatable patient be euthanized due to financial limitations. However, they also recognize that the client's financial constraints are a legitimate factor in decision-making.

To address this ethical dilemma, the technician initiates a compassionate conversation with both the veterinarian and the client, working collaboratively to explore feasible alternatives. They discuss the possibility of a payment plan or financial assistance options offered through the hospital, as well as the potential for support from local rescue organizations or nonprofits that help fund emergency veterinary care. The team also considers whether a limb amputation, rather than a full fracture repair, could serve as a more affordable option while still allowing the dog to enjoy a functional quality of life. Additionally, they evaluate whether the hospital might classify the case as a "Good Samaritan" situation, reserving support for patients with a strong prognosis but financial barriers to care. A conversation is held between the veterinarian, technician, and practice manager to explore what realistic solutions exist while maintaining hospital policies. In the end, the owners opt for limb amputation instead of full fracture repair, allowing their pet to survive within their financial means. The technician, while still feeling the emotional weight of the case, is reassured knowing that an alternative treatment path allowed for a better outcome.

This case study addresses the intersection of medical ethics, financial limitations, and team decision-making. This scenario connects to discussions on client communication, financial ethics, and conflict resolution, showcasing how veterinary teams must balance ideal medical recommendations with real-world financial considerations. It highlights the veterinary technician's role in problem-solving, emphasizing the importance of offering alternatives, discussing client limitations with empathy, and seeking creative solutions to improve patient outcomes. The case also reinforces earlier points on moral distress and emotional resilience, demonstrating how technicians can navigate difficult cases while maintaining their professional integrity.

Addressing Workplace Ethics and Professional Integrity

Veterinary technicians often encounter ethical dilemmas not only in patient care but also within the workplace environment itself. Issues such as whistleblowing, conflicts of interest, and unethical conduct by colleagues present complex challenges that require careful navigation, professional integrity, and adherence to ethical and legal obligations. Addressing these dilemmas requires a strong understanding of ethical decision-making, communication strategies, and the responsibility to uphold both patient welfare and professional standards (Rollin 2018).

Whistleblowing and Reporting Unethical Behavior

One of the most challenging ethical dilemmas a veterinary technician may face is whether to report unethical or illegal behavior within the hospital. This could include animal neglect, falsification of medical records, drug diversion, or violations of veterinary practice laws. Whistleblowing is particularly difficult because it often involves reporting a colleague, supervisor, or even a hospital policy that conflicts with ethical veterinary care. For example, a technician may discover that a fellow staff member is administering expired medications or that a veterinarian is pressuring clients into unnecessary procedures for financial gain. While it may be tempting to avoid confrontation, ignoring such misconduct compromises patient welfare and erodes professional integrity. However, whistleblowing can also come with repercussions, such as workplace retaliation or strained relationships among team members (Yeates and Main 2019).

To navigate these situations, technicians should follow ethical and legal reporting procedures. This typically involves:

1) Documenting the incident thoroughly, noting the date, time, individuals involved, and any supporting evidence.
2) Following internal hospital protocols, such as reporting concerns to a practice manager or hospital director.
3) Consulting regulatory bodies, such as the state veterinary board, if the issue involves legal violations or risks to public safety.
4) Seeking confidential guidance from professional organizations, such as the National Association of Veterinary Technicians in America (NAVTA), to understand reporting options and potential protections.

It is crucial to approach whistleblowing professionally and factually, focusing on patient safety and ethical care rather than personal grievances. Open discussions with leadership and collaborative problem-solving may resolve some issues without the need for formal reporting. However, in cases where unethical behavior endangers animals, clients, or the profession, technicians have a moral and legal duty to act (Rollin 2018).

Conflicts of Interest in Veterinary Practice

Conflicts of interest arise when personal, financial, or professional relationships interfere with ethical decision-making. In veterinary practice, these conflicts can occur in various forms, such as technicians receiving commissions for selling specific products, hospital policies prioritizing profit over patient welfare, or favoritism influencing hiring and promotion decisions. A common example is when a technician is encouraged to upsell unnecessary diagnostic tests or prescription diets, even when they are not medically warranted. While financial sustainability is essential for a hospital, prioritizing profit over ethical patient care creates a conflict of interest that can erode client trust and technician integrity. Similarly, a technician working in a research or pharmaceutical setting may face pressure to endorse a specific drug or treatment protocol, even when objective clinical data does not fully support its efficacy.

To address conflicts of interest, veterinary professionals should prioritize transparency with clients, openly communicating any financial incentives or hospital policies that may influence treatment recommendations. They are ethically obligated to advocate for medical decisions that reflect the patient's needs rather than potential revenue. Consulting ethical guidelines from professional organizations, such as the National Association of Veterinary Technicians in America (NAVTA) or the American Veterinary Medical Association (AVMA), can provide clarity and reinforce the importance of patient-centered care. Additionally, maintaining clear professional boundaries is essential—avoiding personal relationships that could compromise objectivity or create bias in clinical decision-making. Recognizing and addressing conflicts of interest helps maintain professional credibility and ethical responsibility, ensuring that patients receive care based on clinical necessity rather than external pressures (Yeates and Main 2019).

Unethical Conduct by Colleagues and Leadership

Veterinary technicians may also encounter significant ethical challenges when colleagues or hospital leadership engage in practices that violate professional standards or compromise patient and staff welfare. These situations can be particularly difficult to navigate, as they often involve power dynamics, institutional culture, or fear of retaliation. One common example includes the failure to provide adequate pain management for patients, often justified by cost-cutting measures that prioritize financial considerations over humane care. Technicians may also be placed in ethically compromising positions when asked to perform duties that exceed their legal scope of practice—such as diagnosing conditions, formulating treatment plans, or prescribing medications—placing both the patient and the technician's license at risk. Additionally, toxic workplace environments characterized by harassment, discrimination, or poor leadership can erode morale and compromise ethical integrity. These situations not only affect individual well-being but can also diminish the overall standard of care within the hospital. Navigating these situations requires diplomacy, ethical reasoning, and knowledge of veterinary laws. Technicians should first attempt to address concerns internally, speaking with hospital leadership or human resources. If concerns are dismissed or retaliatory actions occur, reporting to state veterinary boards, labor agencies, or professional advocacy groups may be necessary.

Fostering a culture of accountability and ethical integrity within a veterinary hospital starts with open discussions about ethical challenges, continuing education on veterinary ethics, and leadership that prioritizes both patient and employee welfare (Rollin 2018). Hospitals that encourage ethical decision-making and a non-retaliation policy for reporting concerns create a more sustainable, positive, and legally compliant workplace.

Promoting Ethical Integrity in Veterinary Nursing

To uphold ethical integrity, veterinary technicians must commit to ongoing ethical education, professional self-reflection, and open communication within their teams. Engaging in ethical case reviews, participating in continuing education on professional ethics, and fostering a work environment where concerns can be discussed without fear of retaliation are essential steps in strengthening the ethical foundation of veterinary practice. Technicians also play a role in mentoring new team members, helping to set a workplace culture where ethical behavior is valued and reinforced. By leading with transparency, honesty, and professionalism, veterinary technicians contribute to a culture of trust, respect, and accountability, ensuring the highest standards of patient care and workplace ethics.

Case Study 4.7 Reporting a Colleague's Mistake

A veterinary technician is assisting with medication administration during a routine shift when they notice that a colleague administered the wrong dosage of a sedative to a canine patient undergoing a minor surgical procedure. Although the patient does not show immediate adverse effects, the technician is aware that even minor medication errors can have serious consequences. However, the colleague chooses not to report the mistake, downplaying its significance and expressing concern about possible disciplinary action. The technician is now faced with an ethical dilemma: should they prioritize workplace harmony and avoid conflict or uphold professional integrity and report the error?

This scenario presents a classic example of ethical tension between team relationships and patient advocacy. The technician recognizes that ignoring the mistake sets a dangerous precedent, potentially compromising patient safety, legal accountability, and trust within the team. However, they also worry that reporting the mistake may damage their relationship with the colleague, create workplace tension, or lead to retaliation. This case illustrates the moral distress technicians often experience when professional ethics conflict with workplace dynamics (Rollin 2018). To resolve this issue ethically and professionally, the technician takes a structured, nonpunitive approach to address the mistake while maintaining a positive work environment.

The technician's first priority is ensuring patient safety. They immediately assess the patient for any signs of sedation-related complications, such as respiratory depression, prolonged recovery time, or unexpected cardiovascular effects. By closely monitoring the patient and documenting any changes, they ensure that the medical team can intervene if necessary.

Following the clinic's incident-reporting protocol, the technician documents the medication error, ensuring that the mistake is formally acknowledged and addressed. Proper documentation is essential for legal compliance, patient safety, and quality improvement, to help prevent similar errors in the future. The technician carefully avoids placing blame or making accusatory statements in the report, instead focusing on objective details and corrective actions to maintain a constructive approach.

Recognizing the importance of team accountability and ethical transparency, the technician privately approaches their colleague to discuss the mistake in a supportive and nonconfrontational manner. They emphasize that reporting errors is not about punishment but about learning from mistakes and improving patient care. By fostering an open and honest discussion, the technician encourages their colleague to take responsibility for the mistake and recognize the importance of reporting medical errors for the safety of all patients (Yeates and Main 2019).

Fostering a Culture of Ethical Accountability

Rather than treating the situation as an isolated mistake, the veterinary team uses the incident as a learning opportunity. A team meeting is held to discuss medication administration protocols, common sources of error, and strategies for improving accuracy. The discussion is conducted in a nonpunitive manner, reinforcing a culture of accountability, safety, and continuous improvement. By shifting the focus from blame to education, the clinic encourages all team members to report errors without fear of retaliation, ultimately reducing future mistakes and improving patient outcomes.

The technician's ethical actions contribute significantly to the clinic's overall standards of care and professional integrity. By ensuring vigilant monitoring and promptly reporting errors, they enhance patient safety and allow for timely medical intervention if complications arise. Their approach also reinforces a nonpunitive culture, where mistakes are viewed as learning opportunities rather than grounds for punishment, fostering an environment of continuous improvement and ethical responsibility. Additionally, by addressing the situation transparently and constructively, the technician helps strengthen team communication and accountability, ultimately reducing the likelihood of similar errors in the future and promoting a more cohesive and ethically sound workplace.

Managing Emotional and Moral Stress in Veterinary Nursing

Veterinary nursing is a demanding profession, requiring not only technical expertise but also emotional resilience and ethical integrity. The nature of the field exposes veterinary technicians to ethical dilemmas, patient loss, financial constraints, and workplace conflicts, all of which contribute to moral stress—the distress experienced when one is forced to act against their ethical beliefs due to external pressures (Moses et al. 2018). Over time, chronic exposure to moral stress can lead to burnout, a state of emotional, mental, and physical exhaustion that diminishes job satisfaction and can negatively impact patient care. Managing emotional and moral stress is essential for maintaining professional longevity, mental well-being, and ethical decision-making. Strategies such as seeking mentorship and peer support, engaging in professional development, and practicing self-care can help veterinary technicians navigate workplace challenges while preserving their emotional and professional integrity.

Seeking Mentorship and Peer Support: Building a Strong Emotional Network

One of the most effective ways to manage moral stress is by seeking guidance from mentors and engaging with supportive peers. Veterinary technicians often work in emotionally charged environments where ethical dilemmas must be resolved quickly and decisively. According to Moses et al. (2018), moral distress is a significant contributor to burnout in veterinary professionals, particularly when they are forced to act against their ethical beliefs due to external constraints. Without proper support, they may feel isolated in their experiences, leading to increased stress and emotional strain.

Discussing ethical challenges with experienced colleagues, mentors, or professional networks provides a safe space for reflection and reassurance. These conversations can help technicians gain perspective, validate their concerns, and develop coping strategies. For example, when struggling with the emotional weight of euthanasia cases, speaking with a trusted veterinarian or senior technician can offer valuable insights on how to process grief and maintain emotional resilience. A mentor might also help a technician navigate ethical dilemmas, such as conflicts between financial limitations and patient advocacy, by sharing past experiences and effective communication techniques.

Beyond one-on-one mentorship, peer support is crucial in fostering a culture of psychological safety within a veterinary team. Open discussions about ethical dilemmas, emotional distress, and professional challenges create an environment where team members feel heard and valued. Structured team debriefings after difficult cases, compassion rounds, or informal peer-led discussions provide opportunities to share experiences and learn from each other. A workplace that encourages these conversations helps veterinary technicians develop a sense of unity and shared responsibility, reducing the emotional burden of making difficult ethical decisions alone.

Engaging in Professional Development: Strengthening Ethical Reasoning and Coping Skills

Engaging in structured ethics training allows veterinary professionals to explore decision-making models, such as the Four Quadrant Approach, which helps them evaluate medical indications, patient welfare, client preferences, and contextual factors before making a decision. By applying these frameworks to real-world scenarios, technicians can strengthen their ethical reasoning skills and feel more prepared to navigate workplace conflicts.

Professional development also helps veterinary technicians improve communication and conflict-resolution skills, which are essential for addressing ethical disagreements within the team. Learning how to facilitate difficult conversations with veterinarians, clients, and hospital leadership can help technicians advocate for patient welfare while maintaining professional relationships. A technician who has attended a workshop on euthanasia ethics, for example, may feel more confident guiding clients through end-of-life decisions and managing their own emotional responses when faced with terminal patients.

Leadership training provides another avenue for veterinary technicians to play a more active role in shaping the ethical culture of their workplace. By serving on hospital ethics committees, contributing to staff training, or helping develop workplace policies, technicians can influence systemic changes that improve patient care and reduce ethical distress for the entire veterinary team. These opportunities not only enhance professional skills but also empower technicians to create meaningful improvements in their workplace.

Practicing Self-care: Preventing Burnout and Supporting Long-term Well-being

Veterinary technicians often place patient care above their own well-being, making them particularly vulnerable to stress, compassion fatigue, and burnout. To sustain a long-term career in veterinary medicine, it is essential to establish personal boundaries and develop self-care routines that help manage workplace stress. A healthy work-life balance is key to maintaining emotional resilience. Setting limits on overtime, taking regular breaks, and ensuring adequate rest between shifts can prevent exhaustion and improve job satisfaction. Engaging in activities that provide a mental break from work, such as exercise, meditation, creative hobbies, or time spent with family and friends, can help technicians recharge emotionally and reduce feelings of chronic stress.

Seeking professional mental health support when needed is another important aspect of self-care. Veterinary professionals experience high rates of anxiety, depression, and burnout, yet many hesitate to seek help due to stigma or time constraints. Accessing counseling services, participating in support groups, or simply having regular check-ins with a trusted mentor or peer can provide valuable emotional relief. A technician who frequently deals with euthanasia cases, for example, may benefit from debriefing with a counselor or participating in a support group for veterinary professionals who experience compassion fatigue.

Workplace culture also plays a role in supporting technician's well-being. Veterinary hospitals can implement initiatives such as mental health awareness programs, flexible scheduling, or staff appreciation efforts to create a more positive and sustainable work environment. Encouraging team debriefings after emotionally difficult cases allows staff members to process their experiences together, preventing feelings of isolation and reinforcing a sense of team support.

By integrating these self-care strategies into daily practice, veterinary technicians can build resilience against workplace stress and maintain their passion for patient care. Addressing moral stress does not mean eliminating difficult situations but rather developing the skills and support systems needed to navigate them effectively while preserving emotional well-being.

Conclusion

Ethical considerations in veterinary nursing are multifaceted, requiring knowledge, critical thinking, and compassion. Veterinary technicians must balance the well-being of animals with the rights of owners while adhering to professional and legal standards. By understanding ethical principles, utilizing structured decision-making models, and fostering open communication, veterinary technicians can navigate ethical challenges effectively. Ongoing education, teamwork, and emotional resilience are essential in ensuring ethical integrity in veterinary nursing practice.

References

Adams, C. L., & Kurtz, S. (2017). Skills for communicating in veterinary medicine (2nd ed.). Otmoor Publishing.

American Veterinary Medical Association. (2023). *AVMA Accreditation Policies and Procedures of the AVMA Council on Education.*

American Veterinary Medical Association (2024). 2024 AVMA census of veterinarians: survey of the profession. www.avma.org (accessed 4 April 2025).

Baile, W.F., Buckman, R., Lenzi, R. et al. (2000). SPIKES—A six-step protocol for delivering bad news: Application to the patient with cancer. *The Oncologist* 5 (4): 302–311.

Batchelor, C.E. and McKeegan, D.E. (2012). Survey of the frequency and perceived stressfulness of ethical dilemmas encountered in UK veterinary practice. *Veterinary Record* 170 (1): 19.

Beauchamp, T.L. and Childress, J.F. (2019). *Principles of Biomedical Ethics.* Oxford University Press.

Hernandez, J., Fike, D.S., and Rivera, A. (2018). Ethics education in health professions: A systematic review. *Journal of Medical Ethics* 44 (9): 607–614.

Khaghanizadeh, M., Ebadi, A., & Rahmani, M. (2023). The relationship between professional competence and ethical decision-making in healthcare professionals. BMC Medical Education, 23, 112. https://doi.org/10.1186/s12909-023-04112-3

Lincoln Memorial University. (2025). Veterinary medical technology and veterinary nursing academic programs.

Mepham, B. (2005). *Bioethics: An Introduction for the Biosciences.* Oxford University Press.

Moses, L., Malowney, M.J., and Wesley Boyd, J. (2018). Ethical conflict and moral distress in veterinary practice: a survey of North American veterinarians. *Journal of Veterinary Internal Medicine* 32 (7): 2115–2122.

Pride Veterinary Medical Community (2021). Gender identity bill of rights. https://www.pridevmc.org/gibor (accessed 4 April 2025).

Pride Veterinary Medical Community (n.d.). Gender diversity guide: implementation toolkit. [Forthcoming publication]. www.pridevmc.org (accessed 4 April 2025).

Robinson, P. (2020). *Veterinary Nursing Care Plans: Theory and Practice*. CABI.

Rollin, B.E. (2011). *An Introduction to Veterinary Medical Ethics: Theory and Cases*. Wiley-Blackwell.

Rollin, B.E. (2018). *An Introduction to Veterinary Medical Ethics: Theory and Cases*. Wiley-Blackwell.

Shadi, S., Al-Mohaissen, M., & Almutairi, A. (2024). Ethics education and moral reasoning development in healthcare professionals: A cross-sectional study. 105065.

U.S. Bureau of Labor Statistics. (2025). Veterinary technologists and technicians: Occupational outlook handbook.

Yeates, J. (2020). *Animal Welfare in Veterinary Practice*. Wiley-Blackwell.

Yeates, J. and Main, D. (2009). Assessment of companion animal quality of life in veterinary practice and research. *Journal of Small Animal Practice* 50 (6): 274–281.

Yeates, J.W. and Main, D.C. (2019). The ethics of veterinary practice: key concepts and perspectives. *Veterinary Record* 184 (13): 404–408.

Part II

Core Concepts and Models in Veterinary Medicine

5

Nursing Plan Models

Veterinary nursing, a critical component of veterinary medicine, has evolved significantly over the past few decades. This evolution has been driven by advancements in medical science, an increased understanding of animal physiology and pathology, and a growing emphasis on comprehensive patient care. Yet, veterinary nursing is not solely a discipline of science; it is also an art. The science provides the framework—knowledge of anatomy, pharmacology, fluid dynamics, and pathophysiology guides decision-making and clinical interventions. The art, however, lies in the ability to adapt this knowledge to the individual patient, using intuition, empathy, and creativity to meet unique needs.

In this context, the development and implementation of veterinary nursing plans highlight this balance. These plans are systematic and structured, reflecting the scientific rigor necessary for accurate patient assessment, nursing evaluation, planning, and intervention. At the same time, they demand artistry in application, as no two patients are alike. A technician must consider species-specific characteristics, individual health conditions, and environmental influences while tailoring care with sensitivity to the animal's temperament and the client's emotional state.

The integration of such plans into daily practice underscores veterinary nursing as both a science—standardized, evidence-based, and measurable—and an art—fluid, compassionate, and responsive. Together, these dimensions ensure the delivery of high-quality, consistent, and patient-centered care while honoring the individuality of each animal.

Historical Perspective and Evolution

The concept of nursing in veterinary medicine can be traced back to the early 20th century when veterinary assistants were primarily trained on the job (Orpet and Welsh 2011). With the formalization of veterinary nursing education and the establishment of professional bodies, the role of veterinary technicians has expanded significantly. Today, veterinary technicians are indispensable members of the veterinary healthcare team, involved in various facets of patient care ranging from clinical assessments to surgical assistance and rehabilitation.

This evolution has also highlighted the increasing need for structured veterinary nursing care plans. As the responsibilities of veterinary technicians have grown from task-based assistance to autonomous clinical decision-making, the absence of standardized nursing frameworks risks inconsistency in care delivery. Nursing care plans provide a systematic approach that ensures each patient's unique physiological and behavioral needs are identified, documented, and addressed. By drawing from both medical science and the art of patient-centered care, these plans guide veterinary technicians in prioritizing interventions, monitoring progress, and evaluating outcomes.

Moreover, care plans reinforce accountability and continuity across the healthcare team. They allow different professionals—veterinarians, technicians, and assistants—to work from a shared framework, minimizing oversights and optimizing patient welfare. Just as in human nursing, where the nursing process is central to professional practice, veterinary nursing care plans elevate the role of the technician from supportive aide to critical thinker, advocate, and patient-centered practitioner. Their implementation reflects the maturity of veterinary nursing as a profession and underscores its indispensable contribution to modern veterinary medicine.

The Framework of Veterinary Nursing Plans

The nursing process is a systematic, evidence-based framework that guides the delivery of comprehensive patient care in both human and veterinary medicine. It comprises five interrelated steps: assessment, evaluation, planning,

Table 5.1 The nursing process—five interrelated steps.

Step	Description
Assessment	Collecting subjective and objective data, including patient history, physical examination findings, diagnostics, and monitoring results.
Planning	Developing a care plan based on identified problems, prioritizing nursing interventions, and setting measurable goals.
Implementation	Carrying out nursing interventions such as administering medications, monitoring vital signs, providing nutrition, or performing procedures.
Observation	Continuous surveillance of the patient's status, detecting subtle changes, and documenting observations in real time.
Evaluation	Measuring the outcomes of implemented interventions, reassessing patient needs, and adjusting the care plan accordingly.

Source: Schaeffer (2025).

implementation, and observation. Each step is crucial for ensuring that patient care is thorough, effective, and tailored to individual needs. This process is widely adopted in veterinary nursing education, clinical training programs, and inpatient hospital settings across general practice, specialty, and emergency/critical care. Its integration into both academic curricula and clinical protocols ensures that veterinary technicians apply a structured, standardized approach to patient care, reinforcing their role as autonomous, evidence-based practitioners within the veterinary healthcare team. However, the nursing process is particularly geared toward hospitalized patients, where continuous monitoring, dynamic reassessment, and the formulation of a structured care plan are essential. In hospitalized settings, patients often present with acute or complex conditions that require frequent interventions, adjustments in therapy, and collaborative communication among the healthcare team. Here, the nursing process ensures continuity, consistency, and accountability across shifts and caregivers, preventing fragmented or reactive care (Table 5.1).

This differs markedly from the information-gathering process that occurs during wellness care. When obtaining a history from an owner in a preventive or outpatient setting, the focus is primarily on collecting subjective information to support diagnostic reasoning—such as diet, exercise, environmental exposures, and prior medical history. While this interview is critical for identifying risk factors and guiding preventive care recommendations, it does not constitute a nursing care plan. Instead, it serves as a foundation for the veterinarian's medical decision-making and for client education, rather than the ongoing, structured nursing interventions applied in a hospitalized context.

In essence, wellness history-taking is episodic and owner-driven, designed to provide a snapshot of the patient's overall health and lifestyle. In contrast, the nursing process is continuous, patient-driven, and clinician-directed, integrating assessment and intervention into a cycle of care that adapts as the patient's condition evolves. Together, these approaches complement one another: wellness care builds the preventive framework, while the nursing process operationalizes acute and chronic care within the clinical environment.

Assessment: The Foundational Phase of the Nursing Process

Assessment is the foundation of the nursing process, forming the basis upon which subsequent phases—evaluation, planning, implementation, and observation—are built. This critical phase involves the systematic collection, verification, and analysis of data pertaining to the patient's current health status, needs, and responses to potential or actual health problems. Effective assessment enables the formulation of accurate nursing evaluations and the development of tailored care plans, ultimately leading to improved patient outcomes.

Systematic Data Collection

The initial step in the assessment phase involves the meticulous collection of comprehensive data from multiple sources. This data is categorized into subjective and objective data. Subjective data is qualitative data points derived from the patient's owner or caregiver's observations and descriptions of the patient's symptoms, behavior, and history. Subjective data provide insights into how the patient is perceived to feel and act in their environment. Examples include reports of decreased appetite, changes in behavior, or perceived pain levels. This type of data is inherently individualized and relies on effective communication and observational skills. Whereas objective data is quantifiable and observable data obtained

Table 5.2 Subjective vs. objective data in the assessment phase.

Data Type	Definition	Examples	Key Features
Subjective data	Qualitative data derived from owner/caregiver observations and descriptions of the patient's symptoms, behavior, and history.	Reports of decreased appetite, changes in behavior, and perceived pain levels.	Individualized, perception-based, requires effective communication and observational skills.
Objective data	Quantifiable and observable data obtained through direct examination, diagnostic testing, and monitoring.	Vital signs (TPR), laboratory results (CBC, serum biochemistry), diagnostic imaging (radiographs, ultrasounds).	Measurable, standardized, provides physiological indicators, and identifies pathological processes.

Source: Schaeffer (2025).

through direct examination, diagnostic testing, and monitoring. Objective data include vital signs (temperature, pulse, respiratory rate), laboratory results (complete blood count, serum biochemistry), and findings from diagnostic imaging (radiographs, ultrasounds). These data points provide measurable indicators of the patient's physiological status and help identify underlying pathological processes (Table 5.2).

Comprehensive Patient History

A thorough patient history is integral to the assessment process. This includes the animal's medical history, vaccination records, previous illnesses or surgeries, current medications, diet, and environmental factors. The history should be detailed and include the patient's chief complaint or the primary reason for the current visit, as reported by the pet owner. Detailed information about the onset, duration, and progression of the current condition should be discussed. Information on previous medical conditions, treatments, and surgical history as well as a list of current and past medications, including dosages and administration schedules should be included. Information on the type and amount of food consumed, feeding schedules, and any dietary supplements needs to be recorded. Details about the pet's living conditions, exposure to other animals, and travel history often prove to be advantageous. For a more comprehensive exploration of history-taking methods, including structured questioning techniques and clinical reasoning applications, the authors recommend referring to Chapter 3, where this subject is discussed in greater depth (Table 5.3).

The Importance of Nursing Assessment in Conjunction with a Veterinarian's Physical Examination

In veterinary medicine, the integration of a nursing assessment with a veterinarian's physical examination is pivotal for delivering comprehensive and high-quality patient care (Orpet and Welsh 2011). This collaborative approach ensures a thorough understanding of the patient's health status, facilitating accurate diagnoses and the development of effective

Table 5.3 Comprehensive patient history components.

History Component	Details
Medical history	Includes chronic diseases, previous diagnoses, and overall health trends.
Vaccination records	Record of core and elective vaccinations, compliance, and reaction history.
Previous illnesses or surgeries	Documentation of past illnesses, surgical interventions, and recovery outcomes.
Current medications	List of current and past medications, dosages, administration schedules, and responses.
Dietary information	Type and amount of food consumed, feeding schedules, dietary supplements, and changes in appetite.
Environmental factors	Living conditions, household dynamics, exposure to toxins, or the presence of other pets.
Chief complaint	Primary reason for the current visit, as reported by the owner/caregiver.
Condition details	Onset, duration, and progression of the presenting condition.
Exposure and travel history	Travel history, exposure to other animals, and potential zoonotic/environmental risks.

Source: Schaeffer (2025).

treatment plans. The synergy between nursing assessments and veterinary examinations enhances the detection of health issues, optimizes patient outcomes, and supports the holistic care of veterinary patients.

The nursing assessment complements the veterinarian's physical examination by providing a broader, more detailed collection of data. Veterinary technicians gather subjective and objective information, encompassing both clinical signs and behavioral observations that may not be immediately apparent during a physical examination. Veterinary technicians often spend more time with the patient and the owner, enabling them to gather detailed subjective data. This includes the owner's observations about the animal's behavior, appetite, and activity levels, as well as the patient's responses to its environment. Such data provides valuable context to the clinical findings and can reveal subtle changes in the patient's condition. While veterinarians focus on diagnostic tests and physical examination findings, veterinary technicians assist by collecting vital signs, monitoring ongoing health parameters, and performing preliminary diagnostic tests such as blood work or urinalysis. This comprehensive data collection ensures that no aspect of the patient's health is overlooked.

Combining the detailed observations from nursing assessments with the clinical acumen of a veterinarian's physical examination enhances diagnostic accuracy (Baillie 2018). Veterinary technicians are trained to recognize early and subtle signs of illness that may not be immediately evident during a physical examination. For example, changes in eating habits, slight weight loss, or alterations in behavior can be early indicators of underlying health issues. These observations can prompt further investigation by the veterinarian, leading to early diagnosis and intervention. The collaboration between veterinary technicians and veterinarians allows for cross-verification of findings. Technicians can report any discrepancies or concerns noted during their assessment, prompting the veterinarian to conduct a more focused examination or additional diagnostic tests. This collaborative approach minimizes the risk of misdiagnosis and ensures a more accurate understanding of the patient's health (Figure 5.1).

A nursing assessment provides crucial information that informs the development of a comprehensive care plan. This plan is tailored to the patient's unique needs, addressing both medical and nursing care requirements. Veterinary technicians consider the patient's overall well-being, including physical, emotional, and environmental factors. This holistic perspective ensures that the care plan addresses all aspects of the patient's health, from medical treatment to nutritional support and environmental enrichment. The data gathered during the nursing assessment helps in formulating specific nursing interventions. For instance, if a nursing assessment reveals that a patient is experiencing anxiety in a hospital setting, the care plan may include interventions to reduce stress, such as providing a quiet and comfortable environment, pheromone therapy, or gentle handling techniques. These individualized interventions complement the veterinarian's medical treatment, promoting the patient's overall well-being and recovery.

Nursing assessments are integral to the continuous monitoring and evaluation of the patient's progress. Veterinary technicians play a critical role in tracking the patient's response to treatment and identifying any changes in condition that may require adjustment of the care plan. Veterinary technicians frequently monitor the patient's vital signs, pain levels, and behavioral responses, providing real-time data that inform the veterinarian's ongoing clinical decisions. This continuous assessment allows for prompt identification of complications or adverse reactions to treatment, facilitating timely

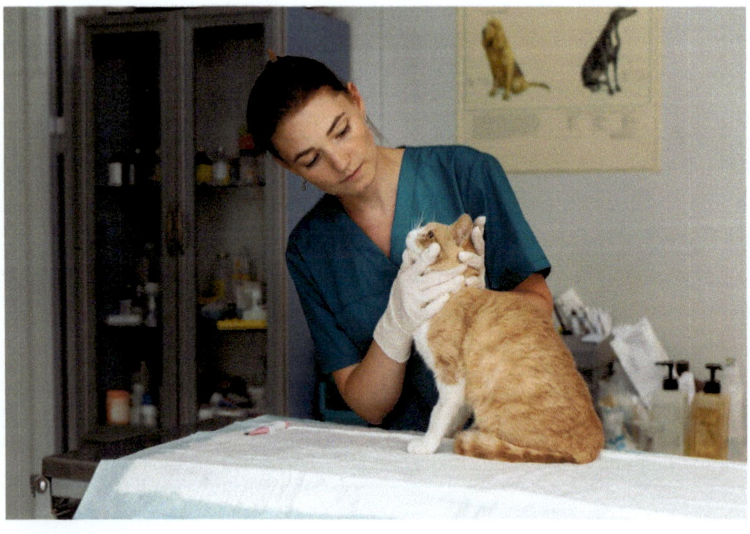

Figure 5.1 Veterinary professional conducting a physical exam on a feline patient. *Source:* Freepik.

interventions. By regularly evaluating the patient's progress against established goals, veterinary technicians ensure that the care plan remains effective and relevant. If the patient is not responding as expected, the nursing assessment provides the necessary information to adjust the interventions or escalate care. This iterative process of evaluation and adjustment is critical for optimizing patient outcomes.

In addition, the integration of nursing assessments with veterinarian-led physical examinations fosters a collaborative, multidisciplinary approach to veterinary care. This teamwork enhances the overall quality of care provided to patients. Effective communication between veterinary technicians and veterinarians ensures that all relevant information is shared and considered in decision-making. Regular case discussions and collaborative planning sessions help align the team's efforts and ensure that care is coordinated and comprehensive. Veterinary technicians and veterinarians bring different but complementary skills to the patient care process. Technicians provide detailed observations and ongoing monitoring, while veterinarians contribute their diagnostic and treatment expertise. This role complementarity maximizes the strengths of both professions, leading to more effective and efficient patient care.

Enhanced Patient and Owner Education

Veterinary technicians play a pivotal role in educating pet owners about their animal's condition, treatment plan, and required home care. The insights gained from the nursing assessment enhance the quality and relevance of this education. Based on the comprehensive data gathered during the assessment, veterinary technicians can provide tailored advice and support to pet owners. This includes instructions on medication administration, dietary modifications, and strategies to manage behavioral issues. Personalized education empowers pet owners to effectively participate in their animal's care, improving adherence to the treatment plan and overall outcomes (Lue et al. 2008). Veterinary technicians often serve as a bridge between the clinical team and the pet owner, providing emotional support and counseling. Understanding the pet owner's perspective and concerns, which are often uncovered during the nursing assessment, enables technicians to address these issues compassionately and effectively.

Improved Patient Outcomes

Ultimately, the integration of nursing assessments with veterinarian physical examinations leads to improved patient outcomes (Orpet and Welsh 2011). The comprehensive and holistic approach to patient evaluation and care planning ensures that all aspects of the patient's health are addressed, from initial diagnosis to long-term management. The detailed data collection and continuous monitoring performed by veterinary technicians enable early detection of health issues, allowing for timely and targeted interventions. Early intervention is often associated with better prognoses and quicker recovery times. By considering the patient's overall well-being and involving pet owners in the care process, the integrated approach promotes patient-centered care. This focus on the individual needs of the patient enhances their quality of life and overall health outcomes.

The importance of nursing assessment in conjunction with a veterinarian's physical examination cannot be overstated in veterinary medicine. This collaborative approach ensures a comprehensive understanding of the patient's health status, leading to accurate diagnoses, effective care planning, and improved patient outcomes. Veterinary technicians' detailed observations, continuous monitoring, and personalized interventions complement the diagnostic and treatment expertise of veterinarians, creating a synergistic partnership that enhances the quality of care provided to veterinary patients. By fostering interdisciplinary collaboration, integrating evidence-based practices, and prioritizing patient-centered care, the combination of nursing assessments and veterinary examinations represents a growing standard in veterinary healthcare.

Diagnostic Testing

Diagnostic tests play a pivotal role in the assessment phase, providing objective data that complement findings from the history and physical examination. Common diagnostic tests include serum biochemistry, complete blood counts with indices, hemogram evaluations, and electrolyte interpretation in conjunction with blood gas and acid-base assessment. Urinalysis, fecal analysis, and cytology help in identifying infections, organ dysfunctions, and other systemic issues. Radiography, ultrasonography, and advanced imaging techniques such as computed tomography (CT) scans and magnetic resonance imaging (MRI) provide detailed views of internal structures, aiding in the diagnosis of conditions not apparent through physical examination alone.

Data Analysis

The final step in the assessment phase is the analysis of the collected data. This involves synthesizing the information to form a comprehensive understanding of the patient's health status. The analysis process includes recognizing trends and correlations in the data, such as persistent symptoms or recurring lab abnormalities, and establishing the patient's normal physiological parameters to detect deviations. This allows the ranking of health problems based on their severity and urgency to guide subsequent phases of the nursing process.

Importance of Accurate Assessment

An accurate and thorough assessment is critical as it directly influences the formulation of nursing evaluations and the overall care plan. Errors or omissions during this phase can lead to inappropriate interventions and suboptimal patient outcomes. Therefore, veterinary technicians must employ a meticulous, systematic approach to assessment, utilizing their clinical knowledge, observational skills, and critical thinking abilities to gather and interpret data effectively. Assessment is the bedrock of the nursing process, providing the essential data needed to understand the patient's health status and guide subsequent care. Through systematic data collection, comprehensive history taking, physical examination, diagnostic testing, and rigorous data verification and analysis, veterinary technicians can develop an accurate and holistic understanding of their patients. This foundational phase ensures that all subsequent steps in the nursing process are informed, precise, and effective, ultimately enhancing the quality of care and improving patient outcomes.

Nursing Evaluation

Nursing evaluations and veterinarian diagnoses serve complementary but distinct roles in the care of veterinary patients (Orpet and Welsh 2011). While both are essential for developing a comprehensive care plan, they differ in focus, scope, and methodology. Understanding these differences is crucial for effective interdisciplinary collaboration and optimized patient outcomes. This discussion will elucidate the distinctions between nursing evaluations and veterinarian diagnoses, exploring their respective definitions, categories, and implications for patient care.

Nursing evaluations are clinical judgments regarding an animal's responses to actual or potential health problems and life processes. These evaluations provide a basis for selecting nursing interventions aimed at achieving specific, desirable outcomes. Nursing evaluations are typically categorized into three types: actual evaluations, risk evaluations, and wellness evaluations (Orpet and Welsh 2011).

Actual nursing evaluations describe existing health problems validated by the assessment data. These evaluations reflect the patient's current state and are substantiated by observable and measurable signs and symptoms. An example of this may be "impaired mobility related to arthritis as evidenced by limping and reluctance to move." This evaluation informs the nursing interventions that aim to improve the animal's mobility and comfort, such as physical therapy, pain management, and environmental modifications to facilitate easier movement.

Risk nursing evaluations identify potential health problems that the animal is at risk of developing. These evaluations highlight vulnerabilities based on the patient's current condition, history, or environment. An example of this may be "risk for infection related to surgical incision." Risk evaluations guide preventive interventions, such as implementing aseptic techniques, monitoring for signs of infection, and educating pet owners on postoperative care to mitigate the identified risks.

Wellness nursing evaluations focus on the patient's readiness to enhance specific health behaviors and achieve higher levels of wellness. These evaluations reflect positive health aspirations rather than problems. An example of this may be "readiness for enhanced nutrition." Wellness evaluations lead to interventions that promote health optimization, such as developing a balanced diet plan, recommending supplements, and providing guidance on healthy feeding practices.

Veterinarian Diagnoses

Veterinarian diagnoses, in contrast, are clinical judgments about specific medical conditions or diseases affecting the animal. These diagnoses are grounded in a pathophysiological understanding of the disease processes and are typically derived from diagnostic tests, physical examinations, and clinical observations. Veterinarian diagnoses identify specific diseases or medical conditions based on clinical signs, diagnostic test results, and imaging studies. An example of this may be "osteoarthritis in the right hip joint." Medical diagnoses inform the treatment plan, including medical or surgical interventions, medication prescriptions, and recommendations for managing the underlying disease.

Differential diagnoses involve identifying multiple potential conditions that could explain the patient's symptoms. This process narrows down the possibilities to arrive at the most accurate diagnosis. Differential diagnoses for a dog presenting with vomiting could include gastroenteritis, pancreatitis, intestinal obstruction, or renal disease. Differential diagnoses

Table 5.4 Nursing evaluation vs. veterinarian diagnosis.

Nursing Evaluation/Nursing Diagnosis	Veterinarian's Diagnosis
Focuses on patient response to illness, injury, hospitalization, or environment.	Focuses on identifying the medical condition or disease causing clinical signs.
Examples: pain, dehydration, hypothermia, anxiety, impaired mobility, risk for infection.	Examples: parvovirus enteritis, osteoarthritis, pancreatitis, chronic kidney disease.
Aims to support patient comfort, optimize nursing care, and anticipate complications.	Aims to define the pathology, prescribe medical treatment, surgery, or diagnostics.
Interventions: warming, analgesia administration, fluid support, environmental modifications, nutritional support.	Interventions: prescribing drugs, performing surgery, ordering diagnostic tests, and confirming pathology.
Guides the nursing care plan, focusing on individualized, holistic patient needs.	Guides the medical treatment plan, focusing on eliminating or controlling the disease.
Performed and documented by veterinary technicians/nurses.	Performed and documented by licensed veterinarians.

Source: Schaeffer (2025).

guide further diagnostic testing and examinations to rule out or confirm specific conditions, ensuring precise and targeted treatment.

Prognostic diagnoses predict the likely course and outcome of a disease based on the current clinical evidence and historical data. An example of this may be "guarded prognosis for a dog with advanced lymphoma." Prognostic diagnoses inform the expectations for treatment outcomes, guide decision-making regarding the aggressiveness of interventions, and support discussions with pet owners about the potential for recovery or palliative care options (Table 5.4).

Distinctions Between Nursing Evaluations and Veterinarian Diagnoses

Nursing evaluations emphasize the animal's holistic responses to health issues, including physical, psychological, and social aspects. They address both actual and potential problems and wellness goals. Whereas a veterinarian diagnosis centers on identifying and managing specific medical conditions and diseases. They focus on pathophysiological mechanisms and treatment of the disease itself. We must also consider the diagnostic methodology of both technicians and veterinarians. A nursing evaluation is often derived from comprehensive nursing assessments, including subjective and objective data, and considers the animal's overall well-being (Orpet and Welsh 2011). The process involves identifying patterns, validating findings, and prioritizing nursing care needs. In contrast, a veterinarian's diagnosis is based on clinical examinations, diagnostic tests (e.g., blood work, imaging), and pathophysiological knowledge (Orpet and Welsh 2011). The process involves forming differential diagnoses, confirming the most likely condition, and determining the appropriate medical treatment. Nursing evaluations ***lead*** to nursing interventions that are typically independent or collaborative, focusing on symptom management, patient education, and preventive care. Outcomes are related to the animal's overall health, comfort, and quality of life. Veterinarian diagnoses lead to medical or surgical treatments, including prescribing medications, performing surgeries, or initiating specialized therapies. Outcomes are primarily related to disease resolution, control, or management.

Collaborative Approach in Veterinary Care

The interplay between nursing evaluations and veterinarian diagnoses is crucial for providing comprehensive and holistic care to veterinary patients. This collaborative approach leverages the unique strengths of veterinary technicians and veterinarians, ensuring that all aspects of the patient's health are addressed. Veterinary technicians contribute detailed observations and data from ongoing assessments, providing a broad understanding of the patient's condition and responses to treatment. Veterinarians provide expertise in diagnosing and treating specific medical conditions, ensuring accurate medical management.

Veterinary technicians develop and implement nursing care plans based on their evaluations, focusing on interventions that support the animal's recovery, comfort, and well-being. Veterinarians create medical treatment plans based on their diagnoses, prescribing medications, performing procedures, and monitoring disease progression. Veterinary technicians continuously monitor the patient's condition, documenting responses to interventions, and reporting any changes to the veterinary team. Veterinarians adjust the medical treatment plan as needed based on the patient's progress and any new diagnostic information.

Case Study: Integrating Nursing Evaluations and Veterinarian Diagnoses

Case Overview

A seven-year-old MN Labrador Retriever presents with a history of lethargy, reduced appetite, and intermittent limping on the right hind leg. The veterinary team undertakes a collaborative approach, integrating both nursing and veterinarian assessments.

1) **Assessment and Initial Findings**
   - **Nursing Assessment:** The veterinary technician conducts a thorough assessment, noting the dog's weight loss, reluctance to bear weight on the right hind leg, and signs of discomfort during palpation of the hip joint.
   - **Veterinarian Examination:** The veterinarian performs a physical examination, observing crepitus and pain on manipulation of the right hip. Radiographs are taken, revealing degenerative joint changes consistent with osteoarthritis.
2) **Diagnoses Formulation**
   - **Nursing Evaluation:**
     - **Actual Evaluation:** "Impaired mobility related to arthritis reported by the veterinarian and as evidenced by limping and reluctance to move."
     - **Risk Evaluation:** "Risk for Infection related to potential skin abrasions from altered gait."
     - **Wellness Evaluation:** "Readiness for enhanced nutrition to support joint health."
   - **Veterinarian Diagnoses:**
     - **Medical Diagnosis:** "Osteoarthritis in the right hip joint."
     - **Differential Diagnoses:** Considered and ruled out other causes of lameness such as hip dysplasia, soft tissue injury, and neoplasia.
     - **Prognostic Diagnosis:** "Chronic but manageable condition with appropriate treatment and lifestyle modifications."
3) **Intervention Planning and Implementation**
   - **Nursing Interventions:**
     - **Impaired Mobility:** Implement a physical therapy regimen, provide supportive bedding, and educate the owner on joint-friendly exercises.
     - **Risk for Infection:** Monitor skin integrity, apply protective barriers as needed, and educate the owner on signs of infection.
     - **Enhanced Nutrition:** Work with the veterinarian to institute a nutritional plan including joint supplements and guide the owner on dietary adjustments.
     - **Environmental Modification:** Work with owners on a home care plan that adjusts the home environment for enhanced mobility.
   - **Veterinarian Interventions:**
     - **Osteoarthritis Management:** Prescribe nonsteroidal anti-inflammatory drugs (NSAIDs) for pain management, recommend weight management strategies, and consider monoclonal injections if needed.
     - **Monitoring Disease Progression:** Schedule follow-up visits to assess response to treatment and adjust the medical plan as necessary.
4) **Evaluation and Follow-Up**
   - **Nursing Role:** The veterinary technician continuously monitors the dog's mobility, comfort, and overall well-being, adjusting the nursing care plan as needed based on the dog's progress.
   - **Veterinarian Role:** The veterinarian evaluates the effectiveness of the medical interventions, making necessary adjustments and addressing any new health issues that arise.

Nursing evaluations and veterinarian diagnoses are both essential for providing comprehensive care to veterinary patients. While nursing evaluations focus on the animal's responses to health issues and guide nursing interventions, veterinarian diagnoses identify specific medical conditions and inform medical treatments. The integration of these diagnoses ensures a holistic approach to patient care, leveraging the strengths of veterinary technicians and veterinarians to achieve optimal health outcomes. This collaborative, interdisciplinary approach enhances patient assessment, care planning, continuous monitoring, and education, ultimately improving the quality of care and the well-being of veterinary patients (Orpet and Welsh 2011).

Planning in the Nursing Process: An Integral Phase Post-assessment and Evaluation

Following the assessment and evaluation phases, the planning phase emerges as a pivotal stage in the nursing process. This phase involves formulating evidence-based strategies and interventions to address the identified health issues, ultimately aiming to achieve optimal patient outcomes.

The Significance of the Planning Phase

The planning phase in the nursing process bridges the gap between the evaluation of a patient's health problems and the actual implementation of interventions. It involves setting realistic and measurable goals, prioritizing nursing evaluations, and selecting appropriate evidence-based interventions (Orpet and Welsh 2011). The thoroughness of this phase directly influences the effectiveness of subsequent care and the achievement of desired health outcomes.

Components of the Planning Phase

This phase is characterized by the development of specific, measurable, achievable, relevant, and time-bound (SMART) goals, the prioritization of nursing evaluations, and the selection of evidence-based interventions (Orpet and Welsh 2011). Figure 5.2 Goals must be clear and specific to guide the nursing interventions effectively. For instance, if a veterinary patient is diagnosed with dehydration, a specific goal would be to restore optimal hydration levels. Goals should be

SMART Goals Example in Veterinary Nursing

This info graphic demonstrates the application of SMART goals in the planning phase of the nursing process, using a dehydrated patient as an example. Each SMART element includes a specific, measurable, achievable, relevant, and time-bound goal that structures patient-centered nursing care.

S **Specific-** **Administer intravenous fluids (Lactated Ringer's solution) at the prescribed maintenance and deficit replacement rate to restore hydration status.**

M **Measurable-** **Monitor and document the dog's hydration parameters every 2 hours, including mucous membrane moisture, capillary refill time, skin turgor, body weight, and urine output. Target:**

normalization of mucous membranes and skin tent within 12–24 hours.

A **Achievable-** **Veterinary technicians will carry out fluid therapy under the veterinarian's orders, with infusion pumps calibrated for accurate delivery and monitoring equipment available in the ICU.**

R **Relevant-** **The goal addresses the dog's primary clinical need—reversing dehydration—which iscritical for restoring perfusion,supporting renalfunction, and improving overall patient stability.**

T **Time-Bound-** **Hydration status will be reassessed every 2 hours, with expected normalization or significant improvement within 24 hours. Fluid therapy will be adjusted at each reassessment based on clinical response and laboratory values (e.g., packed cell volume/total solids, electrolytes).**

Figure 5.2 SMART Goals Example in Veterinary Nursing (Dehydrated patient). *Source:* Schaeffer (2025).

quantifiable to facilitate the assessment of progress. For example, monitoring the intake and urinary output in a dehydrated patient can be a measurable goal. Goals should be realistic and attainable, considering the patient's current health status and resources available. Unrealistic goals can lead to frustration and noncompliance. Goals should be pertinent to the patient's primary health concerns and should address the identified nursing evaluations. Goals should have a clear timeframe to provide a sense of urgency and facilitate timely evaluation. Conditions that pose an immediate threat to life, such as severe hemorrhage or respiratory distress, are prioritized first. Conditions that compromise the patient's safety, such as risk of falls or infection, are addressed next. Considering the owners' preferences and values is crucial in prioritizing care, ensuring that the care plan is patient-centered. This includes acknowledging the owner's financial limitations, cultural beliefs, emotional capacity, and level of understanding, all of which directly influence treatment choices and compliance. By incorporating these factors, veterinary technicians can tailor interventions that are both medically appropriate and realistic for the family, thus avoiding care plans that are unsustainable or misaligned with the owner's expectations. This collaborative approach not only respects the human–animal bond but also fosters trust, shared decision-making, and long-term adherence to the prescribed nursing and medical plan.

Selecting Evidence-based Interventions

The selection of evidence-based interventions is a critical aspect of the planning phase in the nursing process. These interventions are chosen based on scientific evidence, clinical guidelines, and best practices to address the patient's health problems effectively. Evidence-based interventions can be classified into three main categories: independent nursing interventions, dependent nursing interventions, and collaborative interventions (Table 5.5) (Orpet and Welsh 2011).

Independent Nursing Interventions

Independent nursing interventions are actions that nurses can perform autonomously, without requiring a veterinarian's orders (Orpet and Welsh 2011). These interventions are grounded in nursing knowledge and expertise and are essential for promoting patient well-being and addressing routine health needs. Regular monitoring of vital signs, such as temperature, pulse, respiration, and blood pressure, is crucial for detecting early changes in the patient's condition. For example, in a veterinary patient recovering from surgery, technicians can monitor vital signs to identify signs of infection or complications, allowing for timely interventions. Educating the patient's owner is a key independent nursing intervention. This education can cover a wide range of topics, including postoperative care, medication administration, dietary recommendations, and recognizing symptoms that require medical attention. For instance, teaching a pet owner how to monitor their animal's hydration status and signs of dehydration ensures ongoing care at home. Providing basic nursing care, such as wound care, hygiene maintenance, and comfort measures, including stress reduction, is fundamental to patient recovery. In veterinary settings, this might include cleaning and dressing wounds, assisting with mobility, and ensuring the patient is comfortable and free from pain. Independent interventions also encompass health promotion and preventive care activities, such as vaccination reminders, parasite control education, and nutritional counseling. These actions help prevent health issues and promote long-term well-being.

Table 5.5 Types of evidence-based interventions in veterinary nursing.

Intervention Type	Definition	Examples
Independent nursing interventions	Actions that veterinary technicians can initiate based on their professional knowledge, skills, and judgment without direct veterinarian orders.	Providing environmental enrichment, repositioning patients to prevent pressure sores, monitoring comfort levels, and stress reduction techniques.
Dependent nursing interventions	Actions that require a veterinarian's order or prescription before implementation, ensuring compliance with medical directives.	Administering prescribed medications, initiating fluid therapy, and performing diagnostic tests ordered by the veterinarian.
Collaborative interventions	Actions carried out in partnership with veterinarians or other healthcare team members, requiring shared decision-making and coordination.	Developing pain management protocols, implementing nutritional plans, and coordinating physical rehabilitation strategies.

Source: Schaeffer (2025).

Dependent Nursing Interventions

Dependent nursing interventions require orders or instructions from a veterinarian (Orpet and Welsh 2011). These interventions are necessary for managing specific medical conditions and require collaboration with the veterinary team to ensure they are implemented correctly and safely. Administering prescribed medications, such as antibiotics, analgesics, or antiemetics, is a common dependent nursing intervention. Technicians must understand the indications, dosages, potential side effects, and monitoring requirements for each medication. For example, administering intravenous fluids to a dehydrated patient involves precise calculations and monitoring to prevent complications like fluid overhydration. Certain medical procedures, such as catheter insertion, wound suturing, or the application of specific treatments, require a veterinarian's orders. Technicians perform these procedures under the veterinarian's supervision or according to each state's practice act. For instance, placing an intravenous catheter in a veterinary patient requires technical skill and adherence to aseptic techniques to prevent infection. Collecting samples for diagnostic testing, such as blood draws, urine collection, or swabs for culture, often requires a veterinarian's order. Technicians must follow precise protocols to ensure accurate sample collection and handling, which is critical for reliable diagnostic results.

Collaborative Interventions

Collaborative interventions involve the coordinated efforts of multiple healthcare professionals, with veterinary technicians serving as the essential link between patients, clients, and specialists (Orpet and Welsh 2011). Veterinary technicians apply their clinical knowledge and communication skills to integrate specialist recommendations into day-to-day nursing care, ensuring that advanced treatment strategies are practical, consistent, and patient-centered.

For example, when collaborating with physiotherapists, technicians are responsible for carrying out prescribed rehabilitation exercises, monitoring patient tolerance, and recording progress over time. This includes observing subtle changes in mobility, comfort, or behavior that inform adjustments to the physiotherapy plan. Similarly, in partnership with veterinary nutritionists, technicians gather detailed dietary histories, assess body condition scores, educate owners on feeding strategies, and monitor patient responses to specialized diets formulated for conditions such as renal disease, obesity, or gastrointestinal disorders.

Technicians also play a pivotal role when working with veterinary behaviorists. They not only implement behavior-modification strategies but also provide ongoing assessment of patient stress levels and owner compliance. By guiding clients in the consistent application of behavioral interventions, technicians help bridge the gap between clinical recommendations and real-world application in the home environment. Through this collaborative framework, veterinary technicians ensure that specialist expertise is translated into individualized, sustainable care. Their ability to coordinate input from multiple disciplines—while advocating for both the patient's needs and the owner's capacity—allows for the creation of comprehensive care plans. For instance, in a patient with chronic kidney disease, the technician may coordinate regular rechecks, monitor hydration status, administer prescribed treatments, and communicate updates to both the veterinarian and the nutritionist. This integrative role reinforces the technician's value as both a caregiver and a facilitator of interdisciplinary veterinary medicine.

The Process of Planning

Engaging the patient and their caregivers in the planning process ensures that the care plan is aligned with the client's preferences, cultural beliefs, and values. This collaborative approach enhances compliance and fosters a therapeutic technician–patient/client relationship. Veterinary technician engagement with owners must be flexible and responsive to diversity, as each client brings unique perspectives that can shape decision-making. For example, cultural or religious beliefs may influence attitudes toward euthanasia, surgical procedures, or pain management strategies. Socioeconomic status may determine what diagnostic or therapeutic options are financially feasible, while language barriers or differences in health literacy may require technicians to adjust their communication style, use visual aids, or provide translated resources. Additionally, family structure and personal experiences with animals can affect the level of involvement an owner wishes to have in daily care. Recognizing and respecting these differences allows technicians to establish trust and develop realistic, sustainable care plans that honor both medical priorities and client values (Table 5.6).

The selection of interventions should be guided by clinical guidelines and evidence-based practice to ensure that the care provided is based on the best available evidence. This approach enhances the quality of care and improves patient outcomes. The care plan should be meticulously documented, detailing the nursing evaluations, goals, selected interventions, and expected outcomes. This documentation serves as a roadmap for care delivery and facilitates communication among the healthcare team.

Table 5.6 Client diversity in veterinary nursing engagement.

Dimension of Diversity	Influence on Care Planning	Implications for Veterinary Technicians
Cultural and religious beliefs	May shape attitudes toward euthanasia, surgical interventions, or pain management strategies.	Respect and adapt care recommendations to align with client beliefs while ensuring animal welfare.
Socioeconomic status	Determines which diagnostic or treatment options are financially feasible for the client.	Offer tiered or alternative care plans that balance optimal treatment with financial limitations.
Language and health literacy	May require communication adjustments, use of visual aids, or translated resources to ensure understanding.	Ensure clarity and comprehension by tailoring communication methods to the client's needs.
Family structure	Influences the level of involvement different family members wish to have in daily care responsibilities.	Acknowledge varying roles in decision-making and include appropriate stakeholders in discussions.
Personal experiences with animals	Affects expectations for care, willingness to pursue certain treatments, or comfort with medical procedures.	Build trust by validating client experiences and tailoring nursing support to individual perspectives.

Source: Schaeffer (2025).

Case Study: Application in Veterinary Nursing (Figure 5.3)

Case Overview: A five-year-old MN Labrador Retriever presents with symptoms of lethargy, vomiting, and diarrhea. Upon assessment, the dog is diagnosed with acute gastroenteritis and moderate dehydration.

Nursing Evaluations:

1) Fluid volume deficit is related to vomiting and diarrhea.
2) Imbalanced nutrition: Less than body requirements related to decreased oral intake.

Planning Phase:

1) Goal Setting:
   - Restore fluid balance within 24 hours as evidenced by normal skin turgor, moist mucous membranes, and adequate urine output.
   - Improve nutritional status within 48 hours as evidenced by resumed interest in food.

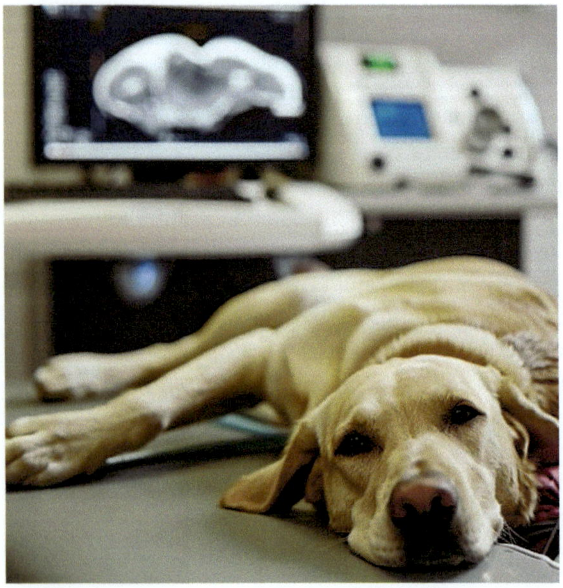

Figure 5.3 Labrador Retriever resting on exam table in a veterinary clinic. *Source:* StockCake / Public Domain.

2) Prioritizing Nursing Evaluations:
   - Address the fluid volume deficit first due to the immediate risk of severe dehydration.
   - Next, focus on balanced nutrition to ensure the patient's energy needs are met.
3) Selecting Evidence-based Interventions:
   - Independent Interventions:
     - Monitor vital signs every two hours.
     - Assess mucous membranes and skin turgor regularly.
     - Ensure IV catheter patency.
   - Dependent Interventions:
     - Administer intravenous fluids as ordered by the veterinarian.
     - Provide antiemetic medications as prescribed.
   - Collaborative Interventions:
     - Collaborate with a nutritionist or veterinarian in charge to develop a suitable diet plan for post-rehydration.
4) Documentation:
   - Document the patient's response to interventions, including fluid intake and output, changes in vital signs, and nutritional intake (Table 5.7).

Challenges in the Planning Phase

Addressing noncompliance requires first identifying and understanding its underlying causes, which may include lack of comprehension, cultural beliefs, or financial limitations. Rather than viewing noncompliance as resistance, veterinary technicians should approach it as an opportunity to adapt the plan to the client's reality. For example, if financial constraints prevent a client from pursuing the gold-standard diagnostic or treatment option, technicians can collaborate with the veterinarian to provide tiered alternatives, focusing on interventions that maximize benefit within the client's means. Similarly, if cultural or personal beliefs affect treatment choices—such as hesitancy about euthanasia, vaccination, or certain medications—technicians can respect those perspectives while providing education and support that aligns medical

Table 5.7 Nursing care plan for a dog with vomiting and diarrhea.

Nursing Diagnosis	Goals/Outcomes (SMART)	Nursing Interventions	Evaluation
Fluid volume deficit related to vomiting and diarrhea	Patient will maintain adequate hydration as evidenced by normal mucous membranes, capillary refill time <2s, and stable body weight within 24 hours.	Administer IV fluids as prescribed; monitor hydration parameters every two hours.	Hydration status maintained; mucous membranes pink/moist; stable body weight achieved.
Risk for electrolyte imbalance related to gastrointestinal losses	Electrolyte levels (Na, K, Cl) will remain within normal ranges on follow-up bloodwork within 24 hours.	Monitor electrolytes via bloodwork; report abnormalities; administer electrolyte supplements as ordered.	Electrolyte values remain stable within reference ranges.
Impaired comfort related to abdominal cramping and nausea	Patient will demonstrate improved comfort, with reduced signs of nausea and restlessness within 12 hours.	Administer antiemetics and analgesics as prescribed; provide a quiet, low-stress environment.	Patient appears comfortable, resting quietly, with minimal nausea behaviors observed.
Risk for malnutrition related to reduced food intake and nutrient loss	Patient will tolerate small, frequent meals or nutritional support within 48 hours.	Introduce an easily digestible diet once vomiting subsides; provide assisted feeding or a feeding tube as required.	Patient tolerates oral intake without vomiting; weight stabilized; improved energy observed.
Anxiety related to hospitalization and illness	Patient will demonstrate reduced signs of anxiety (settled posture, normal heart rate) within 12 hours.	Provide gentle handling, use pheromone therapy, minimize noise, and encourage owner visitation if possible.	Patient calm in kennel; HR normalized; minimal stress behaviors observed.

Source: Schaeffer (2025).

recommendations with the client's values. Adjusting the planning phase in this way transforms potential barriers into opportunities for collaboration and compliance.

Limited resources within the hospital can also challenge the feasibility of a care plan. When equipment, staff, or supplies are constrained, technicians must prioritize interventions based on immediacy, risk, and the potential for patient benefit. For instance, in an emergency or high-census setting, supportive measures such as oxygen therapy or analgesia may take precedence over nonurgent diagnostics. Resourcefulness—such as using alternative monitoring methods, adjusting nursing schedules, or delegating tasks—allows technicians to uphold patient safety and quality of care even in suboptimal circumstances.

Patient health conditions often change rapidly, especially in emergencies or critical care. This reality underscores the need for flexibility and frequent reassessment within the planning phase. Nursing care plans should never be static documents; rather, they are living frameworks that evolve alongside the patient's clinical status. A plan for a stable hospitalized patient may need to be completely restructured if the animal develops respiratory distress or acute decompensation. By integrating reassessment checkpoints and anticipating potential complications, technicians ensure that the plan remains responsive and relevant.

The planning phase, therefore, is not simply about outlining goals and interventions—it is about anticipating obstacles, adapting strategies, and aligning patient care with both medical priorities and client realities. By setting clear, measurable goals, prioritizing nursing evaluations, and integrating evidence-based interventions, technicians can directly influence patient outcomes. Effective planning requires collaboration with veterinarians and specialists, application of clinical guidelines, and meticulous documentation that communicates the evolving needs of the patient. When challenges such as noncompliance, resource limitations, and rapidly changing conditions are addressed proactively within the planning phase, veterinary technicians transform barriers into opportunities to advocate for their patients, ensuring that high-quality, patient-centered care remains achievable under even the most difficult circumstances.

Executing the Care Plan in Veterinary Nursing

Implementation Phase

The implementation phase in veterinary nursing is where planned interventions, based on a comprehensive care plan, are executed. This step is crucial as it involves not only the application of therapeutic measures but also the ongoing assessment of the patient's response to these interventions. The primary goal is to ensure that the patient receives the best possible care to facilitate recovery or manage chronic conditions effectively.

Equally important is the veterinary technician's observational role during implementation. Every intervention—whether administering medication, initiating oxygen therapy, providing nutritional support, or applying wound management techniques—presents an opportunity to gather clinical data in real time. Subtle changes such as alterations in respiratory pattern, mucous membrane color, pain behaviors, posture, vocalizations, or even the patient's willingness to eat and interact can signal either positive progress or early signs of clinical decline.

These observations serve as a guide for adaptive decision-making within the care plan. For instance, if a patient receiving fluid therapy exhibits serous nasal discharge, restlessness, or increased respiratory effort, the technician's careful monitoring may identify early fluid overload, prompting reassessment before a more severe complication occurs. Conversely, noting improved mentation, increased activity, or normalized vital parameters provides evidence that interventions are effective and should be continued. Beyond physical parameters, veterinary technicians also play a pivotal role in behavioral and emotional assessment, recognizing signs of stress, anxiety, or discomfort that may not be immediately apparent to others on the healthcare team. Such findings help guide modifications in handling techniques, analgesia protocols, or environmental enrichment strategies to optimize patient welfare. Ultimately, the veterinary technician's observations bridge planning and evaluation—functioning as a feedback loop that ensures interventions remain appropriate, effective, and patient-centered. By documenting these findings thoroughly and communicating them to the veterinary team, technicians uphold the integrity of the nursing process, transforming the implementation phase into a dynamic and responsive aspect of clinical care.

One of the core responsibilities during this phase is the precise administration of medications. This includes oral, topical, or injectable forms, adhering strictly to prescribed dosages and schedules. Veterinary technicians must understand pharmacokinetics and pharmacodynamics to anticipate potential side effects and interactions, ensuring safe and effective medication administration. Wound management is another critical intervention. It involves cleaning, debriding, dressing, and monitoring wounds for signs of infection or delayed healing. The technician must utilize aseptic techniques to prevent contamination and facilitate optimal healing conditions. For patients requiring rehabilitation, veterinary technicians assist with physical therapy. This may include passive range of motion exercises, hydrotherapy, and other modalities designed to restore function and mobility. Knowledge of musculoskeletal anatomy and the pathophysiology of the condition being treated is essential for effective therapy.

Continuous monitoring of vital signs (e.g., temperature, heart rate, respiratory rate, blood pressure) is paramount. These metrics provide immediate insights into the patient's physiological status, allowing for rapid intervention if abnormalities are detected. This monitoring should be systematic and frequent, especially in critically ill or postoperative patients. Continuous monitoring involves vigilant observation of the patient's clinical status. Veterinary technicians must be adept at recognizing subtle changes in behavior, appetite, activity level, and other indicators that may signal improvement or deterioration. This requires a thorough understanding of the species-specific normal ranges and clinical signs. Accurate and comprehensive documentation is essential. Every intervention, observation, and patient response must be meticulously recorded in the patient's medical record. This documentation serves multiple purposes: it ensures continuity of care, supports clinical decision-making, facilitates communication among the veterinary team, and provides a legal record of the care provided.

A significant aspect of the implementation phase is educating pet owners. Veterinary technicians must communicate complex medical information in an accessible manner, ensuring owners understand the animal's condition, treatment plan, and home care requirements. This education includes demonstrating techniques (e.g., administering medications, wound care), providing written instructions, and addressing any questions or concerns. Effective education is linked to owner compliance and, consequently, to the patient's recovery. Veterinary technicians should employ strategies to enhance understanding and retention of information, such as using visual aids, providing hands-on training, and ensuring follow-up communication.

The implementation phase in veterinary nursing is a dynamic and critical component of patient care. It involves executing planned interventions with precision, continuously monitoring patient responses, and maintaining detailed documentation. Additionally, veterinary technicians play a pivotal role in educating pet owners, ensuring they are equipped to continue care at home.

Observation Phase in Veterinary Nursing

The observation phase represents the culmination of the nursing process, serving as a critical juncture where the efficacy of nursing interventions is systematically reviewed (Orpet and Welsh 2011). This phase is essential for ensuring that the patient's care is continuously optimized and adjusted according to their progress and changing needs.

Assessing Outcomes

During observation, the veterinary technician rigorously compares the patient's current status against the predetermined goals set in the planning phase. This involves a comprehensive reassessment through physical examinations, nursing evaluations, meticulous monitoring of vital signs, and a thorough review of diagnostic test results. The technician must critically appraise whether the goals have been fully met, partially met, or not met. When goals are achieved, nursing interventions are deemed effective. The care plan can be updated to focus on maintaining the positive outcomes or addressing any new or residual issues. This involves setting new goals or reinforcing successful interventions to ensure sustained health and well-being. For goals that are only partially met or not met, the technician must engage in a detailed analysis to identify contributing factors. This may include identifying barriers that impeded progress, such as patient compliance, environmental factors, or unforeseen complications; evaluating the appropriateness and execution of the interventions to ascertain if they were correctly implemented and suitable for the patient's condition. The technician should also take into consideration any changes in the patient's condition that could have influenced the outcomes, such as disease progression, comorbidities, or new health issues.

Revising the Care Plan

Based on the findings from the observation, the care plan may need significant revisions. This is a dynamic and ongoing process aimed at ensuring the care remains aligned with the patient's current needs and promotes the best possible outcomes. Nursing evaluations must be revisited and potentially revised to reflect the current health status and any new insights gained during the observation. Accurate and updated evaluations are crucial for guiding subsequent care. Goals should be adjusted to be realistic and attainable, considering the patient's progress and any new challenges. This may involve setting incremental goals to address complex issues gradually. Interventions must be tailored to better meet the revised goals. This could include introducing new treatments, altering dosages or frequencies of medications, incorporating different therapeutic modalities, or intensifying monitoring protocols.

The observation phase in veterinary nursing is pivotal for determining the effectiveness of nursing interventions and ensuring the patient's care remains appropriate and effective. Through systematic assessment and dynamic adjustment of the care plan, veterinary technicians play a crucial role in promoting optimal health outcomes and adapting to the evolving needs of their patients. This phase underscores the importance of evidence-based practice, critical thinking, and a commitment to continuous improvement in the field of veterinary nursing.

Nursing Care Models in Veterinary Intensive Care Units

In the realm of veterinary nursing, particularly within intensive care units (ICUs), the approach to patient management is crucial for achieving optimal outcomes. Traditional nursing care plans provide a structured framework for individual patient care, but the dynamic and high-pressure environment of an ICU necessitates more flexible and holistic approaches. This has led to the adaptation and adoption of various nursing care models that better align with the complexities of veterinary critical care. These models offer a structured yet adaptable framework that can be tailored to meet the specific needs of each patient.

The primary distinction between traditional nursing care plans and nursing care models lies in their structure and flexibility. Nursing care plans are highly structured and individualized, focusing on detailed documentation and step-by-step execution. In contrast, nursing care models offer more fluid frameworks that can be adapted to the needs of multiple patients simultaneously, often emphasizing teamwork, resource allocation, and patient engagement. In the ICU setting, where conditions can change rapidly, the adaptability and efficiency offered by nursing care models can enhance patient outcomes and improve the overall quality of care. These models encourage collaboration, utilize the diverse skills of the nursing team, and allow for a more rapid response to patient needs. However, they also necessitate robust communication channels, effective leadership, and ongoing observation to ensure consistency and continuity of care.

At the heart of both nursing care plans and nursing care models is the delicate balance of art and science that defines veterinary nursing. The science lies in the evidence-based frameworks, protocols, and clinical knowledge that guide interventions—calculating fluid rates, titrating analgesics, or applying mechanical ventilation settings with precision. The art, however, emerges in the nuanced interpretation of patient signals and the technician's ability to translate objective data into compassionate, individualized care. For example, while monitoring an ICU patient's oxygen saturation is a scientific act, recognizing the subtle behavioral cues of anxiety and adjusting handling techniques to reduce stress reflects the artistry of nursing practice.

This blend becomes especially important in critical care environments. The science ensures safety, accuracy, and consistency, while the art enables flexibility, empathy, and patient advocacy. A nursing care plan without the artistry of observation and interpretation risks becoming rigid and impersonal, while a model applied without scientific rigor risks inconsistency and error. When combined, art and science produce a dynamic approach that not only maintains clinical standards but also elevates the patient experience, ensuring both medical excellence and humane, compassionate care.

Nursing care models provide a more flexible and holistic approach to patient management. These models emphasize adaptability and responsiveness, making them particularly suited for the dynamic environment of veterinary ICUs. Several prominent nursing care models that have been adapted to veterinary medicine include the *Roper, Logan, and Tierney's Model of Nursing, Orem's Model of Self-care,* and the *Orpet and Jeffery Ability Model.*

Roper, Logan, and Tierney's Model of Nursing

The Roper, Logan, and Tierney (RLT) Model of Nursing is a prominent theoretical framework that has been widely adopted in nursing practice. Initially developed by Nancy Roper, Winifred W. Logan, and Alison J. Tierney, this model provides a systematic approach to patient care by focusing on the essential activities of living. It has been adapted for various healthcare contexts, including veterinary nursing, particularly within intensive care units (Roper et al. 2000; Orpet and Welsh 2011).

The RLT Model is grounded in the concept of the activities of living, which are fundamental behaviors that maintain life and promote well-being. This model is underpinned by several key concepts:

1) **Activities of Living (ALs)**: These are the core components of the model, encompassing the daily functions necessary for health and survival.
2) **Lifespan**: This dimension recognizes that an individual's ability to perform ALs changes throughout different stages of life.
3) **Dependence/Independence Continuum**: This continuum acknowledges the varying degrees of dependence and independence individuals experience in performing ALs.
4) **Factors Influencing ALs**: These include biological, psychological, sociocultural, environmental, and politico-economic factors that affect an individual's ability to perform ALs.

The 12 Activities of Living

The RLT Model identifies 12 essential activities of living, which form the basis of patient assessment and care planning:

1) **Maintaining a Safe Environment**: Ensuring the patient is protected from harm and environmental hazards.
2) **Communicating**: Facilitating effective communication to express needs and interact with others.
3) **Breathing**: Managing respiratory function to ensure adequate oxygenation.
4) **Eating and Drinking**: Ensuring nutritional and hydration needs are met.
5) **Eliminating**: Managing excretion processes to maintain homeostasis.
6) **Personal Cleansing and Dressing**: Maintaining hygiene and personal appearance.
7) **Controlling Body Temperature**: Regulating temperature to ensure comfort and prevent hyperthermia or hypothermia.
8) **Mobilizing**: Ensuring the ability to move and maintain physical activity.
9) **Working and Playing**: Balancing occupational and recreational activities.
10) **Sleeping**: Managing rest and sleep patterns to promote recovery and well-being.
11) **Expressing Sexuality**: Recognizing and addressing sexual health and expression.
12) **Dying**: Providing end-of-life care that respects the individual's dignity and comfort.

Application for Veterinary Nursing

In the context of veterinary nursing, particularly in ICUs, the RLT Model can be adapted to assess and address the needs of animal patients. The model's holistic approach ensures comprehensive care that considers all aspects of the animal's well-being.

Example: Application to a Veterinary ICU Patient

Patient: A five-year-old male Labrador Retriever admitted for postoperative care following an orthopedic surgery.

Assessment Using the 12 Activities of Living:

1) **Maintaining a Safe Environment**: Ensure the kennel is secure and free from hazards. Monitor for signs of pain or distress.
2) **Communicating**: Observe vocalizations and body language to assess pain levels and comfort. Use gentle handling and verbal reassurance.
3) **Breathing**: Monitor respiratory rate and effort. Provide supplemental oxygen if needed.
4) **Eating and Drinking**: Assess nutritional intake and hydration status. Administer a balanced diet and fluids, considering any dietary restrictions.
5) **Eliminating**: Monitor urine and fecal output. Ensure the patient can eliminate comfortably, using assistance if necessary.
6) **Personal Cleansing and Dressing**: Keep the surgical site clean and dry. Provide regular grooming to maintain hygiene.
7) **Controlling Body Temperature**: Monitor body temperature and provide blankets or cooling measures as needed.

Table 5.8 Adaptation of Roper, Logan, and Tierney's nursing model to a postoperative orthopedic canine patient.

Activity of Daily Living (ADL)	Considerations for Post-Op Ortho Dog	Nursing Interventions
Maintaining a safe environment	Restricted mobility; risk of slipping, falls, or damaging the surgical site	Confine to a kennel or small padded area; use non-slip flooring; monitor for chewing/licking incision; use E-collar if needed
Communicating	Dogs communicate pain, stress, or needs via behavior (whining, restlessness, vocalizing)	Observe for pain signals, anxiety; provide comfort; update caregivers about progress
Breathing	Post-anesthesia respiratory depression; risk of hypoventilation due to analgesics	Monitor RR, effort, SpO_2; provide oxygen if indicated; ensure patient is positioned to optimize breathing
Eating and drinking	Appetite may be reduced due to anesthesia, pain, or opioids; hydration is important for healing	Offer small palatable meals; monitor water intake; consider syringe feeding if needed; IV fluids if anorexic
Eliminating	Pain and immobility may affect the ability to posture for urination/defecation	Take outside with sling support; monitor for urinary retention/ constipation; provide absorbent bedding if incontinent
Personal cleansing and dressing	Incision hygiene is critical; patient may attempt to lick or soil wound	Clean incision as directed; bandage changes PRN; prevent self-trauma with E-collar or bandaging
Controlling body temperature	Anesthesia can impair thermoregulation; orthopedic procedures often prolonged	Provide warming blankets post-op; monitor temperature closely; avoid overheating
Mobilizing	Restricted weight-bearing; pain limits mobility; risk of implant failure	Support with a sling or harness; restrict exercise to leash walks for elimination only; physiotherapy as indicated
Working and playing	Activity curtailed; frustration possible if the dog is normally active	Provide enrichment (safe chew toys, stuffed Kongs); gentle mental stimulation while confined
Expressing sexuality	Not directly relevant unless intact; stress or frustration may influence behavior	Monitor for mounting or overexcitement that may compromise healing
Sleeping	Pain, stress, or environment may disrupt rest	Provide quiet, comfortable bedding; administer analgesics at regular intervals; maintain routine sleep cycles
Dying	Not directly relevant to elective ortho surgery, but always consider complications	Monitor for complications (infection, implant failure, thromboembolism); prepare for discussions with caregivers if prognosis changes

Source: Schaeffer (2025), Roper et al. (2000).

8) **Mobilizing**: Implement a physiotherapy plan to promote mobility and prevent complications such as muscle atrophy.
9) **Working and Playing**: Provide mental stimulation through toys and interaction to prevent boredom and promote recovery.
10) **Sleeping**: Ensure a quiet and comfortable environment to facilitate rest and recovery.
11) **Expressing Sexuality**: Address any behavioral changes related to the patient's reproductive status, if applicable.
12) **Dying**: If end-of-life care is necessary, provide palliative care that prioritizes comfort and dignity (Table 5.8).

Care Planning and Implementation

Based on the assessment, a comprehensive care plan is developed, outlining specific nursing interventions for each activity of living. For example, the care plan may include administering pain medication and monitoring its effectiveness; providing a specific diet to meet nutritional needs and monitoring intake; implementing a postoperative physiotherapy regimen and ensuring regular grooming and hygiene maintenance. The effectiveness of the care plan is evaluated through continuous reassessment of the patient's condition and abilities. Adjustments to the care plan are made as necessary to address any changes in the patient's needs or responses to interventions.

Influencing Factors

Several factors can influence the ability of veterinary patients to perform the activities of living, including biological factors such as age, breed, genetic predispositions, and medical history. Psychological factors might include stress, anxiety, and

Table 5.9 Influencing factors on the ability of veterinary patients to perform activities of living, adapted to the ICU setting.

Factor	Description in Veterinary Context	Examples/Clinical Relevance
Biological factors	Innate and physical characteristics of the animal that influence ability to perform ADLs	Age (puppy vs. geriatric), breed predispositions (brachycephalic airway syndrome, hip dysplasia), genetic disorders, prior medical history, concurrent diseases (e.g., CKD, heart disease)
Psychological factors	Mental, emotional, and behavioral responses to illness, injury, and hospitalization	Stress from ICU confinement, anxiety from separation, aggression or withdrawal, altered behavior due to pain or sedatives
Sociological factors	Relationship between patient and owner, and impact of social dynamics on care	Level of owner involvement in nursing care, compliance with treatment plans, frequency of visitation, and presence of family dynamics influencing decision-making
Environmental factors	External surroundings and conditions that impact patient comfort, recovery, and safety	ICU noise levels (alarms, barking), lighting cycles (circadian disruption), kennel size and bedding, temperature control, exposure to other patients
Politico-economic factors	Influence of financial, political, and systemic structures on the delivery of veterinary care	Owner's financial resources for diagnostics/surgery, insurance status, availability of advanced care (ventilation, dialysis), and hospital policies shaped by economics

Adapted from the Roper, Logan, and Tierney Nursing Model, this chart outlines the key factors that influence the ability of veterinary patients to perform the activities of living, with emphasis on ICU and critical care contexts.
Source: Schaeffer (2025).

behavioral responses to illness or injury. Sociological factors are often associated with the relationship between the animal and its owner, and cultural attitudes toward veterinary care. Environmental factors include the physical environment of the ICU, including noise levels, lighting, and kennel conditions. We also cannot forget that politico-economic factors or the financial resources available for veterinary care and the impact of economic constraints on the provision of services. The Roper, Logan, and Tierney Model of Nursing provides a comprehensive and holistic framework for assessing and addressing the needs of patients. Its adaptation to veterinary nursing, particularly in the ICU setting, ensures that care is thorough, patient-centered, and responsive to the complex needs of critically ill animals. By focusing on the 12 activities of living, veterinary technicians can deliver high-quality care that promotes recovery, well-being, and overall health outcomes for their patients (Table 5.9).

Orem's Model of Self-care

Orem's Model of Self-care, developed by Dorothea Orem, is a hallmark of human nursing theory that emphasizes the role of the patient in maintaining their own health and well-being (Orem 2001). This model is based on the premise that individuals can recover more effectively if they are encouraged to be as independent as possible in their own care. Although initially designed for human nursing, Orem's Model has been adapted to veterinary care, where the principles of self-care are applied to animals with the support of veterinary professionals.

Orem's Model of Self-care consists of three interrelated theories: *Theory of Self-care, Theory of Self-care Deficit,* and *Theory of Nursing Systems* (Orem 2001). *The theory of Self-Care* posits that individuals can perform activities that maintain their own health and well-being. These activities are referred to as self-care activities or self-care requisites. The *theory of Self-care Deficit* identifies when nursing intervention is needed. It occurs when individuals cannot meet their own self-care needs due to limitations imposed by illness or injury. The *theory of Nursing Systems* outlines the ways in which nursing can support self-care. It includes wholly compensatory, partly compensatory, and supportive-educative systems, depending on the patient's ability to participate in their own care (Table 5.10) (Orem 2001).

Self-care Requisites

Orem identifies three categories of self-care requisites:

1) **Universal Self-care Requisites**: These are common to all individuals and include:
   - Maintenance of sufficient intake of air, water, and food.
   - Provision of care associated with elimination processes.
   - Maintenance of balance between activity and rest, and between solitude and social interaction.

Table 5.10 Summary of Orem's model of self-care.

Component	Description	Application/Example
Theory of self-care	Individuals perform activities (self-care requisites) to maintain their own health and well-being	A person eating a balanced diet, exercising, and adhering to medication to prevent illness
Theory of self-care deficit	Nursing is required when an individual cannot meet their self-care needs due to illness, injury, or limitations	Post-surgical patient unable to bathe or administer their own medication requires nursing support
Theory of nursing systems	Framework for how nursing care is delivered to address self-care deficits. Includes three systems:	
→ Wholly compensatory	The nurse provides total care when the patient is unable to perform any self-care	Unconscious or anesthetized patient
→ Partly compensatory	Nurse and patient share responsibility for self-care activities	Patient is able to feed self with assistance, but the nurse provides mobility support
→ Supportive-educative	A nurse's role is primarily to teach, guide, and support patients to perform self-care independently	Diabetic education on insulin administration and diet management

Orem's Model of Self-care consists of three interrelated theories: Theory of Self-care, Theory of Self-care Deficit, and Theory of Nursing Systems (Orem 2001). The chart below provides a summary.
Source: Adapted from Orem (2001).

- Prevention of hazards to human life, functioning, and well-being.
- Promotion of human functioning and development within social groups.

2) **Developmental Self-care Requisites**: These are associated with developmental processes and events, such as adapting to changes over the lifespan or to life situations.
3) **Health Deviation Self-care Requisites**: These arise from conditions of illness, injury, or disease and include seeking and securing appropriate medical assistance, carrying out prescribed medical regimens, and learning to live with the effects of illness or disability.

Application for Veterinary Nursing

In veterinary nursing, Orem's principles can be adapted to assess and address the self-care capabilities of animals. The focus shifts to the nursing care required to support the animal's health, given that animals cannot perform self-care activities independently without assistance.

Example: Application to a Veterinary ICU Patient

Patient: A four-year-old female Golden Retriever diagnosed with acute pancreatitis.

Assessment Using Orem's Self-care Model:

1) **Universal Self-care Requisites**:
   - **Air**: Ensure the patient has an unobstructed airway and receives supplemental oxygen if needed.
   - **Water and Food**: Monitor and manage fluid therapy to maintain hydration. Adjust diet to a low-fat, easily digestible food appropriate for pancreatitis.
   - **Elimination**: Monitor urinary and fecal output to ensure normal elimination patterns.
   - **Activity and Rest**: Encourage limited, controlled activity to prevent stress on the pancreas while ensuring adequate rest.
   - **Hazard Prevention**: Prevent exposure to potential hazards such as infections or additional stressors.
   - **Functioning and Development**: Support normal functioning through regular monitoring and adjustments to care based on the patient's condition.

2) **Developmental Self-care Requisites**:
   - **Adaptation to Illness**: Assist the animal in adapting to the illness through environmental modifications and supportive care.
   - **Owner Education**: Educate the owner on the condition and how to manage it at home post-discharge.
3) **Health Deviation Self-care Requisites**:
   - **Medical Assistance**: Ensure the patient receives appropriate medical treatments and medications as prescribed.
   - **Medical Regimens**: Administer prescribed medications and treatments consistently and monitor their effects.
   - **Living with Illness**: Provide supportive care to manage symptoms and improve the quality of life during recovery.

Nursing Systems

Depending on the patient's condition and self-care deficit, different nursing systems are applied:

1) **Wholly Compensatory System**:
   - The technician performs all necessary care activities as the patient is unable to participate in their own care. This includes administering medications, providing nutritional support, and performing all hygiene and mobility tasks.
2) **Partly Compensatory System**:
   - The technician and the patient share responsibilities for care activities. For instance, the technician may assist the animal with feeding or mobility, but the animal is encouraged to engage in activities as much as possible.
3) **Supportive-educative System**:
   - The technician provides guidance and support to the owner of the animal, educating them on how to care for their pet at home. This includes teaching about medication administration, dietary management, and recognizing signs of complications (Table 5.11).

Care Planning and Implementation

Based on the assessment, a comprehensive care plan is developed. For example:

- **Hydration Management**: Administer IV fluids and monitor hydration status regularly.
- **Nutritional Support**: Provide a prescribed diet and monitor food intake.
- **Symptom Management**: Administer pain relief and anti-nausea medications as needed.
- **Activity Regulation**: Implement a schedule for controlled activity and rest periods.

Table 5.11 Orem's nursing model applied to a canine patient with pancreatitis.

Component	Description	Veterinary Application—Dog with Pancreatitis
Theory of self-care	Patients (or their caregivers) perform activities that maintain health and well-being	Normally, the dog self-regulates eating, drinking, activity, and elimination. The owner provides balanced nutrition and preventive care.
Theory of self-care deficit	Nursing is needed when the patient cannot meet its own self-care needs due to illness or injury	During acute pancreatitis, the dog cannot eat/drink due to nausea, vomiting, and pain. The owner cannot meet care needs at home → requires hospitalization and nursing interventions.
Theory of nursing systems	Defines how nursing compensates for self-care deficits	Wholly Compensatory: ICU nurses provide IV fluids, analgesia, antiemetics, nutritional support (feeding tubes), and hygiene. The dog is fully dependent.
		Partly Compensatory: As vomiting resolves, the dog begins to take small amounts of water or bland food; nurses assist and monitor tolerance.
		Supportive-educative: Nurses educate the owner on dietary management (low-fat prescription diet), long-term monitoring, and preventing recurrence once discharged.

This chart applies Orem's Model of Self-care to a canine patient with pancreatitis, illustrating the three interrelated theories (Self-care, Self-care Deficit, and Nursing Systems) within a veterinary nursing context.
Source: Schaeffer (2025).

The care plan's effectiveness is evaluated through ongoing reassessment of the patient's condition and abilities. Improvements in hydration, nutritional status, pain levels, and overall well-being indicate successful interventions. If goals are not met, the care plan is adjusted accordingly. Several factors can influence the ability of veterinary patients to achieve self-care requisites. These identified factors include biological (species, age, breed, and genetic predispositions); psychological (stress, anxiety, and behavioral responses to illness or injury); sociocultural factors such as the animal's role in the household, owner's beliefs, and cultural attitudes toward veterinary care; environmental factors such as the physical environment of the ICU, including noise levels, lighting, and kennel conditions. In conjunction with politico-economic factors. This may include financial resources available for veterinary care and the impact of economic constraints on the provision of services. Importantly, these same categories of influencing factors are also reflected in established nursing theories. This mirrors the Roper-Logan-Tierney theory of nursing, which similarly incorporates these domains into its assessment framework. By aligning with these human nursing models, veterinary nursing acknowledges that the multifactorial nature of care applies equally to animal patients, reinforcing a holistic approach to practice.

Orem's Model of Self-care provides a robust framework for nursing practice that emphasizes patient independence and participation in their own care. Its adaptation to veterinary nursing allows for a comprehensive and holistic approach to patient management, particularly in ICU settings. By focusing on the self-care requisites and addressing self-care deficits, veterinary technicians can deliver high-quality care that promotes recovery, well-being, and overall health outcomes for their patients.

The Orpet and Jeffery Ability Model

The Orpet and Jeffery Ability Model (OJAM) is a veterinary-specific adaptation of human nursing models, designed to address the unique needs of animal patients (Orpet and Jeffery 2007). This model, developed by Sue Orpet and Cecelia Jeffery, is grounded in the principles of holistic care and provides a comprehensive framework for assessing and managing veterinary patients, particularly in intensive care settings. OJAM emphasizes the abilities of animals to perform essential functions, ensuring that nursing care is tailored to their specific needs. This is the author's chosen model for veterinary nursing, as it demonstrates a high degree of adaptability to the diverse and often complex needs of animal patients, making it especially suitable for clinical practice across a range of species and conditions.

The OJAM was influenced by existing human nursing models, particularly the Roper, Logan, and Tierney (RLT) Model and Orem's Model of Self-care. It focuses on evaluating the animal's abilities in key areas necessary for maintaining health and well-being. The model's primary components include:

1) **Assessment of Abilities**: Evaluating the animal's capabilities in various functional areas.
2) **Identification of Inabilities**: Recognizing deficits in abilities that require nursing intervention.
3) **Development of a Care Plan**: Formulating a comprehensive care plan based on the assessment.
4) **Implementation of Care**: Delivering appropriate nursing interventions to support and enhance the animal's abilities.
5) **Observation**: Continuously reassessing the animal's condition to determine the effectiveness of the care plan and adjusting as needed.

The 10 Abilities

OJAM identifies 10 essential abilities that are critical for the health and functioning of animal patients. These abilities serve as the foundation for assessment and care planning:

1) **Eating**: The ability to ingest and digest food to meet nutritional needs.
2) **Drinking**: The ability to consume adequate fluids to maintain hydration.
3) **Urination**: The ability to eliminate urine effectively.
4) **Defecation**: The ability to eliminate feces effectively.
5) **Breathing**: The ability to maintain adequate respiratory function.
6) **Maintaining Body Temperature**: The ability to regulate body temperature within a normal range.
7) **Grooming**: The ability to maintain personal hygiene and grooming behaviors.
8) **Mobilization**: The ability to move and perform physical activities.
9) **Sleeping**: The ability to rest and achieve adequate sleep.
10) **Expressing Normal Behavior**: The ability to exhibit behaviors typical of the species and individual animal.

Application for Veterinary Nursing

OJAM is particularly valuable in veterinary intensive care units, where comprehensive and systematic assessments are crucial for managing critically ill patients. The model's holistic approach ensures that all aspects of the animal's health and well-being are considered.

Example: Application to a Veterinary ICU Patient

Patient: A seven-year-old male German Shepherd Dog admitted with severe trauma following a road traffic accident.

Assessment Using OJAM:

1) **Eating**: Assess the animal's ability to eat independently. Determine if assistance with feeding or enteral nutrition is required.
2) **Drinking**: Evaluate hydration status and the animal's ability to drink. Administer intravenous fluids if necessary.
3) **Urination**: Monitor urinary output and ensure the patient can urinate without obstruction. Catheterize if necessary.
4) **Defecation**: Observe for regular bowel movements and assess for any signs of constipation or diarrhea.
5) **Breathing**: Monitor respiratory rate and effort. Provide supplemental oxygen or mechanical ventilation if needed.
6) **Maintaining Body Temperature**: Check body temperature regularly and use warming or cooling devices to maintain normothermia.
7) **Grooming**: Perform regular grooming to maintain hygiene and comfort, especially if the patient is immobilized.
8) **Mobilization**: Assess mobility and implement a physiotherapy plan to prevent complications from immobility.
9) **Sleeping**: Ensure a quiet and comfortable environment to facilitate rest and recovery.
10) **Expressing Normal Behavior**: Provide opportunities for the animal to exhibit natural behaviors, such as chewing or playing, as appropriate for their condition.

Care Planning and Implementation

Based on the assessment, a detailed care plan is developed. For example:

- **Nutritional Support**: Provide a balanced diet through assisted feeding or a feeding tube.
- **Hydration Management**: Administer IV fluids and monitor for signs of dehydration or fluid overload.
- **Respiratory Support**: Use oxygen therapy and monitor blood gases to ensure adequate oxygenation.
- **Temperature Regulation**: Use thermal blankets or cooling pads to maintain a stable body temperature.
- **Physiotherapy**: Implement passive range-of-motion exercises and encourage controlled movement to prevent muscle atrophy and joint stiffness (Table 5.12).

The effectiveness of the care plan is evaluated through continuous monitoring and reassessment of the animal's abilities. Improvements in nutritional status, hydration, respiratory function, and mobility indicate successful interventions. If goals are not met, the care plan is adjusted accordingly to address any ongoing issues.

The Orpet and Jeffery Ability Model provides a structured and holistic approach to veterinary nursing, particularly in intensive care settings. By focusing on the animal's abilities and addressing deficits through comprehensive care planning, veterinary technicians can deliver high-quality care that promotes recovery and well-being. OJAM's emphasis on continuous assessment and individualized care ensures that each patient's unique needs are met, resulting in better health outcomes and improved quality of life for veterinary patients (Orpet and Jeffery 2007).

Nursing care models offer a structured yet adaptable approach to patient management in veterinary ICUs. By utilizing models such as the Orpet and Jeffery Ability Model, veterinary technicians can deliver comprehensive, patient-centered care that addresses the unique needs of each animal. These models facilitate effective communication, continuity of care, and improved patient outcomes, ultimately enhancing the quality of veterinary nursing practice. In the intensive care setting, the environment itself can feel overwhelming—both for patients and for the veterinary team. Constant monitoring demands, the acuity of cases, and the unpredictable nature of critical illness create a high-pressure atmosphere. A structured nursing care model provides a framework to organize interventions, prioritize needs, and ensure that essential aspects of care are not overlooked amidst the complexity. This structure not only supports patient safety and well-being but also promotes technician confidence and resilience by offering clarity and direction in otherwise chaotic circumstances.

Table 5.12 Orpet and Jeffery Ability Model applied to a canine patient with traumatic injuries following a road traffic accident.

Ability	Description	Veterinary Nursing Application—Dog with Traumatic Injuries
Eating	Ability to ingest and process food	The dog may be anorexic due to pain, shock, or trauma; NPO initially until stabilized; nutritional support (IV fluids, feeding tube) may be required
Drinking	Ability to maintain hydration	May be unable/unwilling to drink due to pain; IV fluid therapy critical; monitor hydration via skin turgor, mucous membranes, and urine output
Urinating	Ability to eliminate urine	Trauma may cause bladder rupture or urethral obstruction; urinary catheterization or cystocentesis may be required; strict monitoring of urine output
Defecating	Ability to eliminate feces	Pelvic fractures or neurological injury may impair defecation; stool softeners/enemas PRN; nursing to maintain hygiene and prevent soiling wounds
Breathing	Ability to ventilate and oxygenate	Thoracic trauma may cause pneumothorax, pulmonary contusions; oxygen therapy, thoracocentesis, and close monitoring of respiratory effort
Maintaining Body Temperature	Thermoregulation capacity	Shock and anesthesia predispose to hypothermia; provide warming devices (Bair Hugger, warm IV fluids); monitor closely
Mobilizing	Ability to move and ambulate	Orthopedic and soft tissue trauma impairs movement; strict cage rest, slings/harnesses for support, analgesia to facilitate physiotherapy
Sleeping	Ability to rest and recover	Pain and hospital environment disrupt sleep; provide analgesia, quiet environment, soft bedding
Grooming	Ability to maintain cleanliness	Dog unable to groom; nurses provide hygiene, wound care, clipping, and cleaning around wounds/incisions
Expressing normal behavior	Ability to express species-typical behaviors	Hospitalization and pain limit behavior; enrichment (safe chew toys, gentle handling), owner visits if safe; nursing staff provide reassurance and comfort

This chart applies the Orpet and Jeffery Ability Model (2007) to a canine patient with traumatic injuries after being hit by a car, illustrating the 10 abilities in a veterinary nursing context.
Source: Schaeffer (2025).

Ethical and Legal Considerations

Ethical and legal considerations underpin every phase of the nursing process. Veterinary technicians must adhere to professional standards and codes of ethics, which include principles such as beneficence (doing good), non-maleficence (doing no harm), autonomy (respecting the pet owner's rights and decisions), and justice (providing fair and equal care). Legal considerations involve practicing within the scope of professional regulations, maintaining accurate and confidential patient records, and obtaining informed consent for procedures and treatments.

Conclusion

The domain of veterinary nursing is characterized by its complex, multifaceted nature, requiring a thorough understanding of both clinical and theoretical aspects to provide optimal patient care. The integration of nursing care plans and nursing care models into veterinary practice represents a critical advancement in the systematic and holistic management of animal patients. These frameworks, derived and adapted from human nursing principles, underscore the importance of a structured approach to veterinary nursing, ensuring that each patient receives individualized and comprehensive care.

Nursing care plans are instrumental in organizing and prioritizing patient care activities. They provide a detailed roadmap that guides veterinary technicians through the assessment, evaluation, planning, implementation, and observation phases of patient care. This systematic approach ensures that all aspects of the patient's health and well-being are addressed, from immediate medical needs to long-term recovery and quality of life. At the heart of the nursing care plan is the initial patient assessment, which gathers crucial information about the animal's medical history, current health status, and specific needs.

This assessment forms the basis for identifying nursing evaluations, which pinpoint the patient's health problems and potential complications. By establishing these evaluations, veterinary technicians can formulate targeted interventions aimed at addressing the identified issues. The planning phase involves setting measurable, realistic goals for the patient's care. These goals provide clear benchmarks for evaluating the effectiveness of nursing interventions. Implementation entails carrying out the planned interventions, which may range from administering medications and performing medical procedures to providing nutritional support and engaging in rehabilitative exercises. Throughout this process, the nursing care plan serves as a dynamic document, continually updated to reflect changes in the patient's condition and responses to treatment. The observation phase is crucial for assessing the outcomes of nursing interventions. By comparing the patient's status with the established goals, veterinary technicians can determine the success of their care strategies and make necessary adjustments. This continuous feedback loop ensures that patient care is both effective and responsive to the animal's evolving needs.

Nursing care models provide a theoretical framework that enhances the nursing care plan by offering structured methodologies for patient assessment and intervention. These models, while originally designed for human nursing, have been effectively adapted to the veterinary context, providing a comprehensive approach to animal care. Roper, Logan, and Tierney's Model of Nursing, for instance, focuses on the 12 activities of living, which are essential for maintaining health. This model encourages veterinary technicians to assess the patient's ability to perform these activities and identify areas where nursing intervention is required. The holistic nature of this model ensures that all aspects of the patient's life, from physiological needs to psychological well-being, are considered in the care plan. Orem's Model of Self-care emphasizes the patient's role in maintaining their own health. Adapted for veterinary use, this model helps identify the animal's self-care deficits and guides the formulation of interventions to address these gaps. By promoting the concept of self-care, Orem's model encourages a collaborative approach to patient care, involving both the veterinary team and the pet owner in the recovery process. The Orpet and Jeffery Ability Model (OJAM) is a veterinary-specific model that builds on the principles of human nursing models to create a comprehensive framework for animal care. OJAM focuses on assessing the animal's abilities across ten essential domains, such as eating, drinking, grooming, and expressing normal behavior. This model provides a structured approach to identifying and addressing the patient's needs, ensuring that all aspects of their health and well-being are considered.

Throughout the care process, the nursing care plan serves as a living document, continuously updated to reflect the patient's progress and evolving needs. Regular evaluations ensure that the interventions remain effective and that any necessary adjustments are made promptly. This iterative process, informed by the nursing care model, ensures that patient care is both dynamic and responsive. The adoption of nursing care plans and nursing care models represents a significant advancement in veterinary nursing practice. These frameworks provide a structured, evidence-based approach to patient care, enhancing the quality and consistency of nursing interventions. By ensuring that all aspects of the patient's health are systematically addressed, these tools help veterinary technicians deliver holistic, individualized care. Moreover, the use of nursing care plans and models fosters a collaborative approach to patient care. By involving the entire veterinary team, including veterinary technicians, veterinarians, and pet owners, in the care process, these frameworks promote communication and coordination. This collaborative approach enhances the effectiveness of nursing interventions and ensures that all members of the care team are aligned in their efforts to support the patient's recovery. In addition to improving patient outcomes, the use of nursing care plans and models also benefits veterinary technicians themselves. These tools provide a clear structure for organizing and prioritizing care activities, reducing the risk of oversight and improving efficiency. They also offer a framework for professional development, helping nurses build their skills and knowledge in a systematic way.

References

Baillie, S. (2018). *Developing Practical Skills in Veterinary Nursing*, 3e, 22–24. Edinburgh: Elsevier.

Freepik (2025) *[Title/description of the image]* [Online image]. https://www.freepik.com

Lue, T.W., Pantenburg, D.P., and Crawford, P.M. (2008). Impact of the owner-pet and client-veterinarian bond on the care that pets receive. *Journal of the American Veterinary Medical Association* 232 (4): 531–540. https://doi.org/10.2460/javma.232.4.531.

Orem, D.E. (2001). *Nursing: Concepts of Practice*, 6e. St. Louis: Mosby.

Orpet, H. and Jeffery, A. (2007). *Veterinary Nursing: A Systems Approach*, 3–10. Edinburgh: Elsevier Saunders.

Orpet, H. and Welsh, P. (2011). *Handbook of Veterinary Nursing*, 2e, 1–3. Oxford: Wiley-Blackwell.

Roper, N., Logan, W.W., and Tierney, A.J. (2000). *The Roper-Logan-Tierney Model of Nursing: Based on Activities of Living*. Edinburgh: Churchill Livingstone.

Schaeffer, C. (2025). Nursing plan models and patient-centred frameworks in veterinary practice. In: *Veterinary Nursing Strategy* (ed. C. Schaeffer). Hoboken, NJ: Wiley-Blackwell.

6

Kirby's Rule of 20

Introduction to Rebecca Kirby and the Kirby's Rule of 20 in Veterinary Medicine

Veterinary medicine is a constantly evolving field, where the ability to manage critically ill patients with precision and care is paramount. Among the pioneers who have significantly influenced the discipline of veterinary critical care is Dr. Rebecca Kirby. Her contributions have reshaped how veterinary professionals approach the management of critically ill animals, particularly through her development of Kirby's Rule of 20. This framework has become a foundation in veterinary medicine, offering a systematic approach to clinical decision-making and patient monitoring.

Dr. Kirby is a distinguished veterinarian and academic whose career has been dedicated to advancing the field of veterinary critical care. Her work has been instrumental in bridging the gap between theoretical knowledge and practical application, empowering veterinary professionals to deliver the highest standard of care. Kirby's Rule of 20, a comprehensive checklist that outlines critical parameters for monitoring hospitalized patients, exemplifies her commitment to improving patient outcomes and supporting veterinary teams.

Importantly, the Rule of 20 also embodies the principles of holistic nursing, ensuring that patient care is not limited to single organ systems or isolated conditions, but instead addresses the animal as an integrated whole. By considering parameters ranging from perfusion, oxygenation, and electrolytes to pain, nutrition, and mobility, the framework recognizes the interdependence of physiological, psychological, and environmental factors in recovery. This holistic approach aligns with the nursing philosophy that optimal patient outcomes arise from treating not just the illness, but the entire patient in the context of their lived experience—including their comfort, emotional well-being, and the role of the caregiver. In this way, Kirby's Rule of 20 reflects a model of veterinary critical care that is both scientifically rigorous and compassionately comprehensive, embodying the true essence of nursing as a holistic discipline.

Understanding Kirby's Rule of 20

The Kirby's Rule of 20 is a systematic checklist designed to guide veterinary professionals in assessing and managing critically ill patients. It encompasses 20 critical parameters that should be evaluated daily, or even multiple times a day, in hospitalized patients. These parameters cover various physiological systems, ensuring a holistic approach to patient care. By addressing each parameter, veterinary teams can identify subtle changes in a patient's condition, allowing for timely interventions and reducing the risk of complications.

The Rule of 20 includes the following parameters:

1) **Fluid balance**
2) **Albumin/oncotic pull**
3) **Mentation**
4) **Oxygenation and ventilation**
5) **Blood Pressure**
6) **Heart rate, contractility, rhythm**
7) **Body temperature**
8) **Electrolytes and acid-base**
9) **Glucose**
10) **RBCs and hemoglobin**
11) **Coagulation**
12) **Renal function**

13) **GI motility and integrity**
14) **Nutrition**
15) **Immune status (antibiotics)**
16) **Drug dosage and metabolism**
17) **Wound care and bandages**
18) **Pain control**
19) **Nursing care**
20) **Tender loving care**

Each parameter represents a critical aspect of patient care that requires continuous monitoring and evaluation. The holistic approach embodied by the Rule of 20 ensures that no aspect of patient health is overlooked, making it an invaluable tool in veterinary critical care.

Governing Fluid Balance in Kirby's Rule of 20

Fluid balance is one of the most critical components of Kirby's Rule of 20, emphasizing its essential role in the management of critically ill veterinary patients. Maintaining proper fluid balance involves assessing, managing, and adjusting the body's hydration status, electrolyte levels, and intravascular volume to ensure optimal organ function. In the veterinary setting, fluid balance is particularly challenging due to the diverse physiological needs of different species and the inability of patients to verbalize their symptoms. However, the structured approach provided by Kirby's Rule of 20 equips veterinary professionals with a comprehensive framework for managing this complex and dynamic aspect of patient care.

The Importance of Fluid Balance

Fluid balance underpins the stability of virtually every physiological system. Adequate hydration is necessary to maintain blood pressure, facilitate nutrient transport, regulate body temperature, and support cellular metabolism. Conversely, imbalances in fluid volume—whether due to dehydration, hypovolemia, or fluid overhydration—can result in severe complications. Hypovolemia can lead to inadequate perfusion of vital organs such as the kidneys, liver, and brain, resulting in ischemia and cellular damage. Abnormal fluid shifts can disrupt electrolyte homeostasis, affecting cardiac and neuromuscular function. Fluid overhydration can cause pulmonary edema or ascites, impairing respiratory and gastrointestinal function. In critical care settings, where patients often present with multiple comorbidities, managing fluid balance becomes a cornerstone of therapy. Ensuring precise fluid therapy is not only essential for survival but also for recovery and long-term health (Table 6.1).

Table 6.1 The role of fluid balance in supporting physiological system stability.

Physiological System	Impact of Fluid Balance	Consequences of Imbalance
Cardiovascular	Maintains preload, stroke volume, and blood pressure	Hypovolemia → shock; hypervolemia → edema, hypertension
Respiratory	Supports pulmonary perfusion and oxygen delivery	Pulmonary edema → impaired gas exchange; hypoperfusion → hypoxia
Renal	Regulates water/electrolyte excretion, preserves homeostasis	Hypoperfusion → acute kidney injury; overload → impaired excretion
Neurological	Preserves cerebral perfusion and electrolyte stability	Dehydration → confusion, seizures; overload → cerebral edema
Gastrointestinal	Ensures mucosal perfusion and nutrient absorption	Hypovolemia → ileus, ischemia; overload → gut edema, malabsorption
Musculoskeletal	Maintains perfusion for oxygen/nutrient delivery to muscles	Dehydration → weakness, cramps; overload → compartment syndromes
Immune/Inflammatory	Supports leukocyte transport and tissue repair	Poor perfusion → delayed healing; overload → dilutional coagulopathy

This chart illustrates how fluid balance underpins the stability of multiple physiological systems, emphasizing the consequences of imbalance in critically ill patients.
Source: Schaeffer (2025).

Components of Fluid Balance Assessment

Managing fluid balance begins with a thorough and ongoing assessment. This step requires veterinary professionals to evaluate a combination of clinical signs, diagnostic parameters, and patient history. Key components include a physical assessment of mucous membranes and capillary refill time (CRT). Pale or dry mucous membranes and prolonged CRT may indicate dehydration or hypovolemia. Skin turgor can be utilized as a subjective assessment of dehydration. Reduced skin elasticity is a common sign of dehydration, particularly in cats and dogs. Daily or serial weight measurements provide an objective indicator of fluid loss or retention. It is important to consider that a 0.5 kg weight gain is often equivalent to approximately 0.5 L of fluid accumulation, particularly in hospitalized patients receiving intravenous fluids (Silverstein and Hopper 2014). Thus, a patient who has gained 2 kg while receiving intravenous fluids has potentially retained a total of 2 L of fluids! Another key component to consider includes a patient's vital signs. Tachycardia with weak pulses may suggest hypovolemia, while bounding pulses could indicate fluid overhydration. An increased respiratory effort may result from pulmonary edema due to fluid overhydration. We may also need to consider laboratory diagnostics, including Packed Cell Volume (PCV) and Total Solids (TS). An elevated PCV and TS can indicate dehydration, while decreases may suggest fluid overhydration or blood loss. Sodium, potassium, and chloride levels should be closely monitored to identify imbalances that may exacerbate fluid disturbances. Blood Urea Nitrogen (BUN) and Creatinine assess renal function, which is closely tied to fluid balance. Veterinary technicians should be instructed to monitor urinary output. Adequate urine production indicates sufficient perfusion and renal function.

Normal Urinary Output in Dogs and Cats

Urinary output is a vital indicator of renal function and overall fluid balance. In healthy dogs and cats, normal urinary output typically ranges from **1 to 2 mL/kg/hour**. This value can vary slightly depending on hydration status, activity level, and environmental factors, but persistent deviations from this range warrant further investigation.

Physiology of Urinary Output

The kidneys play a central role in regulating urinary output by filtering blood, reabsorbing essential nutrients and water, and excreting waste products. The processes of glomerular filtration, tubular reabsorption, and tubular secretion collectively determine the volume and composition of urine. Key physiological mechanisms include the Glomerular Filtration Rate (GFR). GFR is the rate at which blood is filtered through the kidneys. It is influenced by factors such as blood pressure, renal perfusion, and the integrity of the glomeruli. The majority of water and electrolytes are reabsorbed in the renal tubules, ensuring that only waste products and excess substances are excreted. Hormones such as antidiuretic hormone (ADH), aldosterone, and atrial natriuretic peptide (ANP) play critical roles in modulating urinary output based on the body's fluid and electrolyte needs.

When to Be Concerned About Urinary Output

Abnormal urinary output can be indicative of underlying medical conditions that require prompt attention. Common concerns include oliguria. Oliguria is defined as a urine output of less than 0.5 mL/kg/hour, and may be an early indicator of hypovolemia, decreased renal perfusion, or acute kidney injury (AKI) (DiBartola 2012; Silverstein and Hopper 2014). Decreased blood volume reduces renal perfusion, impairing filtration. Direct damage to the renal parenchyma disrupts normal filtration and excretion and will often lead to AKI. Anuria is the complete cessation of urine production and is a medical emergency that may result from severe AKI, urethral obstruction, or end-stage renal disease.

Polyuria, defined as urinary output exceeding 2 mL/kg/hour, may be associated with diabetes mellitus, where glucosuria drives osmotic diuresis, increasing urinary output and fluid loss (Nelson and Reusch 2014; DiBartola 2012). Chronic kidney disease (CKD) results in impaired tubular reabsorption, which leads to excessive fluid loss. Other endocrine pathologies, such as Hyperadrenocorticism, result in hormonal imbalances that affect renal water handling.

Monitoring and Assessment

In hospitalized patients, urinary output should be monitored closely using methods such as:

1) **Urinary Catheterization:** Indwelling catheters allow for accurate measurement of urine volume in critical patients.
2) **Weighing Absorbent Pads:** For patients without catheters, weighing pads before and after use provides an estimate of urine output.
3) **Owner Observation:** In outpatient settings, owners can provide valuable insights into changes in urinary habits, such as increased frequency or straining.

Clinical Implications of Abnormal Urinary Output

Abnormalities in urinary output can have serious consequences for fluid balance, electrolyte homeostasis, and overall patient stability. Oliguric and anuric conditions can result in fluid retention, hyperkalemia, and metabolic acidosis, necessitating interventions such as fluid resuscitation, diuretics, or dialysis. Polyuria can result in excessive fluid loss, consequently leading to dehydration, hypovolemia, and electrolyte imbalances, requiring adjustments to fluid therapy and treatment of the underlying cause.

Planning Fluid Therapy

Fluid therapy planning is a critical step that involves determining the type, volume, and rate of fluids to be administered. These decisions are based on the patient's fluid deficit, ongoing losses, and maintenance needs.

Types of Fluids

Crystalloid Fluids: Composition, Isotonicity, and Types

Crystalloid fluids are a fundamental component of fluid therapy in veterinary medicine. These fluids contain water and small molecules, such as electrolytes and glucose, that can pass freely through semipermeable membranes. Crystalloids are categorized based on their molecular composition, isotonicity, and specific applications in clinical settings. Crystalloid fluids are composed of water and solutes that include electrolytes (e.g., sodium, potassium, chloride, and calcium) and other small molecules. The specific composition of a crystalloid fluid determines its clinical indications.

Isotonic Crystalloids

These solutions have an electrolyte composition similar to that of extracellular fluid, making them suitable for volume replacement and maintenance therapy. Isotonicity refers to the osmotic pressure of a solution relative to plasma. The isotonicity of crystalloid fluids influences their distribution within the body's compartments. These solutions remain in the extracellular compartment, making them ideal for treating hypovolemia and dehydration. Examples of isotonic crystalloids include Lactated Ringer's Solution and 0.9% Sodium Chloride.

Hypertonic Crystalloid Fluids

Hypertonic crystalloid fluids are specialized solutions designed for specific clinical scenarios requiring rapid intravascular volume expansion. These fluids have a higher osmolality compared to plasma and extracellular fluid, which allows them to draw water from the intracellular and interstitial compartments into the intravascular space. This osmotic effect makes hypertonic crystalloids particularly effective for managing conditions such as hypovolemic shock and traumatic brain injury (TBI), where rapid intravascular volume expansion and decreased intracranial pressure (ICP) are desired (Mazzaferro and Rudloff 2004; Silverstein and Hopper 2014).

Hypertonic crystalloid solutions are characterized by their elevated concentrations of electrolytes, primarily sodium chloride. 7.5% Sodium Chloride contains 750 mEq/L of sodium and chloride, significantly higher than 154 mEq/L in isotonic saline (0.9%). Hypertonic saline is sometimes combined with other solutes, such as dextran or colloids, to enhance its therapeutic effects. The high sodium and chloride content of these solutions contributes to their ability to shift fluids osmotically into the vascular compartment.

Isotonicity and Osmolality of Hypertonic Crystalloids

Hypertonic crystalloids have an osmolality significantly higher than plasma, which typically ranges from 280 to 300 mOsm/kg. For example, 7.5% sodium chloride has an osmolality of approximately 2,400 mOsm/kg, making it highly hypertonic and effective for rapid plasma volume expansion (DiBartola 2012; Silverstein and Hopper 2014). By creating a strong osmotic gradient, hypertonic crystalloids effectively pull water into the intravascular space, increasing blood volume and improving tissue perfusion.

Types of Hypertonic Crystalloid Fluids

Several formulations of hypertonic crystalloids are used in veterinary medicine, including:

1) **Hypertonic Saline (7.5% Sodium Chloride):**
   - Indications: Hypovolemic shock, severe dehydration, and TBI.
   - Mechanism: Rapidly expands intravascular volume by drawing water from the intracellular and interstitial compartments.

2) **Hypertonic Saline with Dextran:**
- Indications: Similar to hypertonic saline alone, but offers additional colloidal support to maintain intravascular volume.
- Mechanism: Combines the osmotic effects of hypertonic saline with the volume-expanding properties of dextran.

Clinical Applications of Hypertonic Crystalloids

Hypertonic crystalloids are used in various critical care scenarios. Hypertonic saline is particularly effective for treating hypovolemic shock caused by hemorrhage or severe dehydration, as it rapidly expands plasma volume and improves perfusion with smaller infusion volumes (Mazzaferro and Rudloff 2004; Silverstein and Hopper 2014). Its ability to rapidly expand intravascular volume helps restore perfusion and stabilize vital signs. In TBI, hypertonic saline reduces ICP by drawing water out of the brain tissue and into the vascular space. This effect decreases cerebral edema and improves oxygen delivery to the brain. Hypertonic solutions can quickly correct severe dehydration by mobilizing water from intracellular stores, although careful monitoring is required to avoid overcorrection.

Precautions and Monitoring

While hypertonic crystalloids offer significant benefits, their use requires careful monitoring due to the potential for complications. Rapid administration of hypertonic solutions can cause hypernatremia or hyperchloremia, necessitating frequent electrolyte monitoring. Excessive intravascular volume expansion can lead to fluid overhydration and pulmonary edema, particularly in patients with compromised cardiac function. Hypertonic solutions can cause tissue irritation or necrosis if extravasation occurs, highlighting the importance of proper catheter placement.

Hypertonic crystalloid fluids are a powerful tool in the management of critically ill veterinary patients. Their unique molecular composition and osmotic properties enable rapid intravascular volume expansion, making them invaluable in conditions such as hypovolemic shock and TBI. However, their use must be carefully tailored to each patient's needs, with vigilant monitoring to prevent complications. By integrating hypertonic crystalloids into the framework of Kirby's Rule of 20, veterinary professionals can optimize fluid therapy and improve outcomes in challenging clinical scenarios.

Hypotonic Crystalloid Fluids

Hypotonic crystalloid fluids are designed to address free water deficits and promote hydration in situations where intracellular dehydration is a concern. These solutions have a lower osmolality compared to plasma and extracellular fluid, allowing water to move into cells from the extracellular space.

Molecular Composition of Hypotonic Crystalloids

Hypotonic crystalloids are characterized by a lower concentration of electrolytes compared to isotonic solutions, making them particularly effective for intracellular hydration. These solutions facilitate the movement of water into cells without significantly expanding extracellular fluid volume. Notable examples include 0.45% Sodium Chloride (half normal saline) and Dextrose 5% in Water (D5W). Half-Normal Saline contains 77 mEq/L of sodium and chloride, while D5W provides free water along with 50 g/L of glucose but lacks significant electrolytes.

The osmolality of hypotonic crystalloids is lower than that of plasma, which typically ranges between 280 and 300 mOsm/kg. For instance, 0.45% sodium chloride has an osmolality of approximately 154 mOsm/kg, whereas dextrose 5% in water (D5W) is initially isotonic at around 278 mOsm/kg, but becomes hypotonic after metabolism of the dextrose, leaving free water (DiBartola 2012; Silverstein and Hopper 2014). This decrease in osmolality promotes intracellular hydration, making these fluids particularly useful in conditions characterized by intracellular dehydration.

Among the commonly used hypotonic crystalloids, 0.45% Sodium Chloride is indicated for the management of hypernatremia and intracellular dehydration and clinical scenarios necessitating gradual rehydration. It provides free water while maintaining a minimal sodium and chloride concentration to prevent rapid electrolyte shifts. D5W is primarily utilized for treating hypernatremia, dehydration in patients without electrolyte imbalances, and as a vehicle for medication administration. While initially isotonic, its metabolism results in the release of free water, thereby addressing intracellular water deficits.

Clinical Applications of Hypotonic Crystalloids

Hypotonic crystalloids are utilized in various clinical scenarios. Conditions such as diabetes insipidus or osmotic diuresis may lead to hypernatremia and intracellular dehydration. Hypotonic solutions like D5W are ideal for restoring water balance without exacerbating hypernatremia. In cases of pure water loss, such as prolonged fever or inadequate fluid intake, hypotonic solutions rehydrate cells effectively. For patients with low electrolyte needs, such as those with cardiac or renal compromise, hypotonic crystalloids can provide adequate hydration without overloading sodium or chloride.

Precautions and Monitoring

While hypotonic crystalloids are effective in specific situations, their use requires careful consideration. Excessive administration can dilute plasma sodium levels, leading to hyponatremia and associated complications like cerebral edema. Overuse can result in cellular swelling, which is particularly concerning in the brain, where increased ICP can occur. Frequent assessment of hydration status, electrolyte levels, and osmolality is essential to avoid overcorrection or undercorrection.

Hypotonic crystalloid fluids are a vital tool in managing conditions involving intracellular dehydration and hypernatremia. Their low solute concentration and osmolality allow them to effectively rehydrate cells while minimizing risks to the extracellular space. However, their use requires careful monitoring and a clear understanding of the underlying pathology to prevent complications.

Colloid Fluid Therapy in Veterinary Medicine

Colloid fluid therapy plays a crucial role in managing hypovolemia, hypoproteinemia, and conditions that require sustained intravascular volume expansion. Unlike crystalloids, which freely distribute across capillary membranes, colloids contain large molecular weight substances that exert oncotic pressure, promoting fluid retention within the intravascular compartment. These fluids are broadly categorized into natural and synthetic formulations, each possessing distinct physicochemical properties and clinical applications.

Natural colloids primarily include plasma, albumin solutions, and whole blood therapy. Plasma contains albumin, globulins, and clotting factors, making it particularly beneficial for patients with coagulopathies or hypoproteinemia. Albumin solutions, available as species-specific formulations such as canine albumin or as human serum albumin (HSA), provide concentrated oncotic support. However, HSA administration in veterinary patients—particularly in felines and canines—carries a documented risk of hypersensitivity reactions, necessitating cautious use and monitoring (Mathews et al. 2005; Otto et al. 2002; Silverstein and Hopper 2014). Whole blood transfusions serve as another natural colloid option, particularly valuable in patients experiencing significant blood loss or anemia, as they provide not only oncotic support but also oxygen-carrying capacity and clotting factors.

Synthetic colloids, including hydroxyethyl starches (HES), gelatin-based solutions, and dextrans, offer potent oncotic effects by increasing plasma volume. HES such as hetastarch, tetrastarch, and pentastarch vary in molecular weight, molar substitution, and C2:C6 substitution ratio—factors that influence their intravascular retention time and the risk of adverse effects, including coagulopathy and renal dysfunction (Yozova et al. 2016; Silverstein and Hopper 2014). VetStarch, a tetrastarch-based hydroxyethyl starch solution, is a widely used synthetic colloid in veterinary medicine due to its favorable pharmacokinetic profile. With a lower degree of molar substitution compared to hetastarch, VetStarch® (tetrastarch) is associated with a reduced risk of coagulopathy and demonstrates improved hemodynamic stability in critically ill patients, making it a safer synthetic colloid alternative (Yozova et al. 2016; Epstein and Silverstein 2014). Gelatin-based colloids have lower molecular weights and shorter intravascular persistence, whereas dextrans, composed of glucose polymers, can interfere with platelet function and coagulation.

Colloids exert oncotic pressure, influencing fluid dynamics between the intravascular and interstitial compartments. Most colloids are isotonic, with an osmolality approximating 300 mOsm/kg, which helps ensure minimal osmotic shifts across cellular membranes during fluid resuscitation and oncotic support (DiBartola 2012; Silverstein and Hopper 2014). However, their oncotic effects exceed those of plasma, enabling effective plasma volume expansion. HES maintain oncotic pressure for extended durations due to their large molecular structures, while gelatin and dextran solutions exhibit shorter half-lives.

The clinical applications of colloids are diverse and tailored to specific patient needs. They are primarily indicated in conditions requiring rapid and sustained intravascular volume expansion, such as hypovolemic shock, where synthetic colloids restore perfusion by augmenting intravascular volume, particularly in patients unresponsive to crystalloids alone. In cases of hypoalbuminemia, natural colloids such as albumin provide essential oncotic support, particularly in patients with protein-losing enteropathies, nephropathies, or hepatic insufficiency. In septic shock, colloids help maintain vascular integrity and counteract capillary leakage associated with sepsis-induced vasodilation. Additionally, they are utilized perioperatively to stabilize hemodynamics in patients at risk for significant fluid shifts or hypotension. Whole blood therapy is particularly indicated in cases of acute hemorrhage, anemia, and coagulopathies, where the administration of red blood cells (RBCs), plasma proteins, and clotting factors is essential for restoring hemodynamic stability and oxygen delivery.

While colloid therapy provides substantial hemodynamic benefits, careful patient selection and monitoring are imperative to mitigate potential complications. HES, particularly those with higher molar substitution, can impair coagulation by reducing von Willebrand factor (vWF) and factor VIII activity, thereby increasing the risk of bleeding in critically ill patients (Yozova et al. 2016; Epstein and Silverstein 2014). Synthetic colloids may contribute to AKI, particularly in critically ill patients or those with preexisting renal impairment. VetStarch, due to its lower molar substitution, has demonstrated a reduced impact on coagulation compared to older starch formulations such as hetastarch, making it a preferred choice in many clinical scenarios involving fluid resuscitation (Yozova et al. 2016; Epstein and Silverstein 2014). Natural colloids, especially HSA, can elicit hypersensitivity reactions, necessitating pre-administration testing and vigilant monitoring. Excessive administration may lead to fluid overhydration, exacerbating conditions such as congestive heart failure or pulmonary edema. In patients receiving whole blood transfusions, careful crossmatching and monitoring for transfusion reactions, hemolysis, or volume overload are essential to ensure safe administration. Regular assessment of hemodynamic parameters, urine output, and coagulation profiles is essential when administering colloids. Monitoring colloid osmotic pressure (COP) and serum albumin concentrations guides fluid therapy adjustments, optimizing patient outcomes while minimizing risks.

Colloid fluid therapy represents a vital component of veterinary critical care, providing sustained intravascular volume expansion beyond that achievable with crystalloids. Understanding the molecular properties, indications, and potential complications of both natural and synthetic colloids enables precise and effective fluid management in veterinary patients. Through diligent patient monitoring and evidence-based application, colloids serve as a valuable tool in stabilizing critically ill animals and optimizing their recovery (Table 6.2).

Key Aspects of Fluid Monitoring

Regular assessment of mucous membranes, skin turgor, CRT, and body weight provides critical insights into the patient's hydration status. Observing changes in respiratory rate and effort can indicate complications such as pulmonary edema. Monitoring heart rate, blood pressure, and pulse quality helps assess the efficacy of fluid resuscitation and detect early signs of fluid overhydration or hypovolemia. Urine production is a direct indicator of renal perfusion and overall fluid balance. Normal output ranges from 1 to 2 mL/kg/hour, and deviations from this range may require adjustments to fluid therapy. Frequent evaluation of PCV, TS, electrolyte levels, BUN, creatinine, and lactate provides objective data to guide therapy.

Table 6.2 Types of fluids in veterinary medicine with clinical applications, precautions, and monitoring.

Fluid Type	Examples	Clinical Applications	Precautions/Contraindications	Monitoring in Patients
Isotonic Crystalloids	0.9% NaCl, LRS, Normosol-R, Plasmalyte-A	First-line for dehydration, shock, maintenance, perioperative support	Risk of hemodilution, edema if over-administered; NaCl may cause hyperchloremic metabolic acidosis	Body weight, perfusion parameters (HR, CRT, BP), electrolytes, urine output
Hypertonic Crystalloids	7% NaCl, 3% NaCl	Rapid volume expansion in hypovolemic shock; reduces ICP; used in large animals	Contraindicated in dehydration without concurrent isotonic fluid; can cause hypernatremia, osmotic demyelination	Serum sodium, neurologic status, concurrent isotonic fluids, central venous pressure
Hypotonic Crystalloids	0.45% NaCl, D5W (after metabolism acts hypotonic)	Free water replacement for hypernatremia; management of certain renal disorders	Avoid in shock or increased ICP; risk of hyponatremia and cerebral edema	Electrolytes (Na+, K+), mentation, neurologic signs, serum osmolality
Synthetic Colloids	Hetastarch, Pentastarch, VetStarch, Gelatins	Plasma volume expansion in shock, hypoproteinemia	Risk of coagulopathies, renal injury, anaphylaxis; avoid in renal failure, sepsis	Coagulation profile, renal values (BUN/Cr), colloid osmotic pressure, hydration status
Natural Colloids	Plasma (FFP, cryo-poor plasma), Whole blood, Albumin solutions	Replacement in coagulopathy, hypoproteinemia, anemia; oncotic support	Risk of transfusion reaction, volume overload, limited availability	Crossmatching, transfusion monitoring (TP, PCV, HR, BP), allergic reaction signs

This chart outlines the different types of fluids used in veterinary medicine, including isotonic, hypertonic, and hypotonic crystalloids as well as colloids (synthetic and natural). It highlights their clinical applications, precautions, and monitoring requirements.
Source: Schaeffer (2025).

Central venous pressure (CVP) and point-of-care ultrasound (POCUS) can offer additional insights into the patient's fluid status, especially in complex cases.

Volume Calculation in Fluid Therapy

Fluid volume calculation in veterinary medicine is based on three fundamental components: replacement needs, maintenance needs, and ongoing losses. Replacement needs involve correcting existing deficits, typically determined by estimating dehydration as a percentage of body weight. The fluid deficit can be calculated using the formula:

$$\text{Fluid deficit } (L) = \text{Body weight (kg)} \times \frac{\%\text{Dehydration}}{100}$$

For example, a 20 kg dog with 8% dehydration would require 1.6 L of replacement fluid. Maintenance needs encompass the daily fluid requirements necessary for normal physiological functions, generally calculated as 40–60 mL/kg/day. For a 20 kg patient, maintenance fluid requirements would range from 800 to 1200 mL per day. Ongoing losses account for additional fluid depletion due to conditions such as vomiting, diarrhea, or excessive panting. These losses must be estimated and replaced accordingly, often requiring serial assessments and adjustments to maintain adequate hydration and electrolyte balance. Properly calculating and monitoring these components ensures effective fluid therapy tailored to the individual patient's needs. This volume should be administered judiciously over an appropriate timeframe to prevent fluid overhydration or rapid shifts in electrolyte balance. Conversely, in cases of fluid overhydration, reducing administration rates or incorporating diuretics such as furosemide may be necessary to alleviate excessive intravascular volume and mitigate complications such as pulmonary edema.

Tailoring Fluid Therapy to Underlying Pathophysiology

The selection of fluid type, infusion rate, and total volume must align with the patient's primary diagnosis. Hypovolemic patients, for example, require rapid volume expansion through isotonic crystalloids or colloids to restore perfusion, while those with shock may necessitate a more aggressive bolus approach followed by reassessment. Electrolyte imbalances must also be considered; patients presenting with hypernatremia or hyponatremia require carefully calculated fluid adjustments to avoid rapid osmotic shifts, which can lead to neurological complications such as cerebral edema or central pontine myelinolysis.

Dynamic Adjustments in Fluid Therapy Goals

Fluid therapy objectives should be continually reassessed as the patient's clinical status evolves. In critically ill patients, initial resuscitative efforts focus on restoring hemodynamic stability. Once perfusion parameters are stabilized, fluid administration should transition to maintenance therapy, ensuring ongoing homeostasis while preventing iatrogenic complications such as volume overload or electrolyte disturbances.

Challenges in Fluid Monitoring and Adjustment

Critically ill patients frequently experience rapid fluctuations in hydration status, necessitating vigilant monitoring and prompt adjustments to therapy. Species-specific variations further complicate fluid management, as different species exhibit unique physiological responses to fluid therapy. Additionally, resource limitations in certain clinical settings may restrict access to advanced hemodynamic monitoring tools, necessitating reliance on clinical parameters such as mucous membrane color, CRT, urine output, and blood lactate levels to guide fluid therapy decisions.

Clinical Consequences of Inadequate Fluid Monitoring

Failure to appropriately monitor and adjust fluid administration can result in severe complications. Fluid overhydration may lead to pulmonary edema, increased ICP, and peripheral edema, all of which can compromise recovery. Unchecked fluid administration also risks exacerbating electrolyte imbalances, with potential consequences such as hyperkalemia-induced cardiac arrhythmias or hyponatremia-related neurological dysfunction. Prolonged hypovolemia or inadequate fluid resuscitation may further precipitate ischemic injury, ultimately contributing to multi-organ dysfunction and poor clinical outcomes.

Optimizing fluid therapy requires a multifaceted approach that incorporates accurate assessment, tailored intervention, and continuous reassessment to ensure that patients receive appropriate fluid support while mitigating potential adverse effects.

Table 6.3 Clinical signs and laboratory findings of fluid overhydration in dogs and cats.

Category	Clinical Signs	Laboratory Findings
Cardiovascular	Tachycardia, bounding pulses, hypertension, jugular vein distension	Hemodilution → decreased PCV/TP, BNP elevation (if CHF develops)
Respiratory	Tachypnea, increased respiratory effort, moist lung sounds/crackles, dyspnea, pulmonary edema (cough in dogs, open-mouth breathing in cats)	Arterial blood gases: hypoxemia, respiratory alkalosis; thoracic radiographs: interstitial/alveolar pattern
Renal/Urinary	Polyuria initially, oliguria/anuria if concurrent renal compromise	Dilute urine (low USG); electrolyte imbalances (hyponatremia, hypokalemia)
Neurological	Restlessness, disorientation, seizures (secondary to hyponatremia or cerebral edema)	Serum sodium: low (hyponatremia); serum osmolality reduced
Gastrointestinal	Vomiting, nausea, salivation, abdominal distension from ascites	Electrolyte derangements (low Na^+, Cl^-; possible metabolic alkalosis/acidosis depending on cause)
Peripheral/General	Peripheral edema (limbs, dependent regions), chemosis (conjunctival edema), weight gain, serous nasal discharge	Decreased PCV/TS; low albumin if dilutional; possible increased body weight >5% baseline

This chart summarizes the clinical signs and laboratory findings associated with fluid overhydration in dogs and cats, with emphasis on critical care monitoring and veterinary nursing application.
Source: Schaeffer (2025).

Fluid monitoring and therapy adjustment are integral to successful patient management in veterinary medicine. By incorporating continuous assessments and individualized interventions into the framework of Kirby's Rule of 20, veterinary teams can optimize fluid therapy, minimize complications, and improve outcomes for critically ill patients. This dynamic approach ensures that fluid therapy remains responsive to the patient's evolving needs, supporting recovery and long-term health (Table 6.3).

Kirby's Rule of 20 and the Physiology of Oncotic Pressure

Kirby's Rule of 20 provides a structured approach to managing critically ill patients, emphasizing frequent assessment of key physiological parameters, including oncotic pressure. Oncotic pressure is generated primarily by plasma proteins, predominantly albumin, and is responsible for maintaining the balance of fluid distribution between the intravascular and interstitial spaces. The Starling equation describes this balance, incorporating hydrostatic pressure, oncotic pressure, and the integrity of the endothelial glycocalyx in governing capillary exchange.

The Starling equation is defined as:

$$J_v = K_f\ ([P_c - P_i] - \sigma[\pi c - \pi i])$$

where J_v represents the net fluid movement, K_f is the filtration coefficient of the capillary membrane, and P_c and P_i are the hydrostatic pressures in the capillary and interstitial space, respectively; σ is the reflection coefficient, and πc and πi are the oncotic pressures in the capillary and interstitial space, respectively—together comprising the Starling equation for transvascular fluid exchange (DiBartola 2012; Guyton and Hall 2021). This equation governs the movement of fluid across the capillary membrane and highlights the role of oncotic and hydrostatic forces in determining fluid balance (Figure 6.1).

The endothelial glycocalyx is a critical structure that lines the endothelium and serves as a selective barrier regulating fluid and solute movement. Damage to this layer, commonly seen in sepsis, systemic inflammation, or ischemia-reperfusion injury, results in increased vascular permeability and extravasation of fluid into the interstitial space, exacerbating hypo-oncotic states. This pathological shift contributes to the formation of peripheral edema, pulmonary edema, and effusions, particularly in hypoalbuminemic patients (Figure 6.2).

Veterinary technicians must actively assess oncotic pressure by monitoring total protein, albumin levels, and COP. Ensuring adequate oncotic pressure requires tailored fluid therapy incorporating natural or synthetic colloids when indicated. Frequent assessment of hydration status, CRT, and signs of fluid overhydration, such as increased respiratory effort and ascites, is vital in guiding therapeutic interventions. Proper nutritional support, particularly adequate dietary protein intake, is also essential for maintaining albumin synthesis and preventing hypo-oncotic complications (Table 6.4).

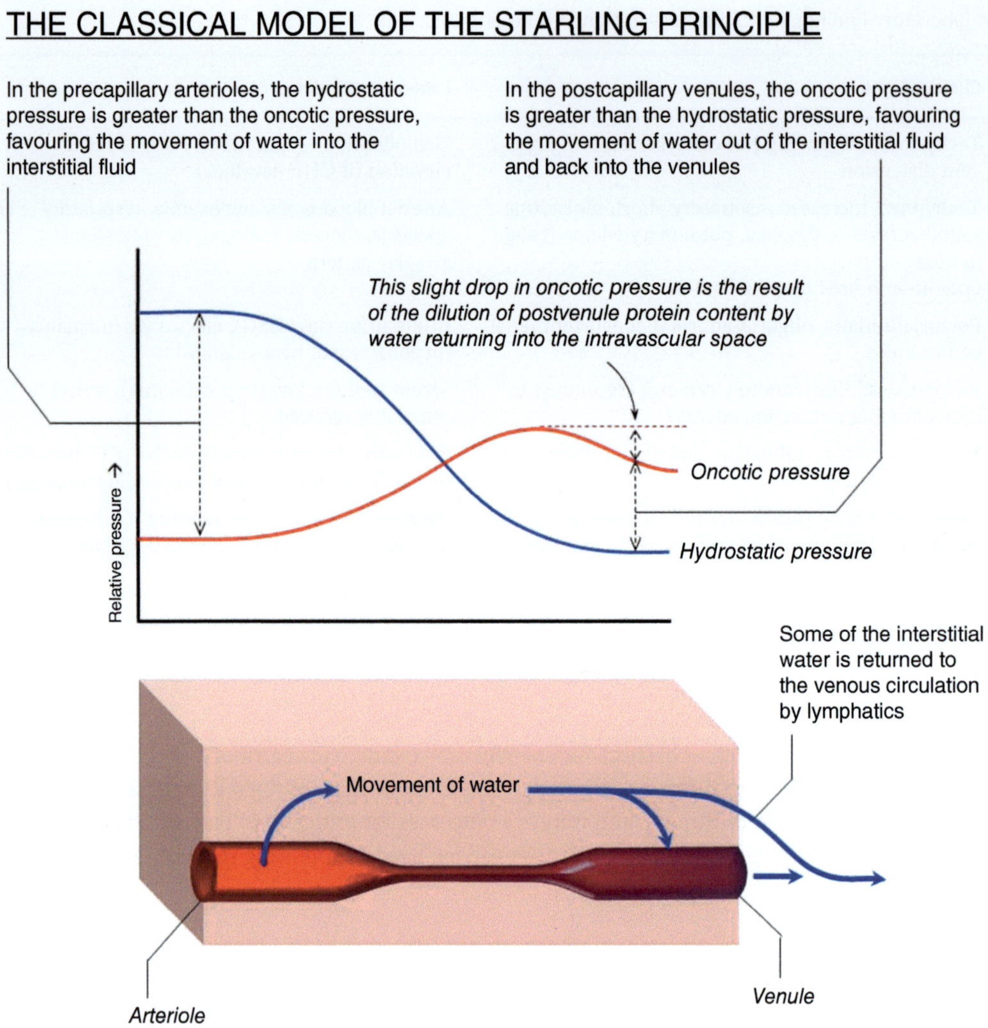

Figure 6.1 Starling principle illustrating the balance of hydrostatic and oncotic pressures determining capillary fluid movement. *Source:* Deranged Physiology, 2025 / Alex Yartsev.

By integrating an understanding of the Starling equation, the role of the endothelial glycocalyx, and vigilant patient monitoring, veterinary technicians play a critical role in oncotic pressure management. Effective interventions, including judicious colloid administration and nutritional support, contribute to improved fluid homeostasis and optimized outcomes in critically ill patients.

Kirby's Rule of 20 and Mentation

Mentation assessment is a crucial component of Kirby's Rule of 20, providing vital insights into the neurological and systemic status of critically ill veterinary patients. Changes in mentation can indicate a wide range of underlying pathophysiological conditions, including metabolic imbalances, intracranial disease, hypoxia, sepsis, or toxin exposure. Close monitoring of mental status is essential for early detection of deteriorating conditions, guiding timely intervention, and optimizing patient outcomes in the intensive care unit (ICU).

Levels of Consciousness and Neurological Status

Assessing mentation requires categorizing a patient's level of consciousness, which reflects both cortical function and brainstem integrity. The primary classifications of mentation include bright and alert, quiet and alert, depression/lethargy, obtundation, stupor, delirium, and coma.

A bright and alert patient exhibits normal cognitive function, is fully responsive to stimuli, and interacts appropriately with the environment and handlers. This level of mentation indicates an intact central nervous system (CNS) and

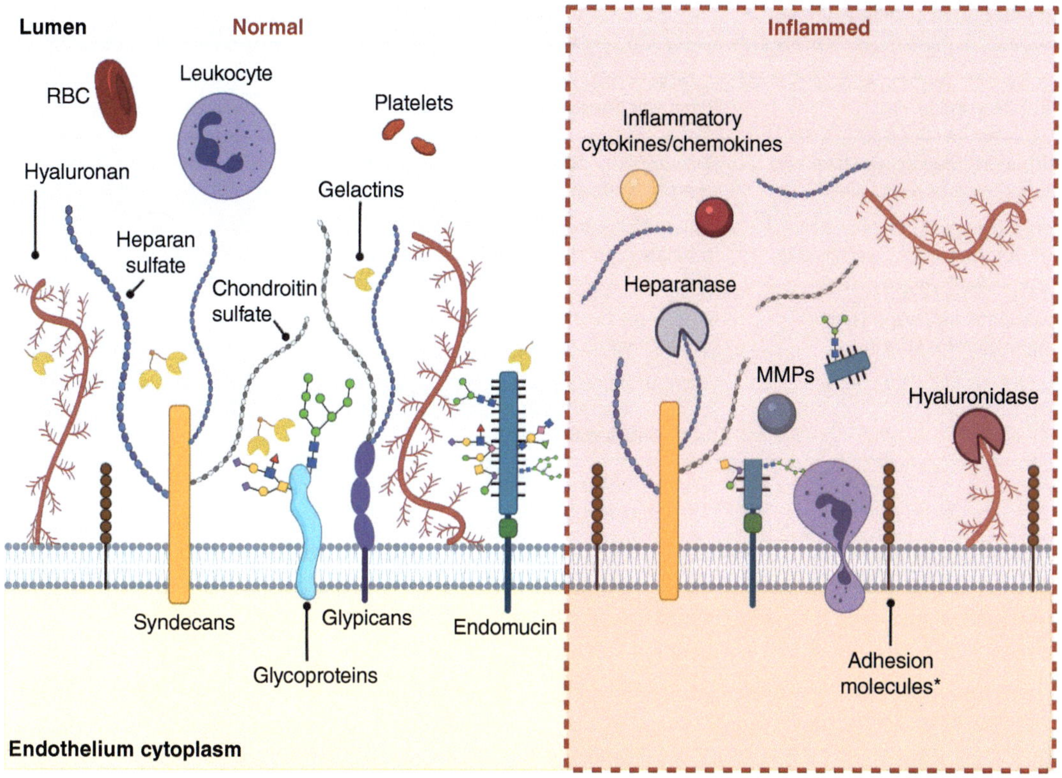

Figure 6.2 Structure of the endothelial glycocalyx under healthy conditions and its degradation during pathological states such as sepsis or inflammation. *Source:* Frontiers in Cell and Developmental Biology, 2024 / Frontiers Media S.A. / CC BY 4.0.

Table 6.4 Measuring oncotic pressure in dogs.

Method	Description	Normal Values (Dog)	Advantages	Limitations
Direct Measurement	Colloid Osmometer: uses a semipermeable membrane to separate plasma from a protein-free solution; pressure read by transducer.	20–25 mmHg	Gold standard; accurate, quantitative.	Expensive, limited availability in practice, requires specialized equipment.
Albumin Concentration	Serum albumin measured on standard chemistry analyzer; major determinant of oncotic pressure.	>2.0 g/dL generally adequate	Widely available; inexpensive.	Only estimates COP; ignores globulin contribution; nonlinear at low albumin.
Total Protein (TP)	Uses TP (albumin + globulins) to approximate colloid osmotic pull.	5.5–7.5 g/dL	Easy to obtain; included in routine diagnostics.	Less precise; different proteins exert different osmotic effects.
Clinical Indicators	Presence of edema, ascites, pleural effusion, pulmonary edema in noncardiogenic disease.	N/A	No equipment needed; clinically relevant.	Subjective; occurs only when COP is already low; does not give quantitative data.

Source: Schaeffer (2025).

homeostatic stability. A quiet and alert patient remains responsive but is less reactive than normal, often due to mild systemic illness, pain, or mild sedation.

Depression or lethargy is characterized by a decreased level of activity and reduced responsiveness to environmental stimuli. These patients may still respond to direct handling but lack interest in their surroundings. This state is commonly associated with systemic illness, metabolic derangements such as hypoglycemia or electrolyte imbalances, early sepsis, or mild intracranial pathology.

Table 6.5 Monitoring mentation in critically ill patients.

Mentation Status	Clinical Description	Diagnostic/Prognostic Significance	Associated Conditions
Normal (BAR/QAR)	Bright, alert, responsive (BAR) or quiet, alert, responsive (QAR).	Baseline; any deviation may suggest early neurologic decline.	Stable patient, mild systemic disease.
Obtunded	Drowsy, decreased response to environmental stimuli; arousable with mild stimulation.	May indicate hypoperfusion, metabolic imbalance, or rising intracranial pressure.	Early sepsis, hypoglycemia, hepatic encephalopathy, TBI.
Stuporous	Unconscious but responsive to strong or painful stimuli.	Significant neurologic compromise; often precedes coma or herniation.	Severe TBI, hypoxemia, toxicities, metabolic crisis.
Comatose	Unconscious and unresponsive even to painful stimuli.	Grave prognosis without rapid intervention; suggests severe brain injury or profound metabolic derangement.	Brain herniation, anoxic brain injury, end-stage encephalopathy.

Source: Schaeffer (2025).

Obtunded patients exhibit significantly decreased responsiveness, requiring stronger stimuli to elicit reactions. These individuals may be difficult to rouse and demonstrate diminished motor activity. This altered mentation suggests moderate to severe systemic illness, more advanced metabolic disturbances, CNS trauma, or increased ICP.

A stuporous patient is in a deeper state of unconsciousness and only responds to noxious stimuli, such as deep pain or aggressive tactile stimulation. Stupor is an ominous sign, typically indicating severe CNS dysfunction, profound metabolic derangements, toxic exposures, or severe hypoxia.

Delirious patients exhibit abnormal behavioral responses, often showing agitation, disorientation, or hyperreactivity to stimuli. This state may result from toxin exposure, hepatic or uremic encephalopathy, hypoxia, or systemic inflammatory response syndrome (SIRS).

A comatose patient is entirely unresponsive to any external stimuli, including pain, and lacks voluntary motor function. Coma indicates severe brainstem dysfunction, advanced intracranial pathology, or profound metabolic derangement and carries a grave prognosis (Table 6.5).

The Importance of Mentation Monitoring in Critical Care Patients

Monitoring mentation in critically ill patients provides critical diagnostic and prognostic information, as even subtle changes may signify worsening disease processes. Neurological deterioration in the ICU may suggest worsening ICP, impending herniation, hypoperfusion, or metabolic decompensation. Mentation changes are particularly significant in patients with TBI, sepsis, hepatic encephalopathy, or acute toxicities.

Frequent reassessment using standardized neurological scoring systems, such as the Modified Glasgow Coma Scale (MGCS), can help quantify mentation and guide therapeutic decisions (Platt and Hall 2014). Serial neurological examinations, including pupil size and reactivity, cranial nerve function, and postural reflex assessments, provide insight into ongoing disease progression and response to therapy. Documentation of mentation trends over time is critical for guiding prognosis, particularly in patients with CNS trauma, inflammatory CNS disease, or metabolic encephalopathies (Figure 6.3).

Physiology of Altered Mentation in Critical Care Patients

Mentation is largely dictated by cerebral perfusion, oxygenation, metabolic substrate availability, and neurotransmitter function. The brain is highly dependent on continuous glucose and oxygen supply, as it lacks substantial energy reserves. Any disruption in cerebral metabolism can lead to altered consciousness, ranging from mild lethargy to coma. The brain's autoregulatory mechanisms maintain cerebral blood flow within a narrow range; however, in critically ill patients, systemic hypotension, hypoxia, hypercapnia, or metabolic acidosis can impair this regulation, resulting in cerebral ischemia and dysfunction.

Hypoxia is a major contributor to altered mentation in ICU patients. Oxygen delivery depends on adequate cardiac output, hemoglobin concentration, and arterial oxygenation. Conditions such as hypovolemic shock, anemia, or respiratory failure can result in cerebral hypoxia, leading to confusion, obtundation, and eventually coma if left uncorrected. Similarly, hypercapnia, commonly observed in patients with respiratory compromise, can cause CNS depression due to CO_2-induced acidosis and cerebrovascular vasodilation, increasing ICP.

Modified Glasgow Coma Scale	
	Score
Motor activity	
Normal gait, normal spinal reflexes	6
Hemiparesis, tetraparesis, or decerebrate rigidity	5
Recumbent, intermittent extensor rigidity	4
Recumbent, constant extensor rigidity	3
Recumbent, constant extensor rigidity with opisthotonus	2
Recumbent, hypotonia of muscles, depressed or absent spinal reflexes	1
Brainstem reflexes	
Normal PLR and oculocephalic reflexes	6
Slow PLR and normal to reduced oculocephalic reflexes	5
Bilateral unresponsive miosis with normal to reduced oculocephalic reflexes	4
Pinpoint pupils with reduced to absent oculocephalic reflexes	3
Unilateral, unresponsive mydriasis with reduced to absent oculocephalic reflexes	2
Bilateral, unresponsive mydriasis with reduced to absent oculocephalic reflexes	1
Level of consciousness	
Occasional periods of alertness and responsive to environment	6
Depression or delirium, capable of responding, but response may be inappropriate	5
Semicomatose, responsive to visual stimuli	4
Semicomatose, responsive to auditory stimuli	3
Semicomatose, responsive only to repeated noxious stimuli	2
Comatose, unresponsive to repeated noxious stimuli	1
MCGS Score	Score
3–8	**Grave**
9–14	**Guarded**
15–18	**Good**

Figure 6.3 The Modified Glasgow Coma Scale (MGCS) is commonly used in veterinary neurology to assess traumatic brain injury in dogs. *Source:* Veterinary Practice, 2020 / Bush Veterinary Neurology Services.

Metabolic imbalances also play a significant role in mentation changes. Hypoglycemia deprives neurons of their primary energy source, leading to disorientation, seizures, and coma. Conversely, hyperglycemia, particularly in diabetic ketoacidosis (DKA), contributes to cellular dehydration, electrolyte shifts, and encephalopathy. Electrolyte abnormalities, including hyponatremia and hypernatremia, affect neuronal excitability, with severe dysnatremia causing cerebral edema or shrinkage, leading to seizures or coma. Hypocalcemia and hypercalcemia disrupt neuromuscular function and may manifest as tremors, tetany, or obtundation.

Toxin accumulation is another critical factor affecting mentation. Uremic encephalopathy, secondary to renal failure, results from the buildup of nitrogenous waste products, leading to lethargy, altered mentation, and seizures. Hepatic encephalopathy, seen in patients with liver dysfunction or portosystemic shunts, occurs due to the accumulation of neurotoxic metabolites such as ammonia, resulting in stupor, disorientation, and abnormal motor function. Sepsis-associated encephalopathy is a multifactorial condition linked to systemic inflammation, cytokine dysregulation, endothelial dysfunction, and impaired cerebral perfusion, often presenting with confusion, agitation, or coma.

The Significance of Mentation Changes in the ICU

Even subtle changes in mentation can indicate deteriorating clinical status, necessitating immediate intervention. A patient transitioning from quiet and alert to obtunded within hours may be experiencing hypovolemia, electrolyte imbalance, or worsening intracranial pathology. Progressive stupor or coma warrants aggressive diagnostics, including arterial blood gas (ABG) analysis, lactate levels, electrolyte panels, imaging, and cerebrospinal fluid (CSF) evaluation when indicated.

Management strategies depend on the underlying cause of altered mentation. Hypoxia requires prompt oxygen supplementation or mechanical ventilation. Hemodynamic stabilization through fluid resuscitation and vasopressor support is critical in patients with systemic hypotension affecting cerebral perfusion. Glucose supplementation must be provided in cases of hypoglycemia, while insulin therapy is necessary for hyperglycemic crises. Electrolyte imbalances should be corrected judiciously to prevent osmotic shifts leading to further neurological deterioration. In patients with increased ICP, interventions such as head elevation, osmotic diuresis (mannitol or hypertonic saline), and controlled ventilation may be required to mitigate secondary brain injury.

Continuous monitoring of neurological status is imperative in critically ill patients, as it provides key prognostic information and facilitates timely medical intervention. Implementing standardized mentation assessment ensures consistency in evaluations, enabling more accurate identification of trends and disease progression. Close collaboration between the veterinary critical care team, including neurologists when needed, enhances patient management and improves overall outcomes in patients experiencing altered mentation in the ICU.

Kirby's Rule of 20 and the Physiology of Oxygenation and Ventilation

Oxygenation involves the uptake of oxygen into the pulmonary system, diffusion across the alveolar-capillary membrane, transport via hemoglobin, and eventual delivery to the tissues. Ventilation, in contrast, refers to the mechanical movement of air into and out of the lungs, ensuring adequate oxygen intake and carbon dioxide removal. Proper assessment and intervention in these areas are crucial for maintaining adequate tissue oxygenation and preventing respiratory failure.

The fraction of inspired oxygen (FiO_2) represents the concentration of oxygen in the air a patient breathes and is a critical consideration in oxygen therapy. Room air has an FiO of approximately 21%, while supplemental oxygen delivery methods can increase FiO substantially. Nasal cannulas, when placed unilaterally, provide an FiO of approximately 30–35% at a flow rate of 1–2 L/min (Silverstein and Hopper 2014). Bilateral nasal cannulas can achieve FiO levels of 40–50% at higher flow rates. Oxygen cages allow for precise control of FiO, typically reaching 40–60% depending on oxygen flow and ventilation within the cage. Flow-by oxygen, with a loosely held mask, provides an FiO of around 25–40%, while a tightly fitting mask can achieve levels up to 60% (King et al. 2014). These methods are useful for short-term oxygen supplementation but may be less effective in patients with severe hypoxemia requiring continuous support (Table 6.6).

High-flow oxygen therapy (HFOT) has emerged as an advanced modality for oxygen supplementation in veterinary patients, offering higher and more stable FiO levels than traditional methods. HFOT delivers heated, humidified oxygen at high flow rates (typically exceeding 20–40 L/min in larger patients), improving oxygenation by washing out dead space, reducing inspiratory effort, and maintaining adequate alveolar ventilation. The benefits of HFOT include improved oxygenation efficiency, enhanced comfort compared to mechanical ventilation, and reduced need for sedation. However, its application requires specialized equipment, including high-flow oxygen delivery systems, humidifiers, and heated circuits, which increase cost and may limit accessibility in some clinical settings. HFOT is particularly useful in patients with moderate to severe hypoxemia who are not yet candidates for mechanical ventilation but require more oxygen than conventional flow methods can provide.

Table 6.6 Oxygen delivery methods and FiO_2 in veterinary patients.

Delivery Method	FIO_2 Range	Flow Rate/Notes	Advantages	Limitations
Room Air	«21%	N/A	Baseline; readily available	Insufficient for hypoxemic patitients
Nasal Cannula (Unilateral)	30–35%	1–2 L/min	Minimally invasive; well-tolerated	Limited FIO, increase; may not meet severs neds
Nasal Cannula (Bilateral)	40–50%	Higher flow rates	Greater FiO_2 than unilateral, usuful im	Discomfort, nasal irritation, not precise
Flow-by Oxygen	25–40%	Loosely held mask	Easy to administer; good for short-term stabilization	Inefficient, wasteful, stress-inducing
Mask (Tightly Fitted)	Up to 60%	Depends on seal	Higher FIO_2 achievable, rapid effect	Poor tolerance, CO_2 rebreathing risk
Oxygen Cage	40–60%	Controlled flow/ ventilation	Allows FIO_2 titration, minimal handling stress	Requires specialized equipment, costly
High-Flow Oxygen Therapy (HFOT)	>60% often >80%	20–40 L/min in larger dogs heated/humidified	Stable FIO_2 washes out dead space, reduces inspiratory	King et al. (2014), Sliverstein and Hopper (2014)

Source: Schaeffer (2025).

Oxygenation Monitoring

The oxygen-hemoglobin dissociation curve serves as a critical tool in understanding oxygen transport and utilization. This sigmoidal curve demonstrates the relationship between arterial oxygen saturation (SaO) and partial pressure of oxygen (PaO). Under normal physiological conditions, the curve follows a predictable pattern, with hemoglobin's affinity for oxygen increasing as PaO rises. However, several factors can shift the curve, altering hemoglobin's ability to bind and release oxygen (Figure 6.4).

A rightward shift of the dissociation curve occurs due to increased temperature, decreased pH (Bohr effect), elevated 2,3-diphosphoglycerate (2,3-DPG) levels, or hypercapnia. 2,3-Diphosphoglycerate (2,3-DPG) is a molecule found in RBCs that plays a critical role in regulating oxygen delivery to tissues (Guyton and Hall 2021). This shift reduces hemoglobin's affinity with oxygen, enhancing unloading at the tissue level. In critically ill patients with high metabolic demand, such as those with sepsis or systemic inflammatory conditions, a rightward shift is beneficial, ensuring adequate oxygenation of peripheral tissues. Conversely, a leftward shift is caused by alkalosis, hypothermia, decreased 2,3-DPG, or carbon monoxide exposure, increasing hemoglobin's affinity for oxygen (Guyton and Hall 2021). This results in impaired oxygen delivery to tissues despite normal PaO levels, which can be detrimental in patients with shock or hypoperfusion.

Blood gas analysis is a fundamental tool for evaluating oxygenation, ventilation, and acid-base balance. ABGs assess PaO, PaCO, pH, bicarbonate (HCO^{-}), and base excess, providing valuable insight into respiratory and metabolic function. A low PaO indicates hypoxemia, necessitating interventions such as oxygen supplementation or ventilation support. Elevated PaCO suggests hypoventilation and respiratory acidosis, while a decreased PaCO may be associated with hyperventilation

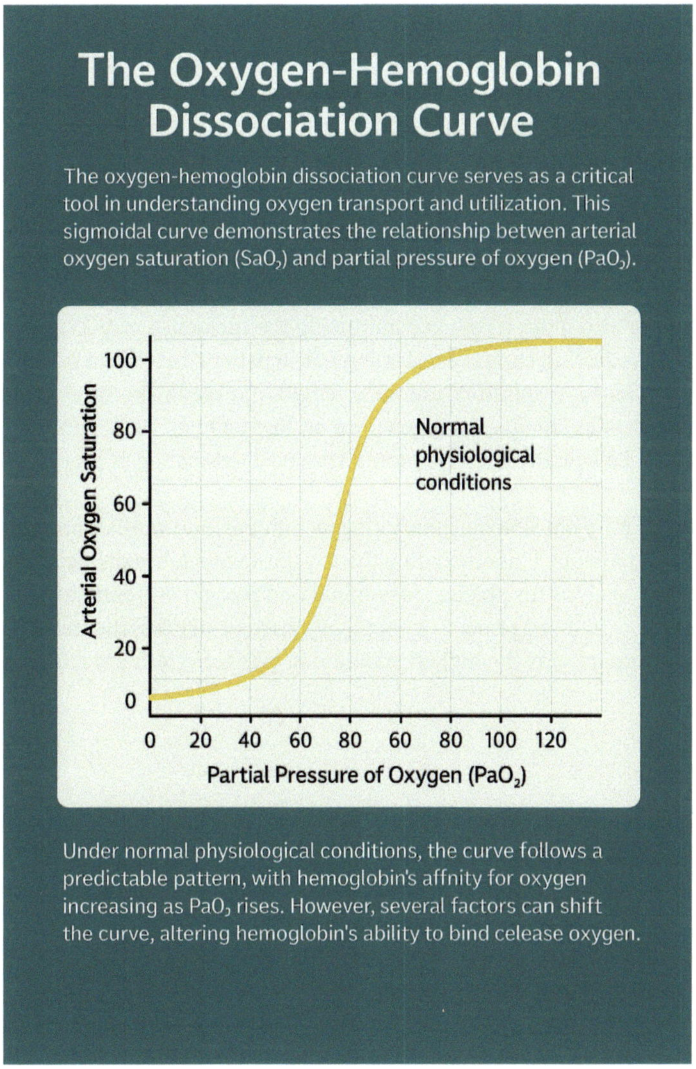

Figure 6.4 Oxygen-hemoglobin dissociation curve. *Source:* Schaeffer (2025).

and respiratory alkalosis. Lactate levels, another critical parameter, reflect anaerobic metabolism and tissue hypoxia, aiding in the assessment of perfusion status.

Pulse oximetry is a noninvasive monitoring tool that estimates arterial oxygen saturation (SpO) using light absorption through capillary beds. While highly useful for continuous monitoring, pulse oximetry has limitations, including inaccuracies in patients with poor peripheral perfusion, hypovolemia, or abnormal hemoglobin variants. In contrast, capnography measures end-tidal CO (EtCO) and serves as a real-time indicator of ventilation efficacy. An elevated EtCO suggests hypoventilation or impaired gas exchange, whereas a low EtCO may indicate hyperventilation, pulmonary embolism, or cardiac arrest.

Mechanical Ventilation

Mechanical ventilation becomes necessary when a patient exhibits severe respiratory failure, defined by a PaO < 60 mmHg on supplemental oxygen, PaCO > 60 mmHg, or evidence of respiratory fatigue. Indications for ventilation include conditions such as acute respiratory distress syndrome (ARDS), pulmonary edema, neuromuscular disorders, or airway obstruction. The goals of mechanical ventilation are to maintain adequate oxygenation and ventilation while minimizing ventilator-induced lung injury (VILI).

Ventilator settings must be tailored to the patient's respiratory status, with adjustments in tidal volume, respiratory rate, fraction of inspired oxygen (FiO), and positive end-expiratory pressure (PEEP). Low tidal volume ventilation (6–8 mL/kg) is recommended to reduce barotrauma and overdistension of alveoli. PEEP prevents alveolar collapse and enhances oxygenation by recruiting collapsed lung units, though excessive PEEP may lead to hemodynamic compromise. FiO should be titrated to maintain SpO between 95% and 98% while minimizing the risk of oxygen toxicity.

Caring for mechanically ventilated patients requires vigilant monitoring of respiratory mechanics, hemodynamic parameters, and gas exchange. Regular assessment of lung compliance, plateau pressures, and inspiratory-to-expiratory (I:E) ratios ensures effective ventilation without causing lung injury. ABG analysis should be performed frequently to evaluate PaO, PaCO, and acid-base status. Additionally, proper sedation and analgesia are critical for patient comfort and synchronization with the ventilator.

Complications associated with mechanical ventilation include ventilator-associated pneumonia (VAP), barotrauma, volutrauma, atelectasis, and oxygen toxicity (Hopper and Powell 2015). Preventative strategies, such as regular endotracheal suctioning, lung-protective ventilation strategies, and appropriate humidification of inspired air, reduce the risk of complications. Proper patient positioning, including head elevation, also plays a role in minimizing the incidence of VAP.

Weaning from mechanical ventilation is a gradual process requiring careful assessment of the patient's ability to sustain spontaneous breathing. Spontaneous breathing trials (SBTs) assess respiratory muscle strength and readiness for extubation. Criteria for successful weaning include stable hemodynamics, adequate oxygenation on low FiO and PEEP, and the ability to generate an appropriate tidal volume (Hopper and Powell 2015). Close monitoring post-extubation is crucial to detect signs of respiratory distress or fatigue.

Veterinary professionals must integrate knowledge of respiratory physiology, monitoring techniques, and ventilation strategies to optimize oxygenation and ventilation in critically ill patients. Understanding the oxygen-hemoglobin dissociation curve as a tool for guiding oxygen therapy, utilizing blood gas analysis for precise assessment, and recognizing early indications for mechanical ventilation are essential skills in critical care management. By applying these principles, the medical team can improve patient outcomes, enhance survival rates, and provide the highest standard of care for veterinary patients experiencing respiratory compromise.

Kirby's Rule of 20 and Blood Pressure Dynamics

Blood pressure is determined by cardiac output and systemic vascular resistance, both of which are influenced by neurohormonal regulation, fluid status, and vascular tone. The maintenance of appropriate mean arterial pressure (MAP) is essential for organ perfusion, and deviations from normal values can result in significant morbidity and mortality in critically ill patients.

The physiology of blood pressure is governed by several key factors. Systolic blood pressure represents the peak arterial pressure during ventricular contraction, while diastolic blood pressure reflects the lowest arterial pressure during ventricular relaxation. MAP, often calculated as diastolic pressure plus one-third of the pulse pressure, is the best indicator of tissue perfusion. Blood pressure is regulated through a complex interplay between baroreceptor reflexes, the renin-angiotensin-aldosterone system (RAAS), and autonomic nervous system input. Baroreceptors located in the carotid sinus and aortic arch detect changes in arterial pressure and mediate compensatory adjustments in heart rate and vascular tone. The RAAS system modulates long-term blood pressure control by influencing sodium retention and vascular resistance through angiotensin II and aldosterone.

Accurate blood pressure measurement is essential for monitoring cardiovascular function in veterinary patients. The selection of an appropriately sized blood pressure cuff is critical for obtaining reliable readings. A cuff width that is approximately 40% of the limb circumference is ideal. Undersized cuffs overestimate blood pressure, whereas oversized cuffs underestimate values. Cuff placement also impacts accuracy. The most reliable measurements are obtained from the tail base and proximal limbs, with the metacarpal and metatarsal arteries providing consistent readings. The coccygeal artery is often used for tail base measurements, while the median and dorsal pedal arteries serve as alternatives. Though auricular artery measurements can be utilized, they are generally less reliable due to variability in vasomotor tone.

Ensuring proper patient positioning during blood pressure assessment enhances accuracy. The patient should be in lateral or sternal recumbency, and the limb or tail used for measurement should be at the level of the heart. Noninvasive blood pressure (NIBP) monitoring, which utilizes oscillometric or Doppler techniques, is commonly employed in clinical practice. Doppler ultrasound is considered the standard in triage and emergency critical care due to its reliability in detecting low-flow states, its ability to provide immediate systolic pressure readings, and its accuracy in small patients where oscillometric readings may be unreliable. The Doppler method involves placing a transducer over an artery distal to the cuff, allowing for real-time assessment of systolic pressure via auditory detection of blood flow. This is particularly advantageous in hypovolemic, hypotensive, or tachycardic patients where oscillometric methods frequently fail due to diminished pulse wave amplitude.

Oscillometric devices estimate systolic, diastolic, and MAPs based on arterial wall oscillations. However, these devices are prone to inaccuracies in small animals and critical patients with weak pulses, arrhythmias, or significant vasoconstriction. While oscillometry may be sufficient for routine monitoring in stable patients, it is not as reliable in the emergency setting where rapid and precise blood pressure assessment is required.

Direct blood pressure measurement via invasive blood pressure (IBP) monitoring is the most accurate method available and is considered the standard for hemodynamic assessment in critically ill patients. IBP monitoring requires arterial catheterization, advanced nursing skills, and specialized equipment, including an arterial catheter, pressure transducer, fluid-filled pressure tubing, and a hemodynamic monitor capable of real-time waveform analysis. Arteries commonly used for catheterization include the dorsal pedal, femoral, and coccygeal arteries, with the choice depending on patient size, accessibility, and clinical status.

The primary advantage of IBP monitoring is its ability to provide real-time, beat-to-beat assessment of arterial pressure, allowing for precise titration of vasoactive drugs and fluid therapy. This continuous data is particularly valuable in patients requiring pressor support, those experiencing hemodynamic instability, or those undergoing prolonged anesthesia. Additionally, waveform analysis can provide further diagnostic insight into cardiovascular performance, including pulse pressure variation and assessment of arterial compliance.

Arterial waveforms in direct blood pressure monitoring provide essential information regarding vascular resistance, stroke volume, and overall perfusion status. The characteristic arterial waveform consists of three primary components: the anacrotic limb, the dicrotic notch, and the diastolic limb. The anacrotic limb represents the rapid upstroke of systolic ejection, corresponding to left ventricular contraction. The dicrotic notch is a distinct deflection in the waveform caused by aortic valve closure and serves as an indicator of diastolic function. The diastolic limb reflects the gradual decline in pressure as blood is distributed to the periphery (Bonagura and Twedt 2021). A dampened waveform suggests catheter obstruction, clot formation, or excessive tubing compliance, while an overly sharp waveform may indicate excessive catheter flushing or overly compliant vessels (Figure 6.5).

Despite its advantages, IBP monitoring carries inherent risks, including infection, thrombosis, hemorrhage, and arterial damage. Strict aseptic technique must be employed during catheter placement, and catheters should be continuously flushed with heparinized saline to prevent clot formation. Frequent monitoring for signs of catheter-related complications, such as local swelling, hemorrhage, or arterial occlusion, is essential to ensuring patient safety. Proper catheter management, including routine line changes and securing of catheters to prevent accidental dislodgement, is critical to reducing adverse effects (Table 6.7).

Normal blood pressure values in veterinary species vary based on size, breed, and clinical status. Generally, systolic pressure should range between 110 and 160 mmHg, diastolic pressure between 60 and 100 mmHg, and MAP between 70 and 120 mmHg. Hypotension, defined as a MAP < 60 mmHg or systolic pressure <90 mmHg, is a common complication in critical care settings and necessitates immediate intervention. Hypotension in critically ill patients arises from multiple

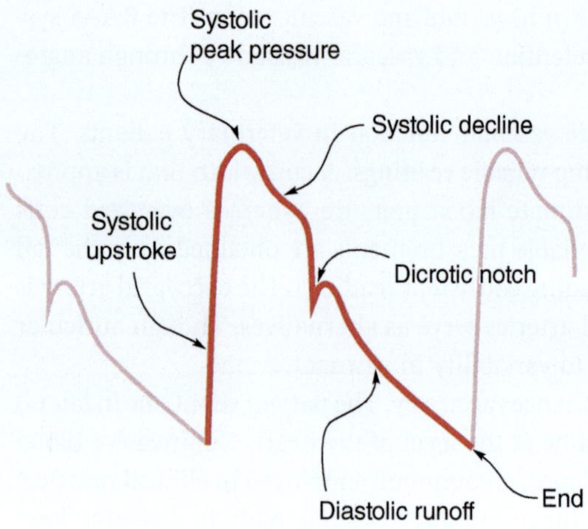

Figure 6.5 Arterial pressure waveform illustrating key components: the anacrotic limb (systolic upstroke), the dicrotic notch marking aortic valve closure, and the diastolic limb indicating vascular runoff and perfusion dynamics. Anacrotic limb = rapid systolic rise due to left ventricular ejection. Dicrotic notch = indicator of diastolic function and valve closure. Diastolic limb = decline in pressure as blood moves peripherally.

Table 6.7 Normal blood pressure values in veterinary patients.

Parameter	Normal Range (mmHg)	Clinical Notes
Systolic Arterial Pressure (SAP)	110–160	Reflects peak pressure during ventricular contraction. Values <90 may indicate hypotension; >180 may indicate hypertension.
Diastolic Arterial Pressure (DAP)	60–100	Reflects lowest arterial pressure during relaxation. Persistent values <50 may compromise organ perfusion.
Mean Arterial Pressure (MAP)	70–120	Represents overall tissue perfusion pressure. MAP < 60 is generally associated with inadequate organ perfusion.

Source: Schaeffer (2025).

etiologies, including hypovolemia, sepsis, anesthesia-induced vasodilation, and myocardial dysfunction. Hypovolemia, caused by hemorrhage, dehydration, or third-spacing of fluids, reduces venous return and cardiac output, leading to a drop in arterial pressure. Sepsis induces widespread vasodilation and endothelial dysfunction due to inflammatory mediators such as nitric oxide and cytokines, impairing vascular tone and cardiac output. Anesthesia-associated hypotension results from anesthetic agents that depress myocardial contractility and reduce sympathetic tone, exacerbating hypotension in volume-depleted patients. Myocardial dysfunction, secondary to conditions such as dilated cardiomyopathy or septic cardiomyopathy, further compromises cardiac output and blood pressure regulation.

Optimizing blood pressure management in critically ill veterinary patients requires a thorough understanding of hemodynamic principles, accurate measurement techniques, and targeted therapeutic interventions. Selecting the appropriate cuff size, placement site, and monitoring modality ensures accurate assessment of arterial pressure. Understanding the physiological mechanisms underlying hypotension and hypertension facilitates appropriate treatment selection, balancing volume resuscitation with vasopressor or antihypertensive therapy.

Kirby's Rule of 20 and Cardiac Rate and Rhythm

The heart's ability to generate and maintain an appropriate rate and rhythm is essential for optimizing cardiac output, oxygen delivery, and systemic perfusion. Any disturbances in heart rate or rhythm can have profound consequences, leading to hemodynamic instability, impaired oxygenation, and organ dysfunction.

The physiology of the heartbeat is governed by an intricate electrical and mechanical interplay. The sinoatrial (SA) node, located in the right atrium, serves as the heart's primary pacemaker, generating action potentials that initiate each heartbeat. These impulses travel through the atria, leading to atrial depolarization and contraction. The electrical signal then passes through the atrioventricular (AV) node, where conduction slows momentarily to allow for ventricular filling. The impulse subsequently propagates through the bundle of His, bundle branches, and Purkinje fibers, resulting in synchronized ventricular depolarization and contraction. This orchestrated electrical activity ensures efficient cardiac function and optimal stroke volume (Figure 6.6).

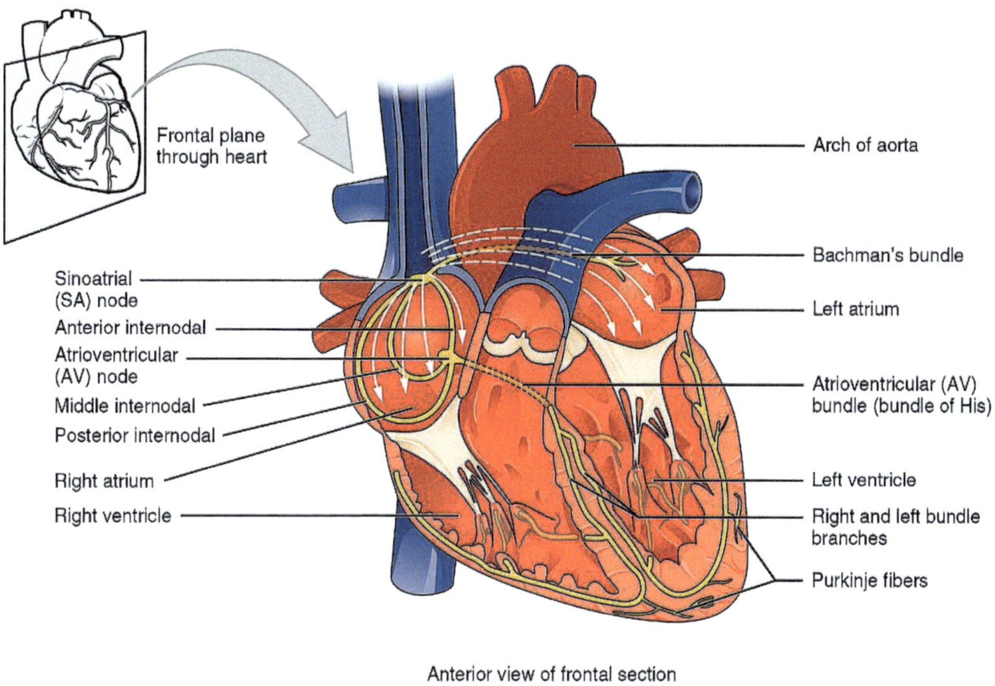

Figure 6.6 The cardiac conduction system: SA node, AV node, bundle of His, bundle branches, and Purkinje fibers. *Source:* OpenStax College / Wikimedia Commons / CC BY 3.0.

Several key parameters influence cardiac function, including preload, afterload, stroke volume, and cardiac output. Preload refers to the volume of blood returning to the heart, affecting ventricular filling and end-diastolic volume. Increased preload enhances stroke volume via the Frank-Starling mechanism, where greater myocardial stretch leads to stronger contraction (Guyton and Hall 2021). Afterload, in contrast, represents the resistance the ventricles must overcome to eject blood. Elevated afterload, as seen in systemic hypertension or aortic stenosis, increases myocardial workload and can reduce cardiac efficiency. Stroke volume, defined as the volume of blood ejected per beat, is directly influenced by preload, afterload, and myocardial contractility. Cardiac output, the total volume of blood pumped per minute, is the product of heart rate and stroke volume and serves as a critical determinant of tissue perfusion.

Electrocardiography (ECG) is the primary diagnostic tool for assessing cardiac rhythm and conduction abnormalities. Proper lead placement is essential for obtaining accurate readings. In veterinary patients, a standard three-lead ECG configuration is commonly used: the right forelimb (RA) lead is placed near the right elbow, the left forelimb (LA) lead near the left elbow, and the left hindlimb (LL) lead near the stifle. The right hindlimb (RL) lead serves as a neutral ground electrode. For continuous telemetry in critical care settings, lead positioning may be adjusted for stability and patient comfort. Proper positioning of the patient in right lateral recumbency is ideal for obtaining a standard six-lead ECG, ensuring optimal waveform morphology and minimizing movement artifacts. Right lateral recumbency provides the most consistent baseline for evaluating conduction disturbances and arrhythmias by reducing motion artifacts and minimizing variability in lead positioning.

The standard ECG tracing consists of distinct waveforms that correspond to electrical events within the heart. The P wave represents atrial depolarization, the QRS complex reflects ventricular depolarization, and the T wave denotes ventricular repolarization. PR interval duration assesses AV node conduction, while the QT interval reflects overall ventricular repolarization. Identifying deviations from normal waveforms is crucial in diagnosing arrhythmias and guiding appropriate therapeutic interventions (Figure 6.7).

Normal heart rates in veterinary patients vary by species, size, and age. In adult dogs, the typical resting heart rate ranges from 60 to 160 beats per minute (bpm), with smaller breeds tending toward the higher end of the spectrum. Large breed dogs generally have lower resting heart rates, while toy breeds and athletic dogs may have naturally higher rates. In cats, the normal resting heart rate is 140–220 bpm. Pediatric patients, particularly neonates, have higher heart rates, with puppies and kittens often exhibiting resting heart rates between 180 and 220 bpm due to increased metabolic demands and immature autonomic regulation (Table 6.8).

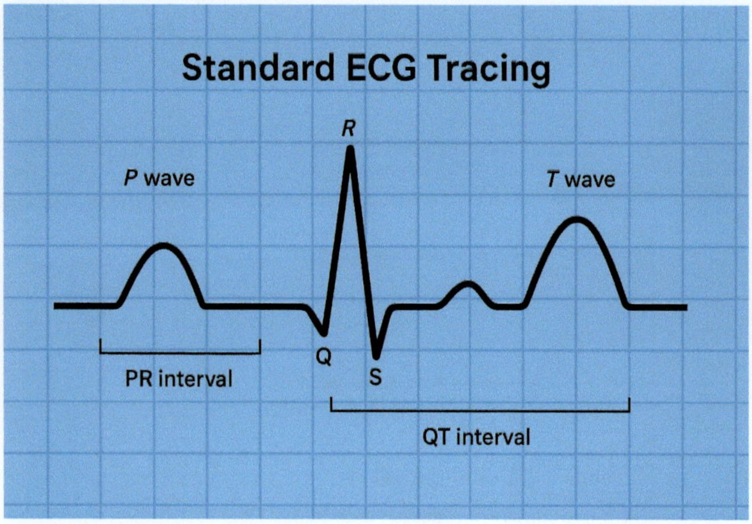

Figure 6.7 Standard ECG tracing with labeled waveforms and intervals. *Source:* Schaeffer (2025).

Table 6.8 Normal resting heart rates in veterinary patients.

Species/Group	Normal Range (bpm)	Clinical Notes
Adult Dogs (General)	60–160	Wide variation based on breed, size, and fitness.
Large Breed Dogs	60–100	Typically lower resting rates due to larger stroke volume.
Small/Toy Breed Dogs	100–160	Higher resting rates; higher metabolic demands.
Athletic Dogs	40–60 (at rest)	Conditioned bradycardia may occur in highly trained dogs.
Adult Cats	140–220	Resting rates are naturally higher than dogs.
Puppies/Kittens (Pediatric)	180–220	Elevated due to immature autonomic control and high metabolic rate.

Source: Schaeffer (2025).

Heart rate disturbances in critically ill patients can be broadly classified as tachyarrhythmias (abnormally fast rhythms) and bradyarrhythmias (abnormally slow rhythms). Sinus tachycardia, characterized by a heart rate exceeding normal physiological ranges, often results from pain, fever, hypovolemia, anemia, or systemic inflammation. More concerning tachyarrhythmias include supraventricular tachycardia (SVT), atrial fibrillation, and ventricular tachycardia (VT), which may compromise cardiac output and necessitate immediate intervention. Conversely, bradyarrhythmias, such as sinus bradycardia, AV block, and atrial standstill, can impair cardiac output and lead to hypotension, syncope, or cardiovascular collapse.

Assessing perfusion parameters is critical in determining whether an arrhythmia requires therapeutic intervention. Heart rate and rhythm abnormalities should not be treated in isolation but rather in conjunction with clinical signs such as mucous membrane color, CRT, pulse quality, mentation, and blood pressure. A patient with an arrhythmia but stable perfusion parameters may not require immediate intervention, whereas a patient with poor perfusion, hypotension, or signs of end-organ dysfunction necessitates prompt treatment. The presence of weak pulses, prolonged CRT, altered mentation, or respiratory distress suggests hemodynamic compromise and the need for therapeutic management.

Telemetry monitoring should be considered for patients with suspected arrhythmias, electrolyte imbalances, or hemodynamic instability. Continuous telemetry is particularly beneficial for patients with a history of collapse, suspected ventricular arrhythmias, or those receiving antiarrhythmic therapy. In the ICU, continuous ECG monitoring is indicated for patients experiencing ongoing cardiac instability, postoperative cardiac patients, or those at high risk for sudden deterioration. Real-time telemetry allows for immediate detection of arrhythmic events and facilitates prompt intervention.

The treatment of cardiac rhythm disturbances depends on the underlying etiology and hemodynamic consequences. Tachyarrhythmias secondary to hypovolemia or anemia often resolve with fluid resuscitation or blood transfusion. SVT may be managed with vagal maneuvers, beta-blockers, or calcium channel blockers, while atrial fibrillation requires rate control and anticoagulation. Hemodynamically unstable VT warrants urgent electrical cardioversion or antiarrhythmic therapy with lidocaine, procainamide, or amiodarone. Bradyarrhythmias may respond to atropine in cases of vagally mediated slowing, though persistent AV block or sick sinus syndrome may necessitate pacemaker placement.

Optimizing heart rate and rhythm in critically ill veterinary patients requires a comprehensive understanding of cardiac physiology, ECG interpretation, and appropriate therapeutic interventions. Early recognition and management of arrhythmias can significantly impact patient outcomes, preserving cardiac function and systemic perfusion. Through vigilant monitoring and evidence-based treatment, veterinary clinicians can ensure the best possible prognosis for patients experiencing cardiac rhythm disturbances in the critical care setting.

Kirby's Rule of 20 and Thermoregulation

Thermoregulation involves maintaining an optimal core body temperature through a balance between heat production and heat loss. This equilibrium is essential for enzymatic reactions, cellular metabolism, and systemic homeostasis. In emergency and intensive care settings, temperature dysregulation can be a significant marker of underlying pathology and often requires immediate intervention to prevent morbidity and mortality.

The physiology of thermoregulation is controlled by the hypothalamus, which acts as the body's thermostat. The hypothalamus establishes a thermoregulatory set point, which represents the body's ideal temperature range and dictates physiological responses to heat gain or loss. The hypothalamus receives afferent input from thermoreceptors located in the skin, spinal cord, and core organs, continuously assessing environmental and internal temperature fluctuations. It modulates heat production through metabolic activity, shivering, and brown adipose tissue metabolism, while heat dissipation is achieved via radiation, conduction, convection, and evaporative cooling through panting or sweating. In veterinary species, particularly dogs and cats, evaporative cooling is predominantly achieved through panting, as sweat glands are limited to paw pads and do not contribute significantly to thermoregulation (Table 6.9).

Hyperthermia results when heat production exceeds the body's ability to dissipate heat, overwhelming the thermoregulatory set point. Unlike pyrexia, which involves an upward adjustment of the hypothalamic set point due to inflammatory cytokines, hyperthermia occurs when excessive heat accumulation disrupts normal homeostatic control. As core temperature rises, vasodilation increases to promote heat dissipation, and panting intensifies to enhance evaporative cooling. However, once body temperature exceeds 41 °C (105.8 °F), compensatory mechanisms become inadequate, leading to systemic endothelial dysfunction, enzymatic failure, and widespread cellular injury (Johnson and McMichael 2015). The severity of hyperthermia determines whether the patient develops heat exhaustion, heatstroke, or SIRS, all of which necessitate rapid intervention.

Immediate intervention is required for hyperthermic emergencies. Active cooling techniques, including tepid water application, evaporative cooling with fans, and intravenous fluid therapy, should be initiated promptly. Wet towels may be applied to vascular regions such as the axilla, groin, and neck, but should be used judiciously to prevent excessive vasoconstriction, which can impede heat dissipation. Cold water immersion is not recommended, as it may trigger peripheral vasoconstriction, trapping heat in the core. The goal of therapy is to reduce body temperature gradually to approximately 39.5 °C (103 °F) to avoid rebound hypothermia. Patients should be monitored for hemodynamic instability, electrolyte disturbances, and secondary complications such as rhabdomyolysis or AKI.

Table 6.9 Heat dissipation mechanisms in dogs, including definitions, examples, and considerations.

Mechanism	Definition	Dog-Specific Example	Notes/Considerations
Radiation	Transfer of heat from the body surface to the environment without direct contact (via infrared waves).	A dog lying in the shade after being in the sun; heat radiates from its skin/fur into the cooler surrounding air.	Works best when ambient temperature is cooler than the dog's body temperature.
Conduction	Direct transfer of heat between the body and objects in contact with it.	A dog lying on a cool tile or concrete floor to release excess body heat.	Efficiency depends on the temperature difference between the dog's body and the surface.
Convection	Heat transfer through movement of air or water across the body.	A fan blowing air across a panting dog's body, carrying heat away.	Airflow is essential; stagnant air limits cooling.
Evaporation	Loss of heat when liquid (water/saliva) converts to vapor.	Panting: water evaporates from the tongue and respiratory tract. Dogs may also sweat slightly through paw pads.	Most effective when humidity is low; limited in high-humidity environments.

Source: Adapted from Guyton and Hall (2021); DiBartola (2012); Speakman and Król (2010); Randall et al. (2002).

Temperature dysregulation in critically ill patients can also present as hypothermia, classified based on severity: mild (99–96 °F), moderate (95–90 °F), and severe (<90 °F) (Boysen and Rozanski 2015). Common etiologies of hypothermia include prolonged anesthesia, environmental exposure, shock, sepsis, metabolic disorders such as hypoadrenocorticism or hypothyroidism, and neuromuscular diseases affecting shivering capacity. In the ICU setting, post-resuscitation patients, neonates, geriatric patients, and those experiencing severe trauma or hemorrhagic shock are at an increased risk of developing hypothermia.

The consequences of hypothermia can be profound, affecting nearly every physiological system. Cardiovascular effects include bradycardia, hypotension, and myocardial depression, while the hematologic system experiences platelet dysfunction and coagulopathies. Metabolic disturbances such as acidosis, electrolyte derangements, and insulin resistance further complicate patient management. Hypothermia also depresses immune function, increasing the risk of secondary infections and delayed wound healing. Severe hypothermia is considered a medical emergency, as patients may develop ventricular arrhythmias, asystole, or refractory shock.

Treatment of hypothermia depends on severity and hemodynamic status. Passive rewarming techniques, including blankets, insulated bedding, and increasing ambient temperature, are appropriate for mild hypothermia. Active external rewarming with forced-air warmers or circulating warm water blankets is indicated in moderate cases, while active core rewarming with warm intravenous fluids, warm water enemas, peritoneal lavage, bladder lavage, or warm humidified oxygen is necessary for severe hypothermia. Aggressive rewarming must be undertaken cautiously to avoid complications such as afterdrop, where cold peripheral blood rapidly returns to the core, precipitating cardiovascular collapse (Boysen and Rozanski 2015). Patients should be monitored continuously for arrhythmias, electrolyte shifts, and evidence of coagulopathy throughout the rewarming process.

In severe hypothermia, rewarming shock and SIRS may occur as the body mounts an inflammatory response during recovery. When hypothermic patients are rewarmed, the release of inflammatory mediators, endothelial dysfunction, and reperfusion injury can lead to systemic inflammation, causing vasodilation, capillary leakage, and hemodynamic instability. This phenomenon mirrors the inflammatory cascade observed in septic shock, with progressive hypotension, tachycardia, and potential progression to multiorgan dysfunction syndrome (MODS). Monitoring for signs of worsening cardiovascular instability, metabolic acidosis, and respiratory distress is essential, and aggressive fluid therapy, vasopressors, and oxygen support may be necessary.

The method of temperature measurement plays a critical role in accurately assessing thermoregulatory status in veterinary patients. Rectal thermometers have traditionally been considered the standard for temperature measurement due to their reliability in reflecting core body temperature. In contrast, aural thermometers, which measure temperature via the tympanic membrane, have been investigated as a less invasive alternative. However, recent research has indicated that aural thermometers in veterinary patients are not as accurate as rectal thermometers, often underestimating or overestimating core temperature due to variability in ear canal anatomy, sensor placement, and ambient temperature influence. A 2022 study published in the *Journal of Veterinary Emergency and Critical Care* found that aural temperatures in dogs and cats were inconsistent compared to rectal temperatures, with variations of up to 1.5 °C, leading to potential misclassification of hypothermia or hyperthermia (Wenger et al. 2022).

Despite their limitations, aural thermometers may be beneficial in certain clinical scenarios. In patients with rectal trauma, severe diarrhea, or risk of iatrogenic injury from repeated rectal probing, aural temperature measurements may provide a safer alternative. Additionally, aural thermometers may offer practical benefits in fractious or aggressive patients where rectal thermometry poses handling challenges. However, given the discrepancies between aural and rectal temperature readings, technicians should interpret aural temperatures with caution and confirm abnormal readings with rectal or esophageal thermometry when precise temperature assessment is critical.

Thermoregulation plays a pivotal role in the survival of critically ill patients, and vigilant monitoring of body temperature should be incorporated into routine ICU assessments. Recognizing early signs of dysregulation and implementing appropriate interventions can prevent severe complications and improve patient outcomes. Integrating knowledge of thermophysiology, understanding the pathophysiological mechanisms underlying hypothermia and hyperthermia, and employing targeted therapeutic strategies will optimize the management of temperature disturbances in emergency and critical care medicine.

Kirby's Rule of 20 and Electrolyte Homeostasis

Electrolyte balance is a fundamental component of physiological stability and an essential aspect of Kirby's Rule of 20 in critically ill veterinary patients. Electrolytes are crucial for maintaining cellular function, neuromuscular activity, acid-base balance, and fluid homeostasis. Any disruption in electrolyte levels can have profound effects on organ function, cardiovascular stability, and metabolic processes. In emergency and intensive care settings, electrolyte derangements are common and often require immediate correction to prevent severe morbidity or mortality.

Physiology of Electrolyte Homeostasis

Electrolytes, including potassium (K^+), sodium (Na^+), chloride (Cl^-), calcium (Ca^{2+}), and magnesium (Mg^{2+}), are tightly regulated by renal function, endocrine control, and cellular transport mechanisms. The kidneys play a central role in electrolyte regulation by adjusting reabsorption and excretion in response to hormonal signals such as aldosterone, ADH, and parathyroid hormone (PTH). The movement of electrolytes across cellular membranes is also influenced by osmoregulation, changes in plasma volume, and acid-base status.

Critically ill patients are at high risk for electrolyte imbalances due to conditions such as dehydration, renal dysfunction, sepsis, trauma, endocrine disease, and the administration of diuretics or fluid therapy. Understanding the pathophysiology and clinical manifestations of electrolyte disturbances is crucial for appropriate intervention.

Major Electrolytes and Clinical Implications

Potassium (K^+) Potassium is the primary intracellular cation and is essential for maintaining resting membrane potential, neuromuscular function, and cardiac excitability. Hypokalemia (<3.5 mEq/L) can result from vomiting, diarrhea, polyuria, diuretic therapy, or anorexia. Clinical signs include muscle weakness, ileus, lethargy, and in severe cases, cardiac arrhythmias such as ventricular premature complexes or atrial fibrillation. Hyperkalemia (>5.5 mEq/L) commonly occurs due to urinary obstruction, AKI, Addison's disease, or reperfusion injury. Severe hyperkalemia (>6.5 mEq/L) may lead to bradyarrhythmias, AV block, atrial standstill, or asystole.

Treatment of hyperkalemia includes calcium gluconate to stabilize myocardial excitability, insulin and dextrose to drive potassium intracellularly, sodium bicarbonate to correct acidosis, and loop diuretics or hemodialysis in refractory cases. Hypokalemia is treated with potassium supplementation, either orally or intravenously. The maximum safe IV potassium infusion rate is **0.5 mEq/kg/h**, as rapid administration can induce fatal arrhythmias.

Sodium (Na^+) Sodium is the major extracellular cation and a critical determinant of plasma osmolality and water balance. Hyponatremia (<135 mEq/L) results from fluid overhydration, Addison's disease, inappropriate ADH secretion, or chronic vomiting and diarrhea. Severe hyponatremia (<120 mEq/L) can lead to cerebral edema, neurological dysfunction, and seizures. Severe hyponatremia results in cerebral edema due to the osmotic gradient that develops between the extracellular and intracellular compartments of brain cells. Sodium is the primary determinant of plasma osmolality, and when serum sodium levels drop significantly, extracellular osmolality decreases. Since the blood-brain barrier limits the rapid movement of large molecules but allows for the movement of water, the relatively hypertonic intracellular environment within neurons and glial cells draws water into the cells, causing swelling.

This cellular swelling in the brain leads to increased ICP, which can result in severe neurological consequences, including altered mentation, seizures, coma, and ultimately brain herniation in extreme cases. The brain attempts to compensate for chronic hyponatremia by downregulating intracellular osmolytes, such as organic solutes (myo-inositol, taurine, and glutamine), to reduce the osmotic gradient and limit swelling (DiBartola 2012). However, in cases of acute or rapidly progressive hyponatremia, the brain does not have sufficient time to compensate, making these patients more susceptible to cerebral edema.

Furthermore, rapid correction of chronic hyponatremia can lead to a dangerous shift in osmolality, resulting in osmotic demyelination syndrome (ODS) (DiBartola 2012). This occurs because the brain, having adapted to a low-sodium environment by decreasing intracellular osmolytes, experiences a rapid osmotic shift when extracellular sodium levels are rapidly increased. The resulting cellular dehydration leads to damage in the myelin sheaths, particularly in the pons, causing neurologic deficits such as quadriparesis, dysphagia, and altered mentation.

The management of severe hyponatremia must be approached cautiously. In cases of acute symptomatic hyponatremia (developing over <24–48 hours), a more aggressive correction rate may be warranted using hypertonic saline to prevent life-threatening cerebral edema. However, in chronic hyponatremia, sodium correction should not exceed 0.5 mEq/L/h or 10–12 mEq/L per 24 hours to reduce the risk of osmotic demyelination (DiBartola 2012). Careful monitoring of serum sodium levels, neurologic status, and fluid balance is essential in critically ill patients to prevent iatrogenic complications.

Hypernatremia (>160 mEq/L) is typically due to dehydration, diabetes insipidus, or excessive sodium administration. Clinical signs include mental dullness, ataxia, and seizures. Treatment involves gradual correction with hypotonic fluids to prevent cerebral edema, with sodium levels reduced by 0.5 mEq/L/h to avoid rapid shifts in brain osmolality (DiBartola 2012).

Chloride (Cl^-) Chloride is an essential extracellular anion involved in acid-base balance and osmoregulation. Hypochloremia (<95 mEq/L) is often secondary to vomiting, diuretic therapy, or metabolic alkalosis. It can lead to neuromuscular dysfunction and hypoventilation. Hyperchloremia (>110 mEq/L) is usually iatrogenic due to excessive saline fluid administration or metabolic acidosis, often presenting with lethargy, tachypnea, and compensatory renal excretion of bicarbonate.

Treatment of hypochloremia involves correcting the underlying cause and providing isotonic saline solutions to restore chloride levels. Hyperchloremia is managed by adjusting fluid therapy, using balanced electrolyte solutions, and addressing acid-base abnormalities.

Calcium (Ca^{2+}) Calcium plays a vital role in neuromuscular excitability, coagulation, and enzymatic reactions. Hypocalcemia (<9 mg/dL) can be caused by hypoparathyroidism, eclampsia, sepsis, or acute pancreatitis. Clinical signs include muscle tremors, facial twitching, tetany, and, in severe cases, seizures. Intravenous calcium gluconate is the treatment of choice, administered slowly over 10–30 minutes with ECG monitoring to prevent bradycardia or arrhythmias.

Hypercalcemia (>12 mg/dL) is most commonly associated with malignancies (lymphoma, anal sac adenocarcinoma), hyperparathyroidism, or renal failure. Clinical signs include polyuria, polydipsia, lethargy, and vomiting. Treatment involves fluid diuresis with saline, loop diuretics, bisphosphonates, or glucocorticoids in cases of malignancy-associated hypercalcemia.

Magnesium (Mg^{2+}) Although often overlooked, magnesium is essential for neuromuscular function and enzymatic processes. Hypomagnesemia can result in refractory hypokalemia or hypocalcemia and should be considered in critically ill patients with persistent electrolyte imbalances. Magnesium sulfate may be supplemented in cases of severe deficiency, particularly in patients with arrhythmias or neuromuscular dysfunction (Table 6.10).

Electrolyte Imbalances and Clinical Manifestations

Electrolyte disturbances can lead to diverse clinical presentations in dogs and cats. Neuromuscular manifestations of electrolyte imbalances include weakness, tremors, altered mentation, and seizures, particularly with hypocalcemia and severe sodium abnormalities. Gastrointestinal signs such as vomiting, diarrhea, and ileus are common with potassium and chloride derangements. Cardiovascular effects are significant in potassium and calcium imbalances, with hyperkalemia predisposing to bradyarrhythmias and asystole, while hypokalemia may result in ventricular ectopy and prolonged QT intervals.

Electrolyte homeostasis is a critical component of managing critically ill veterinary patients. Understanding the mechanisms of electrolyte regulation, recognizing clinical manifestations of imbalances, and implementing appropriate treatments are essential for optimizing patient outcomes. Close monitoring of electrolyte levels, judicious correction strategies, and knowledge of potential complications—such as cerebral edema in hyponatremia or cardiac arrhythmias in potassium

Table 6.10 Key roles of electrolytes in dogs, including primary physiological functions, clinical examples, and relevance. Compiled from established veterinary physiology references.

Electrolyte	Primary Functions	Examples in Dogs	Clinical Relevance
Sodium (Na^+)	Maintains extracellular fluid (ECF) volume and osmotic balance; key in nerve impulse transmission and muscle contraction.	Regulates hydration and blood pressure; critical in neurologic function.	Hyponatremia → seizures, lethargy; Hypernatremia → dehydration, CNS signs.
Potassium (K^+)	Maintains resting membrane potential, neuromuscular function, cardiac rhythm.	Essential for skeletal and cardiac muscle contraction.	Hypokalemia → muscle weakness, arrhythmias; Hyperkalemia → bradycardia, collapse.
Chloride (Cl^-)	Major extracellular anion; maintains acid–base balance; part of gastric acid (HCl).	Supports digestion and buffering systems.	Hypochloremia → metabolic alkalosis (e.g., vomiting); Hyperchloremia → metabolic acidosis.
Calcium (Ca^{2+})	Bone and teeth mineralization, muscle contraction, blood clotting, nerve transmission.	Involved in muscle tone and cardiac contractility.	Hypocalcemia → tremors, seizures, eclampsia; Hypercalcemia → PU/PD, arrhythmias, renal damage.
Magnesium (Mg^{2+})	Cofactor in enzymatic reactions, neuromuscular transmission, stabilizes ATP.	Assists in muscle and nerve function.	Hypomagnesemia → tremors, arrhythmias; Hypermagnesemia → weakness, hypotension.

Source: DiBartola, 2012; Guyton and Hall, 2021; Nelson and Couto, 2020.

imbalances—allow for precise and effective management of these life-threatening disorders in emergency and intensive care settings.

Kirby's Rule of 20 and Blood Glucose Regulation

Blood glucose regulation is a vital component of homeostasis and a critical aspect of Kirby's Rule of 20 in critically ill veterinary patients. Glucose serves as the primary energy source for cellular metabolism, particularly for the brain, RBCs, and renal medulla, which rely on a constant supply due to their limited ability to store glycogen. Glucose homeostasis is tightly regulated by hormonal control, hepatic metabolism, and peripheral glucose utilization. Any dysregulation in glucose levels can significantly impact a patient's prognosis and lead to severe metabolic derangements.

Physiology of Glucose Homeostasis

Glucose homeostasis is maintained through a balance between endogenous production, dietary intake, and cellular utilization. The liver plays a central role in regulating blood glucose through glycogenolysis (breakdown of stored glycogen), gluconeogenesis (synthesis of glucose from noncarbohydrate substrates such as amino acids and lactate), and glycogenesis (storage of glucose as glycogen).

Hormonal regulation is primarily controlled by insulin and glucagon, which are secreted by the pancreas in response to blood glucose fluctuations. Insulin facilitates glucose uptake into cells and promotes glycogenesis and lipogenesis, thereby lowering blood glucose levels. In contrast, glucagon stimulates glycogenolysis and gluconeogenesis during fasting or stress, increasing blood glucose concentrations. Additional counter-regulatory hormones, including cortisol, epinephrine, and growth hormone, play a role in glucose homeostasis, particularly during periods of stress or critical illness.

Glucose Dysregulation in Critical Care Patients

Critically ill patients are susceptible to glucose dysregulation due to metabolic stress, systemic inflammation, sepsis, endocrine dysfunction, and nutritional imbalances. Stress-induced hyperglycemia occurs as a result of excessive counter-regulatory hormone release, while hypoglycemia may develop due to inadequate hepatic glucose production, excessive insulin administration, or increased peripheral glucose consumption.

Normal blood glucose levels in dogs range from 80 to 120 mg/dL, while in cats, they typically range from 70 to 150 mg/dL. Any deviation from these values can indicate underlying metabolic dysfunction and requires clinical intervention.

Hypoglycemia Versus Hypoglycemic Crisis

Hypoglycemia is defined as a blood glucose level below 60 mg/dL in dogs and cats, while a hypoglycemic crisis occurs when glucose levels fall below 40 mg/dL, leading to severe neurological and systemic complications (Feldman and Nelson 2015). Mild hypoglycemia may present with lethargy, weakness, and inappetence, whereas a hypoglycemic crisis can result in seizures, collapse, coma, and potentially death. Neurological signs occur because neurons rely exclusively on glucose for energy, and depletion leads to impaired neuronal function and excitability.

Common causes of hypoglycemia in critical care include sepsis, insulin overdose, hepatic dysfunction, neonatal hypoglycemia, Addison's disease, insulinoma, and severe malnutrition. Immediate treatment involves administering dextrose supplementation via slow IV bolus (0.5–1 mL/kg of 50% dextrose diluted 1:4 with sterile water or saline) followed by a continuous rate infusion (CRI) of 2.5–5% dextrose in maintenance fluids to prevent recurrence (Rozanski and de Laforcade 2015). The underlying conditions must be addressed concurrently to ensure stabilization.

Stress-Induced Hyperglycemia in Cats

Stress hyperglycemia is a well-recognized phenomenon in cats, particularly in hospitalized or fractious patients. It occurs due to excessive catecholamine and glucocorticoid release in response to fear, pain, or handling stress. These hormones promote hepatic gluconeogenesis and glycogenolysis, resulting in transient hyperglycemia that may exceed 250 mg/dL. Unlike pathologic hyperglycemia associated with diabetes mellitus, stress hyperglycemia is typically self-limiting and resolves once the patient is calm and the stressor is removed.

Distinguishing stress hyperglycemia from diabetic hyperglycemia requires serial blood glucose monitoring, assessment of concurrent clinical signs, and measurement of serum fructosamine levels. Fructosamine provides an estimate of average blood glucose concentrations over the preceding 2–3 weeks, with persistently elevated values supporting a diagnosis of diabetes rather than transient stress hyperglycemia. Additionally, patients with diabetes often present with polyuria, polydipsia, weight loss, and persistently high blood glucose readings, whereas stress hyperglycemia lacks these clinical features and normalizes once the cat is no longer stressed.

Hyperglycemia in Critical Care Patients

Hyperglycemia is commonly observed in critically ill patients due to systemic inflammation, pain, sepsis, and administration of glucocorticoids or dextrose-containing fluids. Persistent hyperglycemia (>180 mg/dL in dogs, >250 mg/dL in cats) can lead to osmotic diuresis, electrolyte disturbances, and immunosuppression, increasing susceptibility to infections. While transient stress hyperglycemia does not typically require intervention, prolonged hyperglycemia may necessitate insulin therapy to prevent complications such as DKA or hyperosmolar syndrome. Insulin therapy should be administered cautiously, with close monitoring of blood glucose to prevent iatrogenic hypoglycemia.

Point-of-Care Blood Glucose Correction for Dehydration

Severe dehydration or relative polycythemia can artificially elevate blood glucose readings on point-of-care (POC) devices due to hemoconcentration and alterations in sample viscosity. Recently published discussions governing POC blood glucose correction highlight the importance of adjusting blood glucose measurements in critically ill and dehydrated patients to avoid misinterpretation of blood glucose readings. Research has demonstrated that the AlphaTRAK® glucometer, a commonly used veterinary POC device, underestimates glucose in severely dehydrated patients. The correction formula, supported by research published in the *Journal of Veterinary Emergency and Critical Care*, recommends adjusting blood glucose values based on PCV (Acierno et al. 2014):

$$\text{Corrected POC BG} = \text{POC BG} + (1.6 \times \text{PCV}) - 81.3$$

This formula accounts for the impact of hemoconcentration on blood glucose readings and provides a more accurate assessment of true blood glucose status. By applying this correction in dehydrated patients, clinicians can make more informed decisions regarding glucose management, reducing the risk of unnecessary insulin administration or inappropriate interventions.

Understanding the physiology of glucose homeostasis, recognizing common causes of dysregulation, and implementing appropriate corrective measures are vital for optimizing patient outcomes. Clinicians must differentiate between stress-induced glucose fluctuations and pathological disturbances to avoid unnecessary interventions and improve overall prognosis.

Kirby's Rule of 20 and Acid-Base Status

Acid-base balance is a critical component of homeostasis and plays a fundamental role in maintaining cellular function, enzymatic activity, and metabolic stability. In critically ill veterinary patients, disturbances in acid-base equilibrium are common due to underlying disease processes, respiratory dysfunction, metabolic imbalances, and inadequate tissue perfusion. As part of Kirby's Rule of 20, evaluating and correcting acid-base derangements is essential in optimizing patient outcomes in emergency and critical care settings.

The body maintains acid-base homeostasis through a complex interplay between buffering systems, respiratory compensation, and renal regulation. The primary buffer system is the bicarbonate (HCO^-) and carbonic acid (H_2CO_3) equilibrium, governed by the equation ((DiBartola 2012):

$$CO_2 + H_2O \leftrightarrow H_2CO_3 \leftrightarrow H^+ + HCO_3^-$$

This system functions to minimize pH fluctuations by modulating the ratio of carbon dioxide (CO_2) and bicarbonate (HCO_3^-). The lungs regulate CO_2 elimination through ventilation, while the kidneys maintain acid-base balance by reabsorbing bicarbonate, excreting hydrogen ions (H^+), and generating new bicarbonate as needed (Table 6.11).

Normal arterial blood pH in dogs and cats ranges from 7.35 to 7.45. Any deviation from this range can significantly impact cellular metabolism and systemic function. Acid-base disturbances are classified into four primary categories: metabolic acidosis, metabolic alkalosis, respiratory acidosis, and respiratory alkalosis. Additionally, mixed acid-base disorders can occur when multiple abnormalities exist concurrently.

Metabolic acidosis is characterized by a decrease in bicarbonate (HCO_3^-) and a reduction in blood pH below 7.35. Common causes include lactic acidosis due to hypoxia, sepsis, or shock, ketoacidosis from diabetes or starvation, renal failure, toxin ingestion such as ethylene glycol or aspirin, and severe diarrhea causing bicarbonate loss. Clinical signs may include tachypnea as a compensatory respiratory mechanism, lethargy, weakness, and hypotension. Treatment focuses on addressing the

Table 6.11 Normal arterial blood gas (ABG) ranges in dogs and cats, including pH, $PaCO_2$, PaO_2, bicarbonate, base excess, and oxygen saturation.

Parameter	Dog (Normal Range)	Cat (Normal Range)	Clinical Notes
pH	7.35–7.45	7.30–7.40	Reflects systemic acid–base status; <7.2 = severe acidemia, >7.6 = severe alkalemia.
$PaCO_2$ (mmHg)	35–45	32–38	Reflects adequacy of ventilation; hypercapnia (>45) = hypoventilation, hypocapnia (<30) = hyperventilation.
PaO_2 (mmHg)	80–110 (room air)	80–110 (room air)	Hypoxemia if <80; severe if <60. Must interpret relative to FiO_2.
HCO_3^- (mEq/L)	18–24	17–22	Primary metabolic component of acid–base balance; increased in metabolic alkalosis, decreased in metabolic acidosis.
Base Excess (mEq/L)	−4 to +4	−4 to +4	Assesses metabolic contribution independent of respiratory effects.
SaO_2 (%)	95–100	95–100	<90% indicates significant hypoxemia.

Source: Adapted from DiBartola (2012), Hopper and Epstein (2015), and Rudloff and Kirby (2012).

underlying cause. Sodium bicarbonate therapy may be considered in cases of severe acidosis with a pH below 7.2, but caution is warranted due to the risk of paradoxical intracellular acidosis and electrolyte disturbances (DiBartola 2012).

Metabolic alkalosis occurs when there is an increase in bicarbonate (HCO_3^-) and an elevation in blood pH above 7.45. This disturbance often results from excessive vomiting leading to gastric acid loss, diuretic therapy such as loop or thiazide diuretics, hypokalemia, and hyperaldosteronism. Clinical signs include muscle tremors, weakness, polyuria, polydipsia, and arrhythmias. Treatment involves correcting fluid deficits with chloride-rich fluids such as 0.9% NaCl, replacing potassium when hypokalemia is present, and addressing the primary disease process.

Respiratory acidosis is characterized by an increase in carbon dioxide (CO_2) and a decrease in blood pH below 7.35 due to hypoventilation. Causes include airway obstruction, severe pulmonary disease, neuromuscular disorders such as myasthenia gravis or cervical spinal cord injury, anesthesia-induced respiratory depression, and pleural space disease. Clinical signs may include respiratory distress, cyanosis, obtundation, and hypoventilation. Treatment aims to improve ventilation through oxygen therapy, mechanical ventilation when necessary, and resolution of the underlying cause.

Respiratory alkalosis results from a decrease in CO_2 and an increase in blood pH above 7.45 due to hyperventilation. This condition is commonly associated with pain, anxiety, fever, hypoxemia, sepsis, and excessive mechanical ventilation. Clinical signs may include tachypnea, agitation, muscle tremors, and weakness. Treatment focuses on managing the underlying cause, providing sedation if necessary, and adjusting mechanical ventilation settings to correct excessive ventilation.

Mixed acid-base disorders occur when two or more acid-base abnormalities coexist. Examples include metabolic acidosis with respiratory acidosis, which is often seen in severe sepsis with respiratory failure, and metabolic alkalosis with respiratory alkalosis, which may occur in patients experiencing vomiting in conjunction with pain or anxiety-induced hyperventilation. Diagnosis of mixed disturbances requires ABG analysis and evaluation of pH, CO_2, HCO_3^-, and anion gap. Treatment depends on the dominant abnormality and requires correction of the primary cause or causes.

Acid-base status is best assessed using ABG analysis, which provides critical parameters for evaluating a patient's metabolic and respiratory function. The pH indicates overall acid-base balance, while $PaCO_2$ levels, which range between 35 and 45 mmHg, help determine the respiratory contribution to an imbalance, increasing in acidosis and decreasing in alkalosis. Bicarbonate (HCO_2^-), normally between 18 and 26 mEq/L, reflects the metabolic contribution, decreasing in acidosis and increasing in alkalosis. Base excess, typically ranging from −5 to +5 mEq/L, quantifies the metabolic component, with a negative value suggesting metabolic acidosis and a positive value indicating metabolic alkalosis. Anion gap, calculated as $Na^+ - (Cl^- + HCO_2^-)$, helps differentiate high anion gap acidosis, such as lactic acidosis or ketoacidosis, from normal anion gap acidosis seen in conditions like renal tubular acidosis or diarrhea (DiBartola 2012).

Clinical manifestations of acid-base disturbances vary based on the underlying condition. Acidosis is often associated with lethargy, tachypnea, hypotension, arrhythmias, altered mentation, and respiratory distress when due to respiratory acidosis. Alkalosis can present with muscle tremors, weakness, irritability, arrhythmias, and hypoventilation in cases of respiratory alkalosis.

Treatment modalities for acid-base disturbances focus on addressing the underlying cause. Fluid therapy is a cornerstone of treatment, with balanced electrolyte solutions used for metabolic acidosis and chloride-rich fluids preferred for metabolic alkalosis. Oxygen and ventilation support are critical for respiratory acid-base imbalances, requiring careful adjustments to ventilator settings when managing respiratory acidosis or alkalosis. Sodium bicarbonate therapy should be reserved for cases of severe metabolic acidosis with a pH below 7.2, and its administration must be monitored closely to avoid iatrogenic complications. Electrolyte correction is often necessary, particularly in cases of hypokalemia, hypochloremia, or other imbalances contributing to the acid-base disturbance.

Kirby's Rule of 20 and Renal Function

The kidneys regulate electrolyte levels, acid-base balance, and blood pressure while also contributing to endocrine function through the production of erythropoietin (EPO) and activation of vitamin D. In critically ill veterinary patients, renal function must be closely monitored as kidney dysfunction can significantly impact systemic stability and patient prognosis.

The renal system consists of paired kidneys, which filter blood through a highly specialized network of nephrons. Each nephron contains a glomerulus, proximal tubule, loop of Henle, distal tubule, and collecting duct. The glomerulus is responsible for filtration, while the tubules modulate solute and water reabsorption. The kidneys receive approximately 20–25% of cardiac output, emphasizing their role in maintaining fluid balance and perfusion. The renal system excretes metabolic waste products such as urea and creatinine while conserving essential electrolytes and regulating water balance. Additionally, the kidneys contribute to acid-base homeostasis by excreting hydrogen ions and reabsorbing bicarbonate.

The kidneys also play a major role in systemic blood pressure regulation through the RAAS. When renal perfusion drops, the juxtaglomerular cells in the kidney release renin, which catalyzes the conversion of angiotensinogen to angiotensin I. Angiotensin-converting enzyme (ACE) then converts angiotensin I to angiotensin II, a potent vasoconstrictor that increases blood pressure and stimulates aldosterone release. Aldosterone promotes sodium and water retention to expand circulating blood volume, further supporting renal perfusion. However, in conditions such as congestive heart failure or CKD, excessive RAAS activation can lead to fluid overhydration and systemic hypertension.

Critically ill patients require frequent assessment of renal function to detect early signs of kidney injury or failure. AKI is a sudden decline in renal function due to ischemia, nephrotoxins, infection, or systemic inflammatory disease. In contrast, CKD results from progressive nephron loss over time, leading to a gradual decline in renal function. Some patients may experience an acute-on-chronic kidney injury, where a preexisting renal disease is exacerbated by a secondary insult, such as dehydration, infection, or toxic exposure. AKI can be further classified into stages based on severity, using biomarkers such as creatinine, symmetric dimethylarginine (SDMA), and urine output trends. Early recognition of AKI is essential, as timely intervention can sometimes prevent progression to irreversible renal failure.

Azotemia refers to elevated BUN and creatinine levels due to reduced renal clearance. Uremia, a more severe consequence, involves systemic clinical signs associated with toxin accumulation, including vomiting, anorexia, oral ulcerations, lethargy, and neurologic abnormalities. Differentiating between prerenal, renal, and postrenal azotemia is critical for determining appropriate therapeutic interventions. Prerenal azotemia results from decreased renal perfusion due to dehydration or hypotension, renal azotemia arises from intrinsic kidney dysfunction, and postrenal azotemia occurs secondary to urinary obstruction or leakage. While azotemia is a laboratory finding, uremia indicates a clinical syndrome with systemic manifestations, necessitating aggressive medical management (Table 6.12).

Urine specific gravity (USG) is a valuable diagnostic tool in critically ill patients, reflecting the kidney's ability to concentrate urine. In prerenal azotemia, USG is typically high (>1.030 in dogs, >1.035 in cats) due to intact tubular function, while renal azotemia presents with an isosthenuric USG (1.008–1.012), indicating a loss of concentrating ability. Postrenal azotemia may have variable USG, depending on the underlying cause. Serial USG monitoring, in conjunction with bloodwork, aids in determining whether fluid therapy is improving renal perfusion or if intrinsic kidney injury is present. The presence of hyposthenuria (USG < 1.008) suggests an inability to retain water, commonly seen with conditions such as diabetes insipidus or psychogenic polydipsia (Table 6.13).

Oliguria, defined as urine output less than 0.5 mL/kg/h (Brown 2015), and anuria, the complete absence of urine production, indicate severe renal compromise or obstruction. Persistent oliguria despite adequate fluid resuscitation may warrant diuretic therapy, vasopressor support to improve renal perfusion, or advanced interventions such as dialysis. Monitoring urine output trends provides critical insight into kidney function, and serial measurement of urinary electrolyte concentrations, including fractional excretion of sodium (FENa), can help distinguish between prerenal and intrinsic renal failure (Brown 2015).

Measuring ins and outs is crucial in critically ill patients when assessing fluid balance. Urine output should be closely monitored through catheterization or noninvasive collection methods, and daily body weight assessments provide

Table 6.12 Comparison of azotemia (prerenal, renal, postrenal) and uremia in dogs and cats, including definitions, key features, and clinical relevance.

Condition	Definition	Key Features	Examples/Clinical Relevance
Azotemia	Elevated blood urea nitrogen (BUN) and creatinine due to reduced renal clearance.	Laboratory finding; may be prerenal, renal, or postrenal in origin.	Detected on bloodwork before systemic signs appear. Requires further evaluation to determine the underlying cause.
Pre Renal Azotemia	Decreased renal perfusion (without intrinsic kidney damage).	Causes: dehydration, hypovolemia, hypotension.	Reversible if perfusion restored promptly.
Renal Azotemia	Intrinsic dysfunction of the kidneys.	Causes: acute kidney injury, chronic kidney disease, nephrotoxins, infectious disease.	Typically associated with isosthenuria and requires supportive or long-term management.
Post Renal Azotemia	Secondary to obstruction or leakage of the urinary tract.	Causes: urethral obstruction, bladder rupture, ureteral obstruction.	Rapidly progressive; requires immediate intervention to restore urine flow or repair leakage.
Uremia	Clinical syndrome due to systemic effects of retained uremic toxins.	Vomiting, anorexia, oral ulcerations, lethargy, halitosis, neurologic abnormalities, coagulopathy.	Indicates severe renal dysfunction; requires aggressive medical management (fluids, antiemetics, dialysis, etc.).

Source: Adapted from DiBartola (2012), Polzin (2011), and Grauer (2011).

Table 6.13 Interpretation of urine specific gravity (USG) in dogs and cats, including normal, prerenal, renal, and postrenal azotemia as well as hyposthenuria, with corresponding values, interpretation, and clinical relevance.

Condition	Typical USG Values	Interpretation	Clinical Relevance
Normal/Well-Concentrated Urine	>1.030 in dogs, >1.035 in cats	Normal tubular concentrating ability	Indicates adequate renal function and hydration status.
Pre Renal Azotemia	>1.030 (dogs), >1.035 (cats)	Kidneys concentrate appropriately in response to dehydration or hypoperfusion	Suggests intact renal tubular function; azotemia likely due to reduced renal perfusion.
Renal Azotemia	Isosthenuric (1.008–1.012)	Kidneys unable to concentrate or dilute urine	Indicates intrinsic renal damage; correlates with renal failure.
Post Renal Azotemia	Variable (can be concentrated, isosthenuric, or diluted)	Depends on obstruction or urinary leakage	Interpretation requires correlation with clinical findings and imaging.
Hyposthenuria	<1.008	Active dilution of urine below plasma osmolality	Seen in diabetes insipidus, psychogenic polydipsia, or some endocrine disorders.

Source: Adapted from DiBartola (2012), Grauer (2011), and Polzin (2011).

additional insight into fluid status. Matching fluid intake to output is particularly important in patients receiving aggressive diuresis, those with oliguria or anuria, and those at risk for fluid overhydration. In cases of polyuria, careful assessment of electrolyte losses, hydration status, and osmolar imbalances is required to avoid iatrogenic complications.

Given the kidneys' critical role in homeostasis, early identification and management of renal dysfunction in critical care patients are paramount. Understanding renal physiology, assessing urine production and concentration, and differentiating between azotemia and uremia are essential in guiding appropriate treatment and improving patient outcomes. Comprehensive monitoring strategies, including serial biochemical analysis, urinalysis, and imaging, help determine the progression of renal disease and guide fluid therapy adjustments.

Kirby's Rule of 20 and Red Blood Cells and Hemoglobin

Red blood cell (RBC) and hemoglobin levels are crucial parameters in critical care monitoring. These elements play an essential role in oxygen transport, systemic oxygenation, and overall tissue perfusion. In critically ill patients, assessing RBC count and hemoglobin concentration is vital to detecting and managing conditions such as anemia, hypoxia, and

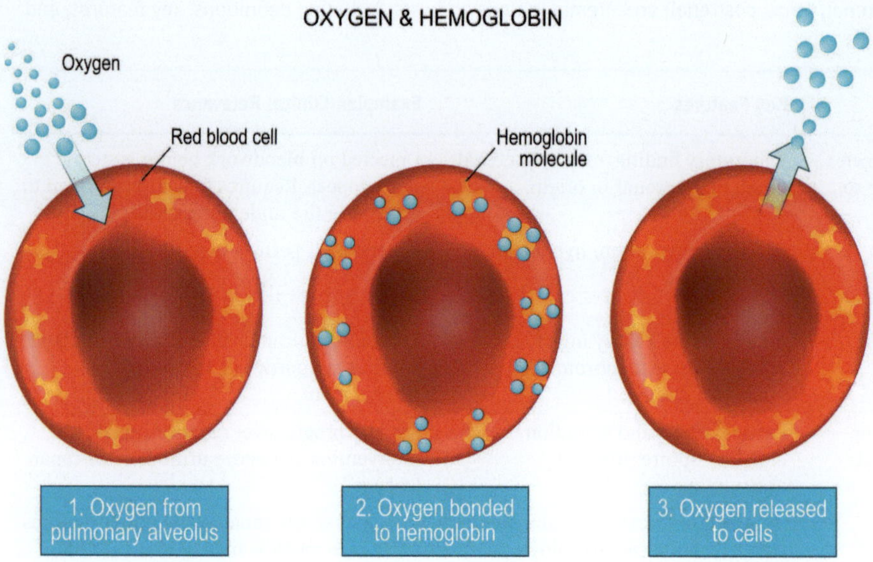

Figure 6.8 Simplified diagram of a red blood cell with hemoglobin binding oxygen molecules, illustrating oxygen transport. *Source:* VectorStock (2024).

impaired oxygen delivery. Without adequate RBCs and hemoglobin, vital organs suffer from oxygen deprivation, leading to metabolic acidosis, organ dysfunction, and, in severe cases, death (Figure 6.8).

Physiology of Red Blood Cells and Hemoglobin

RBCs are specialized cells designed to transport oxygen from the lungs to tissues and facilitate the removal of carbon dioxide. These biconcave, anucleated cells contain hemoglobin, an iron-containing protein that binds to oxygen molecules for delivery to tissues. The efficiency of oxygen transport depends on the number of RBCs, hemoglobin concentration, and hemoglobin's affinity for oxygen.

Hemoglobin exists in several forms, including oxyhemoglobin (oxygen-bound), deoxyhemoglobin (oxygen-released), methemoglobin (oxidized form incapable of oxygen binding), and carboxyhemoglobin (bound to carbon monoxide). The oxygen-carrying capacity of hemoglobin is influenced by factors such as pH, temperature, carbon dioxide concentration, and 2,3-diphosphoglycerate (2,3-DPG) levels, all of which impact the oxyhemoglobin dissociation curve (Guyton and Hall 2021).

Erythropoiesis, the production of RBCs, occurs in bone marrow and is primarily regulated by EPO, a hormone secreted by the kidneys in response to hypoxia. Once produced, RBCs circulate for approximately 100–120 days in dogs and 70–80 days in cats before being removed by the spleen (Harvey 2012). During their lifespan, RBCs are responsible for maintaining oxygen delivery to tissues, buffering blood pH, and ensuring metabolic homeostasis.

The Importance of Monitoring Red Blood Cells and Hemoglobin in Critical Care

In critically ill patients, RBC and hemoglobin abnormalities are common due to blood loss, hemolysis, bone marrow suppression, or systemic disease. Conditions such as hemorrhagic shock, immune-mediated hemolytic anemia (IMHA), sepsis, and renal failure frequently affect RBC production and survival, requiring close monitoring and intervention. Monitoring hematologic parameters, including PCV, hemoglobin concentration, and RBC indices (mean corpuscular volume [MCV] and mean corpuscular hemoglobin concentration [MCHC]), is essential to understanding the cause of anemia or polycythemia.

Oxygen delivery (DO_2) is a function of cardiac output and arterial oxygen content, both of which rely on adequate hemoglobin levels. A decrease in RBCs or hemoglobin concentration reduces oxygen-carrying capacity, leading to compensatory mechanisms such as increased cardiac output, tachycardia, and vasodilation to maintain perfusion. However, these compensatory responses are often insufficient in critical patients, necessitating transfusion therapy or oxygen supplementation.

Clinical Signs of Red Blood Cell and Hemoglobin Abnormalities

Patients with decreased RBCs or hemoglobin may exhibit clinical signs of anemia, including pale mucous membranes, tachycardia, tachypnea, lethargy, weakness, and, in severe cases, collapse. Hypoxia-induced metabolic acidosis can further contribute to tachypnea and altered mentation. In chronic anemia, compensatory mechanisms such as increased 2,3-DPG levels facilitate oxygen unloading at the tissue level, allowing some patients to tolerate lower hemoglobin levels without overt clinical signs (Weiss and Wardrop 2010).

Conversely, an increased RBC count, known as polycythemia, may result from dehydration (relative polycythemia) or primary conditions such as polycythemia vera or chronic hypoxia-induced erythropoiesis (absolute polycythemia). Clinical signs of polycythemia include hyperviscosity syndrome, characterized by neurological abnormalities, seizures, ataxia, and retinal hemorrhages due to increased blood viscosity and impaired microcirculatory flow.

Treatment of Red Blood Cell and Hemoglobin Abnormalities

The treatment of RBC and hemoglobin abnormalities depends on the underlying etiology. In cases of anemia due to hemorrhage, stabilization with intravenous fluid therapy and blood transfusion is often required. Whole blood transfusions or packed red blood cell (pRBC) transfusions may be indicated in patients with severe anemia (PCV < 20%) or evidence of hypoxic tissue injury. The transfusion trigger varies depending on the patient's clinical status, with hemodynamically stable patients often tolerating lower PCV values than unstable patients.

For IMHA, treatment involves immunosuppressive therapy with corticosteroids, azathioprine, cyclosporine, or mycophenolate. In cases of severe hemolysis, transfusions may be required, but these must be administered cautiously due to the risk of exacerbating hemolysis and transfusion reactions.

Polycythemia due to dehydration resolves with appropriate fluid therapy, while absolute polycythemia may require therapeutic phlebotomy or hydroxyurea therapy to reduce RBC mass and prevent hyperviscosity-related complications. Patients with secondary polycythemia due to hypoxia should be assessed for underlying causes such as pulmonary disease or cardiac shunting, with appropriate treatment directed at correcting the hypoxic stimulus.

Methods of Monitoring Red Blood Cells and Hemoglobin in Veterinary Medicine

Monitoring RBC and hemoglobin levels in critically ill patients involves serial evaluation of PCV, hemoglobin concentration, total protein, blood gas analysis, and reticulocyte counts. PCV and TS provide a rapid assessment of anemia and fluid balance but must be interpreted in conjunction with clinical signs and other laboratory values. Hemoglobin concentration, typically measured as a function of PCV, provides insight into oxygen-carrying capacity, with a normal hemoglobin-to-PCV ratio of approximately 1:3 in dogs and cats (Thrall et al. 2012).

Blood gas analysis, particularly venous and ABG, allows for the assessment of oxygen content, lactate levels, and acid-base status. Oxygen saturation (SaO_2) and partial pressure of oxygen (PaO_2) provide further information regarding the efficiency of oxygen transport and tissue oxygenation. Reticulocyte counts differentiate between regenerative and nonregenerative anemia, aiding in the diagnosis of bone marrow disorders or chronic disease-related anemia.

RBCs and hemoglobin are critical components of oxygen transport and systemic homeostasis, making them a fundamental consideration in the management of critically ill veterinary patients. Monitoring RBC count and hemoglobin levels allows clinicians to assess oxygen delivery, identify anemia or polycythemia, and guide appropriate therapeutic interventions. The pathophysiology of RBC and hemoglobin abnormalities varies widely, from acute hemorrhagic anemia to chronic polycythemia, necessitating individualized treatment strategies based on the underlying etiology.

Kirby's Rule of 20 and Coagulation

Coagulation is a critical physiological process that maintains hemostasis by preventing excessive blood loss while ensuring adequate blood flow. In critically ill veterinary patients, coagulation disorders are common due to systemic inflammation, sepsis, trauma, and disseminated intravascular coagulation (DIC). As part of Kirby's Rule of 20, evaluating coagulation status is essential in the ICU to identify, monitor, and manage coagulopathies before they lead to life-threatening hemorrhage or thrombosis.

Physiology of Coagulation

The coagulation system consists of three primary components: the vascular endothelium, platelets, and the coagulation cascade. Hemostasis occurs in three sequential phases: primary hemostasis, secondary hemostasis, and fibrinolysis.

Primary hemostasis begins with vascular injury, leading to endothelial disruption and the exposure of subendothelial collagen and vWF. This exposure promotes platelet adhesion and activation, resulting in the formation of a temporary platelet plug. Platelet activation leads to the release of pro-coagulant factors such as thromboxane A_2 and adenosine diphosphate (ADP), which amplify platelet aggregation (Brooks 2010).

Secondary hemostasis stabilizes the platelet plug through the activation of the coagulation cascade, which involves a series of enzymatic reactions leading to the conversion of fibrinogen to fibrin. The coagulation cascade is divided into the intrinsic, extrinsic, and common pathways. The intrinsic pathway is activated by endothelial injury and involves factors XII, XI, IX, and VIII, while the extrinsic pathway is initiated by tissue factor (factor III) and factor VII. Both pathways converge at the common pathway, where factor X activation leads to the formation of thrombin, which subsequently converts fibrinogen into fibrin, reinforcing the clot.

Fibrinolysis serves as the final stage of coagulation, ensuring clot dissolution and maintaining vascular patency. Plasminogen is converted into plasmin, which degrades fibrin into fibrin degradation products (FDPs), preventing excessive clot formation and thrombosis (Brooks 2010).

Clinical Signs of Coagulopathies

Coagulation abnormalities manifest in various ways depending on the underlying disorder. Platelet disorders, including thrombocytopenia and thrombopathies, result in petechiae, ecchymoses, epistaxis, hematuria, and spontaneous mucosal bleeding. Disorders affecting secondary hemostasis, such as factor deficiencies or anticoagulant rodenticide toxicity, present with more profound bleeding tendencies, including hematomas, hemarthrosis, hemothorax, and intra-abdominal hemorrhage. Hypercoagulable states, such as DIC or immune-mediated diseases, may lead to thromboembolic complications, causing ischemic organ injury, neurologic signs, and respiratory distress (Figure 6.9).

Importance of Coagulation Monitoring in Critical Care

Monitoring coagulation is essential in ICU patients due to the high prevalence of conditions that predispose to either bleeding or thrombosis. Patients with sepsis, SIRS, trauma, pancreatitis, or neoplasia frequently develop coagulation abnormalities that require close monitoring and early intervention. Assessing coagulation status allows for the timely administration of transfusions, anticoagulants, or pro-coagulant therapy as needed.

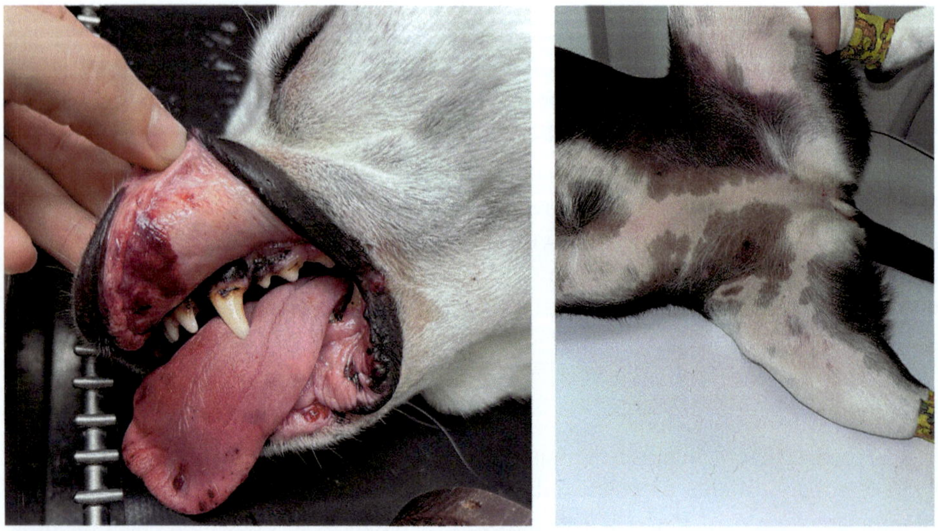

Figure 6.9 Ecchymosis in a coagulopathic patient. *Source:* Photo by Crystal Schaeffer.

Diagnostic Testing for Coagulation Disorders

Several laboratory tests are available to assess coagulation status in veterinary patients. Manual platelet counts are performed using a blood smear and are essential in detecting thrombocytopenia. To perform a manual platelet count, a blood smear is prepared, stained, and examined under oil immersion (100× objective). The number of platelets in 10 fields is averaged and multiplied by 15,000 to 20,000 to estimate the platelet count per microliter. This method is crucial in evaluating platelet clumping, which may falsely lower automated platelet counts (Figure 6.10).

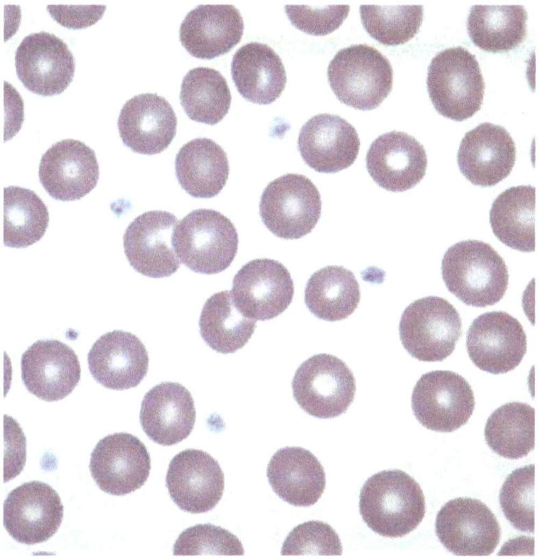

Figure 6.10 Canine blood smear showing red blood cells, and platelets. *Source:* eClinpath / https://eclinpath.com/hematology/hemogram-basics/blood-smear-examination/ / last accessed on 27 Oct, 2025.

Prothrombin time (PT) and activated partial thromboplastin time (aPTT) assess secondary hemostasis. PT evaluates the extrinsic and common pathways, measuring the activity of factors VII, X, V, II, and fibrinogen. A prolonged PT suggests deficiencies in these factors or vitamin K antagonism (e.g., anticoagulant rodenticide toxicity). aPTT evaluates the intrinsic and common pathways, assessing factors XII, XI, IX, and VIII. Prolonged aPTT is observed in conditions such as hemophilia, liver failure, and DIC.

Coagulation profiles are often outsourced to reference laboratories and may include PT, aPTT, fibrinogen concentration, D-dimer levels, FDPs, and thromboelastography (TEG). TEG provides a dynamic assessment of coagulation, including clot formation, stability, and breakdown. It is particularly useful in guiding transfusion therapy and identifying hypercoagulable states.

Coagulation Disturbances in ICU Patients

Critically ill patients are at increased risk for coagulation disturbances due to systemic inflammation, endothelial injury, and alterations in clotting factor production. DIC is a severe coagulopathy characterized by widespread activation of the coagulation cascade, leading to simultaneous thrombosis and hemorrhage. DIC occurs secondary to sepsis, neoplasia, heatstroke, or trauma and is associated with thrombocytopenia, prolonged PT/aPTT, decreased fibrinogen, and increased D-dimer levels.

Patients with anticoagulant rodenticide toxicity develop coagulopathies due to vitamin K antagonism, resulting in deficiencies of factors II, VII, IX, and X. These patients present with spontaneous hemorrhage, prolonged PT and aPTT, and require treatment with vitamin K1 therapy.

Liver failure contributes to coagulopathies due to impaired synthesis of clotting factors, leading to prolonged PT/aPTT and increased bleeding risk. Patients with hepatic dysfunction may require plasma transfusions to restore coagulation factor levels.

Hypercoagulable states are also prevalent in ICU patients, particularly those with IMHA, neoplasia, or sepsis. These conditions predispose patients to thromboembolic complications, requiring anticoagulant therapy with heparin, aspirin, or clopidogrel.

Treatment of Coagulation Disorders

The management of coagulation disorders depends on the underlying etiology. Patients with thrombocytopenia secondary to immune-mediated thrombocytopenia (IMTP) require immunosuppressive therapy with corticosteroids, vincristine, or cyclosporine. Severe thrombocytopenia with active hemorrhage may necessitate platelet-rich plasma or whole blood transfusions. In cases of DIC, treatment focuses on supportive care, addressing the primary disease process, and maintaining adequate perfusion. Fresh frozen plasma transfusions may be administered to replenish clotting factors, while heparin therapy may be considered in hypercoagulable patients. Patients with anticoagulant rodenticide toxicity require vitamin K1 supplementation for at least four to six weeks, with serial PT monitoring to determine treatment duration. In cases of severe hemorrhage, plasma transfusions may be necessary to provide immediate clotting factor replacement. For hypercoagulable patients, anticoagulation therapy is initiated with unfractionated heparin, low-molecular-weight heparin (LMWH), or antiplatelet agents to prevent thromboembolic events. The choice of therapy depends on the patient's risk factors and concurrent medical conditions.

Coagulation monitoring is an essential component of critical care management, as coagulation disorders can lead to severe morbidity and mortality if not identified and treated promptly. Understanding the physiology of coagulation, recognizing clinical signs of coagulopathy, and utilizing appropriate diagnostic tests enable early intervention and improved patient outcomes.

Kirby's Rule of 20: Gastrointestinal Integrity and Motility

Gastrointestinal (GI) integrity and motility play a crucial role in overall patient stability and prognosis. GI dysfunction is a common and often severe complication in critical care patients, frequently resulting from systemic inflammation, hypoperfusion, stress-related mucosal injury, and dysmotility.

Pathophysiology of Gastrointestinal Integrity

The integrity of the gastrointestinal tract relies on a well-coordinated interaction between the mucosal barrier, local immune responses, adequate perfusion, and enteric nervous system regulation. In critically ill patients, multiple pathophysiological processes can compromise these protective mechanisms, leading to increased intestinal permeability, bacterial translocation, and systemic inflammatory responses (Figure 6.11).

Mucosal barrier dysfunction results from damage to the epithelial lining and disruption of tight junctions, which normally regulate selective permeability. Hypoxia, ischemia-reperfusion injury, and inflammatory cytokines such as tumor necrosis factor-alpha (TNF-α) and interleukin-6 (IL-6) compromise these tight junctions, increasing permeability and predisposing the patient to bacterial translocation and endotoxemia (Blikslager et al. 2007). This in turn exacerbates SIRS and can lead to MODS.

Hypoperfusion and ischemic injury contribute significantly to GI dysfunction in critically ill patients. During shock states, whether hypovolemic, septic, or cardiogenic, autoregulatory mechanisms prioritize blood flow to the heart and brain at the expense of the gastrointestinal tract. The resulting ischemic injury leads to sloughing of enterocytes, ulceration, and hemorrhagic gastroenteropathy. When perfusion is restored, ischemia-reperfusion injury can exacerbate damage due to oxidative stress and the release of inflammatory mediators.

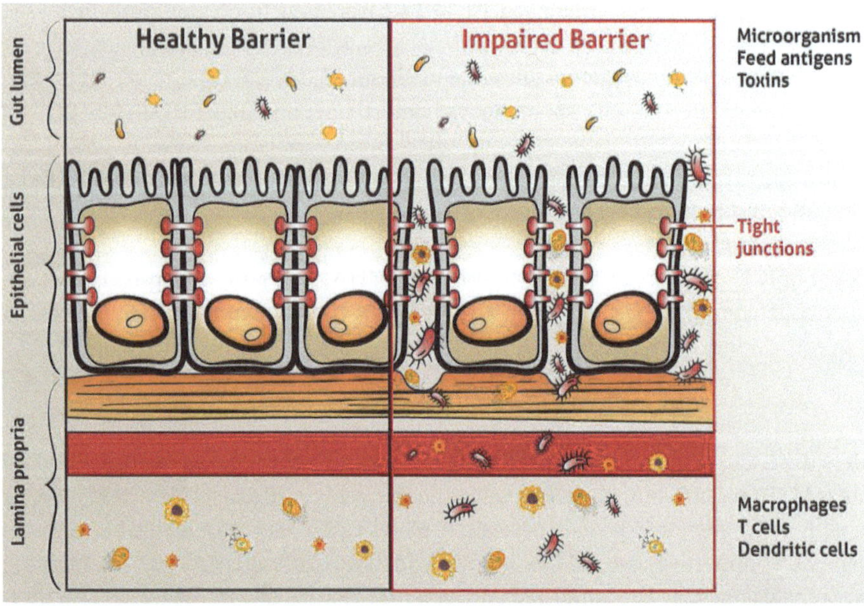

Figure 6.11 Schematic depicting bacterial translocation through an impaired intestinal epithelium compared to a healthy barrier. *Source:* All About Feed / Phytobiotics (2021). / Misset Uitgeverij B.V.

Neuroendocrine and immune dysregulation also play a role in GI pathology. The hypothalamic-pituitary-adrenal (HPA) axis and local immune responses modulate GI function under stress conditions. Elevated cortisol and catecholamines influence motility, mucus production, and immune response. Chronic stress and persistent activation of the HPA axis contribute to dysmotility and stress-related mucosal disease, which can manifest as gastric ulcers and erosions.

Pathophysiology of Gastrointestinal Motility Disorders

GI motility is essential for effective transit of ingesta, prevention of ileus, and maintenance of microbial homeostasis. Critically ill patients often experience impaired motility due to systemic illness, electrolyte imbalances, medication effects, and enteric nervous system dysfunction. Ileus, or functional obstruction of the GI tract, is a common sequela in critically ill patients and is characterized by decreased peristalsis and delayed gastric emptying. The etiology of ileus is multifactorial. Sympathetic overstimulation, which occurs in response to stress, pain, or hypovolemia, inhibits motility. Inflammatory cytokines impair the enteric nervous system, further reducing peristalsis. Electrolyte disturbances, including hypokalemia, hypocalcemia, and hypomagnesemia, contribute to impaired smooth muscle contractility. The administration of opioids, such as morphine and fentanyl, exacerbates dysmotility by binding to μ-opioid receptors in the gut, decreasing acetylcholine release, and inhibiting peristalsis. Sedatives such as benzodiazepines, including midazolam, suppress the enteric nervous system, further reducing gastrointestinal movement. Delayed gastric emptying and paralytic ileus increase the risk of gastroesophageal reflux, aspiration pneumonia, bacterial overgrowth, and malnutrition, worsening the critical state of the patient.

Etiology of Gastrointestinal Dysfunction in Critical Care Patients

Multiple etiological factors contribute to GI dysfunction in critical care patients, including systemic inflammatory conditions, pharmacological influences, and iatrogenic complications. Septic and SIRS-positive patients exhibit profound alterations in GI integrity and motility due to widespread inflammation and circulatory derangements. Endotoxemia from bacterial translocation exacerbates the inflammatory cascade, leading to shock, coagulopathy, and further GI compromise. Patients undergoing major surgical procedures or experiencing polytrauma are at increased risk of GI dysfunction due to pain, blood loss, systemic inflammation, and anesthesia-induced motility suppression. Postoperative ileus is particularly common and can prolong hospitalization and complicate recovery.

Hypovolemia and shock states, whether hypovolemic, distributive, or cardiogenic, reduce splanchnic perfusion and predispose the GI tract to ischemic injury and functional impairment. Fluid resuscitation strategies must balance restoring perfusion with avoiding exacerbation of gut edema and translocation. Endocrine and metabolic imbalances, such as DKA, hypoadrenocorticism, and thyroid dysfunction, alter GI motility and integrity through mechanisms involving electrolyte disturbances, autonomic neuropathy, and altered smooth muscle function.

Pharmacologic management in critical patients often involves medications that impact the GI tract. Nonsteroidal anti-inflammatory drugs (NSAIDs), such as carprofen and meloxicam, increase the risk of gastric ulceration by inhibiting cyclooxygenase (COX) enzymes, reducing prostaglandin-mediated mucosal protection. Proton pump inhibitors (PPIs), including omeprazole, and H2-receptor antagonists, such as famotidine, decrease gastric acid production by blocking the H^+/K^+ ATPase pump and histamine-mediated acid secretion, respectively. While used prophylactically to prevent stress ulcers, long-term use may contribute to dysbiosis and increased infection risk. Broad-spectrum antibiotics, such as enrofloxacin and metronidazole, disrupt gut microbiota, potentially leading to *Clostridioides difficile*-associated diarrhea (Marks and Kook 2021) (Table 6.14).

Clinical Implications and Management

Recognizing and addressing GI integrity and motility concerns in critically ill patients is essential to optimizing patient outcomes. Early enteral nutrition (EEN) maintains mucosal integrity, prevents bacterial translocation, and supports gut motility. Prokinetic agents such as metoclopramide can stimulate GI motility in patients with ileus. Metoclopramide acts as a dopamine D2 receptor antagonist and 5-HT4 receptor agonist, enhancing upper GI motility.

Gastroprotectants such as sucralfate, PPIs, and H2-receptor antagonists mitigate ulcer formation in high-risk patients. Electrolyte correction, ensuring normokalemia, normocalcemia, and normomagnesemia, supports smooth muscle function and peristalsis. Judicious analgesia, including the use of local anesthetics, NMDA receptor antagonists such as ketamine, and gabapentinoids like gabapentin, minimizes opioid-related dysmotility. Antiemetics such as ondansetron and

Table 6.14 Pharmacologic options for maintaining gastrointestinal (GI) integrity in critically ill dogs and cats, including drug classes, mechanisms, and clinical considerations.

Drug Class	Examples	Mechanism of Action	Clinical Use/Considerations
Proton Pump Inhibitors (PPIs)	Omeprazole, Pantoprazole, Esomeprazole	Irreversibly inhibit H^+/K^+-ATPase pumps in gastric parietal cells → reduced gastric acid secretion.	Preferred for stress-related mucosal disease and GI ulcer prophylaxis in critically ill patients. More potent than H2RAs.
H2-Receptor Antagonists	Famotidine, Ranitidine (less common), Nizatidine	Block histamine H2 receptors on parietal cells → decreased acid secretion.	Less effective than PPIs; still used if PPIs contraindicated/unavailable. Ranitidine/nizatidine may enhance motility (prokinetic).
Sucralfate (Mucosal Protectant)	Sucralfate	Forms a protective barrier at ulcer sites, binds bile salts, stimulates prostaglandin and bicarbonate secretion.	Best for existing erosions/ulcers. Must be given separately from other oral meds due to binding interactions.
Prokinetics	Metoclopramide, Cisapride, Erythromycin (low-dose)	Enhance gastric and intestinal motility via dopamine antagonism (metoclopramide), serotonin receptor effects (cisapride), or motilin receptor stimulation (erythromycin).	Useful for ileus, delayed gastric emptying, and reducing risk of reflux/aspiration.
Antiemetics	Maropitant (Cerenia®), Ondansetron, Dolasetron	Block neurokinin-1 (maropitant) or serotonin 5-HT3 (ondansetron, dolasetron) receptors in vomiting pathways.	Control nausea and vomiting, reducing mucosal trauma and aspiration risk.
Prostaglandin Analog	Misoprostol	Synthetic PGE analog → increases mucus and bicarbonate secretion, enhances mucosal blood flow.	Used in NSAID-induced GI injury. Causes diarrhea, cramping; contraindicated in pregnant animals.
Antibiotics (select cases)	Ampicillin, Metronidazole, Broad-spectrum agents	Reduce bacterial overgrowth, control sepsis secondary to bacterial translocation.	Not for routine GI protection—reserved for confirmed/severe risk of bacterial translocation or sepsis.
Nutritional Support (Adjunct)	Enteral nutrition (early feeding)	Maintains mucosal integrity, promotes enterocyte health, prevents villous atrophy.	Not a drug but critical; reduces risk of bacterial translocation and sepsis.

Source: Adapted from DiBartola (2012), Marks and Kook (2021), and Nelson and Couto (2020).

maropitant help prevent nausea and vomiting, reducing the risk of aspiration and improving overall gastrointestinal comfort. Supportive care, including fluid therapy, pain control, and hemodynamic stabilization, remains the basis of GI protection in critically ill patients.

Kirby's Rule of 20: Nutrition

Nutritional support is imperative in critical care management, essential for maintaining cellular metabolism, immune function, and tissue repair. The metabolic demands of critically ill patients are significantly increased due to systemic inflammation, increased protein catabolism, and altered energy metabolism. The provision of adequate nutrition, whether enterally or parenterally, is essential to improving patient outcomes and reducing morbidity and mortality. The failure to provide appropriate nutrition leads to muscle wasting, delayed wound healing, immunosuppression, and prolonged hospitalization.

Pathophysiology of Nutritional Deficits in Critical Care Patients

Critically ill patients frequently experience altered metabolic states due to systemic disease processes, surgical interventions, and inflammatory mediators. In response to stress, there is an increase in counter-regulatory hormones such as cortisol, epinephrine, glucagon, and cytokines, including TNF-α and IL-6, which drive a hypermetabolic, catabolic state (Prittie 2015). This leads to increased protein breakdown, decreased muscle mass, and alterations in glucose and lipid metabolism. When oral intake is insufficient or absent, the body mobilizes endogenous energy stores, leading to depletion of lean body mass, hypoalbuminemia, and progressive immunosuppression.

Malnutrition is further exacerbated by hyporexia, defined as a reduction in appetite leading to decreased caloric intake, and anorexia, characterized by a complete lack of appetite. Hyporexia and anorexia result in prolonged fasting, leading to negative energy balance, gut atrophy, and alterations in intestinal permeability. When enteral nutrition is withheld for an extended period, bacterial translocation occurs as the mucosal barrier function is compromised. This phenomenon facilitates the movement of luminal bacteria into the bloodstream, increasing the risk of sepsis and SIRS. Early and adequate nutritional intervention is crucial in mitigating these risks and maintaining gut integrity.

Refeeding Syndrome: Pathophysiology and Risk Factors

Refeeding syndrome is a life-threatening metabolic disturbance that occurs when nutrition is rapidly introduced to a severely malnourished patient. The hallmark of this condition is severe electrolyte shifts, particularly hypophosphatemia, hypokalemia, and hypomagnesemia, which arise due to insulin-mediated intracellular uptake of these ions. During prolonged fasting or starvation, the body shifts from carbohydrate metabolism to lipolysis and protein catabolism for energy production. Upon refeeding, the sudden influx of glucose stimulates insulin secretion, which promotes cellular uptake of phosphate, potassium, and magnesium, leading to profound systemic depletion. The consequences include cardiac arrhythmias, muscle weakness, hemolysis, respiratory failure, and neurological deficits.

Patients at the highest risk for refeeding syndrome include those with prolonged anorexia, severe cachexia, chronic gastrointestinal disease, and patients with preexisting electrolyte imbalances. Clinical monitoring of electrolyte levels and gradual introduction of nutrition are essential to prevent the onset of refeeding syndrome in at-risk patients. Adequate phosphorus, potassium, and magnesium supplementation should be provided concurrently with nutritional support to mitigate these risks.

The Limitations of Oral Syringe Feeding in Critical Care Patients

Oral syringe feeding, while commonly utilized in stable patients with mild anorexia, is not an appropriate method of nutritional support for critically ill veterinary patients. In the intensive care setting, these patients often have compromised physiological function, altered gastrointestinal motility, and increased risk of aspiration, making forced oral feeding unsafe and potentially harmful. The provision of adequate nutrition in critically ill patients must prioritize safety, efficacy, and physiologic appropriateness, necessitating alternative methods such as enteral tube feeding or parenteral nutrition.

The Risks of Oral Syringe Feeding in Critical Care

Critically ill patients frequently exhibit altered levels of consciousness, impaired swallowing reflexes, or weakened neuromuscular function due to systemic disease, trauma, or sedation. These factors increase the likelihood of aspiration pneumonia when food or liquid is introduced orally without voluntary swallowing coordination. In patients with compromised airway protective mechanisms, the administration of syringe-fed diets can lead to aspiration of food particles into the trachea and lungs, resulting in respiratory distress, infection, and worsening of the patient's critical condition.

Gastrointestinal dysfunction is another significant concern in critical care patients, particularly those with conditions such as ileus, severe pancreatitis, sepsis, or postoperative gastrointestinal recovery. The normal peristaltic activity of the gut is often impaired in these patients due to systemic inflammation, autonomic dysfunction, or medication-induced motility suppression. Forced oral feeding in these cases may exacerbate nausea, induce vomiting, and contribute to abdominal pain and bloating, further worsening the patient's metabolic status and delaying recovery. Unlike controlled enteral nutrition via nasogastric (NG) or esophagostomy tubes, oral syringe feeding does not allow for precise measurement of nutritional intake or ensure continuous nutrient delivery at a tolerable rate.

Stress and Patient Compliance Considerations

Critically ill patients are often in a fragile physiological state and experience heightened stress responses. The act of syringe feeding is inherently stressful, requiring restraint and forced administration, which can lead to increased sympathetic activation, elevated cortisol levels, and resistance to handling. This stress response not only exacerbates metabolic demands but also negatively impacts immune function, increasing the likelihood of nosocomial infections and prolonged hospitalization. Additionally, patient compliance is a major limiting factor in oral syringe feeding. Many critical care patients experience inappetence due to underlying disease processes, pain, or nausea, making them unwilling to accept food voluntarily. Attempting to force-feed an unwilling patient may lead to food aversion, worsening inappetence, and behavioral resistance, which can further delay the transition to voluntary oral intake once the patient stabilizes.

Appropriate Alternatives to Oral Syringe Feeding

Enteral feeding remains the preferred method of providing nutrition in critical care patients when gastrointestinal function is intact. Tube feeding via NG, NE, esophagostomy, gastrostomy, or jejunostomy tubes allows for controlled, measured delivery of nutrition with reduced risk of aspiration and stress. These methods ensure that caloric and protein requirements are met without requiring active participation from the patient, preventing the complications associated with syringe feeding. Tube feeding also allows for administration of liquid diets that can be continuously or intermittently infused at rates that the patient can tolerate, minimizing the risk of gastrointestinal distress.

For patients in whom enteral feeding is contraindicated due to severe gastrointestinal dysfunction, parenteral nutrition (TPN or PPN) provides an alternative means of meeting metabolic demands. This method bypasses the gastrointestinal tract entirely, delivering essential nutrients intravenously in patients with severe malabsorption, prolonged ileus, or nonfunctional gut integrity.

Oral syringe feeding is not an appropriate method of nutritional support in critically ill veterinary patients due to the risks of aspiration, gastrointestinal intolerance, and heightened stress responses. Critically ill patients require precise, controlled, and physiologically appropriate nutritional strategies to support recovery and prevent iatrogenic complications. Enteral feeding via feeding tubes remains the preferred approach when gastrointestinal function is preserved, while parenteral nutrition provides an alternative for patients with severe gastrointestinal dysfunction. The goal of nutritional support in critical care is to optimize patient safety, maintain metabolic stability, and facilitate recovery without exacerbating stress or compromising respiratory and gastrointestinal function.

Feeding Tube Options in Veterinary Medicine

Several types of feeding tubes are available in veterinary medicine, each with specific indications, benefits, and risks. NG and NE tubes are minimally invasive and suitable for short-term feeding in patients who are unable to consume adequate calories orally. These tubes allow for liquid diets and are advantageous due to ease of placement and removal. However, complications such as inadvertent placement in the respiratory tract, nasal irritation, and patient intolerance can occur. Additionally, NE tubes do not allow for gastric decompression, which may be necessary in patients with delayed gastric emptying or ileus.

Esophagostomy (E-tube) tubes are surgically placed through the cervical esophagus and are useful for medium-to-long-term nutritional support. These tubes provide a more stable feeding route compared to NG/NE tubes and allow for the administration of thicker enteral diets. The risks associated with E-tubes include local infection, esophagitis, and accidental tube dislodgement. Patients require appropriate bandaging and routine site maintenance to prevent complications (Figure 6.12).

Gastrostomy (G-tube) tubes provide direct access to the stomach and are indicated for patients requiring prolonged enteral feeding. Percutaneous endoscopic gastrostomy (PEG) tubes are a commonly used variant, allowing for long-term feeding support. These tubes carry a higher risk of peritonitis if displaced prematurely, requiring strict adherence to placement and removal guidelines. Gastrostomy tubes should remain in place for a minimum of 10–14 days to allow for the formation of a mature stoma before removal.

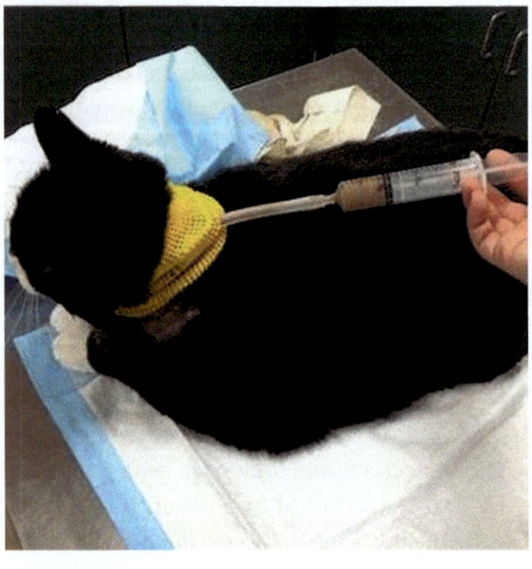

Figure 6.12 Cat receiving enteral nutrition through an esophagostomy feeding tube. *Source:* Photo by University of Missouri Veterinary Health Center (2025).

Jejunostomy (J-tube) tubes provide direct access to the small intestine and are utilized in patients with severe gastric dysfunction, pancreatitis, or high risk of aspiration. These tubes bypass the stomach, reducing the risk of gastroesophageal reflux. However, J-tubes are technically challenging to place, require continuous feeding due to the lack of reservoir capacity, and have a higher risk of clogging and dislodgement.

The selection of a feeding tube must be based on the patient's underlying disease process, anticipated duration of nutritional support, and the risk-benefit profile associated with each method. Nursing care is essential in monitoring tube patency, assessing for signs of infection or inflammation at the insertion site, and ensuring proper nutritional administration. Regular flushing with water prevents clogging, and careful handling reduces the risk of inadvertent displacement. Patient tolerance should be assessed by monitoring for regurgitation, vomiting, diarrhea, or signs of intolerance such as abdominal discomfort and distension.

Total Parenteral Nutrition (TPN) and Partial Parenteral Nutrition (PPN) in Veterinary Critical Care

Parenteral nutrition (PN) is a critical intervention in veterinary medicine for patients who are unable to meet their nutritional requirements through enteral feeding. TPN and PPN serve as essential strategies for providing macronutrients and micronutrients intravenously when gastrointestinal function is compromised or contraindicated. The selection between TPN and PPN depends on the patient's metabolic demands, underlying disease process, and the duration for which parenteral support is required.

Total Parenteral Nutrition (TPN)

TPN is a complete intravenous nutritional support system that delivers all essential macronutrients, including amino acids, dextrose, and lipids, as well as electrolytes, vitamins, and trace elements. It is indicated in patients experiencing severe gastrointestinal dysfunction, such as those with intestinal obstruction, severe pancreatitis, intractable vomiting, malabsorptive disorders, or postoperative ileus. TPN is administered through a central venous catheter to accommodate the hyperosmolar nature of the formulation, which typically exceeds 1,200 mOsm/L (Chan and Freeman 2006). The use of a central line is essential to prevent thrombophlebitis, a complication that arises with peripheral venous administration of highly concentrated solutions.

Metabolic monitoring is critical during TPN administration due to the risk of hyperglycemia, electrolyte imbalances, hepatic dysfunction, and infectious complications. Blood glucose levels should be monitored frequently to prevent insulin resistance or rebound hypoglycemia when discontinuing therapy. Hepatic complications, including cholestasis and hepatic lipidosis, may arise from excessive lipid administration, necessitating careful adjustments in formulation. Strict aseptic techniques are required to reduce the risk of catheter-related bloodstream infections, which are a significant concern in TPN-dependent patients.

Partial Parenteral Nutrition (PPN)

PPN is a less concentrated form of intravenous nutrition that provides partial caloric and protein support, supplementing enteral nutrition when full gastrointestinal function is not yet restored. PPN solutions contain lower concentrations of dextrose and amino acids, allowing for administration through a peripheral vein, as the osmolarity is typically maintained below 900 mOsm/L to minimize the risk of thrombophlebitis (Chan and Freeman 2006). PPN is indicated in patients with mild to moderate gastrointestinal dysfunction who are expected to resume enteral nutrition within a short period or in those requiring supplemental support due to inadequate voluntary intake.

The advantages of PPN include reduced risk of central line-associated infections and lower incidence of metabolic complications compared to TPN. However, its limitations include lower caloric density and the need for higher fluid volumes to meet nutritional demands, which may be contraindicated in patients with fluid-sensitive conditions such as congestive heart failure or renal insufficiency. Since PPN does not provide complete nutrition, it is considered a temporary solution until enteral feeding is feasible or the patient can transition to full nutritional support through TPN.

Clinical Considerations and Monitoring

The selection between TPN and PPN requires careful patient assessment, including evaluation of gastrointestinal function, metabolic status, and vascular access availability. Regular monitoring of serum electrolytes, glucose, liver enzymes, and triglycerides is essential to prevent complications and guide formulation adjustments. Transitioning from parenteral to enteral nutrition should be initiated as soon as gastrointestinal function permits, as enteral feeding preserves intestinal mucosal integrity, reduces bacterial translocation, and promotes a more physiologic nutrient absorption process. Both TPN and PPN require meticulous handling and administration to minimize complications. Strict aseptic techniques in catheter care are essential in reducing the risk of sepsis, a leading concern in parenterally fed patients. Tapering of TPN should be done gradually to prevent hypoglycemia, and close monitoring is needed to identify early signs of metabolic derangements. Veterinary technicians play a vital role in the implementation and monitoring of parenteral nutrition, ensuring that nutritional therapy aligns with the patient's evolving clinical condition and contributes to optimal recovery.

Clinical Considerations in Nutritional Support

Nutritional interventions should be initiated as early as possible in critically ill patients to prevent the consequences of prolonged fasting and malnutrition. Energy requirements should be calculated using resting energy requirements (RER) formulas to prevent underfeeding or overfeeding. RER calculation is used to estimate the energy needs of a patient at rest. It is commonly used in veterinary medicine to determine caloric requirements for hospitalized or critically ill patients.

The standard equation for calculating RER in animals is:

$$\text{RER} = 70 \times (\text{body weight in kg})^{0.75}$$

Alternatively, for animals weighing between **2 and 30 kg**, the simplified equation can be used:

$$\text{RER} = 30 \times (\text{body weight in kg}) + 70$$

Nutrition is a fundamental aspect of critical care medicine, influencing immune function, tissue repair, and overall patient recovery. The metabolic challenges faced by critically ill patients necessitate early and appropriate nutritional intervention to prevent complications associated with malnutrition, bacterial translocation, and metabolic derangements. Refeeding syndrome represents a significant concern in malnourished patients and requires careful electrolyte management during the reintroduction of nutrition. The selection of an appropriate feeding tube depends on the patient's clinical status, disease process, and anticipated duration of nutritional support.

Kirby's Rule of 20: Immune Status and Antibiotic Stewardship

Antibiotic stewardship is a fundamental aspect of critical care medicine, ensuring the judicious use of antimicrobial agents to combat infections while mitigating the risk of resistance development, adverse reactions, and dysbiosis. In critically ill veterinary patients, bacterial infections are often secondary to systemic disease, immunosuppression, invasive procedures, or prolonged hospitalization. The timely administration of appropriate antibiotics is crucial, but the goal should always be to transition to oral medications as soon as the patient is clinically stable and capable of tolerating enteral administration. Transitioning to oral therapy reduces the risk of catheter-associated infections, minimizes hospitalization duration, and supports improved patient comfort. To optimize antibiotic therapy, it is imperative to adhere to the principles of appropriate administration, ensuring the right patient receives the right dose at the right time via the right route.

Antibiotic Therapy in Critical Care: Pathophysiology and Indications

Critically ill patients frequently develop infections due to breaches in immune function, impaired mucosal barriers, and systemic inflammation. Common infections include bacterial pneumonia, sepsis, pyothorax, peritonitis, urinary tract infections, and surgical site infections. The SIRS and sepsis trigger widespread activation of pro-inflammatory cytokines such as TNF-α, interleukin-1 (IL-1), and IL-6, which exacerbate vascular permeability, leukocyte activation, and endothelial dysfunction (DeClue and Sharp 2015). These changes increase the risk of bacterial translocation, where pathogens from the gastrointestinal tract cross into systemic circulation, contributing to secondary infections and MODS.

Empirical antibiotic therapy is initiated based on the suspected infection site, patient history, and cytological findings. Whenever possible, bacterial culture and sensitivity testing should be performed to guide antibiotic selection and prevent unnecessary exposure to broad-spectrum agents. Inappropriate or excessive antibiotic use fosters antimicrobial resistance, disrupts normal microbiota, and increases the risk of complications such as *C. difficile* overgrowth and antibiotic-associated diarrhea. The right patient should be assessed based on clinical presentation and diagnostic findings before initiating antimicrobial therapy, ensuring that antibiotics are only prescribed when a bacterial infection is suspected or confirmed.

Common Parenteral Antibiotics in Critical Care

Several parenteral antibiotics are routinely used in critically ill veterinary patients. Understanding their mechanism of action, indications, pharmacokinetics, administration parameters, and potential adverse effects is essential for optimizing therapeutic outcomes (Table 6.15).

Ampicillin is a broad-spectrum beta-lactam antibiotic that inhibits bacterial cell wall synthesis by binding to penicillin-binding proteins (PBPs), leading to bacterial lysis. It is commonly used to treat respiratory infections, urinary tract infections, and soft tissue infections. Ampicillin should be diluted in sterile saline and administered slowly over 15–30 minutes to minimize the risk of anaphylactic reactions. Adverse effects include hypersensitivity reactions, gastrointestinal disturbances, and, rarely, neurotoxicity in high doses. It is contraindicated in patients with known penicillin allergies. The right dose must be calculated based on patient weight and severity of infection, ensuring therapeutic efficacy while minimizing toxicity.

Ampicillin-sulbactam is a combination of ampicillin and sulbactam, a beta-lactamase inhibitor that enhances ampicillin's efficacy against beta-lactamase-producing bacteria. It is commonly indicated for polymicrobial infections, aspiration pneumonia, and complicated soft tissue infections. This drug requires dilution prior to administration and should be infused

Table 6.15 Common intravenous (IV) antibiotics administered in critically ill dogs, including typical dosages, administration rates, and common drug interactions.

Drug	Typical IV Dose (Dog)	Administration Notes	Common Drug Interactions/Precautions
Ampicillin-Sulbactam	22–30 mg/kg IV q6–8h	Administer slowly over 3–5 minutes or dilute and infuse over 15–30 minutes to reduce GI upset.	Synergistic with aminoglycosides; avoid mixing in same syringe.
Cefazolin (1st Gen Cephalosporin)	20–25 mg/kg IV q8h	Administer IV over 3–5 minutes or dilute and infuse over 20–30 minutes.	Avoid concurrent aminoglycosides or loop diuretics due to nephrotoxicity risk.
Ceftriaxone (3rd Gen Cephalosporin)	20–25 mg/kg IV q24h	Give over 30 minutes; dilute in compatible fluids.	May displace protein-bound drugs (NSAIDs, warfarin); avoid with calcium solutions (risk of precipitation).
Enrofloxacin (Fluoroquinolone)	5–10 mg/kg IV q24h	Infuse slowly over ≥30 minutes to reduce risk of seizures and hypotension.	Avoid with theophylline, cyclosporine (↑ toxicity); do not combine with cation-containing fluids. Contraindicated in young dogs.
Marbofloxacin	2–5 mg/kg IV q24h	Administer over 30 minutes.	Same cautions as enrofloxacin; may prolong QT interval with certain drugs.
Metronidazole	10–15 mg/kg IV q12h	Infuse over ≥30 minutes; rapid IV can cause hypotension and neurologic signs.	Avoid with phenobarbital (↓ efficacy) and warfarin (↑ bleeding risk).
Clindamycin	10–15 mg/kg IV q12h	Dilute and give slowly over 10–30 minutes to reduce risk of arrhythmias/hypotension.	Antagonistic with erythromycin; may enhance neuromuscular blockade.
Gentamicin (Aminoglycoside)	4–6 mg/kg IV q24h (single daily dosing preferred)	Infuse over 20–30 minutes; never IV bolus. Monitor trough levels and renal function.	Nephrotoxic with NSAIDs, cephalosporins, amphotericin B; ototoxic risk with loop diuretics.
Tobramycin (Aminoglycoside)	4–6 mg/kg IV q24h	Infuse over 30 minutes; similar to gentamicin.	Same cautions as gentamicin.
Imipenem-Cilastatin	5 mg/kg IV q6–8h	Infuse over 20–30 minutes; rapid infusion ↑ risk of seizures.	Avoid with ganciclovir (↑ seizure risk); potential cross-reactivity with penicillin allergy.

Source: Adapted from Plumb (2023), Boothe (2012), and Papich (2016).

slowly over 30 minutes to reduce the risk of adverse effects. Potential side effects include vomiting, diarrhea, and hypersensitivity reactions. Administration should be performed at the right time, maintaining a dosing interval that ensures sustained antimicrobial activity without inducing resistance.

Enrofloxacin, a fluoroquinolone antibiotic, exerts its bactericidal effects by inhibiting bacterial DNA gyrase and topoisomerase IV, enzymes essential for DNA replication. It is highly effective against Gram-negative pathogens, including *Pseudomonas* spp., and is commonly used in cases of septicemia, pneumonia, and urinary tract infections. Enrofloxacin should not be administered as a rapid intravenous (IV) bolus, as it can cause seizures and hypotension. It should be given slowly over 30–60 minutes. It is contraindicated in growing animals due to its potential to cause cartilage damage and should be used cautiously in patients with known CNS disorders. The right route of administration should be chosen based on patient status, as enrofloxacin has excellent oral bioavailability and may be transitioned to oral therapy once feasible.

Cefazolin is a first-generation cephalosporin with excellent Gram-positive coverage, including *Staphylococcus* and *Streptococcus spp*. It inhibits bacterial cell wall synthesis, leading to cell lysis. Cefazolin is frequently used as a perioperative prophylactic antibiotic and for treating pyoderma, osteomyelitis, and bacterial endocarditis. It should be administered over 5–10 minutes via slow IV push or diluted for infusion over 20–30 minutes. Adverse effects include hypersensitivity reactions, gastrointestinal upset, and, rarely, nephrotoxicity in patients with compromised renal function. Ensuring the right route and correct administration technique is essential to minimize adverse effects and maximize efficacy.

Metronidazole is a nitroimidazole antibiotic that disrupts bacterial DNA synthesis, making it particularly effective against anaerobic bacteria and protozoal infections. It is commonly used for bacterial peritonitis, *C. difficile* infections, and inflammatory bowel disease. Metronidazole should be infused over 30–60 minutes to reduce the risk of neurological toxicity, which may manifest as ataxia, nystagmus, or seizures. It is contraindicated in patients with severe hepatic dysfunction and should be used cautiously in those with preexisting neurological conditions.

Transitioning to Oral Antibiotics: Clinical Considerations

The transition from intravenous to oral antibiotic therapy should be considered once the patient demonstrates clinical improvement, including resolution of fever, improved leukocyte count, and hemodynamic stability (Weese and Blondeau 2013). Oral antibiotic therapy offers several advantages, including reduced hospital stay, lower risk of catheter-associated infections, and improved patient comfort. Most antibiotics have oral formulations with comparable bioavailability to their IV counterparts, allowing for seamless transition without loss of efficacy.

Monitoring for tolerance to oral medications is essential. Patients recovering from gastrointestinal disease or those with delayed gastric emptying should be assessed for vomiting, diarrhea, or inappetence before oral antibiotics are introduced. When transitioning from IV to oral therapy, clinicians must ensure appropriate dosing adjustments based on pharmacokinetic differences between formulations. Some antibiotics, such as enrofloxacin and metronidazole, maintain high oral bioavailability and can be directly substituted, while others, such as ampicillin, may require increased dosing frequency due to lower systemic absorption (Papich 2016).

Antibiotic stewardship in critical care settings requires a balance between effective infection control and minimizing the risks associated with overuse or inappropriate antimicrobial selection. Ensuring the right patient receives the right antibiotic at the right dose, at the right time, and via the right route is essential in achieving optimal therapeutic outcomes. Parenteral antibiotics are essential for managing severe infections, but transitioning to oral therapy as soon as tolerated is crucial to reducing hospitalization time, improving patient comfort, and minimizing iatrogenic complications.

Kirby's Rule of 20: Drug Dosage and Metabolism

Drug dosage and metabolism in critically ill patients are profoundly altered by pathophysiological changes that impact pharmacokinetics and pharmacodynamics. Understanding these alterations is essential for ensuring appropriate drug efficacy while minimizing toxicity. Critical illness frequently results in hemodynamic instability, altered protein binding, modified enzymatic activity, and disruptions in renal and hepatic function, all of which affect drug absorption, distribution, metabolism, and excretion. These changes require careful consideration in drug selection, dosing adjustments, and therapeutic monitoring to optimize clinical outcomes.

Pathophysiology of Altered Drug Metabolism in Critical Illness

Pharmacokinetics, which encompasses drug absorption, distribution, metabolism, and excretion, is significantly affected by the systemic derangements seen in critical care patients. Hypoperfusion due to shock, sepsis, or cardiovascular compromise impairs blood flow to the liver and kidneys, reducing drug metabolism and clearance. Hepatic metabolism, which primarily occurs via cytochrome P450 enzymes, is suppressed in states of hypoxia, metabolic acidosis, or inflammation. As a result, drugs that rely on hepatic metabolism, including opioids, benzodiazepines, and many anesthetic agents, may accumulate to toxic levels or exhibit prolonged duration of action (Papich 2016).

Drug distribution is also affected by alterations in plasma protein levels. Hypoalbuminemia, common in critically ill patients due to systemic inflammation and protein loss, decreases protein binding of highly protein-bound drugs such as furosemide, enrofloxacin, and propofol. This results in an increased free drug fraction, enhancing drug effects but also increasing the risk of toxicity. Conversely, fluid shifts and capillary leak syndrome, particularly in sepsis and SIRS, increase the volume of distribution for hydrophilic drugs such as aminoglycosides and beta-lactam antibiotics, necessitating higher loading doses to achieve therapeutic concentrations.

Renal function is often compromised in critically ill patients due to AKI, hypovolemia, or nephrotoxic insults. Drugs eliminated through renal clearance, including aminoglycosides, penicillins, and NSAIDs, require careful dose adjustments to prevent accumulation and nephrotoxicity. Renal replacement therapies such as hemodialysis or continuous renal replacement therapy (CRRT) further alter drug elimination, necessitating individualized dosing strategies based on filtration rates and dialysis modalities.

Pharmacodynamics and Drug Response in Critical States

Pharmacodynamics, which describes the effect of a drug on the body, is equally impacted by critical illness. Receptor sensitivity, signal transduction, and tissue perfusion play pivotal roles in drug efficacy. Hypotension and hypoxia reduce drug delivery to target tissues, particularly for vasopressors and sedatives, leading to altered responses. Catecholamine resistance, commonly observed in septic shock, necessitates higher doses of vasopressors such as norepinephrine or dopamine to achieve hemodynamic stabilization (DeClue and Sharp 2015). Similarly, opioid tolerance and increased inflammatory pain pathways in critically ill patients may require multimodal analgesic approaches, incorporating ketamine or lidocaine infusions to optimize pain control.

Nursing Considerations and Drug Administration in Critical Care

Nursing care plays a vital role in ensuring proper drug administration, therapeutic monitoring, and adverse event recognition in critically ill patients. Accurate dosing calculations based on patient weight, renal function, and hepatic metabolism must be performed to prevent under- or overdosing. Infusion rates and dilution protocols are critical for drugs with narrow therapeutic indices, such as propofol, fentanyl, and neuromuscular blockers, where improper administration can lead to significant adverse effects.

Monitoring for signs of drug toxicity, including CNS depression, respiratory compromise, cardiac arrhythmias, and nephrotoxicity, is essential for early intervention. Therapeutic drug monitoring (TDM) should be employed for medications with variable pharmacokinetics, including aminoglycosides, vancomycin, and anticonvulsants, to ensure appropriate plasma concentrations. Adjustments in dosing regimens based on serial blood levels can prevent drug accumulation and improve efficacy.

Enteral versus parenteral drug administration must also be considered in critical care patients. Gastric motility is often impaired due to ileus, sepsis, or opioid administration, affecting oral drug absorption. Intravenous administration may be preferred in unstable patients to ensure predictable pharmacokinetics, but transitioning to enteral formulations as soon as tolerated is advantageous for reducing intravenous catheter complications and hospital-associated infections. When enteral administration is resumed, careful assessment of gastrointestinal function is required to ensure proper drug bioavailability and absorption.

Drug metabolism and dosage are significantly influenced by the physiological alterations occurring in critically ill patients. Changes in hepatic and renal function, protein binding, and drug distribution necessitate individualized pharmacotherapeutic approaches to optimize treatment efficacy and minimize toxicity. Nursing care is integral to ensuring appropriate drug administration, therapeutic monitoring, and patient safety in the critical care setting.

Kirby's Rule of 20: Wound Care and Bandages

Wound care is a critical component of patient management in the intensive care setting, where delayed healing and complications are common. The healing process is influenced by multiple factors, including perfusion, infection, systemic disease, and nutritional status. In critically ill patients, these factors are frequently compromised, leading to prolonged healing times and increased susceptibility to secondary infections. Proper wound management, including the selection of appropriate dressings, aseptic handling, and bandage maintenance, is essential to promote optimal healing and prevent further complications.

Wound Healing in the Critical Care Patient

Wound healing is a complex and dynamic process involving hemostasis, inflammation, proliferation, and remodeling. The hemostatic phase begins immediately after injury, as platelets aggregate to form a fibrin clot and release cytokines that recruit inflammatory cells. The inflammatory phase, which follows within hours to days, involves neutrophils and macrophages that clear debris and bacteria while releasing additional signaling molecules to promote tissue repair. The proliferative phase is characterized by fibroblast migration, angiogenesis, and extracellular matrix deposition, while the final remodeling phase strengthens the newly formed tissue through collagen cross-linking and reorganization.

In critically ill patients, wound healing is frequently delayed due to systemic derangements. Hypoperfusion, common in shock states and sepsis, deprives tissues of oxygen and nutrients essential for cellular function and repair. Hypoxia impairs fibroblast activity, collagen synthesis, and angiogenesis, slowing the progression from inflammation to proliferation. Inflammatory mediators such as TNF-α and IL-6, which are elevated in sepsis and SIRS, further disrupt healing by perpetuating a pro-inflammatory state that inhibits normal cellular function (Glass 2012).

Hyperglycemia, which is often present in critically ill patients due to stress-induced insulin resistance, exacerbates wound healing delays by impairing leukocyte function, reducing phagocytosis, and increasing the risk of infection. Malnutrition, particularly deficiencies in protein, vitamins A and C, and zinc, further contributes to impaired tissue repair. Inadequate protein intake reduces fibroblast proliferation and collagen deposition, weakening the structural integrity of new tissue.

Additionally, chronic conditions such as renal disease, hepatic dysfunction, and endocrinopathies further impair the body's ability to mount an effective healing response.

Aseptic Wound Care in the Intensive Care Unit

Strict aseptic technique is paramount in wound care to prevent nosocomial infections, which can significantly increase morbidity in critical care patients. The compromised immune function of these patients makes them particularly susceptible to opportunistic infections that can lead to abscess formation, wound dehiscence, and systemic sepsis.

Wound cleansing should be performed using sterile saline or balanced electrolyte solutions, as harsh antiseptics such as hydrogen peroxide or povidone-iodine can cause cytotoxic damage to healing tissues. Debridement of necrotic tissue is necessary to prevent bacterial colonization and promote granulation tissue formation. Sharp debridement using sterile instruments is preferred in cases of significant necrosis, whereas enzymatic debridement may be utilized for nonsurgical candidates. Dressings should be selected based on wound characteristics, with hydrocolloid or foam dressings used for exudative wounds and alginate or hydrogel dressings employed to maintain moisture in dry wounds. Frequent assessment for signs of infection, such as increased exudate, erythema, malodor, or delayed granulation, is necessary to initiate appropriate interventions before systemic involvement occurs.

Bandage and Splint Care in the Critical Care Patient

Bandages and splints serve multiple functions in wound management, including protection from environmental contaminants, support for healing structures, and reduction of patient interference. However, improper bandage application or maintenance can lead to significant complications, including pressure sores, circulatory compromise, and infection.

Bandage changes should be performed under sterile conditions, with careful inspection of the underlying tissue to assess for pressure-induced necrosis, excessive moisture accumulation, or signs of infection. Overly tight bandages can impede lymphatic and venous return, leading to distal limb edema and ischemia. Conversely, loose bandages may fail to provide adequate support and protection, allowing for wound contamination. The use of padded layers beneath compression dressings helps to prevent pressure-related injuries while maintaining adequate support for the wound.

Splints are commonly employed for orthopedic injuries, postoperative stabilization, and immobilization of fractures or soft tissue injuries. The application of splints must ensure that proper limb alignment is maintained while avoiding excessive pressure on bony prominences. Monitoring for changes in limb temperature and swelling is essential to detect early signs of vascular compromise. Splints should be adjusted as necessary to accommodate changes in swelling and tissue positioning over time, ensuring continued therapeutic benefit without contributing to secondary complications.

Critical care patients often have reduced mobility, necessitating additional precautions in bandage and splint care. Prolonged recumbency increases the risk of decubitus ulcers and moisture-associated dermatitis, requiring frequent repositioning and assessment of pressure points. Soft padding materials and pressure-relief bedding can aid in preventing ischemic injuries, while diligent hygiene and wound monitoring reduce the risk of secondary infections.

Wound healing in critically ill patients is influenced by multiple systemic factors, including hypoperfusion, inflammation, hyperglycemia, and malnutrition, all of which contribute to delayed tissue repair and increased risk of infection. Aseptic wound care is essential in preventing nosocomial infections and ensuring optimal conditions for healing. Proper selection and maintenance of bandages and splints play a critical role in wound protection and stabilization, but they require diligent monitoring to prevent complications such as pressure sores, circulatory compromise, and secondary infections.

Kirby's Rule of 20: Pain Control

Pain management is a critical aspect of patient care in veterinary medicine, particularly in the ICU, where patients often experience severe and multifaceted pain. Untreated or poorly managed pain has profound physiological and psychological consequences, contributing to increased morbidity, prolonged hospitalization, and diminished quality of life. The pathophysiology of pain involves complex interactions between peripheral nociceptors, the spinal cord, and higher brain centers, and its perception is modulated by neurochemical and inflammatory mediators. In critically ill patients, pain is often exacerbated by systemic disease, surgical interventions, or prolonged immobility, necessitating a multimodal approach to analgesia to ensure effective and compassionate management.

Physiology of Pain and Its Impact on Critical Care Patients

Pain perception, or nociception, begins when noxious stimuli activate primary afferent nociceptors in peripheral tissues. These nociceptors transduce mechanical, thermal, and chemical stimuli into electrical signals, which are transmitted along

A-delta and C fibers to the dorsal horn of the spinal cord. Within the spinal cord, these signals undergo modulation before being relayed to the brainstem, thalamus, and higher cortical centers, where pain is consciously perceived. The CNS processes these signals through excitatory neurotransmitters such as glutamate and substance P, while descending inhibitory pathways modulate the pain response via endogenous opioids, gamma-aminobutyric acid (GABA), and serotonin.

In critically ill patients, pain pathways become dysregulated due to prolonged nociceptive input and systemic inflammation, leading to a phenomenon known as central sensitization. Central sensitization amplifies pain perception, reducing the threshold for nociceptor activation and causing allodynia, where normally nonpainful stimuli elicit pain. This heightened pain response not only contributes to patient distress but also exacerbates systemic stress responses. Activation of the HPA axis results in increased cortisol production, hyperglycemia, immunosuppression, and delayed wound healing (Hopper and Epstein 2015). Additionally, persistent pain can impair respiratory function, increase cardiovascular workload, and lead to muscle atrophy due to prolonged immobility.

The Pain Pathway, Centralization, and Multimodal Analgesia

The pain pathway consists of four primary components: transduction, transmission, modulation, and perception. Transduction occurs at the site of tissue injury, where nociceptors detect and convert noxious stimuli into electrical impulses. Transmission involves the propagation of these signals along peripheral nerves to the dorsal horn of the spinal cord. Modulation occurs at various levels within the CNS, where excitatory and inhibitory mechanisms either amplify or suppress pain signals. Finally, perception takes place in the cerebral cortex, where the pain experience is consciously recognized (Figure 6.13).

In critically ill patients, pain pathways become maladaptive due to sustained nociceptive input, leading to hyperalgesia and central sensitization. This maladaptive response necessitates a multimodal analgesic approach, which targets multiple points along the pain pathway to enhance pain relief while minimizing adverse effects. Multimodal analgesia combines various drug classes, including opioids, NSAIDs, local anesthetics, NMDA receptor antagonists, and gabapentinoids, to disrupt pain signaling at multiple levels. This approach not only improves analgesic efficacy but also reduces the reliance on high-dose opioids, thereby decreasing the risk of opioid-induced adverse effects such as respiratory depression, ileus, and dysphoria.

Recognizing Pain in Dogs and Cats

Effective pain management requires accurate assessment and recognition of pain behaviors, which can vary significantly between species. Dogs experiencing pain may exhibit overt signs such as vocalization, restlessness, panting, guarding behavior, and reluctance to move. In contrast, cats often display more subtle indicators of pain, including withdrawal, decreased grooming, flattened ears, dilated pupils, and decreased social interaction. Cats are particularly prone to stress-induced analgesia, which can mask signs of pain and lead to underestimation of their discomfort.

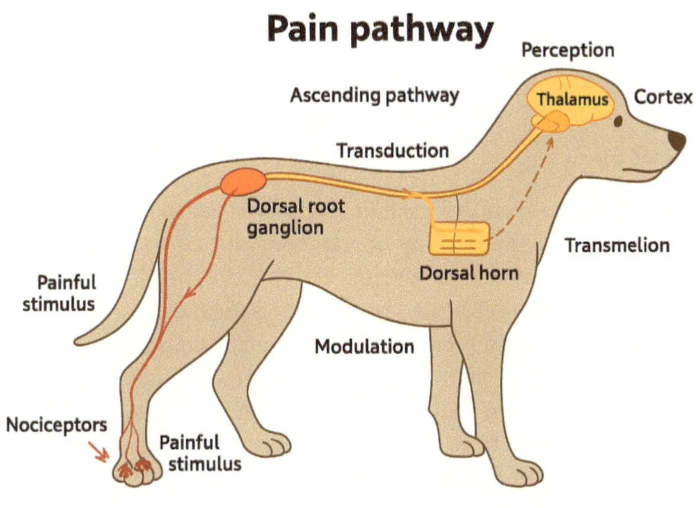

Figure 6.13 Illustration of the nociceptive (pain) pathway in a dog, including transduction at nociceptors, transmission through the dorsal root ganglion and dorsal horn, modulation at the spinal cord, and perception in the thalamus and cortex. *Source:* Created with OpenAI (2025).

Several validated pain scales have been developed to standardize pain assessment in veterinary patients. The Glasgow Composite Measure Pain Scale (CMPS) and the Colorado State University (CSU) Acute Pain Scale are widely used in dogs to quantify pain severity based on behavioral and physiological parameters (Reid et al. 2007; Hellyer et al. 2007). The Feline Grimace Scale is a species-specific tool that evaluates pain in cats by assessing changes in facial expressions, including ear position, eye aperture, and muzzle tension (Evangelista et al. 2019). These objective pain assessment tools are essential for guiding analgesic interventions and monitoring treatment efficacy. Readers are encouraged to review pain scales in detail in Chapter 8, where their structure and application are discussed further.

The Importance of Patient Advocacy in Pain Management

Veterinary professionals play a critical role in advocating for effective pain management, ensuring that patients receive appropriate analgesic care tailored to their individual needs. Pain is often under-recognized or undertreated in veterinary medicine due to the challenges of objective pain assessment, reliance on subjective interpretation, and concerns over drug side effects. However, untreated pain has far-reaching consequences, contributing to prolonged recovery, increased stress, and diminished patient well-being.

Advocacy in pain management involves proactive identification of pain sources, timely administration of analgesics, and regular reassessment of pain control measures. It also requires education of pet owners regarding pain recognition and the importance of continued pain management at home. By prioritizing patient comfort and implementing evidence-based analgesic protocols, veterinary professionals can enhance patient outcomes and improve the quality of life in critically ill and recovering animals.

Pain control is a fundamental component of critical care, requiring a comprehensive understanding of pain physiology, recognition of pain behaviors, and the implementation of multimodal analgesia. The pain pathway involves transduction, transmission, modulation, and perception, all of which can become dysregulated in critically ill patients, leading to central sensitization and heightened pain responses. Multimodal analgesia is essential for targeting multiple points in the pain pathway, reducing reliance on single-agent therapy, and improving overall analgesic efficacy. Recognizing pain in dogs and cats requires careful observation of behavioral cues, supplemented by validated pain scales such as the Glasgow CMPS and the Feline Grimace Scale. Veterinary professionals must act as patient advocates, ensuring timely and appropriate pain management to minimize suffering and enhance recovery. Through diligent assessment, tailored analgesic protocols, and ongoing monitoring, pain control can be optimized, ultimately improving clinical outcomes and patient welfare in the intensive care setting.

Kirby's Rule of 20: The Role of Nursing Care

Kirby's Rule of 20 is an essential framework for the assessment and management of critically ill veterinary patients, ensuring that fundamental physiological parameters are continuously monitored and optimized. This structured approach allows for early identification of clinical deterioration and timely intervention, which is critical in an intensive care setting. Veterinary nursing care is a crucial component of Kirby's Rule of 20, as technicians are responsible for ongoing patient assessments, the implementation of therapeutic interventions, and patient advocacy. Understanding and applying this rule enhances nursing efficiency, improves patient outcomes, and ensures the highest standard of care in critical care medicine.

Why Nursing Care is an Essential Part of Kirby's Rule of 20

Veterinary technicians act as the frontline providers, responsible for identifying subtle changes in patient status that may indicate hemodynamic instability, respiratory distress, metabolic imbalances, or emerging infections. The nursing process—comprising assessment, planning, implementation, and evaluation—mirrors the principles of Kirby's Rule of 20, ensuring that each critical parameter is consistently addressed and reassessed to optimize patient care.

Veterinary technicians play a central role in executing the medical plan prescribed by clinicians, administering medications, adjusting fluid therapy, providing nutritional support, and ensuring pain control. In addition to technical proficiency, technicians must apply critical thinking skills to anticipate complications, adapt interventions, and advocate for evidence-based treatment modifications. Without vigilant nursing care, deviations from normal physiological function may go unnoticed, delaying interventions that could prevent deterioration or organ failure.

This emphasis on vigilance and continuous reassessment echoes the foundational principles established by Florence Nightingale, widely regarded as the founder of modern nursing. Nightingale revolutionized healthcare by emphasizing systematic observation, not only of the patient's physical condition, but also of the external environment—light, ventilation, hygiene, and noise—which she recognized as integral to recovery (Nightingale 1860; Dossey et al. 2005). Her belief that nursing extended beyond medical treatment to encompass the totality of the patient's surroundings was groundbreaking in the 19th century, shifting the perception of nursing from a task-oriented role to a profession grounded in science, critical thinking, and patient advocacy (Nightingale 1860).

Nightingale's meticulous collection of observational data, often quantified through statistics and innovative infographics, established the importance of evidence-based practice long before the term entered modern healthcare (Nightingale 1860; McDonald 2001). She demonstrated that careful monitoring and recording of patient responses, environmental variables, and treatment outcomes could directly influence survival rates (Dossey 2010). This methodological rigor not only elevated nursing as a discipline but also created a template for structured, holistic patient care that remains relevant today (Nightingale 1860; Dossey et al. 2005).

In veterinary nursing, her principles find renewed significance. Just as Nightingale recognized that environmental conditions could dictate outcomes for soldiers in wartime hospitals, veterinary technicians appreciate how the kennel environment, noise levels, sanitation, and stress can directly affect the recovery of critically ill animals. Her insistence that "the most important practical lesson...is to teach nurses what to observe" resonates deeply within the veterinary ICU, where subtle cues—a change in posture, appetite, respiratory effort, or behavioral demeanor—often provide the earliest warning signs of clinical decline.

When viewed through the lens of Kirby's Rule of 20, Nightingale's environmental model becomes strikingly modern. Her focus on ventilation and fresh air aligns with the Rule's emphasis on oxygenation and ventilation. Her insistence on cleanliness and infection prevention is echoed in the parameters monitoring sepsis and immune function. Her priority on nutrition and hydration resonates with the Rule's monitoring of fluid balance, electrolytes, and nutritional support. Even her concern for light and noise levels, which influence sleep and recovery, mirrors the modern recognition of stress, comfort, and analgesia as critical to patient outcomes.

Together, Nightingale's environmental philosophy and Kirby's Rule of 20 illustrate a continuum of nursing knowledge: from holistic observation of environment and patient to the structured, evidence-based monitoring of critical parameters. For veterinary technicians, this synthesis reinforces that nursing is both an art and a science—rooted in Nightingale's tradition of observation and compassion, while elevated by Kirby's systematic framework for critical care (Table 6.16).

The Importance of Veterinary Technicians Understanding Kirby's Rule of 20

A thorough understanding of Kirby's Rule of 20 empowers veterinary technicians to provide more effective and proactive care. Critical care patients experience rapid physiological changes, necessitating continuous reassessment of their cardiovascular status, respiratory function, fluid balance, metabolic state, and neurologic health. Technicians trained in Kirby's Rule of 20 can systematically evaluate these parameters, recognize abnormalities, and respond appropriately to stabilize the patient.

Knowledge of Kirby's Rule of 20 allows veterinary technicians to anticipate patient needs and implement preemptive care strategies. For example, in a patient with SIRS, the technician must closely monitor hypoperfusion, coagulopathy, and electrolyte disturbances, discussing potential adjustments in intravenous fluid therapy and ensuring timely laboratory assessments. Similarly, for a patient with respiratory compromise, the technician must evaluate oxygen saturation, end-tidal carbon dioxide, and ventilatory effort, making necessary adjustments to oxygen therapy or mechanical ventilation settings.

Moreover, understanding the interconnectivity of physiological systems is critical. A disruption in one system often affects multiple others, requiring a holistic nursing approach. A patient experiencing hypovolemia, for instance, may not only have altered perfusion but also experience delayed drug metabolism, impaired renal function, and altered mental status. Technicians who are proficient in Kirby's Rule of 20 can recognize these interdependencies and advocate for interventions that address the full spectrum of the patient's condition.

Kirby's Rule of 20: Tender Loving Care

Tender Loving Care (TLC) is a foundational element of veterinary critical care, earning its place in Kirby's Rule of 20 due to its profound impact on patient recovery, stress reduction, and overall well-being. While medical and physiological parameters are essential to stabilizing critically ill patients, the human–animal bond, emotional support, and compassionate care contribute significantly to patient outcomes. Veterinary technicians and clinicians must recognize that, beyond medical intervention, the provision of comfort, familiarity, and reassurance plays a crucial role in the healing process. TLC embodies the essence of veterinary nursing, integrating technical skills with empathy and patient-centered care.

This balance highlights the intersection of art and science in nursing practice. The *science* of TLC is demonstrated through measurable outcomes—reduced cortisol levels, improved wound healing, normalized heart rates, and enhanced immune response when stress is minimized. These physiological improvements are rooted in evidence-based studies that validate the medical necessity of comfort and stress management. The *art* of TLC, however, lies in the ability of veterinary technicians to

Table 6.16 Comparison of the Nursing Process, Kirby's Rule of 20, and Florence Nightingale's ideologies, including their core focus, key components, and applications in veterinary and human nursing.

Framework	Core Focus	Key Components	Application in Practice
Nursing Process	Systematic, patient-centered approach to care.	1) Assessment—data collection (history, physical exam, diagnostics). 2) Diagnosis—nursing diagnoses/identifying patient problems. 3) Planning—setting goals, prioritizing interventions. 4) Implementation—carrying out interventions. 5) 5. Evaluation—reassessing outcomes and adjusting care.	Provides a cyclical framework for individualized care, critical thinking, and adaptation to patient changes. Used in both human and veterinary nursing models.
Kirby's Rule of 20	Critical care checklist to ensure comprehensive monitoring and treatment in ICU patients.	20 parameters to be evaluated daily in critical patients, including: • Oxygenation/ventilation • Fluid balance • Electrolytes and acid–base • Nutrition • Analgesia/sedation • Renal function • Coagulation • GI integrity, etc.	Functions as a structured ICU checklist to avoid overlooking critical parameters. Guides consistent monitoring, intervention, and interdisciplinary communication in veterinary critical care.
Florence Nightingale's Ideologies	Holistic, environment-based model of nursing; foundation of modern nursing ethics and philosophy.	• Environment as therapy—clean air, water, light, warmth, nutrition. • Hygiene—infection control through cleanliness and sanitation. • Observation—systematic patient observation to guide interventions. • Holism—caring for the whole patient (body, mind, environment). • Advocacy—compassion and patient-centered focus.	Laid the groundwork for nursing ethics, sanitary practice, and holistic care. Many of her principles are embedded in modern veterinary and human nursing, especially infection control and patient advocacy.

Source: Adapted from Doane and Varcoe (2021), Kirby and Rudloff (2012), and Nightingale (1860).

perceive the subtle emotional needs of each patient, interpret nonverbal cues, and tailor interventions that foster trust and reduce fear. A gentle touch, a calm voice, or providing a patient's favorite toy may not appear in medical charts, yet these interventions are as vital as fluid therapy or analgesia in promoting recovery.

In this way, TLC demonstrates that veterinary critical care is never exclusively technical nor purely emotional—it is the fusion of scientific precision with the art of compassion. By combining measurable medical interventions with individualized, empathetic care, veterinary nurses uphold the holistic philosophy of nursing: treating the patient not just as a clinical case, but as a sentient being whose physical and emotional states are inseparably linked.

The Role of TLC in Critical Care Medicine

Critically ill patients experience significant physiological and psychological stressors, including pain, anxiety, disorientation, and separation from their owners. These stressors activate the HPA axis, leading to elevated cortisol levels, increased sympathetic tone, and systemic inflammation. Prolonged stress can exacerbate disease states, delay healing, and contribute to maladaptive behaviors such as inappetence, self-trauma, and aggression. The implementation of TLC mitigates these effects by providing a sense of security, reducing fear, and promoting relaxation, all of which are critical for recovery.

Veterinary technicians serve as the primary providers of TLC in the ICU. Their role extends beyond technical proficiency to include emotional support, environmental management, and individualized patient care. Simple interventions such as gentle handling, soft bedding, quiet surroundings, and minimizing excessive stimulation can significantly impact patient comfort and reduce stress-induced complications. Additionally, incorporating familiar items, such as a patient's blanket or a worn t-shirt from the owner, can provide a source of comfort and familiarity (Figure 6.14).

Equally important is the thoughtful integration of owners into the TLC framework. While ICU environments often limit physical interaction, strategic involvement of owners can profoundly influence recovery. Supervised visitation, when feasible, allows the patient to receive reassurance from their primary attachment figure, helping to normalize the ICU experience and attenuate stress responses. Even brief periods of contact, such as gentle petting or speaking in a familiar voice, can lower heart rate and cortisol levels while reinforcing the human–animal bond.

When physical presence is not possible, owners can still contribute meaningfully to TLC. Supplying personal items that carry their scent, recording voice messages, or providing videos can create familiarity in an otherwise sterile environment. Involving owners in care planning, educating them on stress-reducing interventions, and validating their role as an essential part of the healing team not only benefits the patient but also strengthens the owner's trust in the veterinary team. Ultimately, by incorporating owners into the delivery of TLC, veterinary technicians extend the reach of compassionate care beyond the clinic walls, reinforcing the holistic principle that healing occurs most effectively when the patient, caregiver, and medical team are all engaged in the process.

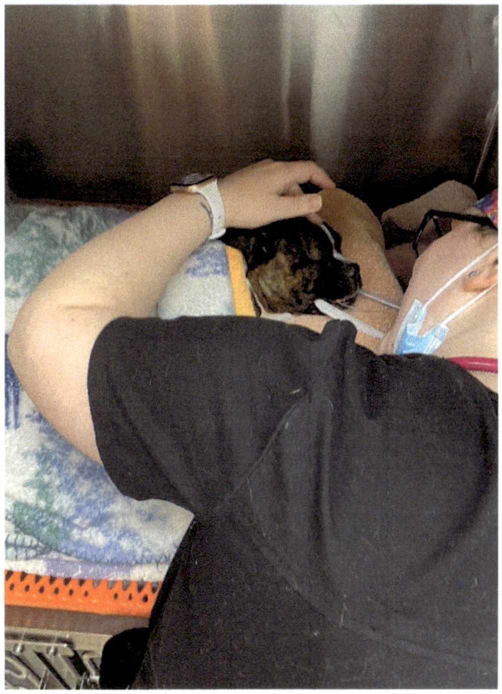

Figure 6.14 Veterinary technician providing TLC to a hospitalized patient [Photograph]. Photo by Crystal Schaeffer.

TLC as a Core Nursing Principle

Veterinary nursing is inherently centered on the principles of TLC. Technicians provide not only medical interventions but also holistic patient care, addressing the emotional and psychological needs of critically ill animals. This patient-centered approach ensures that care is not solely dictated by clinical parameters but also by the overall well-being and comfort of the patient.

TLC in nursing care involves:

- Gentle and compassionate handling to minimize stress and pain.
- Recognizing nonverbal cues of discomfort and intervening promptly.
- Ensuring clean, dry, and comfortable bedding to prevent pressure sores and enhance rest.
- Maintaining a quiet and calm ICU environment to reduce stress-related agitation.
- Providing frequent, low-stress human interaction to reassure patients.
- Individualizing care plans based on each patient's temperament, history, and needs.

Critically ill patients, particularly feline patients, are highly susceptible to stress-related complications. Cats experiencing prolonged hospitalization often develop stress-induced anorexia, exacerbating metabolic imbalances and delaying recovery. TLC-focused interventions, such as offering palatable diets, using feline pheromone diffusers, and maintaining minimal handling approaches, can greatly improve their response to care (Table 6.17).

The Physiological Impact of TLC on Healing

Scientific research supports the role of emotional well-being in physiological recovery, emphasizing that reducing fear, anxiety, and stress (FAS) in hospitalized animals enhances healing, immune function, and overall outcomes (Mathews et al. 2014). Stress reduction through TLC has been shown to lower cortisol levels, reducing systemic inflammation and enhancing immune function, and promoting parasympathetic nervous system activation, aiding in digestion, rest, and recovery. TLC has been cited as improving cardiovascular stability by reducing tachycardia and hypertension associated with fear and distress (Landsberg et al. 2013). It enhances appetite stimulation, reducing the need for forced feeding and improving nutritional outcomes. TLC and human interaction can also encourage voluntary movement and interaction, preventing muscle atrophy and facilitating physical rehabilitation. Pain perception is also closely linked to emotional well-being. Fear and anxiety can heighten pain sensitivity, making pain management less effective. Veterinary technicians play a vital role in recognizing these interactions and implementing interventions that combine multimodal analgesia with environmental and emotional support.

Table 6.17 Ways veterinary technicians provide TLC to critical care patients.

Category	Examples of TLC Interventions	Clinical Considerations
Physical Comfort	Soft, clean bedding; gentle repositioning to prevent pressure sores; warm blankets or heat support (with monitoring); hygiene care (bathing, peri-care, cleaning soiled patients)	Monitor for hypothermia/hyperthermia, skin breakdown, and patient tolerance during handling
Emotional Support	Calm, reassuring voice; gentle petting or therapeutic touch; presence at bedside during stressful procedures; minimizing fear by reducing loud noises and bright lights	Recognize patient's stress signals, avoid overstimulation in painful or anxious animals
Pain and **Anxiety Relief**	Prompt recognition and communication of pain signs; use of pheromone sprays (e.g., Feliway®, Adaptil®); nonpharmacologic comfort (gentle massage, quiet environment)	Coordinate with DVM for analgesic or anxiolytic adjustments; use validated pain scales
Nutrition and **Hydration Support**	Hand-feeding when safe; Offering highly palatable diets; oral care for patients with decreased appetite; hydration support via assisted drinking or monitoring IV/feeding tubes	Monitor aspiration risk, caloric intake, hydration status, and weight trends
Environmental Enrichment	Providing toys or familiar items from home; playing soft, soothing music; allowing visual contact with staff or other calm animals	Ensure enrichment is appropriate for the patient's medical status and infection control protocols
Human–Animal Bond Advocacy	Facilitating safe visitation from owners; using owner's clothing/blanket for scent comfort; encouraging owner participation in gentle care when possible	Balance infection control, patient stability, and visitation policies with the benefits of client presence
Monitoring and **Vigilance**	Staying attentive to subtle behavioral or physiological changes; documenting patient comfort interventions; advocating for adjustments in care when the patient appears distressed	Continuous reassessment to ensure interventions remain beneficial and safe

Source: Schaeffer (2025).

The Ethical Imperative of TLC in Critical Care

Providing compassionate care is not merely a supplementary aspect of veterinary medicine; it is an ethical obligation. Veterinary professionals are entrusted with the well-being of their patients, and ensuring comfort, dignity, and a reduction in suffering is fundamental to humane medical practice. Kirby's Rule of 20 acknowledges TLC as a necessity rather than a luxury, reinforcing the idea that true critical care extends beyond physiological stabilization to include comprehensive, patient-centered care.

The ethical principle of beneficence underscores the responsibility of veterinary professionals to maximize patient welfare. In cases where medical interventions are extensive or aggressive, incorporating TLC into daily care routines ensures that patient comfort is prioritized. Euthanasia decisions, palliative care, and end-of-life discussions must also incorporate TLC principles, ensuring that patients experience minimal distress and that owners are guided with empathy and support.

TLC is a fundamental component of critical care, earning its place in Kirby's Rule of 20 due to its profound impact on patient recovery, stress reduction, and overall well-being. Veterinary technicians are at the forefront of providing TLC, integrating compassionate handling, environmental modification, and emotional support into patient care. The human–animal bond remains a critical factor in the ICU, influencing patient stability and owner confidence in veterinary decision-making. TLC is not an optional component of veterinary medicine; it is a core principle that enhances healing, reduces suffering, and fosters a holistic approach to patient care. Through the dedicated efforts of veterinary professionals, TLC ensures that even the most critically ill patients receive compassionate, dignified, and humane care throughout their recovery journey.

Kirby's Rule of 20: Practical Application, Challenges, and Integration into Clinical Decision-Making

Kirby's Rule of 20 is an essential framework in veterinary critical care, systematically addressing key physiological and clinical parameters necessary for stabilizing and managing critically ill patients. This structured approach ensures that no critical aspect of patient care is overlooked, facilitating a comprehensive and methodical strategy for assessment and intervention. The integration of Kirby's Rule of 20 into clinical practice is both a challenge and an opportunity, requiring seamless coordination among veterinary professionals and a deep understanding of its application in real-world scenarios. Veterinary nursing plays a pivotal role in its execution, as technicians are responsible for patient monitoring, intervention, and advocacy to ensure optimal clinical outcomes.

Practical Application of Kirby's Rule of 20 in Critical Care

The practical application of Kirby's Rule of 20 is evident in various critical care scenarios. For instance, a patient presenting with sepsis requires vigilant monitoring of perfusion parameters, electrolyte balance, acid-base status, and immune function. Early detection of hypotension and hypoperfusion allows for timely fluid resuscitation and vasopressor support, while metabolic monitoring ensures correction of electrolyte and glucose imbalances. Similarly, in a trauma patient with polytrauma, Kirby's Rule of 20 guides comprehensive assessment of oxygenation, ventilation, pain control, coagulation status, and neurologic function to prevent secondary complications such as hypoxemia, shock, or coagulopathies.

Veterinary technicians serve as the frontline providers in these cases, continuously evaluating patient responses to interventions and ensuring timely adjustments. A postsurgical patient, for example, requires diligent pain assessment, nutritional support, and wound care monitoring, all of which fall within the framework of Kirby's Rule of 20. By systematically addressing each of the 20 parameters, veterinary technicians and clinicians can detect deviations from normal physiology early, preventing deterioration and improving overall survival rates.

Challenges and Opportunities in Implementation

Despite its value, implementing Kirby's Rule of 20 in a high-paced clinical setting presents challenges. Time constraints, staffing shortages, and limited resources can make a thorough assessment difficult, requiring efficient prioritization and delegation among veterinary teams. Some parameters, such as advanced hemodynamic monitoring or comprehensive metabolic profiling, may be difficult to perform in general practice settings due to financial or technological limitations.

Additionally, variability in patient responses necessitates individualized treatment approaches, making it challenging to apply standardized protocols across all cases. A septic patient may require aggressive fluid therapy and antibiotic administration, whereas a patient with congestive heart failure may need judicious fluid management and diuretics, demonstrating the need for clinical flexibility when implementing Kirby's Rule of 20.

Opportunities for improved implementation include leveraging technology such as continuous patient monitoring systems, POC diagnostics, and electronic medical record alerts that flag abnormalities in real time. Education and training programs for veterinary technicians and clinicians further enhance competency in applying Kirby's Rule of 20, ensuring that all team members can systematically evaluate and manage critically ill patients.

Integration with the Nursing Process

The nursing process—comprising assessment, planning, implementation, and evaluation—aligns seamlessly with Kirby's Rule of 20. Veterinary technicians initiate patient assessment by systematically evaluating each parameter, ensuring that critical issues such as oxygenation, fluid balance, and pain control are promptly identified. This structured approach enables the formulation of individualized nursing care plans that prioritize patient stability and recovery.

During the implementation phase, technicians execute prescribed treatments while continuously monitoring patient responses. Whether adjusting fluid therapy based on urine output and lactate clearance or modifying analgesic plans to optimize pain control, veterinary technicians play a key role in real-time clinical adjustments. The evaluation phase is ongoing, requiring reassessment of vital parameters, laboratory values, and overall patient demeanor to ensure that interventions remain effective.

Furthermore, veterinary technicians serve as patient advocates, identifying subtle clinical changes that may precede significant deterioration. By integrating Kirby's Rule of 20 into daily patient care, technicians ensure that every aspect of critical care management is systematically addressed, improving patient outcomes and reducing morbidity and mortality.

Kirby's Rule of 20 in Clinical Decision-Making

Incorporating Kirby's Rule of 20 into clinical decision-making provides a structured framework that supports the veterinarian's diagnosis and guides the treatment of critically ill patients. It serves as a reference for prioritizing interventions, particularly in complex cases where multiple organ systems are compromised. Decision-making guided by this framework ensures that all relevant physiological parameters are assessed, preventing oversight and enhancing diagnostic accuracy.

For example, a patient with ARDS requires an integrated approach, balancing oxygenation strategies with fluid management, acid-base stabilization, and immune support. Kirby's Rule of 20 helps clinicians and veterinary technicians determine whether the patient requires positive-pressure ventilation or immunomodulatory therapy based on continuous reassessment of respiratory parameters and systemic inflammatory markers.

In cases of polytrauma, the rule ensures that immediate life-threatening conditions such as hypovolemic shock and TBI are prioritized, followed by secondary assessments of pain control, coagulation status, and nutritional support. By systematically addressing each parameter, clinicians can make informed decisions that optimize patient survival and long-term recovery.

Kirby's Rule of 20 is an indispensable tool in veterinary critical care, providing a structured approach to patient assessment and management. Its practical application spans a wide range of critical scenarios, ensuring that essential physiological parameters are continuously monitored and addressed. Despite challenges in implementation, opportunities for improvement through technology, education, and interdisciplinary collaboration continue to enhance its effectiveness (Table 6.18).

Table 6.18 Application of Kirby's Rule of 20 to a canine IMHA case.

Parameter (Rule of 20)	Assessment of IMHA Patient	Veterinary Technician Interventions
Perfusion Parameters	Pale MM, CRT 2.5s, weak pulses	Monitor HR, CRT, BP, lactate; notify DVM of deterioration
Fluid Balance	Risk of hypovolemia with hemolysis and GI losses	IV fluid therapy per plan; strict input/output charting
Oncotic Pull (Colloid Osmotic Pressure)	Risk of hypoalbuminemia from hemolysis/IV fluids	Monitor TP/albumin; prep for plasma transfusion if ordered
Oxygenation/Ventilation	Tachypnea, anemia reduce oxygen carrying capacity	O_2 supplementation via nasal cannula or flow-by
Hematocrit/Hemoglobin	PCV 14%; hemolysis ongoing	Serial PCVs/TS every four to six hours; assist with blood transfusion
Electrolytes	Risk of hypokalemia with anorexia/hemolysis	Monitor electrolytes; replace as needed
Acid–Base Status	Risk of metabolic acidosis from hypoxia/shock	Collect venous/arterial blood gases; monitor trends
Blood Pressure	Hypotension secondary to anemia/shock	Doppler/oscillometric monitoring; titrate fluids
Heart Rate/Rhythm	Tachycardia 180 bpm; possible arrhythmia	Continuous ECG monitoring; report arrhythmias
Temperature	Febrile (103.9°F) from inflammation/hemolysis	Monitor q4–6h; apply cooling if >104.5°F
Coagulation	IMHA predisposes to DIC/thrombosis	Monitor PT/aPTT, D-dimer; assess for petechiae/bleeding
Renal Function/Urine Output	Risk of pigment nephropathy (hemoglobinuria)	Measure UOP (closed collection); monitor for hematuria
Glucose	At risk for hypoglycemia with sepsis/DIC	Monitor BG q4–6h
GI Motility	Stress/anemia can cause ileus, melena possibly	Monitor feces; administer GI protectants
Nutrition	Anorexic >24 hours	Initiate assisted feeding/NG tube if safe
Wound Healing	Delayed healing with anemia/hypoxia	Protect catheter sites; aseptic technique
Pain Assessment	Discomfort from IV catheters, hematuria, +/− thromboembolic events	Regular pain scoring; provide analgesia per DVM
Nursing Care/TLC	Separation anxiety, stress worsen hypercoagulability	Provide soft bedding, quiet environment, owner's shirt
Drugs/Dosing	On prednisolone, heparin, gastroprotectants, transfusion	Double-check dosing; monitor for ADRs (PU/PD, GI upset)
Patient's Attitude/ Mentation	Obtunded, lethargic, weak	Monitor mentation q2–4h; report acute changes immediately

Signalment: Six-year-old female spayed Cocker Spaniel
Presenting Complaint: Lethargy, pale mucous membranes, tachypnea, and collapse at home
Diagnosis: Immune-mediated hemolytic anemia (IMHA) confirmed via Coombs' test and spherocytosis on blood smear
Source: Schaeffer (2025).

The Legacy of Dr. Rebecca Kirby

The Kirby's Rule of 20 is a transformative tool that embodies the essence of veterinary critical care. By providing a structured framework for patient monitoring and decision-making, it empowers veterinary teams to deliver comprehensive, evidence-based care. Integrating the Rule of 20 with the veterinary nursing process enhances its effectiveness, creating a cohesive approach to managing critically ill patients.

Dr. Kirby's contributions to veterinary medicine extend far beyond the Rule of 20. Her work has inspired generations of veterinary professionals to pursue excellence in critical care. By emphasizing the importance of systematic assessment and holistic care, she has left an indelible mark on the profession. The Kirby's Rule of 20 remains a testament to her vision and dedication. It serves as a guiding light for veterinary teams, ensuring that critically ill patients receive the highest standard of care. As veterinary medicine continues to evolve, the principles underlying the Rule of 20 will remain relevant, adapting to new challenges and opportunities while upholding Dr. Kirby's legacy of excellence. As veterinary professionals continue to embrace the principles championed by Dr. Rebecca Kirby, they carry forward her legacy of compassion, innovation, and excellence. The Rule of 20 not only improves patient outcomes but also strengthens the profession, ensuring that critically ill animals receive the care they deserve.

References

Acierno, M.J., Schnellbacher, R.W., Ray, A.C., and Panciera, D.L. (2014). Evaluation of four portable blood glucose meters in dogs. *Journal of Veterinary Emergency and Critical Care* 24 (3): 335–343. https://doi.org/10.1111/vec.12149.

Blikslager, A.T., Moeser, A.J., Gookin, J.L. et al. (2007). Restoration of barrier function in injured intestinal mucosa. *Physiology* 22 (5): 266–275. https://doi.org/10.1152/physiol.00010.2007.

Bonagura, J.D. and Twedt, D.C. (2021). *Kirk's Current Veterinary Therapy XV*, 15e. St. Louis: Elsevier.

Boothe, D.M. (2012). *Small Animal Clinical Pharmacology and Therapeutics*, 2e. Elsevier.

Boysen, S.R. and Rozanski, E.A. (2015). Hypothermia. In: *Small Animal Critical Care Medicine*, 2e (ed. D.C. Silverstein and K. Hopper), 435–438. Elsevier Saunders: St. Louis.

Brooks, M.B. (2010). Disorders of hemostasis. In: *Schalm's Veterinary Hematology*, 6e (ed. D.J. Weiss and K.J. Wardrop), 576–589. Wiley-Blackwell: Ames, IA.

Brown, S.A. (2015). Acute kidney injury. In: *Small Animal Critical Care Medicine*, 2e (ed. D.C. Silverstein and K. Hopper), 649–654. Elsevier Saunders: St. Louis.

Chan, D.L. and Freeman, L.M. (2006). Nutrition in critical illness. In: *Veterinary Emergency and Critical Care Manual*, 2e (ed. K. Wingfield and M. Palmer), 319–326. Lifelearn: Guelph.

DeClue, A.E. and Sharp, C.R. (2015). Sepsis. In: *Small Animal Critical Care Medicine*, 2e (ed. D.C. Silverstein and K. Hopper), 747–752. Elsevier Saunders: St. Louis.

Deranged Physiology (2025) *The classical model of the Starling principle*. derangedphysiology.com (accessed 26 August 2025).

DiBartola, S.P. (2012). *Fluid, Electrolyte, and Acid-Base Disorders in Small Animal Practice*, 4e. St. Louis: Elsevier Saunders, 292–297; 300–303; 306–308; 318–323; 364–367.

Doane, G.H. and Varcoe, C. (2021). *How to Nurse: Relational Inquiry With Individuals and Families in Changing Health and Health Care Contexts*. Wolters Kluwer.

Dossey, B.M. (2010). *Holistic Nursing: A Handbook for Practice*, 6the. Sudbury, MA: Jones and Bartlett Publishers.

Dossey, B.M., Keegan, L., Guzzetta, C.E., and Kolkmeier, L.G. (2005). *Holistic Nursing: A Handbook for Practice*, 4e. Sudbury, MA: Jones and Bartlett.

eClinpath, 2024. *Blood smear examination – Hemogram basics*. https://eclinpath.com/hematology/hemogram-basics/blood-smear-examination/

Epstein, S.E. and Silverstein, D.C. (2014). Colloid therapy: controversies and considerations in veterinary critical care. In: *Small Animal Critical Care Medicine*, 2e (ed. D.C. Silverstein and K. Hopper), 338–342. Saunders Elsevier: St. Louis.

Evangelista, M.C., Watanabe, R., Leung, V.S.Y. et al. (2019). Facial expressions of pain in cats: the development and validation of a Feline Grimace Scale. *Scientific Reports* 9 (1): 19128. https://doi.org/10.1038/s41598-019-55693-8.

Feldman, E.C. and Nelson, R.W. (2015). *Canine and Feline Endocrinology*, 4e, 66–70. St. Louis: Elsevier Saunders.

Frontiers in Cell and Developmental Biology (2024) *Update on the Role of the Endothelial Glycocalyx in*. (accessed 26 August 2025).

Glass, G.E. (2012). The molecular mechanisms of impaired wound healing in diabetes: a review. *Wound Repair and Regeneration* 20 (3): 352–365. https://doi.org/10.1111/j.1524-475X.2012.00772.x.

Grauer, G.F. (2011). Early detection of renal damage and disease in dogs and cats. *Veterinary Clinics of North America: Small Animal Practice* 41 (1): 261–281.

Guyton, A.C. and Hall, J.E. (2021). *Textbook of Medical Physiology*, 14e. Philadelphia: Elsevier.

Harvey, J.W. (2012). *Veterinary Hematology: A Diagnostic Guide and Color Atlas*, 15–18. St. Louis: Elsevier Saunders.

Hellyer, P.W., Uhrig, S.R., and Robinson, N.G. (2007). *Canine Acute Pain Scale*. Colorado State University College of Veterinary Medicine and Biomedical Sciences https://vetmedbiosci.colostate.edu/vth/diagnostic-and-support/pain-management/.

Hopper, K. and Epstein, S.E. (2015). Stress response and critical illness. In: *Small Animal Critical Care Medicine*, 2e (ed. D.C. Silverstein and K. Hopper), 305–311. Elsevier Saunders: St. Louis.

Hopper, K. and Powell, L.L. (2015). Mechanical ventilation. In: *Small Animal Critical Care Medicine*, 2e (ed. D.C. Silverstein and K. Hopper), 1043–1049. Elsevier Saunders: St. Louis.

Johnson, L.R. and McMichael, M.A. (2015). Heatstroke. In: *Small Animal Critical Care Medicine*, 2e (ed. D.C. Silverstein and K. Hopper), 441–444. Elsevier Saunders: St. Louis.

King, L.G., Boag, A., and Hughes, D. (2014). *Textbook of Small Animal Emergency Medicine*. Ames, IA: Wiley-Blackwell.

Kirby, R. and Rudloff, E. (2012). *Small Animal Emergency and Critical Care Medicine*, 2e. Wiley-Blackwell.

Landsberg, G.M., Hunthausen, W., and Ackerman, L. (2013). *Behavior Problems of the Dog and Cat*, 3e, 43–45. Edinburgh: Elsevier Saunders.

Marks, S.L. and Kook, P.H. (2021). Gastrointestinal pharmacology. In: *Kirk's Current Veterinary Therapy XV*, 15e (ed. J.D. Bonagura and D.C. Twedt), 519–525. St. Louis: Elsevier.

Mathews, K.A., Barry, M., Taylor, S.M., and Gilroy, C. (2005). A retrospective study of human albumin use in critically ill dogs. *Journal of Veterinary Emergency and Critical Care* 15 (2): 110–116.

Mathews, K.A., Kronen, P.W., Lascelles, D. et al. (2014). Guidelines for recognition, assessment and treatment of pain. *Journal of Small Animal Practice* 55 (6): E10–E68. https://doi.org/10.1111/jsap.12200.

Mazzaferro, E.M. and Rudloff, E. (2004). Fluid therapy for the emergent small animal patient: crystalloid and colloid resuscitation. *Clinical Techniques in Small Animal Practice* 19 (2): 83–87.

McDonald, L. (2001). Florence nightingale: statistics and the crimean war. *Journal of the Royal Statistical Society: Series A (Statistics in Society)* 164 (2): 321–329.

Nelson, R.W. and Couto, C.G. (2020). *Small Animal Internal Medicine*, 6e. St. Louis: Elsevier.

Nelson, R.W. and Reusch, C.E. (2014). Classification and pathogenesis of diabetes mellitus. In: *Canine and Feline Endocrinology*, 4e (ed. E.C. Feldman, R.W. Nelson, C.E. Reusch, and J. Scott-Moncrieff), 751–768. Elsevier Saunders: St. Louis.

Nightingale, F. (1860). *Notes on Nursing: What It is, and What It is Not*. London: Harrison & Sons.

OpenAI, 2025. *Pain pathway in a dog* [digital illustration]. Generated with AI image tools, 28 August 2025.

Otto, C.M., Crowe, D.T., and Glaus, T.M. (2002). Use of human serum albumin in critically ill dogs and cats: 100 cases (1998–2000). *Journal of the American Veterinary Medical Association* 221 (9): 1421–1427.

Papich, M.G. (2016). *Saunders Handbook of Veterinary Drugs: Small and Large Animal*, 4e. St. Louis: Elsevier, 1–5, 16–18, 366–368, 541–543.

Platt, S.R. and Hall, S. (2014). *Small Animal Neurological Emergencies*. CRC Press.

Plumb, D.C. (2023). *Plumb's Veterinary Drug Handbook*, 10e. Wiley-Blackwell.

Polzin, D.J. (2011). Chronic kidney disease in small animals. *Veterinary Clinics of North America: Small Animal Practice* 41 (1): 15–30.

Prittie, J. (2015). Nutritional support. In: *Small Animal Critical Care Medicine*, 2e (ed. D.C. Silverstein and K. Hopper), 325–330. Elsevier Saunders: St. Louis.

Randall, D., Burggren, W., French, K., and Eckert, R. (2002). *Eckert Animal Physiology: Mechanisms and Adaptations*, 5e. New York: W.H. Freeman.

Reid, J., Nolan, A.M., Hughes, J.M.L. et al. (2007). Development of the short-form Glasgow Composite Measure Pain Scale (CMPS-SF) and derivation of an analgesic intervention score. *Animal Welfare* 16 (S1): 97–104.

Rozanski, E.A. and de Laforcade, A.M. (2015). Endocrine emergencies. In: *Small Animal Critical Care Medicine*, 2e (ed. D.C. Silverstein and K. Hopper), 691–696. Elsevier Saunders: St. Louis.

Schaeffer, C. (2025). *Veterinary Nursing Strategy*. Hoboken, NJ: Wiley-Blackwell.

Silverstein, D.C. and Hopper, K. (2014). *Small Animal Critical Care Medicine*, 2e. St. Louis: Saunders Elsevier. 324–327; 331–333.

Speakman, J.R. and Król, E. (2010). Maximal heat dissipation capacity and hyperthermia risk: neglected key factors in the ecology of endotherms. *Journal of Animal Ecology* 79 (4): 726–746.

Thrall, M.A., Weiser, G., Allison, R.W., and Campbell, T.W. (2012). *Veterinary Hematology and Clinical Chemistry*, 2e. Ames: Wiley-Blackwell.

University of Missouri Veterinary Health Center 2025. *Esophagostomy tube feeding in cats* [photograph]. Veterinary Health Center – Wentzville.

Veterinary Practice (2020) *Traumatic brain injury in companion animals.* Veterinary Practice. https://www.veterinary-practice.com/article/traumatic-brain-injury-in-companion-animals

VectorStock (2024) https://www.vectorstock.com (accessed: 26 August 2025).

WagWalking (n.d.) *Stupor and coma in dogs.* https://wagwalking.com/condition/stupor-and-coma

Weese, J.S. and Blondeau, J.M. (2013). Antimicrobial therapy. In: *Kirk's Current Veterinary Therapy XV*, 15e (ed. J.D. Bonagura and D.C. Twedt), 1271–1279. Elsevier Saunders: St. Louis.

Weiss, D.J. and Wardrop, K.J. (2010). *Schalm's Veterinary Hematology*, 6e, 152–154. Ames, IA: Wiley-Blackwell.

Wenger, S., Musulin, S., Shepherd, K. et al. (2022). Comparison of aural and rectal temperature measurements in dogs and cats presenting to an emergency service. *Journal of Veterinary Emergency and Critical Care* 32 (5): 531–538. https://doi.org/10.1111/vec.13197.

Yozova, I.D., Howard, J., and Adamik, K.N. (2016). Use of synthetic colloids in veterinary critical care: a review of the current literature. *Journal of Veterinary Emergency and Critical Care* 26 (5): 591–605.

Part III

Advanced Nursing Practices

7

Practical Nursing Techniques

Veterinary nursing is a discipline deeply rooted in both the art and science of clinical care. Up to this point in our exploration of veterinary nursing, we have laid a comprehensive foundation. We began with a historical overview, tracing the evolution of veterinary nursing from its informal origins to its current, increasingly professionalized form. We examined the fundamental principles, core knowledge, and foundational skills essential for every veterinary technician, delving into the importance of ethics, critical thinking, and case management. We have explored the nursing cycle as a systematic framework for patient care and integrated nursing care plans to optimize outcomes across various settings, including general practice and intensive care units. Additionally, we introduced Dr. Rebecca Kirby's "Rule of 20," a cornerstone in critical care that has advanced observational nursing and encouraged a vigilant, holistic approach to patient evaluation. Now, we turn to the practical application of this extensive body of knowledge: hands-on skills and clinical procedures that bring the theory of veterinary nursing into living practice.

Chapter 7 marks the transition from theoretical knowledge to the precise and purposeful application of clinical skills. This chapter explores, in comprehensive detail, the techniques, protocols, and standard operating procedures that underpin competent and confident veterinary nursing practice. It is the assumption of the authors that the reader has already established a foundational level of theoretical understanding and clinical acumen necessary to engage with the material presented. For those in need of guidance on fundamental skills, it is strongly recommended to consult introductory veterinary nursing textbooks or pursue continuing education opportunities designed for the developing technician. Whether supporting aseptic procedures in the surgical suite, stabilizing critically ill patients in the emergency department, performing advanced intravenous catheterization, administering enteral or parenteral nutrition, or monitoring anesthetic depth, the procedures in this chapter represent the essential competencies expected of the proficient veterinary technician.

What distinguishes the exceptional veterinary technician is not merely technical proficiency but an unrelenting commitment to observation. Observation is the cornerstone of effective veterinary nursing, arguably the most critical skill a technician can possess. It encompasses much more than visual assessment. It is the integration of all sensory input, coupled with clinical knowledge, intuition, and pattern recognition. It is the ability to recognize subtle shifts in a patient's demeanor, respiratory rate, mucous membrane color, posture, or behavior that may precede significant clinical decline or signal recovery. The skilled veterinary technician is constantly attuned to these nuances, functioning as the vigilant eyes and ears of the attending veterinarian. Indeed, observation is not passive but an active and engaged process, demanding both presence and interpretation.

Moreover, observation is inherently tied to collaboration. Veterinary nursing is not a solitary profession. It flourishes in the context of interdisciplinary teamwork, where the technician and veterinarian work in tandem to deliver comprehensive, high-quality patient care. The veterinarian may diagnose and direct, but the veterinary technician executes, monitors, evaluates, and adjusts in real time. A successful veterinary team is one in which communication is fluid, roles are respected, and the shared goal of patient welfare drives every action.

In this chapter, the reader will find a series of case studies and real-world applications, drawn from diverse practice settings, that demonstrate the critical role of practical nursing techniques. These case studies are more than illustrative—they are instructive. They provide the reader with scenarios that integrate theoretical principles, ethical decision-making, critical thinking, and tactile, procedural action. By dissecting these cases, readers will be challenged to consider not just the "how" of clinical procedures, but the "why"—why we choose one intervention over another, why timing matters, and why patient temperament and signalment influence our technique.

Table 7.1 Chapter domains in veterinary nursing.

Domain	Focus Areas
Veterinary Nursing Assessment	Systematic patient evaluation, documentation, prioritization of care, and application of the nursing process.
Advanced Catheterization	Placement techniques, anatomical landmarks, complication management, and catheter maintenance protocols.
Anesthetic Monitoring and Analgesic Techniques	Intraoperative monitoring parameters, pain scoring systems, and multimodal analgesia strategies for stability and comfort.
Fluid Therapy and Nutrition	IV and SQ fluid delivery, enteral and parenteral nutrition, and recognition of fluid imbalance or nutritional compromise.
Wound Management and Bandaging	Management of acute and chronic wounds, dressing selection, infection control, and techniques to promote healing.
Urinary Catheterization	Technical considerations, aseptic protocols, and prevention of catheter-associated urinary tract infections.
Blood Pressure Dynamics	Accurate measurement, interpretation of values, and clinical significance in health and disease.
Blood Gas Analysis	Collection methods, assessment of acid–base status, oxygenation, and ventilation indices.
Fecal Microbiota Transplantation	Indications, donor material handling, patient preparation, and nursing responsibilities.
Neonatal Resuscitation	Airway management, thermoregulation, cardiovascular stabilization, and neonatal monitoring.
Blood Product Administration	Compatibility testing, transfusion protocols, monitoring for reactions, and post-transfusion care.
Recognition and Management of Shock	Identification of shock states, triage, stabilization, and ongoing nursing management.
Oxygen Delivery Techniques and Respiratory Support	Oxygen supplementation methods, patient monitoring, and escalation to mechanical ventilation.
Cardiopulmonary Arrest and Resuscitation (CPA)	RECOVER guidelines for BLS and ALS, pharmacologic interventions, and post-resuscitation nursing care.

The chapter will be structured to guide the reader through various domains of veterinary nursing, including but not limited to (Table 7.1):

Each section is designed not only to describe procedural techniques but to embed them within the broader context of nursing care and patient advocacy. Step-by-step procedures will be accompanied by annotated diagrams, evidence-based guidelines, and highlighted clinical tips that reflect the collective wisdom of seasoned veterinary technicians and medical professionals.

Throughout the chapter, particular emphasis will be placed on understanding patient individuality. A brachycephalic dog undergoing anesthesia requires a markedly different approach than a fractious feline needing wound care. A geriatric patient with concurrent renal insufficiency cannot be managed in the same way as a robust, young canine with a simple fracture. This recognition—that each patient is a unique constellation of physiology, psychology, and environment—is at the heart of clinical nursing excellence. The skilled veterinary technician recognizes that every action taken—every injection, every restraint hold, every treatment delivered—has ethical weight. Patient autonomy, comfort, and dignity must be preserved to the greatest extent possible, even in the face of clinical urgency.

Finally, this chapter underscores the idea that veterinary nursing is a dynamic, evolving practice. Best practices change as new evidence emerges, technologies evolve, and the expectations of both pet owners and regulatory bodies shift. The veterinary technician must remain curious, adaptive, and committed to lifelong learning. The techniques you learn in this chapter are not static; they are the current standard, subject to refinement and review as the profession continues to grow.

By the end of this chapter, readers will have not only a refined skill set but a deeper appreciation for the complexity and significance of advanced practical nursing interventions. These are the techniques that stabilize the critically ill, soothe the frightened, and contribute to the healing process in tangible, measurable ways. In mastering them, the veterinary technician affirms their role as a vital, indispensable member of the veterinary healthcare team.

Welcome to the applied heart of veterinary nursing. Let us now put knowledge into practice.

The Veterinary Nursing Physical Assessment

Veterinary nursing is rooted not only in compassionate care and critical thinking but in direct, hands-on patient assessment. While the physical examination conducted by a veterinarian is vital for diagnosis and treatment planning, and the primary survey during emergency triage is essential for rapid stabilization, the veterinary nursing physical assessment serves a distinct and equally critical role. It is a methodical, tactile, and observational process that bridges the gap between history-taking and clinical diagnostics. Veterinary technicians must be proficient in performing thorough, systematic physical assessments as a cornerstone of patient advocacy, monitoring, and nursing care planning.

The veterinary nursing physical assessment should not be conducted from a distance or in the back of the hospital away from the client. Instead, it begins in the examination room, with the client present, creating a transparent and collaborative environment. This practice fosters trust and encourages client participation, while also allowing technicians to observe the animal's behavior in the presence of its owner—a vital consideration for animals that present differently under stress or in unfamiliar environments.

Touching the patient is nonnegotiable. Veterinary technicians must engage their senses—sight, touch, smell, and hearing—to collect essential clinical data. Visual inspection alone is inadequate. Palpation can reveal lymphadenopathy, pain, masses, or abnormalities in muscle tone or body condition that might be missed during visual observation. Auscultation using a stethoscope is imperative to detect cardiac murmurs, arrhythmias, pulmonary abnormalities, or gastrointestinal sounds. The veterinary technician must be confident and competent in these techniques (Figure 7.1).

A systematic approach to physical assessment ensures consistency and comprehensiveness. The head-to-tail method, also referred to as a cephalocaudal assessment, is a logical and reproducible format (Bassert et al. 2021). This approach begins with evaluation of the patient's general demeanor and mentation—are they BAR (bright, alert, responsive), QAR (quiet, alert, responsive), or displaying signs of obtundation, stupor, or coma? Gait and posture should be noted as the patient enters the exam room. From there, the technician systematically examines the head, including the eyes (for discharge, corneal clarity, pupil symmetry, menace response), ears (odor, discharge, pinna integrity), and oral cavity (mucous membrane color, capillary refill time, dental status, masses, ulceration).

The cervical area is palpated for lymph nodes and tracheal sensitivity. Thoracic auscultation must include both sides of the chest, with attention paid to rate, rhythm, and quality of both heart and lung sounds. The abdominal region should be assessed with gentle palpation, identifying pain, organomegaly, or masses, and evaluating tense or doughy consistency that may indicate gastrointestinal pathology.

Urogenital assessments vary by species and sex but should include evaluation of mammary tissue, vulva, penis, scrotum, and prepuce for discharge, swelling, or neoplasia. Limbs should be examined for muscle tone, joint swelling, crepitus, or lameness. The integumentary system is evaluated for ectoparasites, alopecia, masses, wounds, or lesions throughout. Finally, a complete weight and Body Condition Score (BCS) must be recorded, using species-specific guidelines.

As a vital part of the physical assessment, a complete and accurate TPR—temperature, pulse, and respiratory rate—must be obtained. The order in which these parameters are assessed is of paramount importance, both for the accuracy of the data and for minimizing patient stress. Respiratory rate should be assessed first, and whenever possible, this should be done using a hands-off approach. Observing the patient undisturbed allows for an accurate assessment of resting respiratory effort and rate, which can be significantly altered by touch or stimulation. Noting the rate, depth, and pattern of respiration while the animal is calm provides baseline data and helps to detect early signs of dyspnea or respiratory compromise.

Following the respiratory assessment, the pulse should be palpated. This is generally performed using the femoral artery in small animals, though other peripheral pulses (such as the dorsal pedal) may also be evaluated in certain situations. Palpation of the pulse provides important information on pulse quality, rhythm, and synchronization with the heartbeat.

The heart rate should then be auscultated using a stethoscope. Performing pulse palpation and heart auscultation concurrently allows the technician to detect pulse deficits—instances where a heartbeat is heard but not palpable as a peripheral pulse—which may suggest arrhythmias or reduced cardiac output.

Finally, the temperature should be taken rectally. Rectal thermography remains the gold standard in veterinary medicine due to its superior reliability and consistency compared to aural methods (Zanghi 2016). A rectal temperature provides a direct and relatively accurate assessment of core body temperature, which is critical in diagnosing fever, hypothermia, or systemic inflammation. Aural temperatures, though less invasive and more tolerable to some patients, can be influenced by environmental temperature, ear canal anatomy, cerumen accumulation, or infection, leading to unreliable readings. Despite the development of improved infrared tympanic thermometers, current evidence continues to support rectal thermometry as the clinical standard.

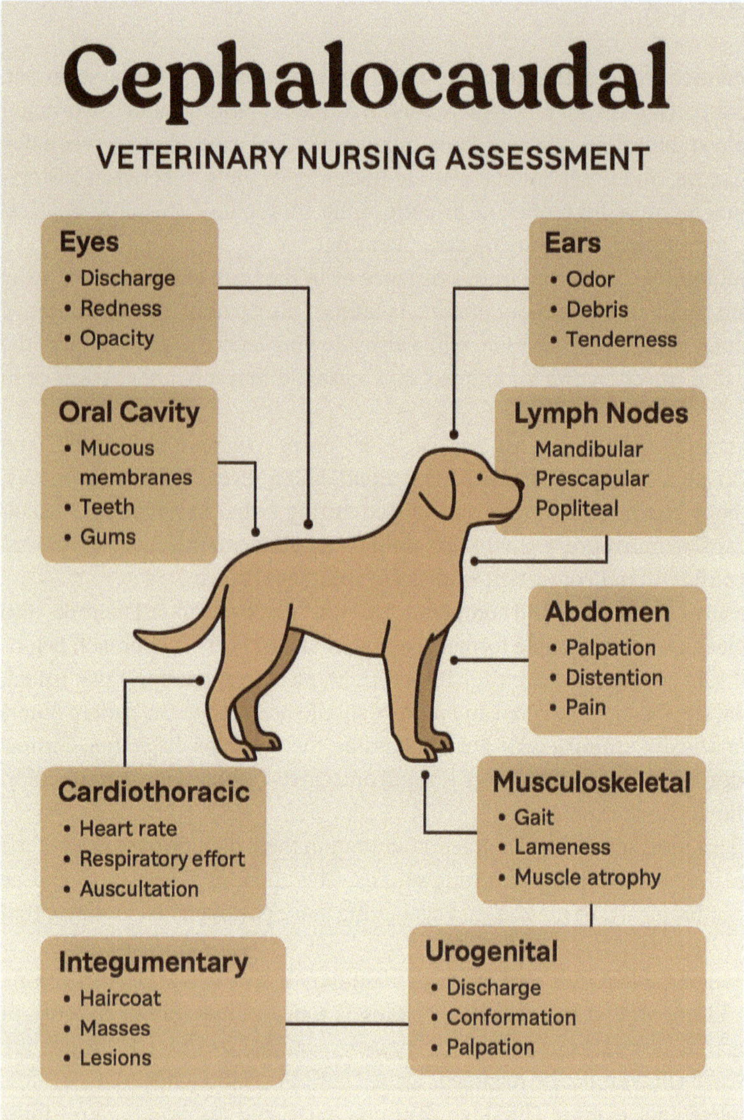

Figure 7.1 Cephalocaudal veterinary nursing assessment. A schematic representation of a cephalocaudal veterinary nursing assessment in the dog. Systematic evaluation progresses from head to tail, encompassing ocular, aural, oral, lymphatic, cardiothoracic, abdominal, integumentary, musculoskeletal, and urogenital systems. This structured approach ensures comprehensive patient evaluation and accurate documentation of clinical findings. *Source:* OpenAI (2025).

In conjunction with TPR, evaluation of mucous membrane (MM) color and capillary refill time (CRT) is an indispensable component of the veterinary nursing assessment. These parameters provide real-time information about a patient's cardiovascular and perfusion status. Normal mucous membranes are moist and pink, reflecting adequate perfusion and oxygenation. Pale mucous membranes may indicate anemia, peripheral vasoconstriction, or hypovolemia and often signify the need for immediate medical intervention. Hyperemic, or brick-red, mucous membranes may be indicative of sepsis, systemic inflammation, or heatstroke, suggesting vasodilation and possible cardiovascular compromise. Icteric, or yellow-tinged, mucous membranes suggest hepatic dysfunction or hemolysis, warranting further diagnostic investigation.

Capillary refill time is assessed by applying gentle pressure to the gingival tissue and observing the time taken for color to return after blanching. A normal CRT is less than two seconds. Prolonged CRT suggests poor peripheral perfusion, often due to hypovolemia, low cardiac output, or vasoconstriction. A shortened CRT, though less commonly discussed, may be indicative of hyperdynamic circulatory states such as early sepsis or systemic vasodilation. Both prolonged and shortened CRTs are clinically significant and warrant additional assessment.

While gingival tissue is the most commonly used site for evaluating MM color and CRT, there are alternative locations that may be employed when oral examination is not feasible due to patient temperament, oral trauma, or other clinical limitations. These include the conjunctival mucosa, the vulvar mucosa in females, and the preputial mucosa in males. In neonates, the digital pad or the inner aspect of the pinna may also provide useful information. However, the veterinary team must consider pigmentation, lighting, and mucosal moisture at these alternative sites, which can affect the accuracy of assessment.

Pain has rightfully earned recognition as the fourth vital sign in veterinary medicine (Mathews et al. 2014). This designation underscores the necessity of integrating pain assessment into every physical evaluation. Pain, both acute and chronic, is a complex physiological and psychological response to actual or potential tissue injury. It involves nociceptive pathways beginning at peripheral receptors, transmitting through the spinal cord, and ultimately processing in the brain. In animals, pain manifests through behavioral, postural, and physiological changes. Because animals cannot verbalize their discomfort, veterinary professionals must rely on careful observation and validated pain scoring systems.

Commonly used pain scoring tools include the Colorado State University Canine and Feline Acute Pain Scales, the Glasgow Composite Measure Pain Scale, the Feline Grimace Scale, and the UNESP-Botucatu Multidimensional Composite Pain Scale for cats (Colorado State University n.d.; Reid et al. 2017; Steagall et al. 2022; Brondani et al. 2013). These tools evaluate parameters such as posture, facial expression, response to palpation, vocalization, and physiological indicators like heart rate and respiratory rate.

Veterinary technicians must be adept at recognizing subtle signs of pain and applying these scales consistently. Pain should be scored as part of the initial physical assessment, as well as throughout hospitalization and following surgical or invasive procedures. A change in pain score necessitates prompt action. When a moderate to high pain score is identified, the technician must advocate for the patient by initiating a discussion with the attending veterinarian. Actions may include the administration or adjustment of analgesic protocols—such as opioids, NSAIDs, local anesthetics, or adjunctive agents like gabapentin—as well as the implementation of nonpharmacologic interventions such as gentle handling, low-stress housing, heat or cold therapy, and physical positioning.

Pain is not simply a welfare concern—it has direct physiological consequences, including increased cortisol release, immunosuppression, delayed healing, anorexia, and cardiovascular strain. Failure to address pain adequately impairs recovery and diminishes the quality of life. As such, technicians must treat pain assessment with the same clinical urgency as abnormal TPR values or CRT abnormalities.

The author strongly encourages continued learning in the realm of animal pain management and recommends reviewing current veterinary literature and attending continuing education opportunities focused on this critical area of practice. Mastery of pain recognition and response positions the veterinary technician as a true patient advocate and integral member of the medical team.

Together, MM color, CRT, TPR, and pain scoring form a comprehensive foundation of clinical evaluation. These vital signs allow veterinary technicians to monitor trends, detect abnormalities early, initiate timely interventions, and advocate for the well-being of every patient in their care.

In addition to these, the American Animal Hospital Association (AAHA) has designated nutrition as the fifth vital sign (American Animal Hospital Association 2010). This recognition emphasizes the critical role of nutritional status in the overall health and recovery of veterinary patients. Nutritional evaluation should be performed as part of every physical assessment, not merely reserved for underweight or critically ill animals. Malnutrition, whether from inadequate intake, malabsorption, or increased metabolic demand, can profoundly affect immune function, wound healing, tissue regeneration, and medication metabolism.

During a nursing assessment, evaluation of nutrition includes determining body weight, Body Condition Score (BCS), and in some cases, Muscle Condition Score (MCS). These metrics should be compared with prior values to detect subtle trends in weight gain or loss. Further inquiry with the client should explore the type of diet, amount fed, feeding frequency, treats, supplements, and recent changes in appetite or gastrointestinal signs.

The veterinary technician plays a pivotal role in identifying patients at risk of nutritional compromise and initiating a plan for nutritional support. This may include recommending specific therapeutic diets, adjusting feeding methods (e.g., feeding tubes), or collaborating with the veterinarian for a formal nutritional consult. In hospitalized patients, timely initiation of nutritional therapy is associated with improved outcomes, particularly in those with systemic illness, trauma, or undergoing surgery.

By incorporating nutrition into the core set of vital signs, veterinary technicians are empowered to assess and act on nutritional concerns with the same clinical rigor as pain, temperature, or mucous membrane abnormalities. This holistic approach ensures comprehensive patient care and supports optimal recovery and long-term health.

Advanced Catheterization

Intraosseous Catheters

Intraosseous (IO) catheters are used in critical patients or neonates with collapsed veins. Preferred sites include the proximal humerus, femur, or tibia. After aseptic preparation and local anesthesia, a bone marrow needle, IO needle, or a hypodermic needle is inserted at a 45–90° angle until a "pop" or decreased resistance is felt, indicating entry into the medullary cavity. Confirm placement by aspirating marrow or flushing easily. These catheters should be removed within 24–72 hours to avoid osteomyelitis (Table 7.2).

The advantages of intraosseous catheterization include rapid vascular access when peripheral veins are inaccessible, particularly during cardiopulmonary resuscitation or shock. The medullary cavity provides a noncollapsible venous plexus, allowing for the administration of fluids, medications, and blood products with systemic absorption comparable to intravenous routes. Intraosseous (IO) access can be lifesaving in neonates, small exotic species, and profoundly hypotensive patients.

However, disadvantages include a higher risk of infection (osteomyelitis), pain upon infusion, potential damage to the growth plate in immature animals, and the technical difficulty associated with accurate placement. Complications may also include fracture, extravasation of fluids, compartment syndrome, and failure to achieve adequate flow due to malposition or obstruction.

Table 7.2 Intraosseous (IO) catheterization—quick reference.

Section	Details
Indications	Emergency access in hypovolemic or shock patients; neonates and small exotics when veins are inaccessible; temporary vascular access until IV catheter is possible; administration of fluids, medications, and blood products.
Contraindications	Fractures at/near intended site; infection or osteomyelitis at insertion site; osteoporosis or other bone pathology; recent IO access in the same bone.
Common IO Sites	Dogs and Cats: Proximal humerus, proximal tibia, femur, iliac crest. Neonates: Proximal tibia (most common), femur. Exotics: Distal femur, proximal tibia, proximal humerus.
Supplies	Clippers and antiseptic scrub materials; sterile gloves; local anesthetic (e.g., lidocaine) for conscious patients; 16–22 g spinal needle or bone marrow IO needle (Jamshidi, EZ-IO, Cook); T-connector or extension set with Luer lock; heparinized saline flush; securement materials (suture, tape, bandage); infusion pump or gravity set (if fluids administered).
Technique—Preparation	Clip and aseptically prep chosen IO site; if conscious, infiltrate local anesthetic SC and into the periosteum; position patient in lateral or dorsal recumbency according to site.
Technique—Positioning (Proximal Tibia)	Flex stifle; palpate tibial tuberosity; insert needle slightly caudal and distal to tuberosity, directed parallel to tibial shaft.
Technique—Insertion	Advance with firm, rotating motion through cortex; feel a "pop"/reduced resistance entering medullary cavity; needle stands upright without lateral motion; remove stylet.
Technique—Confirmation	Attempt to aspirate marrow/blood (may be difficult in dehydrated/hypovolemic patients); flush sterile saline with minimal resistance; if high resistance or swelling, remove and select another site; placement of radiographs are standard for affirmation.
Technique—Securement	Suture or tape the hub; apply a light bandage to stabilize/protect; label site with time/date.
Monitoring and **Maintenance**	Flush sterile saline every two hours to maintain patency; change IO catheter every 24–72 hours or sooner if complications; monitor for extravasation/swelling, local infection/inflammation, and dislodgement.
Complications	Infection (cellulitis, osteomyelitis); extravasation/compartment syndrome; bone fracture; fat embolism; dislodgement or occlusion.
Advantages	Rapid, reliable access in emergencies; direct access to central circulation; useful in neonates, exotics, and critical patients.
Disadvantages	Short-term use only; risk of bone/soft-tissue complications; requires skill and anatomical familiarity.

Peripherally Inserted Central Catheters (PICC)

PICC lines are placed via the cephalic or saphenous vein and advanced into the cranial or caudal vena cava. Measure externally from the insertion point to the third intercostal space (cranial vena cava) or last rib (caudal vena cava). After sterile placement, confirm the location radiographically. PICC lines can remain in place for up to 14 days (Table 7.3).

The advantages of PICC catheterization include the ability to maintain long-term venous access without the need for repeated venipuncture, thereby reducing patient discomfort and vessel trauma. PICC lines are ideal for patients requiring frequent blood sampling, extended fluid therapy, or administration of irritant drugs, such as chemotherapeutics or hyperosmolar solutions. Placement in peripheral veins makes them technically easier and safer than central venous catheters, particularly in unstable or fractious patients.

Table 7.3 PICC line placement in veterinary medicine—quick reference.

Section	Details
Indications	Long-term IV therapy (chemotherapy, antibiotics, total parenteral nutrition); repeated blood sampling in critical care or research; poor peripheral venous access; need to minimize multiple venipunctures.
Contraindications	Local infection or phlebitis at insertion site; coagulopathies or thrombocytopenia (relative); uncorrected vascular anomalies or severe dehydration; fractures or injuries to the limb used for placement.
Supplies Needed	Sterile gloves, cap, and mask; clippers and antiseptic scrub; sterile drapes; 4–6 Fr single- or multi-lumen polyurethane catheter (60–80 cm for large dogs, shorter for smaller animals); catheter introducer set (modified Seldinger technique); vascular access kit (guidewire, dilator, scalpel, catheter); sterile saline and flushes; sterile T-connector or extension set; sutures or securement device; radiographs for confirmation; ultrasound optional for vein visualization.
Common Insertion Sites	Dogs and Cats: Cephalic or lateral saphenous vein → tip advanced to cranial or caudal vena cava. Exotics: Saphenous or femoral vein → caudal vena cava.
Procedure: Patient Preparation	Patient in lateral or sternal recumbency; clip wide margin over vein; perform sterile surgical scrub; drape for asepsis.
Procedure: Vein Identification and **Local Anesthesia**	Palpation or ultrasound guidance; lidocaine infiltration in conscious patients.
Procedure: Vessel Cannulation	Introducer needle (20–22G) into vein; confirm blood return; insert guidewire; remove needle, leaving guidewire.
Procedure: Vessel Dilation	Small skin nick with scalpel; advance dilator over guidewire to enlarge tract; remove dilator, guidewire remains.
Procedure: Catheter Insertion	Advance catheter over guidewire toward central vein; remove guidewire once fully inserted; estimate catheter length by measuring insertion site to thoracic inlet or abdomen landmarks.
Procedure: Verification	Aspirate for blood return; flush saline to check patency; radiograph to confirm tip in cranial or caudal vena cava.
Procedure: Securement and **Bandaging**	Suture hub or use securement device; apply sterile gauze and light bandage; label with date and time.
Catheter Maintenance	Flush q6–8h with sterile saline if not in continuous use; change extension tubing and ports every 72 hours; change bandage every 48–72 hours or if soiled; use aseptic technique for all access.
Complications	Phlebitis, thrombosis, local infection or catheter-related bloodstream infections, occlusion or kinking, malposition or dislodgement, air embolism (rare), extravasation if catheter backs out.
Advantages	Provides long-term venous access; less invasive than jugular central lines; may be placed without sedation in some cases; reduces stress for patients with frequent drug administration or sampling.
Disadvantages	Requires advanced skill; strict sterility essential; risk of tip migration or malposition; radiographic confirmation required.

However, disadvantages include the potential for malpositioning, thrombus formation, and catheter occlusion. Because the catheter traverses a long venous path, there is an increased risk of mechanical complications and biofilm development along the catheter tract. Infection remains a concern, particularly if aseptic technique is compromised. Complications may also include phlebitis, catheter-associated bloodstream infection (CABSI), or catheter embolization if the line is inadvertently sheared or damaged. Vigilant monitoring and strict adherence to catheter care protocols are essential to reduce these risks.

Central Venous Catheters

Central venous catheters placed using the Seldinger technique involve insertion into the jugular vein with an introducer needle, guidewire, dilator, and catheter. External measurement follows the vein path to the third intercostal space or the point of the shoulder in dorsal recumbency. The guidewire is advanced, a dilator is used, and the catheter is inserted over the guidewire. Suture and secure the catheter with a sterile bandage. Central lines allow for CVP monitoring, blood sampling, and long-term fluid administration Table 7.4; Figure 7.2).

The advantages of central venous catheterization include reliable access to central circulation, the ability to monitor central venous pressure, and the facilitation of administration of hypertonic or vesicant solutions that may be damaging to peripheral veins. Central lines are particularly beneficial in critically ill patients, those requiring parenteral nutrition, or those undergoing long-term drug therapy. The Seldinger technique allows for precise placement and minimizes trauma to vascular structures during insertion.

Disadvantages include the increased technical complexity of the procedure and a higher risk of complications compared to peripheral or PICC lines. Infections such as catheter-associated bloodstream infections (CABSIs) and thrombosis are also

Table 7.4 Central venous catheter (CVC) placement—quick reference.

Section	Details
Indications	Critically ill patients requiring central venous access; administration of irritating drugs (e.g., hypertonic saline, chemotherapy); total parenteral nutrition (TPN); repeated blood sampling; central venous pressure (CVP) monitoring.
Contraindications	Coagulopathy or severe thrombocytopenia (relative); local infection at insertion site; thrombosis or stenosis of target vein; uncorrected hypovolemia or severe hypotension (relative).
Common Insertion Sites	Internal jugular vein (most common); external jugular vein (some large dogs); femoral or lateral saphenous veins (less common). Right jugular preferred to reduce risk of thoracic duct puncture.
Required Supplies	Central line kit (catheter, guidewire, introducer needle, dilator); chlorhexidine scrub and 70% isopropyl alcohol; sterile gloves, gown, and drapes; local anesthetic (lidocaine); scalpel blade (#11 or 15); syringe (3–5 mL); sterile flush (heparinized or normal saline); suture material (e.g., 2-0 nylon); bandaging material; ultrasound optional; radiography for confirmation.
Patient Preparation	Positioning: Lateral or dorsal recumbency, neck extended, head turned away, towel under neck to distend jugular. Site prep: Clip wide margin, aseptically scrub, don sterile attire, drape field.
Seldinger Technique	1. Locate vein (palpation or ultrasound).2. Venipuncture with introducer needle (18–20G), confirm blood return.3. Advance guidewire 10–20 cm; never force resistance.4. Dilate tract with scalpel nick and dilator.5. Insert catheter to ~1/3 body length; tip ideally in cranial vena cava at 3rd intercostal space.6. Remove guidewire, aspirate and flush ports, suture catheter, apply sterile bandage, label ports and date.
Confirm Placement	Lateral thoracic radiograph (preferred) to confirm catheter tip in cranial vena cava. Ultrasound can confirm intraoperatively.
Catheter Maintenance	Flush every 6–8 hours if not in continuous use; replace injection caps q72h; change bandage q48–72h or sooner if soiled; strict aseptic technique for all access and medication administration.
Complications	Malposition (tip in azygos or subclavian vein, or coiled); thrombosis; air embolism; infection (sepsis); hemorrhage/hematoma; cardiac arrhythmia (rare, from over-insertion).
Advantages	Provides long-term venous access (1–2 weeks if maintained); reduces peripheral vein trauma; allows central monitoring and CVP measurement.
Disadvantages	Requires advanced skill and strict sterility; complications are possible with incorrect placement; requires imaging confirmation.

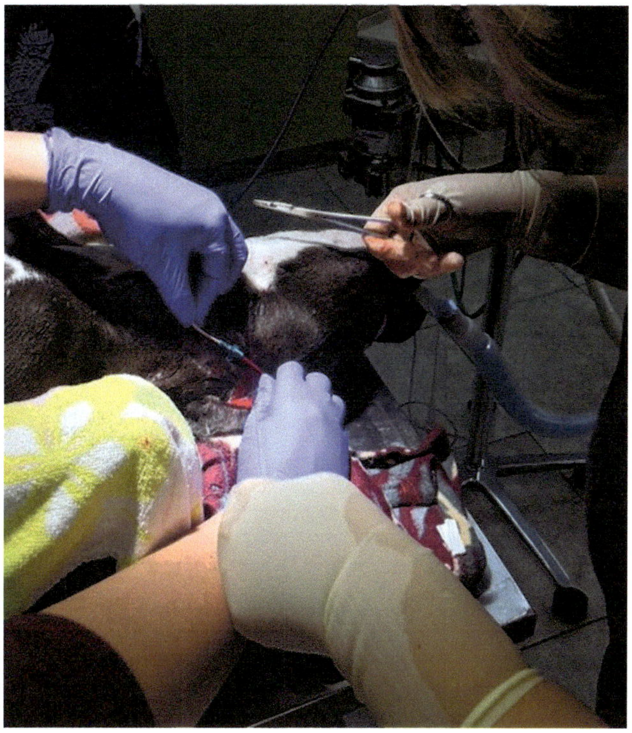

Figure 7.2 Central venous catheter being sutured in a canine patient. *Source:* Schaeffer (2025).

notable concerns. Strict aseptic technique, continuous monitoring, and timely removal when clinically appropriate are crucial for minimizing these risks and optimizing patient outcomes.

Catheter Maintenance

Peripheral catheters should be flushed every four to six hours with sterile saline to maintain patency. Central and PICC lines also require sterile saline after use. Dressings must be inspected for moisture or debris every shift and changed every 24–48 hours. All access points must be cleaned with alcohol or chlorhexidine prior to use. Document all flushes, dressing changes, and observed changes.

Signs of complications include localized swelling, erythema, discharge, resistance to flushing, and systemic signs (fever, tachycardia). If resistance occurs during flushing, do not apply force. Attempt gentle aspiration and limb repositioning; replace if unsuccessful. Infections require immediate removal and potential tip culture. Suspected CABSI may warrant blood cultures and empiric antibiotics. Thrombophlebitis should be treated with warm compresses and anti-inflammatories. Extravasation requires stopping infusions and possibly administering antidotes or compresses. Dislodged or leaking catheters must be replaced, and all complications must be recorded. All venous catheter interactions must maintain aseptic technique. Wear gloves and use sterile supplies. Central and PICC lines benefit from transparent dressings for visual inspection. Adhering to these protocols minimizes the risk of infection and ensures the success of vascular access (Table 7.5).

Arterial Catheters

Arterial catheterization, also known as arterial line or "art line" placement, is an advanced vascular access procedure utilized in veterinary medicine for direct arterial access. This technique is particularly useful in settings where real-time hemodynamic monitoring or repeated arterial blood sampling is required. While less frequently performed than venous catheterization in general practice, arterial catheterization is indispensable in the context of anesthetic monitoring and intensive care for critically ill patients.

The primary rationale for arterial catheterization lies in its ability to provide continuous, beat-to-beat monitoring of arterial blood pressure. Unlike noninvasive methods such as Doppler or oscillometric systems, arterial catheters allow for direct measurement of systolic, diastolic, and mean arterial pressures. This real-time data is essential for titrating vasoactive drugs

Table 7.5 Recognition and management of venous catheter complications.

Complication/Sign	Recognition	Management
Infection	Localized swelling, erythema, discharge; systemic signs (fever, tachycardia).	Immediate catheter removal, culture catheter tip, obtain blood cultures if CABSI suspected, begin empiric antibiotics.
Resistance to Flushing	Increased resistance when flushing catheter.	Do not apply force. Attempt gentle aspiration and reposition limb. Replace catheter if unsuccessful.
Thrombophlebitis	Pain, erythema, swelling along vein.	Warm compresses, anti-inflammatory medications, and catheter removal if severe.
Extravasation	Swelling, pain, or leakage around insertion site during infusion.	Stop infusions immediately, administer antidotes if applicable, apply compresses, replace catheter.
Dislodgement/ Leakage	Catheter is visibly displaced or leaking.	Remove and replace catheter. Document event.
General Protocols	Risk of contamination or mismanagement of line.	Maintain aseptic technique for all catheter interactions; wear gloves, use sterile supplies; transparent dressings allow visual inspection of central and PICC lines.

and detecting rapid changes in cardiovascular status. In addition to pressure monitoring, arterial lines facilitate serial blood sampling for arterial blood gas (ABG) analysis. This is particularly valuable in patients requiring ventilatory support or undergoing treatment for acid-base disturbances and metabolic derangements.

Clinical situations that commonly necessitate arterial catheterization include shock states such as septic, hemorrhagic, or cardiogenic shock, and cases involving patients on continuous infusions of inotropes or vasopressors. High-risk anesthetic procedures, such as those classified under ASA IV or V, benefit from invasive pressure monitoring to improve intraoperative management. Furthermore, any patient with significant pulmonary pathology that requires serial arterial blood gas analysis—such as those with acute respiratory distress syndrome (ARDS) or on mechanical ventilation—should be considered for arterial access. Patients undergoing major surgeries associated with rapid fluid shifts, substantial blood loss, or cardiovascular instability also stand to benefit from the use of arterial catheters. In these cases, invasive monitoring facilitates dynamic assessment of fluid responsiveness through parameters such as pulse pressure variation.

Several anatomical sites may be utilized for arterial catheter placement. The dorsal pedal artery is the most frequently used site in dogs and cats due to its ease of access, consistent anatomy, and relatively low complication rate. The femoral artery is another common location, offering strong pulsatility and vessel diameter but with a higher associated risk of infection and hematoma (Davis and Jensen 2006). The coccygeal artery may be utilized in certain large animals or unique clinical cases.

Arterial catheterization should be performed using sterile technique and appropriate equipment. The patient is positioned in lateral recumbency, and the selected site is clipped and aseptically prepared. In the case of dorsal pedal access, the hind limb is gently restrained to expose the medial dorsal surface of the paw. Local anesthesia, such as a subcutaneous bleb of 1% lidocaine, should be administered in awake or lightly sedated patients to minimize discomfort (Table 7.6).

Following preparation, the artery is palpated carefully, and a short, over-the-needle catheter (typically 20–24 gauge) is introduced at a 30- to 45-degree angle to the skin. Upon entry into the vessel, pulsatile blood will appear in the catheter hub, indicating successful arterial puncture. The catheter is then advanced slightly before threading it fully into the lumen. It is connected to a sterile extension set primed with heparinized saline or to a pressure transducer system for continuous monitoring. The catheter is secured using a sterile adhesive dressing and light bandaging, with careful attention paid to avoid occlusion or kinking of the line. The placement should be documented, including the time and date, and the site should be inspected regularly for signs of complications (Figure 7.3).

While arterial catheterization is highly beneficial, it is not without contraindications. Patients with coagulopathies or severe thrombocytopenia are at increased risk of hemorrhage and may not be ideal candidates. Arterial catheterization should also be avoided in patients with peripheral vascular disease, thrombosis of the intended vessel, or local infection at the insertion site. Poor perfusion to the limb, often seen in shock or peripheral vasoconstriction, can make placement technically challenging and may increase the risk of distal ischemia.

Table 7.6 Arterial line placement—quick reference.

Section	Details
Indications	Continuous direct blood pressure monitoring in unstable or anesthetized patients; frequent arterial blood gas (ABG) sampling; monitoring during critical illness or major surgery.
Contraindications	Severe coagulopathy or thrombocytopenia (risk of hemorrhage); infection at insertion site; peripheral vascular disease or compromised perfusion of target limb; hypotension with poor peripheral pulses.
Common Insertion Sites	Dogs and Cats: Dorsal pedal artery, femoral artery. Less common: coccygeal artery, auricular artery (large animals).
Required Supplies	Arterial catheter (20–24G depending on patient size); introducer needle; sterile gloves and drapes; chlorhexidine scrub; heparinized saline flush; pressure transducer system or heparinized fluid line with pressure bag; securement materials (sutures, tape, bandage).
Patient Preparation	Positioning depends on site (dorsal recumbency for pedal, lateral for femoral); clip and aseptically prepare site; apply local anesthetic if conscious.
Placement Technique	1. Palpate arterial pulse at chosen site.2. Insert introducer needle/catheter at shallow angle until bright red pulsatile blood appears.3. Advance catheter into artery, remove needle.4. Connect catheter to heparinized flush line or transducer.5. Aspirate and flush to ensure patency.
Verification	Bright red, pulsatile flow confirms arterial placement; transducer tracing confirms arterial waveform; ABG sample analysis for confirmation if needed.
Securement and Bandaging	Suture or tape hub to skin; apply light padded bandage to protect line; ensure limb immobilization if needed to reduce movement.
Maintenance	Continuous heparinized flush at 1–2 mL/h to prevent clotting; inspect insertion site frequently; change dressings every 48–72 hours; monitor waveform for damping.
Complications	Thrombosis or embolism leading to distal ischemia; hematoma; infection; hemorrhage; inadvertent venous placement; line dislodgement or kinking.
Advantages	Provides accurate, continuous blood pressure monitoring; allows repeated ABG sampling without multiple needle sticks.
Disadvantages	Invasive; requires specialized monitoring equipment; higher risk of complications compared to venous access.

Potential complications associated with arterial lines include hematoma formation, which is particularly common if the site is not compressed adequately upon removal of the catheter. Thrombosis may occur with prolonged catheter dwell times or if the catheter is of an inappropriate size for the vessel. This may result in ischemic injury to distal tissues. Infection is another risk, especially in sites with less skin coverage or high bacterial load, such as the femoral region. Rare but serious complications include exsanguination due to accidental dislodgement of the catheter and embolic events resulting from the introduction of thrombi or air into the arterial circulation. False pressure readings may occur if the transducer is improperly zeroed or if air bubbles are present in the line, emphasizing the importance of vigilant maintenance and calibration.

In conclusion, arterial catheterization is a powerful tool in the management of critically ill or anesthetized veterinary patients. Its ability to provide continuous, accurate cardiovascular data and facilitate blood sampling makes it an essential component of advanced veterinary care. When performed with skill and precision, and when patients are selected appropriately, the benefits of arterial catheterization far outweigh the potential risks. It is imperative that veterinary professionals possess both theoretical knowledge and clinical acumen to utilize arterial lines effectively and safely.

Urinary Catheterization in the Small Animal Patient

Urinary catheterization is a fundamental procedure in veterinary clinical practice, performed to achieve diagnostic, therapeutic, and supportive care objectives. Indications include sterile urine collection for analysis and culture, decompression of the urinary bladder in cases of obstruction, quantification of urinary output in critically ill patients, radiographic contrast studies, and management of urinary incontinence or detrusor atony. Safe and effective catheterization requires a comprehensive understanding of lower urinary tract anatomy, appropriate catheter selection, strict adherence to aseptic technique, and species- and sex-specific technical adaptations.

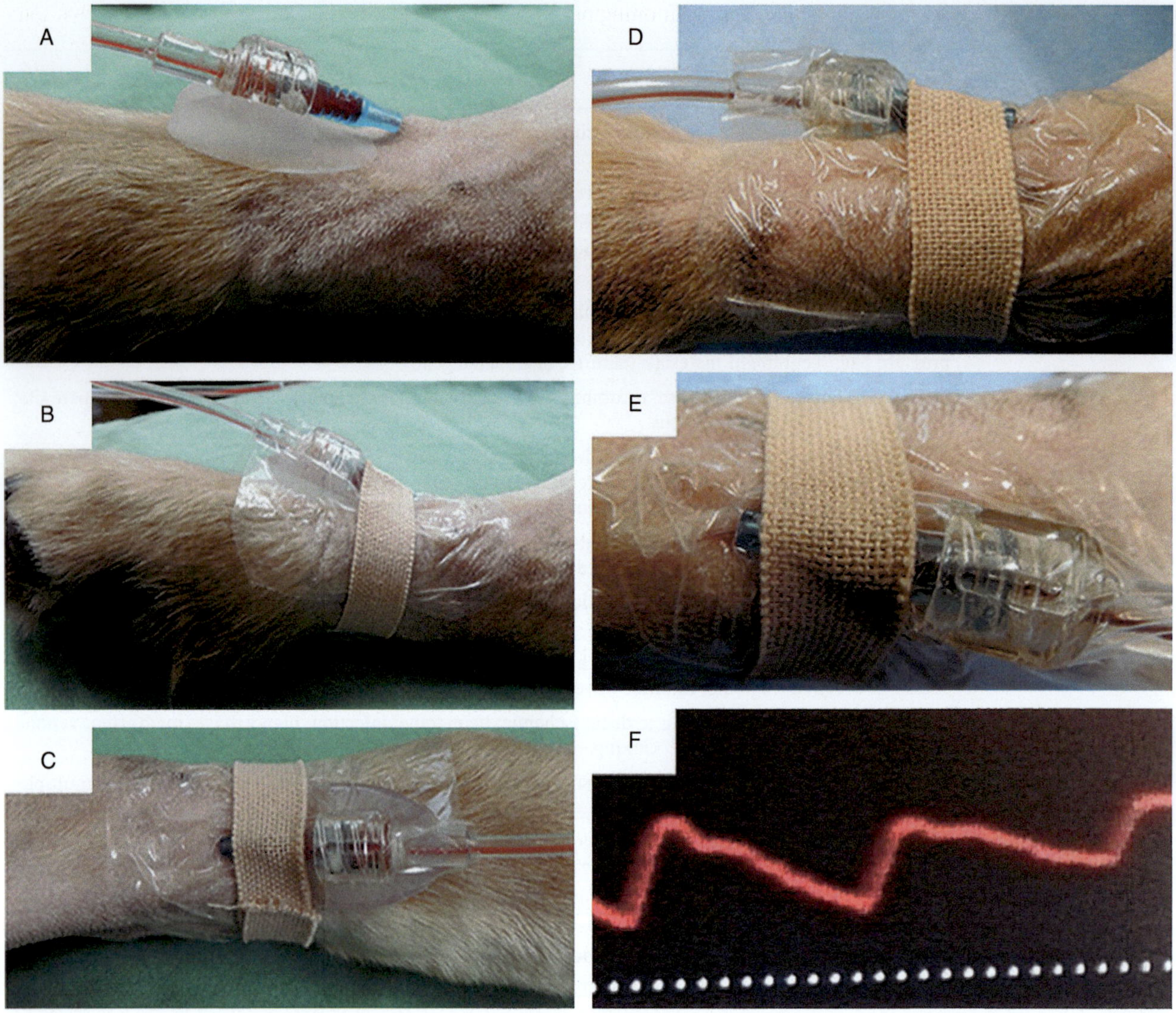

Figure 7.3 Arterial catheterization in the dorsal pedal artery of a canine patient, connected to a pressure transducer for invasive blood pressure monitoring. *Source:* Iizuka et al., (2019) / Frontiers Media S.A. / CC BY 4.0. Picture A-D provide different angles for securing a dorsal pedal arterial line. Picture F is the pleth form indicating proper placement of the arterial catheter, transducer, and functioning of the multisystem parameter unit.

Urinary Tract Anatomy

In male dogs, the urethra originates at the neck of the bladder and courses caudally through the pelvic canal, curving around the ischial arch, and continues distally within the os penis to terminate at the tip of the glans penis. The presence of the os penis and the curvature at the ischial arch introduces some degree of resistance during catheter advancement. In female dogs, the urethra is relatively short and straight, extending from the bladder neck and terminating at the urethral tubercle on the ventral floor of the vaginal vestibule. Its location, in close proximity to the vulva and rectum, requires meticulous hygiene to reduce iatrogenic infection risk.

In male cats, the urethra extends from the bladder neck and follows a caudal path through the pelvic canal and into the penis. The penis of the male cat has a sigmoid shape, with a ventral flexion in its resting state. Successful catheterization requires complete extrusion and full extension of the penis to straighten the sigmoid urethral curve and allow for unobstructed catheter passage. The distal urethra is narrow and encased in the os penis, increasing the risk for trauma during catheterization. In sexually intact males, the presence of keratinized penile spines can further complicate catheter advancement. In female cats, the urethra is short and narrow, opening into the vestibule just cranial to the vaginal opening. Due to the small size of the external genitalia and deep positioning of the urethral papilla, visualization can be difficult without specialized instrumentation or digital guidance.

Types of Urinary Catheters

Selection of the appropriate catheter is dictated by patient size, sex, species, duration of use, and clinical indication. The most common catheter types include:

- **Polypropylene Catheters**: These semirigid, sterile catheters are useful for initial decompression or to relieve obstruction. Their stiffness facilitates passage through strictured areas, but they are not recommended for long-term use due to increased risk of urethral trauma.
- **Red Rubber Catheters**: Constructed of flexible latex or silicone-based material, red rubber catheters are preferred for intermittent catheterization or short-term placement. Their pliability minimizes urethral irritation, although they lack a retention mechanism.
- **Tomcat Catheters**: Typically made of rigid polyethylene, these are designed for use in obstructed male cats. Available in open- or closed-ended formats, they facilitate rapid bladder decompression but should be replaced with softer materials for long-term use to reduce urethral trauma.
- **Slippery Sam™/Polyurethane Catheters**: These flexible, hydrophilic-coated catheters are well suited for indwelling use in male cats. Their softness minimizes mucosal irritation, and many are radiopaque to facilitate imaging confirmation.
- **Foley Catheters**: Constructed of silicone or latex, Foley catheters contain a distal balloon that can be inflated with sterile saline to retain the catheter within the bladder. They are the author's preferred choice for indwelling catheterization in dogs, particularly in patients requiring accurate urine output monitoring or long-term drainage. Their compatibility with closed collection systems reduces ascending urinary tract infection risk and allows secure placement.

Patient Preparation and Aseptic Technique

Patient preparation is critical to minimizing iatrogenic infection and urethral trauma:

1) **Physical Assessment**: All patients should be evaluated for urethral patency, urinary bladder distension, and overall health status. Sedation or general anesthesia is recommended, particularly for female patients and fractious animals.
2) **Clipping and Scrubbing**: The perineal area must be clipped and aseptically prepared using applications of 2% chlorhexidine solution and sterile saline. The external genitalia must be cleansed thoroughly to remove debris and microbial contaminants. Veterinary technicians must exercise particular diligence when performing the clipping process to avoid iatrogenic trauma. Excessive pressure, inappropriate blade angle, or repeated passes over delicate tissue may result in clipper burn or abrasions to the perineal region. Such disruptions of the epidermal barrier not only compromise patient comfort but also create a nidus for bacterial proliferation, predisposing the patient to ascending urinary tract infections. Equally important is the avoidance of instilling chlorhexidine solution directly into the vestibule or internal vulvar structures, as this can result in significant mucosal irritation. Proper technique therefore requires a balance of thorough decontamination while maintaining the integrity of perineal tissues to minimize postoperative complications.
3) **Positioning**:
    - **Male dogs**: Lateral recumbency with the upper hindlimb abducted.
    - **Female dogs**: Standing, sternal, or lateral recumbency with hindlimbs elevated to expose the vulva.
    - **Male cats**: Dorsal or lateral recumbency with gentle caudal retraction of the penis.
    - **Female cats**: Sternal recumbency with hindlimbs flexed cranially and the tail elevated.
4) **Aseptic Technique**: Sterile gloves, lubricants, catheterization kits, and closed collection systems must be utilized. Catheters should be lubricated generously with sterile, water-soluble jelly to reduce friction and urethral irritation (Table 7.7).

Complications and Considerations

Excessive force or improper alignment during catheter placement can result in urethral trauma, including mucosal abrasions, hematuria, or, in severe cases, urethral rupture—an outcome particularly concerning in feline patients due to their narrow urethral lumen. Iatrogenic urinary tract infections are another potential complication, mitigated by adherence to

Table 7.7 Catheterization techniques by species and sex.

Species/Sex	Technique
Male Dog	• Retract the prepuce to expose the glans penis and clean with sterile saline or antiseptic solution. • Insert a lubricated catheter into the urethral orifice and gently advance toward the bladder, noting mild resistance at the ischial arch. • Bladder entry is confirmed by urine flow. • For Foley catheters, inflate the balloon with sterile saline per manufacturer recommendations. • Secure the catheter to the prepuce with suture or adhesive anchoring device and attach it to a sterile closed collection system.
Female Dog	• A vaginal speculum or otoscope may be used to visualize the urethral opening on the ventral vestibular floor, though many technicians prefer the blind digital palpation technique. • Clean the vulva with dilute antimicrobial solution. • Insert a well-lubricated catheter into the urethral orifice under direct visualization or digital guidance, advancing gently until urine flow is observed. • For indwelling use, secure the catheter and connect to a collection system.
Male Cat	• Retract the prepuce and fully extend the penis to straighten its sigmoid curvature. • Clean the glans penis and apply sterile lubricant to the catheter. • Insert into the urethral orifice and advance with gentle, controlled pressure; slight rotation of the catheter and traction on the penis may assist passage. • Initial decompression may require a Tomcat catheter, which should later be replaced with a flexible indwelling catheter once patency is restored. • Confirm bladder entry with urine flow, secure externally to the perineum with suture, and attach to a closed collection system.
Female Cat	• Position in sternal recumbency with hindlimbs flexed cranially and tail elevated. • Cleanse the vulva and perineum aseptically with dilute antimicrobial solution. • Due to the narrow vaginal vault, visualization with a speculum or otoscopic cone is often impractical. Instead, gently part the vulvar labia and direct a lubricated catheter into the central vestibule, advancing passively until the urethral orifice is entered on the ventral floor, cranial to the vaginal opening. • Advance until urine flow is observed, then secure and connect to a collection system if indwelling.

strict aseptic techniques and the use of closed urine collection systems. Indwelling catheters should be assessed daily for signs of bacterial colonization or ascending infection. In Foley catheters, balloon misplacement is a critical concern; inflating the retention balloon prior to verified intravesicular placement may result in urethral obstruction, mucosal tearing, or ischemic necrosis. Therefore, confirmation of urine flow prior to balloon inflation is essential. Catheter displacement, tubing kinking, or excessive bladder distension may lead to urinary leakage around the catheter or complete outflow obstruction. Additionally, behavioral signs such as vocalization, restlessness, abnormal posturing, or dysuria should prompt immediate reevaluation of catheter positioning and adequacy of analgesia.

Urinary Catheter Maintenance and Nursing Considerations

The maintenance of an indwelling urinary catheter requires vigilant nursing care to preserve catheter patency, minimize patient discomfort, and prevent iatrogenic complications—most notably, ascending urinary tract infections. These infections are a significant risk associated with prolonged catheterization, often arising from contamination during placement, manipulation of the catheter or collection system, or bacterial migration along the catheter's external surface (Weese et al. 2011). Rigorous adherence to aseptic technique and meticulous nursing oversight are paramount in mitigating these risks.

Once the catheter is placed and secured, it should be connected to a sterile, closed urine collection system without disconnection unless medically indicated. Any necessary disconnection—for example, for urine sampling or system replacement—must be performed using aseptic technique, including the use of gloves and disinfectant swabbing of all ports and connection points. Breaks in the closed system substantially increase the likelihood of bacterial ingress into the bladder.

Medical staff must ensure that the catheter and collection tubing remain free of kinks, dependent loops, or tension points that may impede urine flow or encourage backflow. The collection bag should be positioned below the level of the urinary bladder at all times to maintain unidirectional drainage by gravity and prevent retrograde contamination. The catheter insertion site should be monitored at regular intervals for signs of inflammation, discharge, erythema, or leakage. The perineal area should be gently cleaned using sterile saline or an approved antiseptic solution to remove residual urine or exudate that may serve as a nidus for infection. Cleaning should always proceed in a proximal-to-distal direction—moving from the area closest to the vulva or prepuce outward toward the anus or hindlimbs—to prevent the inadvertent transfer of bacteria from more contaminated regions to cleaner areas. This directional technique minimizes the risk of introducing urogenital or fecal contaminants into the urethral orifice, thereby reducing the potential for ascending infections and iatrogenic urinary tract contamination during subsequent procedures such as re-catheterization.

Careful documentation of urinary output, catheter appearance, urine character (including color, turbidity, and presence of hematuria or debris), and patient behavior is an essential component of ongoing assessment. Any changes suggestive of infection or catheter malfunction should prompt immediate clinical reevaluation. The use of prophylactic antibiotics is not routinely recommended for catheterized patients, as it may promote the development of antimicrobial resistance and mask early signs of infection (Weese et al. 2011).

Urinary catheters should be removed as soon as clinically appropriate to reduce infection risk, and patients with indwelling catheters require individualized nursing care plans that prioritize hygiene, comfort, and surveillance for complications. Through proactive and informed nursing intervention, the risks associated with urinary catheterization can be significantly reduced, thereby enhancing patient outcomes and supporting the broader goals of veterinary intensive care.

Urinary catheterization is a core nursing and medical procedure in small animal practice, requiring technical skill, anatomical knowledge, and attention to detail. Foley catheters are typically preferred for indwelling use due to their ability to maintain bladder drainage and prevent accidental removal. Incorporating aseptic technique, species-specific anatomy, and gentle catheter manipulation ensures optimal outcomes while minimizing iatrogenic complications. Mastery of this technique is essential for all veterinary professionals involved in the care of hospitalized or critically ill patients.

Blood Pressure Assessment in the Canine and Feline Patient

Arterial blood pressure is a critical physiological parameter that reflects the force exerted by circulating blood upon the walls of the arteries. It is a fundamental component of cardiovascular assessment, offering insights into perfusion status, systemic vascular resistance, and cardiac output. In both canine and feline patients, maintaining adequate blood pressure is essential for oxygen and nutrient delivery to tissues. Deviations from normal blood pressure ranges may signify underlying pathology or anesthetic complications, necessitating prompt recognition and intervention.

Blood pressure is determined by the product of cardiac output and systemic vascular resistance. Cardiac output itself is influenced by stroke volume and heart rate. Mean arterial pressure (MAP) is the most clinically relevant component during anesthetic monitoring and critical care, as it reflects the average perfusion pressure to vital organs during the cardiac cycle. The MAP is calculated using the formula:

$$\text{MAP} = (1/3 \times \text{Systolic BP}) + (2/3 \times \text{Diastolic BP})$$

This calculation accounts for the fact that diastole occupies a longer duration in the cardiac cycle than systole. A MAP greater than 60 mmHg is typically required to maintain adequate perfusion to the kidneys, brain, and other vital organs in both dogs and cats.

Blood pressure in veterinary patients may be assessed via direct (invasive) or indirect (noninvasive) methods. Direct measurement involves placement of an arterial catheter, typically into the dorsal pedal or femoral artery, connected to a calibrated pressure transducer. This method is considered the gold standard for accuracy and is commonly utilized in critical care and during high-risk anesthetic events.

Indirect measurement techniques include Doppler ultrasonic sphygmomanometry and oscillometric devices. The Doppler method involves placement of an ultrasonic probe distal to a sphygmomanometer cuff, allowing detection of blood flow via audible signals. It is especially reliable in small or hypotensive patients but primarily yields systolic pressure values. Oscillometric devices estimate systolic, diastolic, and mean pressures through analysis of oscillations generated within the cuff during arterial flow. However, their accuracy may diminish in small patients, patients with arrhythmias, or those with low perfusion states (Acierno et al. 2018) (Table 7.8).

Accurate blood pressure readings require proper cuff selection and placement. The cuff should be approximately 40% of the limb circumference in dogs and 30–40% in cats. An improperly sized cuff—either too narrow or too wide—can result in falsely elevated or diminished readings, respectively. Appropriate cuff placement sites include the cranial aspect of the antebrachium (forelimb distal to the elbow), distal to the hock on the pelvic limb, the base of the tail, and occasionally the

Table 7.8 Comparison of blood pressure monitoring methods in veterinary medicine.

Method	Advantages	Disadvantages	When to Utilize
Doppler Blood Pressure	Provides reliable systolic pressure readings, especially in small patients. Inexpensive and portable.Useful in hypotensive states where oscillometric may fail.	Does not provide diastolic or mean arterial pressure reliably.Requires trained personnel and is operator-dependent.Background noise may make detection difficult.	Preferred in small dogs, cats, and exotics.Hypotensive or unstable patients.Situations requiring accurate systolic pressure monitoring.
Oscillometric Blood Pressure	Provides systolic, mean, and diastolic pressure.Automated, requires less operator training.Can provide continuous monitoring.	Less accurate in small animals (<5–7 kg).Unreliable in hypotension, arrhythmias, or patient movement. More expensive than Doppler.	Suitable for medium to large dogs. Patients with stable cardiovascular status.In anesthetized or sedated patients with regular rhythms.
Direct (Invasive) Blood Pressure	Gold standard: continuous, real-time monitoring of systolic, diastolic, and mean arterial pressure.Most accurate in unstable or critical patients.Allows waveform analysis for advanced hemodynamic assessment.	Invasive and technically demanding. Requires arterial catheterization and specialized monitoring equipment. Risk of infection, hematoma, or thrombosis.	Critical care and unstable patients. Major surgeries require tight BP control.Research settings and cases need precise hemodynamic monitoring.

metacarpal or metatarsal regions in very small patients. In long-eared dogs, the auricular artery may be used as an alternative site. The limb or tail must be maintained at heart level during measurement, and the patient should be calm, minimally restrained, and in lateral or sternal recumbency. Under general circumstances, a total of five readings should be obtained in sequence. To improve accuracy and minimize artifact, the lowest and highest values should be discarded, and the remaining three averaged to provide the most reliable estimate of the patient's blood pressure. It is also prudent to obtain a heart rate simultaneously, as this can assist in identifying pulse deficits or arrhythmias that may influence interpretation. In addition, the patient's temperament and mentation should be documented at the time of measurement, as stress, anxiety, or altered mental status can directly affect cardiovascular parameters and confound clinical assessment.

Normal systolic blood pressure in dogs and cats ranges between 110 and 160 mmHg, with MAP values typically between 70 and 120 mmHg. Diastolic values range from 60 to 100 mmHg. Interpretation of these values must consider the patient's clinical condition, with particular attention paid to hypotension (MAP < 60 mmHg) or hypertension (systolic > 160 mmHg or diastolic > 100 mmHg).

Hypotension is defined as a systolic pressure below 90 mmHg or a MAP below 60 mmHg. These thresholds indicate insufficient tissue perfusion, requiring immediate reassessment of volume status, anesthetic depth, and cardiac function. Hypertension is classified as systolic pressure consistently exceeding 160 mmHg or MAP above 120 mmHg. Persistent hypertension should prompt investigation into underlying systemic disease, as it poses risks for renal, ocular, and cardiovascular damage.

Indications for Veterinary Notification

The veterinary technician must alert the attending veterinarian under the following circumstances:

- Systolic pressure <90 mmHg or MAP < 60 mmHg (hypotension)
- Systolic pressure >180 mmHg or MAP > 130 mmHg (hypertensive crisis)
- Rapid decline in pressure (>20% from baseline) even if within normal limits
- Inconsistent or nonrepeatable readings despite correct technique
- Clinical signs incongruent with pressure readings, such as altered mentation, prolonged capillary refill time, or weak pulses

Timely communication facilitates appropriate intervention, including fluid therapy, vasoactive agents, analgesia adjustment, or further diagnostics (Table 7.9).

Persistent hypertension can lead to end-organ damage (EOD), including hypertensive retinopathy, glomerular sclerosis, and left ventricular hypertrophy, warranting timely diagnosis and management.

Assessment of arterial blood pressure is a vital component of patient monitoring and clinical decision-making. Accurate technique, knowledge of normal and abnormal ranges, and understanding of the physiological principles governing blood pressure are essential competencies for the veterinary technician. Early recognition of abnormal readings and prompt communication with the veterinarian contribute significantly to patient safety, especially in anesthetized or critically ill animals.

Table 7.9 Common causes of hypotension and hypertension in dogs and cats.

Condition	Hypotension (↓ BP)	Hypertension (↑ BP)
Cardiovascular	Cardiogenic shock (dilated cardiomyopathy, severe valvular disease, arrhythmias).Hemorrhage leading to hypovolemia.Sepsis-induced vasodilation.	Chronic kidney disease (secondary hypertension). Hyperthyroidism (cats).Hyperadrenocorticism (dogs). Pheochromocytoma.
Anesthetic/ Drug-Related	Excessive anesthetic depth (inhalants, propofol, alfaxalone).Vasodilators or overdose of acepromazine. Acute adverse reactions to opioids or alpha-2 agonists.	Alpha-2 agonists (e.g., dexmedetomidine, xylazine) cause transient hypertension.Glucocorticoids with chronic use.NSAIDs in susceptible patients (renal hypertension).
Metabolic/ Endocrine	Addisonian crisis (hypoadrenocorticism).Severe hypoglycemia.Sepsis or systemic inflammatory response syndrome (SIRS).	Diabetes mellitus (secondary hypertension due to renal changes).Hyperaldosteronism.Acromegaly (cats).
Volume/Fluid Status	Dehydration and hypovolemia.Severe vomiting/diarrhea. Third spacing (effusions, severe burns, pancreatitis).	Iatrogenic fluid overload.Excessive IV fluids in hospitalized patients.
Other Causes	Anaphylaxis.Trauma with internal bleeding.Heat stroke (vasodilation).	Pain or stress (sympathetic activation).Intracranial disease (Cushing's reflex).Primary/idiopathic systemic hypertension (esp. in older cats).

As veterinary medicine continues to advance, the role of the technician in hemodynamic monitoring remains indispensable in promoting optimal patient outcomes.

Techniques for Fluid Administration, Nutritional Delivery, and Recognition of Early Fluid or Nutritional Compromise

The ability to maintain and restore fluid and nutritional homeostasis is a fundamental component of comprehensive veterinary nursing care. In both acute and chronic disease states, prompt intervention to correct fluid deficits and ensure adequate caloric intake is essential for recovery. Veterinary technicians play a critical role in implementing both parenteral and enteral delivery systems, monitoring the efficacy of therapeutic interventions, and recognizing the early indicators of physiological compromise.

Intravenous fluid therapy remains the foundation of supportive care in hospitalized and anesthetized patients. It is used for the correction of dehydration, restoration of circulating blood volume, management of electrolyte disturbances, and facilitation of drug delivery. Catheter selection is dictated by patient size, venous accessibility, therapeutic goals, and urgency. In large or unstable canine patients, 14- to 18-gauge catheters are often indicated to facilitate high-volume or bolus administration. In cats and small dogs, 20- to 22-gauge catheters are preferred due to the smaller vessel diameter, minimizing the risk of trauma or thrombosis (Table 7.10).

Catheters are most commonly placed in the cephalic or lateral saphenous veins, though the jugular vein may be utilized when central access is required for hyperosmolar fluids or central venous pressure monitoring. The selected site must be prepared with aseptic technique to reduce the risk of catheter-associated bloodstream infections. After placement, the catheter is secured and connected to a calibrated fluid administration system, with continuous evaluation for signs of infiltration, phlebitis, or displacement. Further guidance regarding fluid selection, resuscitation strategies, and electrolyte management can be found in Chapter 5.

Subcutaneous (SQ) fluid administration is an appropriate and commonly used route for treating mild to moderate dehydration in stable, normovolemic patients. It is particularly valuable in outpatient and home-care management of chronic conditions, such as feline chronic kidney disease, where frequent intravenous access is neither feasible nor necessary. The intrascapular region and dorsolateral thorax are preferred sites due to the relative looseness and extensibility of subcutaneous connective tissue in these areas, which allows for comfortable deposition and gradual absorption of fluid.

Warmed isotonic crystalloids, such as 0.9% NaCl or lactated Ringer's solution, are delivered using an 18- to 22-gauge needle, selected based on patient size, temperament, and viscosity of the fluid. A visible and palpable fluid bleb should form beneath the skin, indicating proper placement. A gentle digital massage can be employed after administration to facilitate even distribution and absorption across the tissue planes.

Table 7.10 IV catheter gauge size and fluid bolus flow rate.

Catheter Gauge (Length ~1 in)	Approx. Internal Diameter (mm)	Estimated Flow Rate (Gravity, mL/min)	Clinical Use
24 G	0.7 mm	~20 mL/min	Neonates, small exotics, very small/fragile veins
22 G	0.9 mm	~35 mL/min	Cats, small dogs, fluid therapy with moderate flow needs
20 G	1.1 mm	~60–65 mL/min	Medium-sized dogs, rapid fluid therapy in stable patients
18 G	1.3 mm	~90–100 mL/min	Large dogs, effective for shock boluses and resuscitation
16 G	1.7 mm	~150–160 mL/min	Giant breed dogs, massive resuscitation, trauma patients
14 G	2.1 mm	~250–270 mL/min	Very large/critical dogs; rapid volume resuscitation in severe shock

Clinical Context Notes:

- Flow rate follows Poiseuille's law: proportional to the fourth power of the radius and inversely proportional to catheter length.
- Short, wide-bore catheters deliver the fastest flow.
- Pressure bags or syringe-push techniques can dramatically increase delivery rate compared to gravity flow.
- In emergencies, always select the largest bore catheter the vein can accommodate.

However, there is a physiological and structural limit to how much fluid a single subcutaneous pocket can safely accommodate. In general, no more than 10–20 mL/kg of fluid should be infused into a single site. For an average-sized adult cat, this equates to approximately 100 to 150 mL per location. In small dogs and cats, exceeding these volumes can lead to overdistension of the subcutaneous tissue, which impairs lymphatic drainage and capillary blood flow. When this limit is approached, the technician should redirect the needle to an adjacent site, ideally at least a few centimeters away, to avoid excessive mechanical pressure on the same fascial plane.

Overfilling a subcutaneous space beyond its physiological tolerance can result in pressure necrosis, particularly if the patient is cachectic, geriatric, or has compromised dermal integrity. Pressure necrosis occurs when persistent tension on the tissue impairs microvascular perfusion, leading to ischemia and eventual tissue breakdown. In some cases, this may present initially as firm, nonresolving edema, followed by erythema, skin sloughing, or even abscess formation due to secondary infection. These complications can be painful, delay healing, and significantly impact the patient's quality of life—especially in patients already managing chronic disease (Figure 7.4).

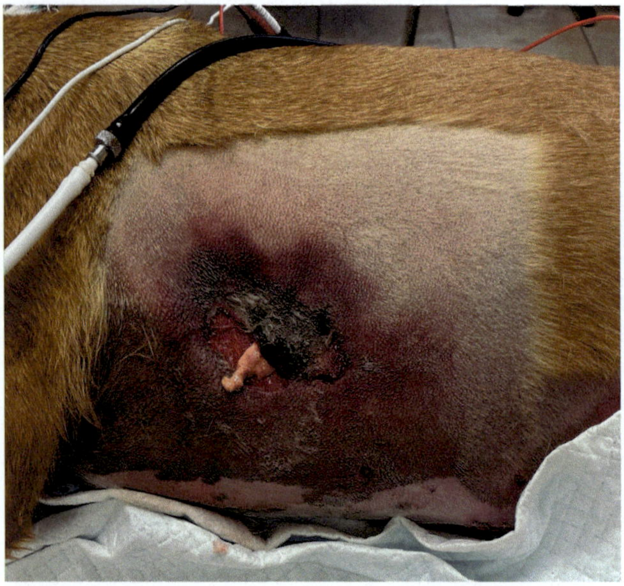

Figure 7.4 Subcutaneous necrosis in a canine patient following administration of 700 mL of subcutaneous fluids into a single site. *Source:* Schaeffer (2025).

It is also critical to recognize the limitations of subcutaneous absorption. Subcutaneous fluids should never be administered to patients exhibiting signs of hypovolemia, hypotension, peripheral vasoconstriction, or poor perfusion, as the efficacy of fluid uptake is directly dependent on intact subcutaneous perfusion and lymphatic drainage. In such cases, intravenous or intraosseous fluid administration is the preferred and clinically appropriate route.

Finally, fluid composition is a key consideration. Hypertonic saline, colloidal solutions, or fluids containing dextrose are strictly contraindicated for subcutaneous use due to their high osmolality, which can induce tissue irritation, inflammation, and necrosis. Only isotonic crystalloids should be used for SQ administration, and all fluids should be warmed to approximate body temperature to minimize vasoconstriction and improve patient comfort.

In summary, proper technique, volume control, and site selection are essential for the safe administration of subcutaneous fluids. Veterinary technicians must monitor for overfilling, assess tissue integrity, and ensure that patients receiving SQ fluids are appropriate candidates for this route, with an understanding of the physiologic and anatomical constraints that govern safe absorption.

Supplemental Nutrition

When gastrointestinal function is intact, enteral nutrition is strongly preferred. It maintains mucosal integrity, preserves intestinal immunity, and supports gut motility. Nutritional intervention should begin early—ideally within the first 24–48 hours of hospitalization—to prevent muscle catabolism and immune compromise. If voluntary intake is inadequate or absent, assisted feeding must be initiated through the appropriate route.

Short-term nutritional support may be provided via nasoesophageal or nasogastric tubes, which can be placed with minimal sedation. These tubes must be measured accurately and placement confirmed radiographically to ensure appropriate position and avoid aspiration. For longer-term support, esophagostomy tubes offer greater stability and are indicated in patients with orofacial trauma, prolonged anorexia, or mechanical dysphagia. Gastrostomy tubes, placed surgically or endoscopically, are suitable for patients requiring bypass of the esophagus or pharynx.

Nasogastric Tube Placement and Utilization in Small Animal Patients

Nasogastric (NG) tube placement is a minimally invasive, versatile technique used to facilitate enteral nutrition, administer medications, and decompress the stomach in small animal patients. It is especially valuable in critical care, postoperative management of gastrointestinal surgery, and in patients with anorexia, nausea, or gastrointestinal dysmotility. Due to its relatively straightforward placement in most patients, the nasogastric route is widely utilized in both emergency and general practice settings.

Indications and Anatomical Considerations

Indications for NG tube placement include short-term nutritional support in anorexic patients, delivery of medications to patients unable to tolerate oral intake, gastric decompression following surgery, and management of nausea, delayed gastric emptying, or ileus. It is particularly beneficial in patients recovering from upper gastrointestinal surgeries, such as gastrotomy, gastropexy, or resection procedures, in which oral feeding may be contraindicated during early postoperative periods.

The nasogastric tube traverses the external nares, ventral nasal meatus, nasopharynx, oropharynx, and esophagus, terminating in the gastric lumen. The route must be carefully navigated to avoid trauma to delicate nasal structures and to prevent inadvertent intubation of the trachea.

Measurement and Landmarks for Proper Placement

Accurate external measurement of the nasogastric tube is critical to ensure proper positioning within the gastric lumen, particularly in dogs that have undergone gastropexy. In these patients, the stomach has been surgically affixed to the right abdominal wall—usually the right ventrolateral body wall near the 13th intercostal space—to prevent volvulus and rotation of the stomach. This anatomical modification can alter the normal gastric position, particularly the pyloric antrum, and must be considered during tube measurement.

For dogs without a gastropexy, the tube should be measured from the tip of the nares to the caudal margin of the 13th rib, which typically corresponds to the gastric body. However, in dogs with a gastropexy, the author recommends extending the measurement slightly beyond the 13th rib (approximately one to two intercostal spaces caudally) to ensure the tube traverses the esophagus and reaches the gastric body or antrum where decompression or feeding is desired. This accounts for the slightly altered orientation and reduced gastric motility commonly observed post-gastropexy. The external measurement should be marked with a sterile marker prior to insertion to guide appropriate advancement.

Topical Anesthesia and Analgesia Considerations

Placement of a nasogastric tube, particularly in awake or minimally sedated patients, can elicit discomfort and resistance. To minimize this, topical local anesthesia should be instilled into both nares and each conjunctival sac. A few drops of 0.5–2% proparacaine ophthalmic solution in each eye anesthetize the nasolacrimal duct, which opens into the ventral nasal meatus. Additionally, instillation of 0.05–0.1 mL of 2% lidocaine or lidocaine-lubricant gel into each naris desensitizes the nasal mucosa and improves patient tolerance.

The relevance of ocular anesthesia lies in the anatomical connection between the conjunctiva and the nasal cavity via the lacrimal apparatus, which consists of the lacrimal puncta, canaliculi, lacrimal sac, and nasolacrimal duct. This system drains the tear film into the nasal cavity, allowing anesthetic agents applied to the eye to reach the rostral nasal mucosa, where they reduce nociceptive stimulation during catheter insertion.

Placement Technique

For nasogastric tube placement, the patient should be positioned in sternal recumbency with the head held in a neutral or slightly extended position. Prior to insertion, the premeasured and lubricated tube should be prepared, and topical anesthesia instilled into both nares and conjunctival sacs to desensitize the nasal mucosa and associated lacrimal structures.

To facilitate passage of the tube through the ventral nasal meatus, the nurse should employ a technique colloquially referred to as "pigging the nose"—gently tilting the patient's nasal planum dorsally so that the nose is angled upward. This maneuver aligns the long axis of the nasal cavity with the operator's hand and the advancing tube, creating a more linear trajectory through the ventral nasal meatus. Anatomically, this path runs beneath the dorsal and middle turbinates and provides the most patent and least resistive route into the nasopharynx.

Pigging the nose upwards is particularly advantageous because it reduces the likelihood of inadvertently directing the tube dorsally toward the ethmoid turbinates or cribriform plate, structures that are highly vascular and delicate. Passage through these areas increases the risk of epistaxis, discomfort, and, in rare cases, intracranial penetration. By orienting the nose upward, the ventral floor of the nasal passage becomes more accessible, allowing the tube to advance with minimal resistance and improved patient tolerance.

The tube should be gently advanced through the ventral meatus until it reaches the oropharynx and then into the esophagus. Steady advancement continues until the external marker reaches the level of the nares. If resistance is encountered or the patient exhibits signs of coughing, retching, or respiratory distress, the tube must be withdrawn immediately, as this may indicate inadvertent tracheal intubation. In most patients, this technique enables successful, atraumatic placement of the nasogastric tube into the gastric lumen (Table 7.11).

Care must be taken to avoid tracheal misplacement. If resistance is encountered or if the patient begins to cough, gag, or exhibit signs of respiratory distress, the procedure should be immediately halted and the tube withdrawn. In some cases, light sedation with agents such as dexmedetomidine or butorphanol may facilitate placement.

Table 7.11 Nasogastric tube placement reference guide.

Step	Key Points
Patient Positioning	Hold head in a neutral or slightly extended position.
Preparation	Premeasure and lubricate the tube. Instill topical anesthesia (lidocaine or proparacaine) into both nares and conjunctival sacs to desensitize the nasal mucosa and lacrimal structures.
"Pigging the Nose" Technique	Gently tilt the nasal planum dorsally so the nose points upward. This maneuver aligns the nasal cavity with the operator's hand and tube, creating a linear path through the ventral nasal meatus.
Anatomical Pathway	Tube advances via the ventral nasal meatus beneath the dorsal and middle turbinates → nasopharynx → oropharynx → esophagus. This route avoids fragile ethmoid turbinates and cribriform plate, reducing risk of trauma or epistaxis.
Advancement	Advance gently until tube reaches oropharynx, then continue into esophagus and stomach until external marker aligns with the nares.
Warning Signs	If resistance, coughing, retching, or respiratory distress occurs → immediately withdraw (possible tracheal intubation).
Outcome	Technique generally enables atraumatic placement into the gastric lumen with minimal resistance and improved patient tolerance.

In dogs with a prior gastropexy, careful consideration must be given to ensure the tube reaches the gastric body or pyloric region, which may be slightly displaced cranially and laterally. Radiographic confirmation is especially important in these cases to ensure that the tube is not coiled in the esophagus or terminating prematurely in the cardia.

Placement Confirmation

Verification of correct nasogastric tube placement is imperative prior to administration of fluids, nutrition, or medications. This can be performed by aspiration of gastric contents, auscultation of the stomach while injecting air through the tube, or—preferably—lateral radiography. The tube should be visualized within the esophageal lumen and terminating within the gastric shadow, extending caudally and ventrally in the abdominal cavity. In post-gastropexy patients, the tube tip may appear more cranially located relative to the stomach's new position but should still lie within the gastric lumen.

Enteral Nutrition and Trickle Feeding

Once confirmed, the nasogastric tube can be utilized for enteral nutrition, typically through a method known as trickle feeding, in which small volumes of liquid diet are delivered continuously via an intravenous fluid pump. This technique mimics normal physiological feeding patterns, supports mucosal integrity, reduces the risk of gastric overload, and is particularly well tolerated in critically ill or postoperative patients.

The most commonly employed diets for trickle feeding include Clinicare®, Liquid EN, or other commercially available, isotonic, enteral nutritional formulas designed for veterinary use. These formulations provide complete, balanced nutrition in a form that is easily absorbed and minimizes risk of aspiration or delayed gastric transit. Trickle feeds are typically initiated at 1–2 mL/kg/h, titrated gradually as the patient tolerates. Close monitoring for regurgitation, nausea, or abdominal discomfort is essential. Residual gastric volume checks may be performed periodically to evaluate gastric motility and ensure ongoing tolerance. The author reminds the reader to refer to Chapter 6 for comprehensive energy requirement calculations, including methods for determining Resting Energy Requirement (RER) in the intensive care patient.

Enteral feeding protocols typically begin at 25–33% of the patient's resting energy requirement and advance as tolerated. Diet selection should account for the patient's disease state, nutrient digestibility, and gastrointestinal tolerance. Technicians must monitor for vomiting, regurgitation, bloating, diarrhea, or tube occlusion, all of which may signal feeding intolerance. Tube patency and stoma site hygiene are also critical to reduce the risk of infection or displacement.

Parenteral nutrition (PN) is employed when enteral routes are contraindicated due to gastrointestinal pathology such as severe ileus, uncontrolled vomiting, or gastrointestinal perforation. Partial parenteral nutrition (PPN) may be delivered via a peripheral vein, but due to osmolarity limitations, it provides only a fraction of the patient's nutritional needs. Total parenteral nutrition (TPN), administered via a centrally placed venous catheter, delivers complete macronutrient and micronutrient support.

Placement of a jugular central line for TPN requires stringent aseptic technique. The catheter must be dedicated to parenteral nutrition only to minimize contamination risk. Nutritional solutions are ideally compounded under sterile pharmacy conditions and administered using an infusion pump. Frequent laboratory monitoring is essential, including serum glucose, electrolytes, triglycerides, and hepatic enzymes. One of the most serious complications of TPN is refeeding syndrome, which results from sudden shifts in phosphate, potassium, and magnesium in chronically malnourished patients. It must be prevented by gradually introducing calories and closely monitoring electrolyte levels during the first 72 hours.

Iatrogenic Overhydration

Serial body weights are a critical component of ongoing monitoring, particularly in the intensive care unit (ICU). Weight changes in critically ill patients provide valuable insight into fluid status, nutritional adequacy, and treatment efficacy. Weights should be recorded at the same time each day, using the same scale, and documented with precision.

An acute increase in body weight—especially in the absence of increased caloric intake—may indicate fluid retention and signal early fluid overhydration. When associated with chemosis, increased respiratory effort, or serous nasal discharge, weight gain may support the diagnosis of interstitial or pulmonary edema. Conversely, progressive weight loss may reflect dehydration, caloric deficit, catabolism, or worsening disease status. In patients receiving enteral or parenteral nutrition, a stable or increasing weight trend is a desired outcome, but it must be interpreted alongside other clinical signs to differentiate between lean mass gain and fluid accumulation (Table 7.12).

Veterinary technicians must be adept at interpreting these trends and correlating them with the patient's overall status. Sudden or unexpected weight shifts should be promptly reported to the attending veterinarian, as they may necessitate changes to fluid therapy, diuretic administration, or nutritional plan.

Table 7.12 Signs of Iatrogenic fluid overhydration in dogs and cats.

System	Clinical Signs	Diagnostic Findings
General	Lethargy, restlessness, weight gain over a short period (hours–days).	Acute increase in body weight, positive fluid balance calculations.
Cardiovascular	Tachycardia, bounding pulses, and hypertension (may occur in early stages).	Elevated central venous pressure (CVP); changes in blood pressure trends.
Respiratory	Tachypnea, dyspnea, increased respiratory effort, orthopnea.	Crackles on auscultation, pulmonary edema on thoracic radiographs, hypoxemia on blood gas analysis.
Renal/Urinary	Polyuria (if renal function intact), or oliguria in renal compromise.	Dilute urine despite dehydration signs, decreased urine specific gravity, and worsening azotemia in renal patients.
Gastrointestinal	Vomiting, serous nasal discharge, and hypersalivation.	Abdominal distension, ascites, and effusions visible on ultrasound or abdominocentesis.
Neurological	Restlessness, seizures, altered mentation in severe cases due to cerebral edema.	Dilutional hyponatremia, changes in serum osmolality.
Peripheral Tissues	Peripheral edema (limbs, dependent regions), chemosis (conjunctival edema).	Increased skin turgor without dehydration, soft tissue swelling visible on exam or imaging.

Clinical Note:
Fluid overload occurs when infusion rates exceed the patient's cardiovascular and renal compensatory capacity. Small patients (cats, toy-breed dogs, neonates, geriatrics, or those with cardiac/renal disease) are at highest risk. Frequent reassessment of body weight, respiratory rate/effort, auscultation, urine output, and laboratory parameters is essential to prevent and detect overhydration.

Early signs of dehydration and hypovolemia include prolonged capillary refill time, tachycardia, dry mucous membranes, decreased skin turgor, and sunken eyes. Pulse quality may be weak or thready, and mental dullness may be noted. Laboratory values often show hemoconcentration, azotemia, or elevated lactate levels in severe cases. Conversely, signs of early fluid overload include serous nasal discharge, chemosis, increased respiratory rate, and the onset of pulmonary crackles upon auscultation. Jugular vein distension and peripheral edema may also occur. Increases in body weight over a short period may be the first or only visible sign of iatrogenic overhydration.

The veterinary technician must remain alert for signs of caloric insufficiency, which often manifest subtly in the early stages. These include decreased voluntary food intake, reduced fecal output, weight loss, poor coat condition, muscle atrophy, and hypoalbuminemia. Patients with poor intake for more than three consecutive days are at high risk of developing negative energy balance, leading to protein catabolism, delayed wound healing, immune dysfunction, and prolonged recovery. Body Condition Score (BCS) and Muscle Condition Score (MCS) should be assessed on admission and at regular intervals throughout hospitalization. These scores are valuable tools for identifying sarcopenia or cachexia, particularly when weight loss is masked by concurrent fluid therapy.

Veterinary technicians must demonstrate a high level of competency in the techniques of fluid and nutritional support. Knowledge of intravenous and subcutaneous administration, coupled with the technical proficiency to initiate enteral or parenteral nutrition, allows the veterinary technician to sustain life and support recovery in critically ill patients. Serial body weights serve as an indispensable tool in the ICU, providing objective data to guide fluid and nutritional therapy. Recognizing the subtle signs of fluid imbalance or nutritional compromise ensures timely intervention and improved clinical outcomes. For an expanded discussion on intravenous fluid selection and resuscitation protocols, the reader is encouraged to refer to Chapter 6.

Blood Gas Analysis

Blood gas analysis is a critical diagnostic modality in veterinary medicine, offering comprehensive insight into a patient's respiratory function, acid-base balance, and overall metabolic status. Particularly valuable in emergency and critical care, as well as anesthetic monitoring, the evaluation of arterial or venous blood gases enables veterinary professionals to make informed clinical decisions grounded in the physiological needs of the patient. We will examine the physiological principles of blood gas dynamics, the techniques for appropriate sample collection, best practices for handling, and a structured framework for interpreting results in both dogs and cats.

Physiological Foundations of Blood Gas Analysis

Blood gas analysis encompasses the measurement of arterial or venous pH, partial pressure of oxygen (PaO_2), partial pressure of carbon dioxide ($PaCO_2$), bicarbonate concentration (HCO_3^-), and base excess. Each of these parameters reflects a component of systemic homeostasis and can illuminate disruptions in respiratory or metabolic function.

Oxygenation status is primarily assessed through PaO_2 and oxygen saturation (SaO_2). PaO_2 quantifies the amount of dissolved oxygen in the arterial blood, while SaO_2 measures the proportion of hemoglobin molecules bound to oxygen. Effective oxygenation requires intact pulmonary diffusion, adequate ventilation, normal cardiac output, and sufficient hemoglobin concentration. Hypoxemia may result from ventilation-perfusion mismatch, diffusion impairment, or alveolar hypoventilation and typically requires arterial sampling for accurate assessment.

Carbon dioxide homeostasis is evaluated through $PaCO_2$. This parameter serves as a surrogate for alveolar ventilation. Elevations in $PaCO_2$, or hypercapnia, indicate hypoventilation and are commonly associated with conditions such as airway obstruction, neurologic impairment, or anesthetic overdose. In contrast, hypocapnia is indicative of hyperventilation and may occur in scenarios involving pain, anxiety, or compensation for metabolic acidosis.

The acid-base status of the patient is represented by pH, HCO_3^-, and base excess. In dogs and cats, normal pH ranges from 7.35–7.45. Deviations outside of this range are considered acidemic or alkalemic, depending on directionality. Respiratory contributions to acid-base balance are mediated through $PaCO_2$. An increase in $PaCO_2$ leads to respiratory acidosis due to carbonic acid accumulation, whereas a decrease in $PaCO_2$ results in respiratory alkalosis secondary to excessive carbon dioxide elimination. The metabolic component is primarily represented by bicarbonate. A reduction in HCO_3^-, often seen in lactic acidosis, renal tubular acidosis, or diabetic ketoacidosis, signifies metabolic acidosis. Conversely, metabolic alkalosis is marked by elevated HCO_3^- levels, frequently due to vomiting-induced hydrogen ion loss or diuretic therapy. Base excess serves as a calculated index reflecting the nonrespiratory component of acid-base disturbance and is particularly useful in identifying complex or mixed acid-base disorders. While compensatory mechanisms do exist, such as renal regulation of bicarbonate or pulmonary adjustments in ventilation, they are often incomplete and time-dependent, making early detection and intervention essential.

Collection Techniques

Accurate interpretation of blood gas values is contingent upon proper collection technique. Arterial blood samples are necessary for evaluating true oxygenation parameters such as PaO_2 and SaO_2. Commonly used arterial sites in small animal patients include the dorsal pedal artery, femoral artery, and, under anesthesia, the lingual artery. The dorsal pedal artery is particularly accessible in both dogs and cats and is generally well-tolerated in conscious or lightly sedated patients.

To collect from the dorsal pedal artery, the patient should be placed in lateral or dorsal recumbency with the limb appropriately extended. Sedation or local anesthetic blocks may be used to minimize stress, which can artificially alter blood gas values. Once the artery is palpated, the area is clipped and aseptically prepared. A heparinized syringe, preferably precoated with dry heparin to avoid sample dilution, is used to puncture the artery at a shallow angle. Once pulsatile blood flow is observed filling the syringe spontaneously, the needle is withdrawn, and direct pressure is applied for at least two minutes to prevent hematoma formation. The sample must be promptly capped to prevent atmospheric contamination, which can alter gas tensions, particularly PaO_2.

Venous blood gas analysis may be performed using samples collected from peripheral veins, with the jugular or cephalic veins being the most commonly accessed sites in canine and feline patients. While venous samples are not suitable for accurately assessing oxygenation—given the substantial variability in local tissue oxygen extraction—they can provide meaningful information regarding acid-base balance, bicarbonate concentration, and $PaCO_2$ trends, particularly in scenarios where arterial access is impractical or poses added risk.

Among peripheral sites, jugular venipuncture yields the most physiologically reliable venous blood gas values (Hopper and Haskins 2015). This is due to the anatomical proximity of the jugular vein to the central venous circulation, which reflects systemic rather than localized metabolic activity. Venous blood sampled from the jugular vein is less influenced by regional variations in tissue perfusion and oxygen extraction, which are common in distal peripheral sites such as the saphenous or cephalic veins. In these distal vessels, the local metabolic demands of the surrounding musculature and connective tissue may result in exaggerated desaturation, altered pH, and falsely elevated $PaCO_2$ or lactate levels. Jugular blood, conversely, is drawn from a large central vessel that receives drainage from the head and upper thorax—regions with relatively stable and representative metabolic profiles under most physiological and pathological conditions.

In critically ill or hypotensive patients, especially those experiencing peripheral vasoconstriction, arterial sampling may be technically challenging or poorly tolerated. Under such circumstances, jugular venous blood gas analysis offers a more practical and safer alternative for monitoring global metabolic status, identifying trends in carbon dioxide retention, and assessing the adequacy of perfusion through surrogate markers such as venous lactate. While PaO_2 cannot be assessed using venous samples, the ability to evaluate acid-base derangements, ventilation adequacy (via trends in $PvCO_2$), and the presence of anaerobic metabolism remains highly valuable in the acute setting.

Sample Handling

Blood gas samples must be handled with precision to avoid artifactual changes. Samples should be immediately placed on ice to minimize cellular metabolism, which continues post-collection and may lead to falsely decreased PaO_2 and increased $PaCO_2$. Analysis should ideally occur within 10–15 minutes of collection. Air bubbles introduced into the syringe must be expelled without delay, as the presence of room air can drastically affect PaO_2 and $PaCO_2$ readings. Heparin must be used in appropriate quantities, as over-anticoagulation may dilute the sample and distort bicarbonate and pH measurements.

Interpretation of Blood Gas Values

Interpretation requires a methodical approach. Begin by evaluating the pH to determine if the patient is acidemic or alkalemic. Then assess the $PaCO_2$ and HCO_3^- to determine the primary origin of the disturbance—respiratory or metabolic. A low pH with a high $PaCO_2$ suggests primary respiratory acidosis, whereas a low pH with a low HCO_3^- points to metabolic acidosis. Compensation should then be evaluated. In respiratory acidosis, the kidneys should increase bicarbonate reabsorption if the condition is chronic. Conversely, in metabolic acidosis, the respiratory system should reduce $PaCO_2$ through hyperventilation.

A simplified approach involves using the Henderson-Hasselbalch equation to understand the relationship between pH, HCO_3^-, and $PaCO_2$, and to assess the adequacy of compensation. Anion gap calculations may be required in metabolic acidosis to differentiate between loss of bicarbonate and addition of acids. In dogs, a normal anion gap ranges from 12–24 mEq/L, and in cats, 13–27 mEq/L. An increased anion gap indicates the presence of unmeasured acids, such as lactate, ketones, or toxins, whereas a normal gap in metabolic acidosis suggests bicarbonate loss through gastrointestinal or renal routes.

The interpretation of blood gas values should follow a consistent, stepwise algorithm to accurately identify primary disorders and assess the presence and extent of compensation. The following six-step method is widely used in both veterinary and human critical care settings:

1) **Evaluate the pH:**
   Determine if the patient is acidemic ($pH < 7.35$), alkalemic ($pH > 7.45$), or within the reference range.
2) **Assess $PaCO_2$ and HCO_3^-:**
   Identify which parameter is consistent with the pH change.
   - If $PaCO_2$ is abnormal in the direction of the pH, the disorder is respiratory.
   - If HCO_3^- is abnormal in the direction of the pH, the disorder is metabolic.
3) **Determine the primary disturbance:**
   Match the abnormality ($PaCO_2$ or HCO_3^-) that aligns with the direction of the pH shift. This is the **primary acid-base disorder**.
4) **Assess for compensation:**
   - In **respiratory disorders**, the kidneys adjust HCO_3^-, which occurs over hours to days.
   - In **metabolic disorders**, the lungs adjust $PaCO_2$ via respiratory rate changes, typically within minutes to hours.

   Use expected compensation formulas to determine if the compensation is appropriate (i.e., not over- or under-compensated).
5) **Evaluate PaO_2 and SaO_2 (if arterial sample):**
   Assess oxygenation. Hypoxemia is present if $PaO_2 < 80$ mmHg on room air. Adjust expectations if supplemental oxygen is in use.
6) **Calculate the Anion Gap (for metabolic acidosis):**
   Anion gap = $([Na^+] + [K^+]) - ([Cl^-] + [HCO_3^-])$
   An increased anion gap suggests the presence of unmeasured acids (lactic acid, ketones, ethylene glycol, etc.) (Tables 7.13 and 7.14).

Table 7.13 Normal Arterial Blood Gas (ABG) parameters in dogs and cats.

Parameter	Dog (Normal Range)	Cat (Normal Range)	Clinical Notes
pH	7.35–7.45	7.30–7.40	Reflects acid–base balance; acidosis <7.35, alkalosis >7.45.
$PaCO_2$ (mmHg)	35–45	32–38	Indicator of ventilatory status; $\uparrow PaCO_2$ = hypoventilation (respiratory acidosis).
PaO_2 (mmHg)	80–110 (room air)	80–110 (room air)	Hypoxemia if <80 mmHg; severe if <60 mmHg.
HCO_3^- (mmol/L)	18–24	16–22	Reflects metabolic component of acid–base status.
Base Excess (BE, mmol/L)	−4 to +4	−4 to +4	Indicates metabolic contribution; negative = metabolic acidosis, positive = alkalosis.
SaO_2 (%)	>95%	>95%	Percent hemoglobin saturation with O_2; hypoxemia if <90%.
Lactate (mmol/L)	<2.0	<2.0	Elevations indicate tissue hypoperfusion/anaerobic metabolism.

Clinical Note (ABG):
Always interpret ABG values in conjunction with patient signalment, clinical signs, and perfusion parameters. Hypothermia, anesthesia, and sampling/handling errors (e.g., venous contamination, air bubbles, delayed analysis) can alter results. Dogs and cats may show species-specific variations under anesthesia, stress, or critical illness.

Table 7.14 Normal Venous Blood Gas (VBG) parameters in dogs and cats.

Parameter	Dog (Normal Range)	Cat (Normal Range)	Clinical Notes
pH	7.30–7.40	7.25–7.35	Venous samples are slightly more acidotic compared to arterial.
$PvCO_2$ (mmHg)	40–50	38–48	Higher than arterial due to tissue CO_2 production; reflects ventilation and perfusion.
PvO_2 (mmHg)	35–45	30–40	Lower than arterial due to O_2 extraction in tissues; not reliable for oxygenation assessment.
HCO_3^- (mmol/L)	20–26	18–24	Represents metabolic component; closely correlates with arterial values.
Base Excess (BE, mmol/L)	−4 to +4	−4 to +4	Useful for metabolic acid–base evaluation.
SvO_2 (%)	65–75%	65–75%	Mixed venous oxygen saturation; indicates balance between O_2 delivery and consumption.
Lactate (mmol/L)	<2.5	<2.5	Venous lactate is commonly measured; elevations suggest hypoperfusion/anaerobic metabolism.

Clinical Note (VBG):
Venous blood gas analysis is useful for evaluating acid–base balance and trends in CO_2 and bicarbonate but is not reliable for assessing oxygenation. Arterial samples should be used when evaluating pulmonary function, oxygenation, or precise acid–base disturbances. VBG is often easier and less invasive to obtain, making it valuable for serial monitoring in critical care patients.

Case Study Example: Mixed Acid-Base Disorder in a Canine Patient

Signalment

6-year-old neutered male Labrador Retriever, 34 kg, presented to the emergency department for acute onset of vomiting, lethargy, and collapse. The patient is obtunded, tachypneic, and hypotensive on presentation. Blood gas was obtained via a dorsal pedal arterial catheter.

Arterial Blood Gas Results (on room air)

- pH: 7.12
- $PaCO_2$: 55 mmHg
- PaO_2: 63 mmHg
- HCO_3^-: 17 mEq/L
- Base Excess: –10
- Lactate: 6.8 mmol/L
- Na^+: 150 mEq/L
- K^+: 4.5 mEq/L
- Cl^-: 115 mEq/L

Step 1: Evaluate pH
The pH is 7.12, indicating significant acidemia.
Step 2: Assess $PaCO_2$ and HCO_3^-
$PaCO_2$ is elevated (55 mmHg), which would cause acidemia.
HCO_3^- is decreased (17 mEq/L), which would also cause acidemia.
Both are contributing to the low pH.
Step 3: Determine the primary disorder
Since both $PaCO_2$ and HCO_3^- are abnormal in the acidemic direction, this suggests a **mixed disorder**: both respiratory and metabolic acidosis are present.
Step 4: Assess compensation
This step reveals that the metabolic acidosis has not been adequately compensated by respiratory alkalosis—$PaCO_2$ should have been decreased, not elevated, in compensation. Therefore, this is a **concurrent primary respiratory acidosis** with **primary metabolic acidosis**.
Step 5: Evaluate PaO_2
PaO_2 is 63 mmHg on room air, which indicates **mild hypoxemia**. This may reflect poor ventilation-perfusion matching or alveolar hypoventilation. Given the elevated $PaCO_2$, hypoventilation is likely contributing.
Step 6: Calculate Anion Gap
Anion Gap = (150 + 4.5) – (115 + 17) = 154.5 – 132 = **22.5 mEq/L**
The reference range in dogs is 12–24 mEq/L, so this is **borderline elevated**, and in conjunction with a markedly elevated lactate, suggests a **high anion gap metabolic acidosis**.

Interpretation

This patient is suffering from a **mixed acid-base disorder**:

- **Primary high anion gap metabolic acidosis**, likely due to lactic acidosis from hypoperfusion.
- **Primary respiratory acidosis**, likely from hypoventilation secondary to CNS depression or fatigue.
- **Mild hypoxemia**, likely due to hypoventilation.

Clinical Response and Outcome

The patient was immediately placed on supplemental oxygen and initiated on intravenous fluid resuscitation using isotonic crystalloids. Given the high lactate and hypotension, a diagnosis of hypovolemic shock was made. A central venous catheter was placed for continued monitoring and advanced resuscitation. Mechanical ventilation was considered due to progressive hypercapnia and declining neurologic status. Repeat blood gas analysis after fluid therapy showed gradual improvement in pH and lactate, suggesting improved perfusion and oxygen delivery.

Blood gas analysis provides invaluable information in both acute and chronic clinical scenarios involving respiratory compromise, metabolic derangement, or anesthetic monitoring. Mastery of physiologic principles, correct sample handling, and algorithmic interpretation empowers the veterinary technician and clinician alike to identify subtle disturbances early, initiate appropriate intervention, and closely monitor patient trajectory in critical care environments.

Fecal Microbiota Transplantation in Small Animal Veterinary Medicine

Fecal microbiota transplantation (FMT), also referred to as fecal transfaunation, is an emerging therapeutic modality in veterinary medicine aimed at restoring intestinal microbial diversity and function (Sugita et al. 2019). It involves the administration of fecal material, rich in commensal bacteria, from a healthy donor to a recipient patient with gastrointestinal dysbiosis. This intervention has gained traction due to its success in treating recurrent *Clostridium difficile* infections in human medicine, and mounting evidence suggests similar potential in dogs and cats suffering from microbiota-associated diseases (Chaitman et al. 2020; Cammarota et al. 2017). When executed with careful donor screening and appropriate technique, FMT is a safe, cost-effective, and biologically rational approach to manipulating the enteric microbiome for therapeutic benefit.

Physiologic Basis of FMT

The gastrointestinal tract houses a complex ecosystem of bacteria, viruses, fungi, and protozoa that contribute to digestion, nutrient absorption, immune modulation, and mucosal barrier integrity. Disruption of this ecosystem—termed dysbiosis—can result from antibiotic exposure, dietary indiscretion, infectious agents, chronic inflammation, or systemic illness. FMT aims to reintroduce a balanced and diverse microbial population capable of outcompeting pathogenic organisms, restoring metabolic function, and re-establishing immune homeostasis (Figure 7.5).

Clinical Indications for Fecal Transplantation

The following conditions are believed to be mediated, in part, by intestinal dysbiosis and may benefit from FMT:

- **Chronic enteropathies**, including antibiotic-responsive enteropathy, food-responsive diarrhea, and idiopathic inflammatory bowel disease (IBD)
- **Acute or chronic diarrhea** associated with antibiotic administration or hospitalization
- **Recurrent *Clostridium perfringens* or *C. difficile* infection**
- **Parvoviral enteritis**, as an adjunctive therapy to restore mucosal integrity and accelerate microbial repopulation
- **Exocrine pancreatic insufficiency (EPI)**, in which chronic maldigestion alters the intestinal microenvironment
- **Geriatric patients** with age-associated microbial shifts contributing to anorexia or altered bowel habits

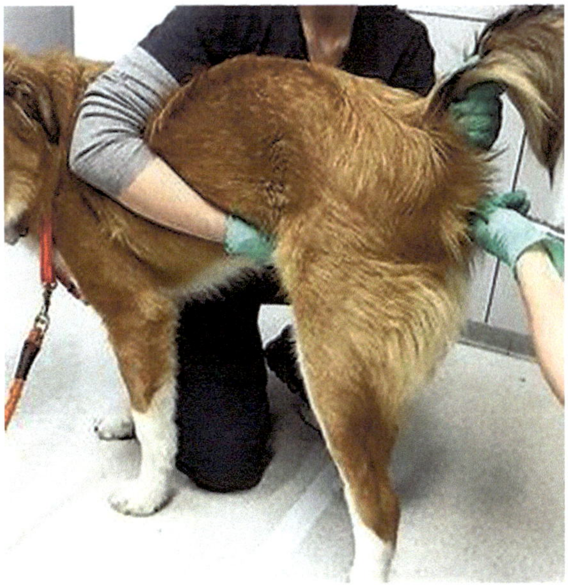

Figure 7.5 The gastrointestinal microbiome in health versus dysbiosis. A diverse microbial ecosystem (bacteria, viruses, fungi, protozoa) contributes to digestion, nutrient absorption, immune modulation, and mucosal barrier integrity. Disruption of this ecosystem—due to antibiotics, diet, infection, chronic inflammation, or systemic illness—leads to dysbiosis, impaired barrier function, and immune dysregulation. *Source:* Educational Concepts, LLC. / https://www.cliniciansbrief.com/article/intestinal-dysbiosis / last accessed on Oct 27, 2025

While the evidence in veterinary species remains largely anecdotal or extrapolated from human literature, clinical outcomes in select patient populations have demonstrated improvement in stool consistency, appetite, energy level, and reduced dependence on immunosuppressants or antibiotics.

Donor Selection and Fecal Material Collection

Donor selection is paramount to minimizing the risk of transmitting infectious agents or undesirable microbial populations. Donors should be healthy, age-matched where possible, and free of any history of gastrointestinal, dermatologic, allergic, or autoimmune disease. The donor should not have received antibiotics, probiotics, or other microbiome-altering agents for a minimum of three to six months.

A comprehensive health screening should include:

- Fecal flotation and direct smear (including *Giardia* and *Tritrichomonas*)
- Fecal PCR panel for enteric pathogens (e.g., *Clostridium*, *Salmonella*, *Campylobacter*)
- Fecal ELISA or antigen testing for *Giardia*, *Cryptosporidium*
- Parvovirus antigen testing in canine donors, especially in multi-dog environments
- General health screening including CBC, chemistry panel, and urinalysis

Fresh fecal samples should be collected within six hours of transplantation to maximize bacterial viability. Ideally, feces should be collected directly from the rectum or immediately after defecation using a clean, sterile container. Samples should be transported on ice and processed as soon as possible.

Preparation of Fecal Suspension

In a sterile environment, approximately 10–30 g of fresh donor feces are homogenized with 30–60 mL of sterile, nonbacteriostatic saline or isotonic Hartmann's solution. The mixture is blended using a syringe-to-syringe technique, vortexed in a sterile container, or processed in a blender dedicated exclusively for this purpose. The homogenate is then filtered through gauze, a tea strainer, or a sterile mesh sieve to remove large particulate matter. The resulting solution should be smooth, injectable consistency, and used immediately or stored refrigerated for no more than 6 hours. Freezing at −80 °C is possible for long-term storage but may reduce efficacy; cryopreservatives such as glycerol (10%) may be added to protect anaerobic bacteria (Kelly et al. 2015; Chaitman et al. 2020) (Table 7.15).

Routes and Techniques of Transplantation

Several routes have been described for fecal microbiota transplantation, with the method selected based on the clinical condition, patient temperament, and available equipment (Figure 7.6).

Table 7.15 Preparation of fecal microbiota transplantation (FMT) solution in dogs.

Step	Details	Notes/Precautions
Donor Material	10–30 g fresh donor feces	Screen donor for pathogens prior to collection. Must be fresh, preferably <6 hours old.
Diluent	30–60 mL sterile, nonbacteriostatic saline or isotonic Hartmann's solution	Avoid bacteriostatic fluids, which can kill beneficial microbes.
Homogenization Methods	• Syringe-to-syringe technique • Vortex in sterile container • Blender (dedicated to FMT only)	Maintain sterility at all times. Use PPE and a biosafety cabinet when possible.
Filtration	Filter homogenate through gauze, tea strainer, or sterile mesh sieve	Removes large particulate matter, producing smooth, injectable consistency.
Final Product	Smooth slurry-like suspension	Should be easily passable through syringe or catheter.
Storage (Short-term)	Use immediately or refrigerate ≤6 h.	Microbial viability decreases with time at room temperature.
Storage (Long-term)	Freezing at −80°C is possible	Add 10% glycerol as a cryoprotectant to preserve anaerobic bacteria. Efficacy may be reduced after thawing.

Source: Adapted from Kelly et al. (2015) and Chaitman et al. (2020).

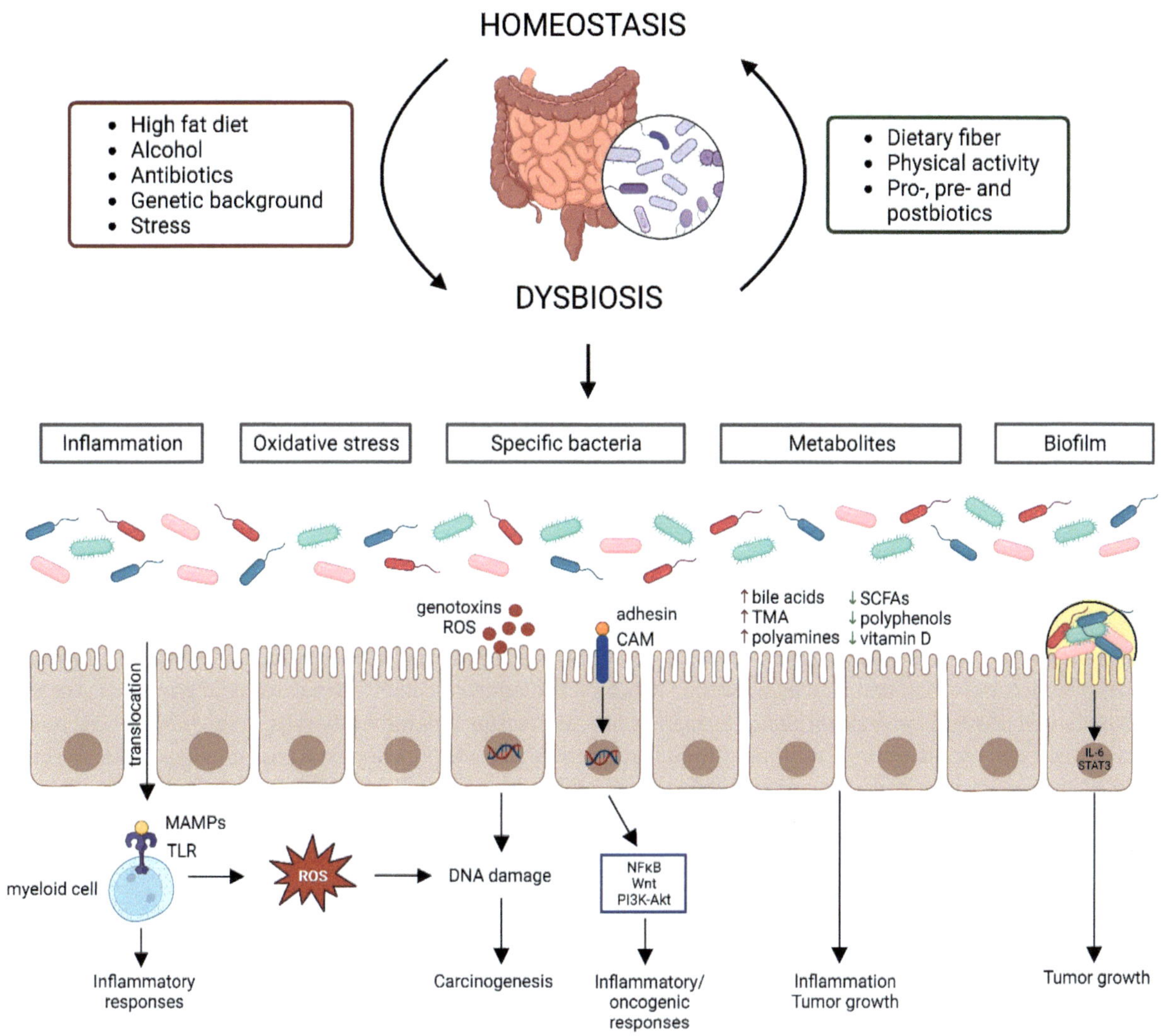

Figure 7.6 Canine receiving fecal microbiota transplantation via rectal enema (Clinician's Brief 2019).

1) **Rectal Enema (Most Common):**
   After evacuating the distal colon with a warm water enema, a lubricated red rubber or feeding tube is inserted into the rectum and advanced to the descending colon (approximately 5–15 cm, depending on patient size). The fecal slurry is slowly infused (5–10 mL/kg) and the patient's hindquarters are elevated slightly for 10–15 minutes post-procedure to reduce expulsion. This route provides direct delivery to the large intestine, making it ideal for colonic dysbiosis.
2) **Oral Capsule Administration:**
   Fecal capsules contain freeze-dried or frozen fecal material encased in acid-resistant gelatin capsules. This method is noninvasive and better tolerated in conscious patients, though it may bypass upper GI dysbiosis and requires specialized preparation and storage.
3) **Endoscopic-Guided Infusion:**
   In specialized centers, fecal suspension may be delivered through the working channel of an endoscope into the proximal or distal colon. This allows for visual assessment of mucosa and precise placement but requires anesthesia and specialized equipment.

Post-Transplant Considerations and Monitoring

Following FMT, patients should be monitored for clinical response over 48–72 hours. Improvement in stool consistency, appetite, and demeanor may be evident within days. It is advised to avoid antibiotics, antiparasitics, or microbiome-altering therapies during this period unless clinically necessary, as these may negate the effects of the transplant. Repeat transplantation may be necessary in chronic cases or when only partial improvement is observed. In some cases, FMT is administered serially—daily for three consecutive days or once weekly for three to four weeks.

Potential adverse effects are rare but may include transient flatulence, soft stools, or nausea. There is a theoretical risk of pathogen transmission, autoimmune disease induction, or microbial imbalance if improper donor screening is performed.

Fecal microbiota transplantation offers a novel, biologically targeted therapeutic intervention for patients suffering from enteric dysbiosis. Its success depends on rigorous donor screening, appropriate preparation and administration, and careful selection of cases where FMT may offer distinct advantages over traditional pharmacologic therapies. As the understanding of the microbiome evolves, FMT may become an integral component of gastrointestinal disease management, with applications extending into immunology, oncology, and neurology.

Wound Management and Bandaging

The management of wounds in veterinary patients represents a critical domain in clinical nursing care that demands not only technical proficiency but also a deep understanding of tissue physiology, microbiology, and pharmacologic support. Both acute and chronic wounds present distinct challenges, and the veterinary technician must integrate knowledge of wound healing dynamics, dressing technologies, and infection control principles to create and maintain an optimal environment for recovery. Evidence-based wound care is not a static protocol but rather a fluid, adaptive process that responds to the wound's appearance, stage, and underlying cause, as well as to the patient's systemic health.

Wound healing is a complex biological process that unfolds through four overlapping but distinct phases: hemostasis, inflammation, proliferation, and maturation. The initial phase, hemostasis, begins within seconds of tissue injury and is characterized by vasoconstriction and platelet activation. These activated platelets release a cascade of growth factors that not only mediate vasoconstriction and fibrin clot formation but also recruit inflammatory cells to the wound bed. As the inflammatory phase begins, neutrophils infiltrate the site and initiate microbial clearance through phagocytosis, reactive oxygen species release, and cytokine production. Macrophages later replace neutrophils and play a critical dual role—continuing phagocytic activity while secreting angiogenic and fibroblast-stimulating growth factors that signal the transition into the proliferative phase. During proliferation, fibroblasts synthesize extracellular matrix proteins, particularly type III collagen, while endothelial cells establish neovascularization, and keratinocytes begin to re-epithelialize the wound margins. The final stage, maturation or remodeling, involves the conversion of type III to type I collagen, reorganization of the collagen lattice, contraction of the wound margins by myofibroblasts, and progressive strengthening of the tissue over time. This final phase may take weeks to months, and its quality determines the tensile strength and long-term durability of the repaired tissue (Figure 7.7).

To initiate appropriate wound management, the veterinary technician must conduct a meticulous and systematic assessment. This begins with determining the etiology—whether the wound was caused by mechanical trauma, thermal injury, pressure necrosis, surgical incision, or underlying disease. The degree of contamination must be accurately classified as clean, clean-contaminated, contaminated, or infected, with recognition that infection exists only when bacterial colonization exceeds the host's local immune defenses and results in tissue injury. The presence of foreign material, necrotic tissue, devitalization, or desiccation should be noted, as these factors may inhibit progression through the healing cascade. The characteristics of wound exudate—including quantity, color, and odor—provide vital diagnostic cues, as do patient-level factors such as immunosuppression, malnutrition, endocrine dysfunction, or concurrent infection. Wounds exhibiting purulent discharge, malodor, increasing pain, or delayed granulation may benefit from cytology and microbial culture with sensitivity testing, especially when antibiotic therapy is being considered.

Wounds are often broadly categorized as acute or chronic, though this dichotomy should not be oversimplified. Acute wounds, such as those resulting from recent lacerations, bite wounds, or surgical incisions, typically follow a predictable and timely healing process when managed appropriately. Immediate goals in managing acute wounds include thorough lavage with isotonic, sterile fluids, sharp debridement of devitalized or necrotic tissues, and determination of whether the wound is amenable to primary closure, delayed primary closure, or healing by second intention. Conversely, chronic wounds—those persisting longer than three to four weeks without progression through normal healing stages—are more frequently associated with comorbidities such as diabetes mellitus, hyperadrenocorticism, neoplasia, or immune-mediated disease. These wounds may become arrested in the inflammatory or proliferative stages, often due to hypoxia, repeated trauma, foreign body presence, or biofilm development. Chronic wounds demand an integrative management approach, emphasizing the removal of inhibitory factors, enhancement of perfusion, and promotion of granulation through the strategic use of topical agents and advanced dressings.

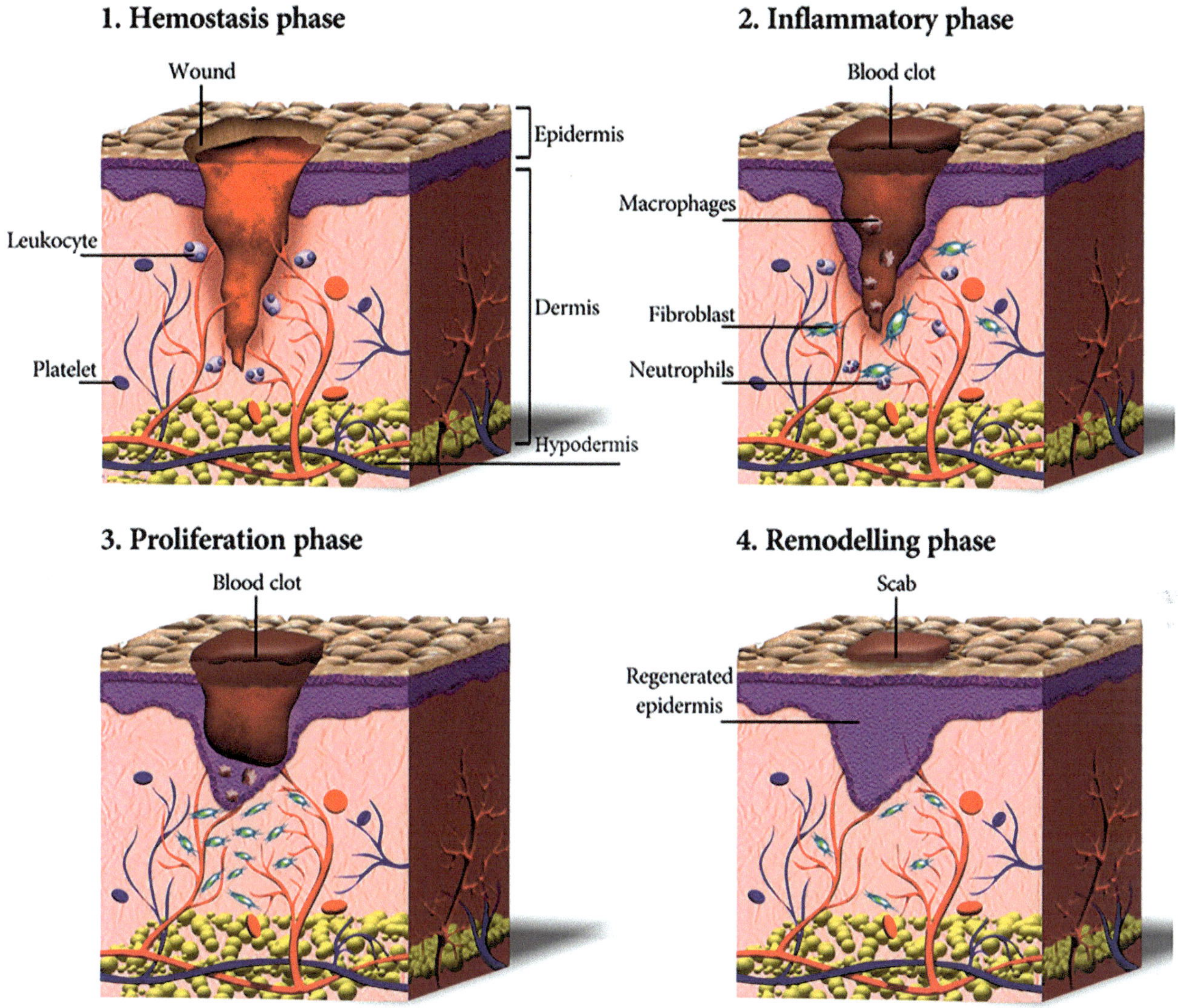

Figure 7.7 Four phases of wound healing: hemostasis, inflammation, proliferation, and remodeling. *Source:* Adapted from Tavakoli and Klar (2020).

Selecting an appropriate dressing is a cornerstone of evidence-based wound management and should be guided by the wound's moisture balance, bioburden, depth, and exudative nature. Contrary to earlier beliefs that favored dry wound environments, contemporary veterinary nursing practice supports the principle of moist wound healing, which has been shown to accelerate epithelial migration, reduce pain, and minimize scar formation (Hewson and McCready 2019). Non-adherent primary dressings, including silicone-coated gauze or petroleum-impregnated meshes, are frequently used in superficial, epithelializing wounds to prevent iatrogenic trauma upon dressing changes. Hydrogels, composed of cross-linked polymers capable of absorbing moisture, are well suited for dry, necrotic, or sloughing wounds and encourage autolytic debridement by facilitating enzymatic breakdown of nonviable tissue. For wounds with moderate to high levels of exudate, hydrocolloids or foam dressings may be employed to absorb fluid while maintaining a sealed, occlusive environment that promotes fibroblast proliferation. Calcium alginate dressings, derived from seaweed, exhibit excellent absorptive and hemostatic properties and are ideal for wounds with hemorrhagic exudate or fragile capillaries. In wounds at risk for infection or in which biofilm formation is suspected, dressings impregnated with antimicrobial agents such as silver, polyhexanide, iodine, or medical-grade honey are often beneficial. The use of negative pressure wound therapy (NPWT), wherein subatmospheric pressure is applied via a sealed foam dressing, has gained traction in managing deep, complex, or dehisced wounds, as it promotes granulation tissue formation, reduces edema, and enhances local perfusion (Radlinsky 2016) (Table 7.16).

Infection control remains paramount in all stages of wound management. While bacterial contamination is common in open wounds, not all colonization warrants intervention. True infection is characterized by evidence of host compromise,

Table 7.16 Primary layer options for wound management in dogs and cats.

Primary Layer Type	Examples	Indications	Advantages	Disadvantages/Precautions
Adherent (Wet-to-Dry/Dry-to-Dry)	Dry sterile gauze; saline-moistened gauze	Initial wound debridement; contaminated or infected wounds with necrotic tissue	Mechanical debridement; inexpensive; widely available	Painful removal; non-selective (removes viable tissue); delays healing if prolonged use; requires frequent changes
Non-Adherent, Semi-Occlusive	Telfa pads, Adaptic, Melolin	Clean wounds in proliferative phase; surgical wounds	Maintains moisture; reduces trauma at dressing changes; allows exudate absorption	Less effective for heavily exudative wounds; requires secondary absorptive layer
Non-Adherent, Occlusive	Hydrocolloids (DuoDERM), Hydrogels (Intrasite), Semi-permeable films (Opsite, Tegaderm)	Granulating or minimally exudative wounds; promote moist wound healing	Maintain moist environment; enhance autolytic debridement; reduce infection risk; decrease pain	May trap exudate and cause maceration if overused; not for infected wounds; can be costly
Impregnated Dressings (Antimicrobial / Medicated)	Silver-impregnated dressings, Honey-coated gauze, Iodine-based dressings	Contaminated, infected, or high-risk wounds	Antimicrobial action; reduce bacterial load; promote healing	Potential cytotoxicity (iodine, silver) with prolonged use; honey may attract insects if not covered
Biologic Dressings/ Advanced Therapies	Collagen matrices, Amnion, Platelet-rich plasma (PRP) gels	Chronic non-healing wounds; surgical adjuncts	Promote growth factor activity; enhance granulation and epithelialization	Expensive; availability limited; specialized handling required

Clinical Notes

- Primary layer selection is phase-dependent:
  - Inflammatory/debridement phase → Adherent dressings may be appropriate short-term.
  - Proliferative phase → Switch to non-adherent, occlusive/semi-occlusive dressings to maintain a moist environment.
  - Chronic wounds → Advanced/biologic options may be required.

Source: Adapted from Pavletic (2018) and Fossum (2019).

such as erythema, increased exudate, pain, fever, or cytologic detection of intracellular bacteria. In the early phases of wound contamination, topical antimicrobials may be preferred to minimize systemic drug use. Medical-grade honey, for example, exhibits osmotic bactericidal action while promoting autolysis and neovascularization. Silver-based dressings provide broad-spectrum antimicrobial activity and may help in disrupting biofilms, which are notoriously resistant to both immune clearance and systemic antimicrobials. Biofilm management often necessitates repeated mechanical or enzymatic debridement, combined with the use of surfactant-based wound cleansers and antiseptic agents to disrupt the extracellular matrix protecting sessile bacteria. When systemic antibiotics are indicated—such as in cases of deep tissue infection, cellulitis, osteomyelitis, or systemic inflammatory response—the choice of antimicrobial must be based on culture and sensitivity whenever feasible, as empirical therapies may not penetrate necrotic or ischemic tissues effectively (Figure 7.8).

Bandaging is both an art and a science in veterinary wound management. A well-applied bandage not only protects the wound from environmental contamination but also controls edema, immobilizes the affected area, and supports tissue apposition. Most veterinary bandages follow a three-layer construct. The primary wound layer, which lies in direct contact with the wound bed, should not be selected arbitrarily but rather treated as a prescribed medical intervention under the direction of a veterinarian. Its selection must be based on the specific clinical needs of the wound—whether to absorb exudate, retain moisture, deliver antimicrobial agents, or provide a non-adherent interface. Like any pharmacologic treatment, the primary dressing exerts a biological effect on the wound environment and can significantly influence the trajectory of healing. Inappropriate selection may delay epithelialization, exacerbate infection, or contribute to maceration or desiccation. Therefore, the veterinary technician must regard the primary layer with the same clinical precision and accountability as any prescription, adhering to the veterinarian's treatment plan while providing feedback based on the wound's response over time. The secondary layer, typically composed of cast padding or absorbent gauze, provides cushioning and pressure distribution. Finally, the tertiary layer, such as cohesive elastic wrap or adhesive tape, secures the bandage while offering a protective barrier against soiling. Proper application technique is critical. Bandages must be snug but not constrictive, as excessive tension may impair venous return or lymphatic drainage, leading to distal swelling, ischemia, or pressure necrosis.

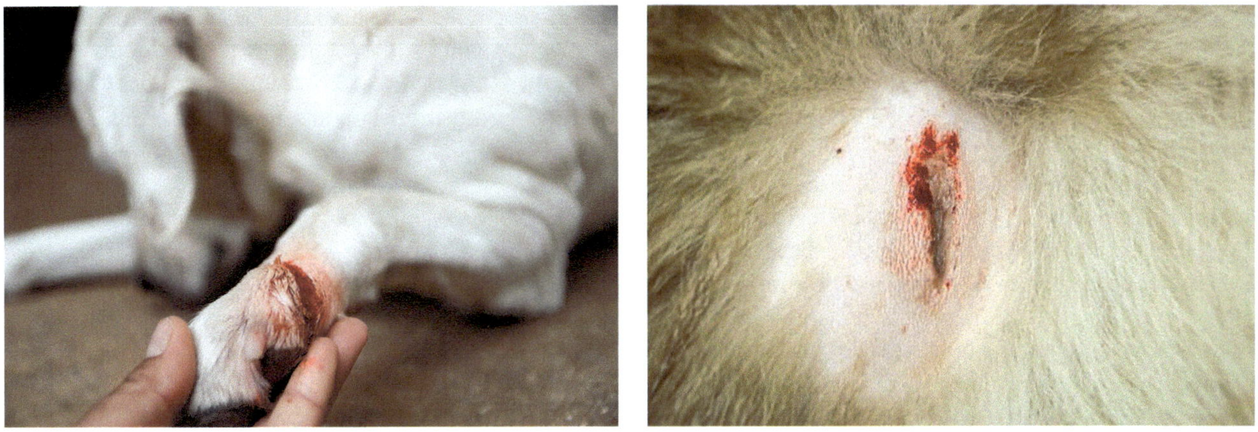

Figure 7.8 Examples of infected wounds in dogs: (L) An infected paw lesion showing erythema and tissue breakdown, (R) An open skin lesion with signs of active inflammation. *Source:* lovelyday12 / Adobe Stock Photos (left) Rarin Lee / Shutterstock (Right).

Veterinary technicians must perform daily evaluations of all bandaged limbs or regions, assessing for changes in skin temperature, color, swelling, odor, discharge, or evidence of bandage slippage (Table 7.17).

Promoting wound healing requires an integrative approach beyond topical and mechanical interventions. Nutritional support is essential; protein malnutrition is directly linked to impaired fibroblast function, delayed angiogenesis, and compromised collagen deposition. Micronutrients such as zinc, vitamin A, vitamin C, and essential fatty acids are vital cofactors in tissue repair processes and should be supplemented in patients with known deficits or chronic wounds (Pavletic 2010). Adequate analgesia is another cornerstone of wound care, as uncontrolled pain induces sympathetic vasoconstriction and increases cortisol levels, both of which delay tissue regeneration. Multimodal pain management, utilizing opioid analgesics,

Table 7.17 Reference guide outlining proper bandaging technique in dogs and cats.

Step	Action	Key Points/Precautions
Preparation	Clip hair around wound/area, clean and dry skin, apply sterile wound dressing (primary layer if needed).	Avoid excessive shaving (can irritate skin). Ensure wound is fully debrided and disinfected before bandaging.
Apply Primary Layer	Select based on wound phase (e.g., adherent for debridement, non-adherent for proliferative phase, medicated for infected wounds). Place directly in contact with wound.	Maintain sterility. Dressing should conform to wound without leaving dead space.
Apply Secondary Layer	Add absorbent cotton or cast padding over the primary layer to absorb exudate, provide cushioning, and distribute pressure.	Wrap evenly with 50% overlap, avoiding wrinkles to prevent pressure sores.
Apply Tertiary Layer	Secure with conforming bandage (e.g., Kling, VetRap). Provides compression and protection.	Apply with uniform tension—should be snug but not tight. Check distal circulation (toe swelling, cyanosis, coldness).
Immobilization (if needed)	For orthopedic/splint bandages, insert splints between secondary and tertiary layers.	Ensure splint does not extend beyond padding—edges can cause pressure necrosis.
Finishing	Seal proximal and distal edges with tape; leave 2 toes exposed for monitoring.	Allows for observation of swelling, color, and circulation.
Aftercare/ Monitoring	Check bandage daily for swelling, slippage, foul odor, or strike-through. Replace if soiled or wet.	Educate owner: use e-collar, cover bandage outdoors, never allow moisture penetration.

Clinical Notes

- Always select the primary layer based on wound healing stage.
- Bandages should be changed every 24–72 hours, depending on wound exudate and dressing type.
- Complications of improper bandaging include vascular compromise, pressure necrosis, infection, and delayed wound healing.
- Use light, even pressure—bandages applied too tightly risk ischemia, while loose bandages slip and cause friction.

Source: Adapted from Pavletic (2018), Fossum (2019), and Tobias and Johnston (2017).

NSAIDs, local anesthetics, and even adjunctive agents like gabapentin or amantadine, should be employed to improve both comfort and healing. Where indicated, immobilization strategies such as splints, slings, or activity restriction may be necessary to protect fragile granulation tissue or prevent wound dehiscence. Lastly, veterinary technicians must be adept at educating pet owners about proper wound care at home, including bandage integrity, signs of complications, and the importance of follow-up evaluations.

In conclusion, the successful management of acute and chronic wounds in veterinary patients demands a comprehensive understanding of wound pathophysiology, evidence-based dressing technologies, infection mitigation strategies, and effective client communication. Veterinary technicians are indispensable in this continuum of care, bridging clinical knowledge with compassionate nursing to support the animal's healing journey from injury to recovery.

Proper Wound Cleaning and Lavage: Technique, Solutions, and Antiseptic Considerations

Wound lavage is a foundational intervention in veterinary wound management, designed to reduce the microbial burden, remove debris, dilute toxins, and prepare the wound bed for healing or closure. The efficacy of lavage is dependent not only on the selection of solution but also on the delivery method, pressure, angle of irrigation, and total fluid volume used. Evidence from both veterinary and human surgical literature underscores that mechanical cleansing via high-volume, low-cytotoxicity lavage is more effective in reducing bacterial contamination than antimicrobial irrigation alone (Brown and Kowalewich 2012; Hosgood 2006).

Before initiating lavage, the surrounding skin must be thoroughly prepared. This begins with the removal of hair from the periwound region, which serves several critical purposes. Hair can harbor bacteria, interfere with the visualization of wound margins, and contribute to delayed healing or foreign body reactions if introduced into the wound bed. Clipping must extend generously beyond the wound margins until normal, unabraded skin is visualized, often at least 2–3 cm from the visible edge of the wound. This allows for full assessment of undermining, tunneling, or peripheral tissue trauma that may not be apparent on initial inspection.

To prevent hair and particulate debris from entering the wound during clipping, a sterile, water-based lubricant should be applied directly over the open wound bed prior to clipping. Products such as sterile KY jelly or medical-grade surgical lubricants serve as a protective physical barrier, entrapping hair and particulate matter. After clipping is completed, the lubricant and any trapped debris can be removed by gentle lavage with sterile isotonic fluids or saline-soaked gauze. This simple intervention significantly reduces iatrogenic contamination and is especially important in heavily contaminated or traumatic wounds.

Lavage Pressure and Delivery Technique

Optimal lavage pressure is critical to achieve mechanical decontamination without causing additional tissue trauma. Pressures between 7 and 15 pounds per square inch (psi) are widely accepted as the therapeutic window for both veterinary and human patients. Pressures below 7 psi are often inadequate for removing bacteria and particulate matter, while pressures exceeding 15 psi have been shown to drive bacteria deeper into tissue planes, damage granulating tissue, and potentially disrupt capillary networks essential for healing (Pavletic 2010; Brown and Kowalewich 2012).

The most commonly recommended method for achieving appropriate pressure in clinical settings is the use of an 18-gauge needle attached to a 35-mL syringe, which generates approximately 8–12 psi (Pavletic 2010; Brown and Kowalewich 2012). This setup allows for directional control and consistent force. An alternative and highly effective method utilizes a pressurized IV fluid bag enclosed in a pressure cuff inflated to 300 mmHg. When connected to standard IV extension tubing and a lavage set or stopcock, this system delivers lavage fluid at approximately 8.5 psi, which falls comfortably within the therapeutic range (Pavletic 2010; Hosgood 2006). This technique allows for sustained, hands-free lavage over large wound surfaces, is reproducible, and is ideal for wounds requiring copious irrigation, such as bite wounds, degloving injuries, or abscess cavities (Figure 7.9).

Lavage should be applied perpendicular or slightly oblique (15–45 degrees) to the wound bed, as direct perpendicular streams may cause tissue trauma, and highly oblique angles may inadequately penetrate recesses or undermine necrotic tissue. Commercially available pressure irrigation devices or gravity-fed lavage systems with pressure regulators may also be used, particularly in referral or surgical settings, to deliver more controlled and continuous flow.

Lavage Volume and Repetition

There is no universally established volume of fluid required to adequately cleanse a wound, as volume should be titrated based on wound size, contamination severity, and chronicity. However, literature supports the use of at least 500–1000 mL

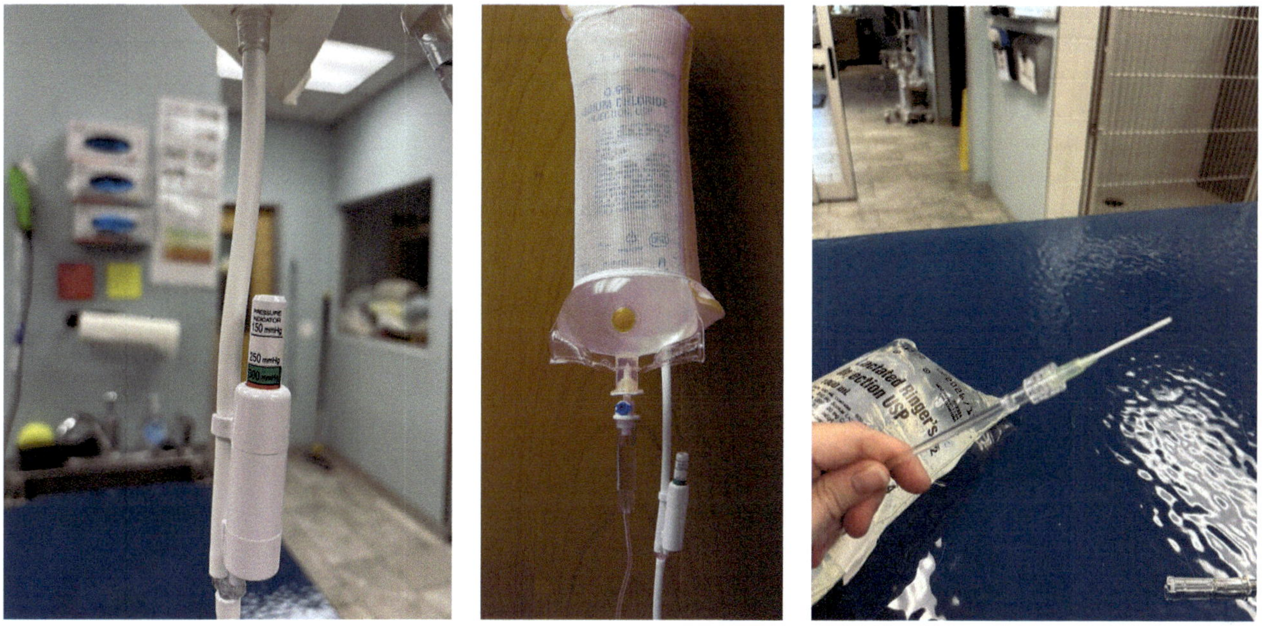

Figure 7.9 Pressurized sleeve inflated to 300 mmHg in preparation for wound lavage, yielding 7–15 psi IV fluid bag for wound management (Veterinary Practice News 2016); and 18-gauge catheter without stylet attached to an IV fluid line in preparation for wound lavage.

for small wounds, and 3–5 L or more for large, contaminated, or infected wounds, especially those resulting from bite trauma or vehicular injury (Pavletic 2010; Hosgood 2006). The key is copiousness: "dilution is the solution to pollution." Lavage should continue until gross contaminants are removed and the effluent fluid appears macroscopically clear.

In highly exudative, necrotic, or biofilm-producing wounds, repeated lavage over multiple dressing changes may be required. In these cases, instillation therapy—where the wound is filled with solution and left to dwell before removal—may be beneficial and is often paired with negative pressure wound therapy.

Selection of Lavage Solutions

The ideal lavage solution should be isotonic, noncytotoxic, readily available, and cost-effective. Sterile isotonic saline (0.9% NaCl) remains the gold standard for initial lavage due to its compatibility with living tissues and lack of antimicrobial or cytotoxic properties. Lactated Ringer's Solution (LRS) is a suitable alternative, particularly when large volumes are needed, though it may be less bacteriostatic than saline.

While plain sterile fluids are generally preferred for initial gross decontamination, antiseptic solutions may be employed cautiously in wounds with heavy bioburden or necrotic debris, particularly when surgical debridement is delayed or not possible. However, antiseptics must be used at proper dilutions to avoid cytotoxic effects on fibroblasts, keratinocytes, and endothelial cells, which are critical for granulation and epithelialization.

Dilution Guidelines for Antiseptics

1) **Chlorhexidine Gluconate**: Chlorhexidine possesses broad-spectrum antimicrobial activity and is effective against Gram-positive and Gram-negative bacteria, as well as some fungi and viruses. The commonly available 2% or 4% surgical scrub or solution must never be used undiluted on open wounds, as concentrations above 0.05% have been shown to induce significant cytotoxicity. The evidence supports diluting 2% chlorhexidine solution 1:40 with sterile saline or LRS to achieve a 0.05% solution, which maintains antimicrobial efficacy with minimal cellular toxicity.
2) **Povidone-Iodine (Betadine®)**: Iodine-based solutions are effective against a broad array of pathogens, including resistant Gram-negative organisms and spores. However, their cytotoxicity is significant unless properly diluted. A 1% solution of povidone-iodine, prepared by diluting a 10% stock solution 1:10 in sterile saline, has been shown to preserve antimicrobial activity while minimizing toxicity. Caution must be exercised in wounds with significant exudate or organic matter, as iodine's effectiveness may be reduced in the presence of proteinaceous debris.

Contraindicated or Restricted Lavage Agents

The use of certain household or veterinary antiseptics, while historically common, is now discouraged due to overwhelming evidence of cytotoxicity and delayed wound healing.

Hydrogen Peroxide (H_2O_2) has no place in wound management. Despite its effervescence and visual appeal, hydrogen peroxide induces oxidative injury to fibroblasts, delays angiogenesis, and has been implicated in gas embolism when introduced into subcutaneous tissues or closed cavities. Studies have shown that chlorhexidine and other cytotoxic antiseptics contribute more to tissue damage than to bacterial clearance, and their antimicrobial effect is transient at best (Brown and Kowalewich 2012; Cooper and Bowler 2003).

Sodium Hypochlorite (Diluted Bleach, Dakin's Solution), while possessing bactericidal properties, is highly cytotoxic to mammalian cells even at diluted concentrations (e.g., 0.025%). Although it may still have limited roles in managing infected cavitary lesions under strict dilution and time-controlled exposure protocols, its use in open, healing wounds is discouraged unless no other options exist. The contemporary veterinary standard favors less cytotoxic agents unless guided by culture sensitivity and under direct supervision by a DVM.

Proper Technique and Clinical Considerations

Regardless of solution choice, lavage must be performed under aseptic conditions to prevent iatrogenic contamination. Gloves, masks, and sterile delivery systems should be used whenever possible, especially in wounds that are being prepped for primary closure or that overlay joints, tendons, or thoracic/abdominal cavities. Reusable equipment such as syringes and needles should be sterile, and pressure-generating devices should be properly cleaned between uses.

Wounds should be thoroughly debrided—mechanically, enzymatically, or surgically—before or during lavage to expose viable tissue and enhance contact between the irrigant and microbial colonies. Following lavage, the wound bed should be blotted dry using sterile gauze prior to dressing application. Dressings should be selected to complement the chosen solution—some agents, such as silver-based antimicrobials, may interact negatively with iodine-based products.

In summary, proper wound cleaning through lavage is not merely a preparatory step but a therapeutic intervention that significantly impacts healing trajectory. Veterinary technicians must understand the principles governing effective lavage pressure, antiseptic selection, and fluid volume to minimize cellular injury, reduce infection risk, and optimize the healing environment. The scientific literature strongly supports the use of isotonic fluids and diluted antiseptics over cytotoxic agents, and proper technique must be upheld with every dressing change or reassessment.

Anesthetic Monitoring and Analgesic Techniques: Ensuring Physiological Stability and Patient Comfort

Intraoperative anesthetic monitoring and analgesic support are inseparable pillars of perioperative veterinary care. They exist not only to prevent patient morbidity and mortality, but also to uphold the highest standards of physiological stability, humane intervention, and ethical responsibility. The veterinary technician, as the primary operator of intraoperative monitoring equipment and the sentinel of patient comfort, must possess an advanced understanding of physiological parameters, nociceptive pathways, pharmacologic interventions, and how these elements intersect within the anesthetized patient.

Preanesthetic Risk Stratification: Comorbidities and ASA Physical Status

The foundation of any anesthetic event begins with a comprehensive assessment of the patient's systemic health and surgical risk. The American Society of Anesthesiologists (ASA) Physical Status Classification System, though originally developed for human medicine, remains a valuable stratification tool in veterinary anesthesia. It assigns a score from I (healthy) to V (moribund), based on the presence and severity of systemic disease. An additional designation of "E" (Emergency) may be appended in urgent surgical cases.

A patient classified as **ASA I** presents with no discernible systemic disease, whereas **ASA II** patients possess mild systemic conditions such as controlled hypothyroidism or early-stage periodontal disease. **ASA III** encompasses animals with moderate systemic disease that may affect anesthetic tolerance, including diabetes mellitus, early congestive heart failure, or chronic kidney disease (CKD). **ASA IV** includes patients with severe systemic dysfunction, such as decompensated cardiomyopathy or hepatic failure, which poses a constant threat to life under anesthesia. **ASA V** patients are not expected to survive without immediate surgical intervention and may be experiencing terminal shock, multi-organ failure, or exsanguination (Table 7.18).

The presence of comorbidities—whether cardiovascular, pulmonary, endocrine, or renal—directly influences anesthetic drug choice, fluid strategy, monitoring intensity, and analgesic planning. For instance, in patients with hypertrophic

Table 7.18 ASA Physical Status Classification adapted for veterinary patients, with examples in dogs and cats.

ASA Status	Description	Examples in Dogs and Cats
ASA I	Normal healthy patient with no systemic disease, good exercise tolerance.	Young, healthy dog or cat for elective spay/neuter; Healthy patient undergoing minor, elective procedure
ASA II	Mild systemic disease that does not limit normal activity; no clinical signs.	Mild heart murmur without clinical signs; Well-controlled diabetes or hypothyroidism; Obese but otherwise healthy patient
ASA III	Severe systemic disease that limits activity but is not incapacitating; clinical signs present but stable.	Anemia (PCV ~20%); Moderate dehydration; Chronic heart disease with mild exercise intolerance; Controlled seizures
ASA IV	Severe systemic disease that is a constant threat to life.	Severe congestive heart failure; Advanced renal or hepatic disease; Shock; Severe electrolyte derangements
ASA V	Moribund patient not expected to survive without surgery; critical condition.	Severe trauma with massive hemorrhage; Advanced sepsis; GDV with shock and organ dysfunction
E (Emergency Modifier)	Any patient requiring immediate anesthesia to preserve life, regardless of underlying status. Added as a suffix (e.g., ASA II-E).	GDV requiring emergency surgery; Cesarean section; Severe trauma requiring immediate stabilization

Clinical Notes

- ASA classification is not a direct predictor of anesthetic complications, but it correlates with risk.
- Use ASA status to help guide drug selection, monitoring intensity, and client communication about anesthetic risks.

Source: Adapted from American Society of Anesthesiologists (2014); Grimm et al. (2017).

cardiomyopathy, the use of alpha-2 agonists may precipitate significant increases in afterload and myocardial oxygen demand, whereas in animals with CKD, drugs primarily cleared renally such as ketamine or NSAIDs may accumulate and worsen nephron injury. A vigilant anesthetist must not only anticipate these risks but proactively alter protocols to maintain perfusion and homeostasis.

Intraoperative Monitoring: A Multisystem Physiological Perspective

Anesthetic monitoring must be performed at a frequency and depth appropriate for the patient's ASA status, comorbidities, and procedure type. Key physiological systems assessed intraoperatively include the cardiovascular system, oxygenation status, ventilatory function, and thermoregulatory integrity. These are not static variables but dynamic, interrelated processes that must be continually interpreted in the context of anesthetic depth, drug interactions, surgical stimuli, and patient-specific response.

Cardiovascular Monitoring

Cardiovascular monitoring aims to ensure adequate tissue perfusion and oxygen delivery (DO_2), which is a function of cardiac output (CO) and arterial oxygen content (PaO_2). Cardiac output is defined as the product of heart rate (HR) and stroke volume (SV) and is sensitive to anesthetic-induced alterations in preload, afterload, contractility, and autonomic tone. Heart rate and rhythm should be continuously assessed using electrocardiography (ECG), with attention to the presence of arrhythmias such as ventricular premature complexes (VPCs), atrioventricular blocks, or sinus bradycardia—all of which may signify excessive anesthetic depth, vagal stimulation, electrolyte derangement, or primary myocardial disease (Table 7.19).

Blood pressure is a critical determinant of tissue perfusion and organ function during anesthesia. In the anesthetized patient, it serves as both a surrogate for global perfusion pressure and a dynamic reflection of the interplay between cardiac output, systemic vascular resistance (SVR), and intravascular volume status. Due to the profound effects that anesthetic drugs have on autonomic tone, myocardial contractility, and vascular smooth muscle, vigilant monitoring of blood pressure is essential to prevent ischemic injury to vital organs such as the brain, kidneys, myocardium, and gastrointestinal tract.

Table 7.19 Cardiovascular physiology definitions outlining key hemodynamic parameters.

Term	Definition
DO_2 (Oxygen Delivery)	The total amount of oxygen delivered to tissues per minute. Calculated as: DO_2 = Cardiac Output (CO) × Arterial Oxygen Content (CaO_2). Units: mL O_2/min.
CO (Cardiac Output)	The volume of blood the heart pumps per minute. CO = Heart Rate (HR) × Stroke Volume (SV). Normal adult dog: ~3–6 L/min.
PaO_2 (Arterial Partial Pressure of Oxygen)	The measure of oxygen dissolved in arterial blood plasma. Reflects efficiency of pulmonary oxygen exchange. Normal: ~80–100 mmHg (species-dependent).
HR (Heart Rate)	The number of times the heart beats per minute. Contributes directly to cardiac output.
SV (Stroke Volume)	The volume of blood ejected from the left ventricle with each contraction. Influenced by preload, afterload, and contractility.
SVR (Systemic Vascular Resistance)	The resistance the left ventricle must overcome to pump blood through systemic circulation. Determined by vessel diameter and blood viscosity.
Preload	The degree of myocardial fiber stretch at the end of diastole, primarily determined by venous return and end-diastolic volume. Often equated with "filling pressure."
Afterload	The pressure the heart must overcome during systole to eject blood, largely dependent on systemic vascular resistance and arterial pressure.
Contractility	The intrinsic strength of the myocardium independent of preload and afterload. Influenced by sympathetic stimulation, inotropes, and myocardial health.
Autonomic Tone	The balance of sympathetic and parasympathetic nervous system activity regulates HR, contractility, vascular tone, and overall cardiovascular function.

Source: Adapted by Schaeffer (2025).

Pathophysiology of Blood Pressure Under Anesthesia

The maintenance of systemic arterial pressure during anesthesia relies on the balance between cardiac output (CO) and systemic vascular resistance. Cardiac output is the product of heart rate and stroke volume, both of which may be altered by anesthetic agents. For instance, volatile anesthetics such as isoflurane and sevoflurane induce dose-dependent vasodilation and myocardial depression, which reduce preload and afterload while blunting baroreceptor reflexes. Opioids, though largely cardiovascularly stable, may cause bradycardia through enhanced vagal tone. Alpha-2 adrenergic agonists (e.g., dexmedetomidine) produce biphasic blood pressure responses, with an initial vasoconstrictive hypertension followed by reflex bradycardia and a subsequent hypotensive phase due to reduced sympathetic outflow and diminished cardiac output.

In the face of these pharmacologic effects, mean arterial pressure (MAP) becomes the most clinically relevant value, as it approximates the average pressure driving blood through the vascular system during the entire cardiac cycle. In small animal patients, a MAP above 60 mmHg is typically required to maintain adequate perfusion of high-demand organs, such as the brain and kidneys. However, patients with chronic hypertension, intracranial pathology, or reduced autoregulatory capacity may require higher perfusion pressures (MAP $\geq$ 70–80 mmHg) to prevent cerebral or renal hypoperfusion.

Systolic arterial pressure (SAP) reflects the maximal pressure during ventricular systole and is influenced primarily by stroke volume and aortic compliance. Diastolic arterial pressure (DAP) reflects arterial tone and is the dominant determinant of coronary perfusion. The MAP, calculated as DAP + 1/3 (SAP – DAP), represents the perfusion pressure available to end organs and should be the primary target during anesthetic management.

Direct vs. Indirect Blood Pressure Measurement

Direct arterial catheterization, also known as invasive blood pressure monitoring, is the gold standard for real-time and beat-to-beat measurement of SAP, DAP, and MAP. It involves placement of an over-the-needle catheter into a peripheral artery (commonly the dorsal pedal, femoral, or coccygeal artery) connected via a fluid-filled pressure line to a calibrated transducer. This system allows for precise assessment of hemodynamic trends and responsiveness to therapeutic interventions such as fluid boluses or inotropes. Direct monitoring is particularly indicated in hemodynamically unstable, hypotensive, hypertensive, or critically ill patients, as well as in those undergoing prolonged or complex surgical procedures.

The arterial waveform, displayed on a multiparameter monitor, provides additional information beyond pressure values. The dicrotic notch within the arterial pressure waveform represents aortic valve closure, and its presence and morphology reflect systemic vascular resistance (SVR) and arterial compliance. A flattened or absent dicrotic notch may indicate low

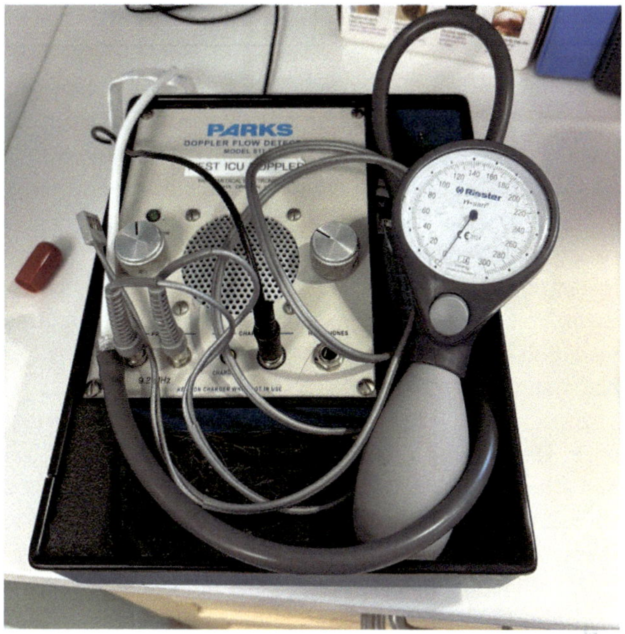

Figure 7.10 A veterinary Doppler blood pressure unit used for noninvasive blood pressure measurement in small animal patients. *Source:* Courtesy of Schaeffer (2025).

SVR or dampened wave transmission, while a tall, narrow waveform with a high dicrotic notch may suggest vasoconstriction or a hyperdynamic state (Haskins 2015; Duke-Novakovski et al. 2016).

When direct monitoring is not feasible, indirect methods such as oscillometric or Doppler-based systems are employed. Oscillometric monitors use an inflatable cuff placed around a limb or tail to detect pressure oscillations within the artery during cuff deflation. They provide SAP, MAP, and DAP values, but may become unreliable in patients with low cardiac output, small body size (<5 kg), bradycardia, or vasoconstriction, which can interfere with oscillation detection and cuff cycling. In such cases, a Doppler ultrasonic sphygmomanometer is preferred. The Doppler method uses a piezoelectric crystal to detect changes in blood flow velocity, providing an audible signal that corresponds to SAP when the cuff is deflated. While Doppler units do not provide mean arterial pressure (MAP) or diastolic arterial pressure (DAP), they are more accurate and sensitive in small patients, hypotensive states, and under conditions of peripheral vasoconstriction (Grosenbaugh and Muir 1998; Duke-Novakovski et al. 2016). In cats, where oscillometric monitors frequently underperform due to small vessel size and rapid HR, Doppler remains the technique of choice. Additionally, Doppler devices allow for continuous auditory feedback, which enhances situational awareness of perfusion during dynamic anesthetic changes (Figure 7.10).

Plethysmographic Waveform and Hemodynamic Trends

Though often associated with pulse oximetry, the plethysmographic waveform (pleth form) can provide indirect hemodynamic information analogous to arterial pressure waveforms. The pleth form reflects the optical detection of pulsatile arterial blood volume changes in peripheral tissue and can demonstrate pulse amplitude, rhythm regularity, and waveform morphology.

When well defined, a strong pleth waveform with regular pulsations suggests adequate cardiac output and peripheral perfusion. A blunted or low-amplitude pleth may signify hypotension, hypovolemia, or vasoconstriction. Some monitors display a visible dicrotic notch on the pleth waveform, which—like in arterial waveforms—represents aortic valve closure and can be used to monitor vascular tone and fluid responsiveness. The pleth waveform may also be used to evaluate pulsus paradoxus or respiratory variation in patients receiving mechanical ventilation, which can inform preload dependency and fluid responsiveness. However, because the pleth is sensitive to motion artifact, ambient light, and probe malposition, it should not replace invasive or Doppler measurements, but rather be used as a supporting trend tool in multimodal hemodynamic assessment.

The Impact of IPPV on Blood Pressure

Intermittent positive pressure ventilation (IPPV)—a cornerstone of anesthetic management for ensuring adequate oxygenation and ventilation—can significantly decrease blood pressure in anesthetized animals. The reduction in arterial blood pressure observed during intermittent positive pressure ventilation (IPPV) is primarily attributable to two interrelated hemodynamic mechanisms. First, IPPV significantly impairs venous return to the heart by altering the normal intrathoracic pressure gradient. During spontaneous respiration, negative intrathoracic pressure generated on inspiration facilitates the return of systemic venous blood to the right atrium by creating a favorable pressure gradient across the great veins, particularly the cranial and caudal vena cava. However, when IPPV is employed, the application of positive pressure during inspiration increases intrathoracic pressure, thereby compressing the great veins and raising the pressure surrounding them. This diminishes the venous return gradient, resulting in a decrease in right ventricular preload. A reduction in preload leads directly to a decrease in stroke volume via the Frank-Starling mechanism, culminating in a lower cardiac output and systemic hypotension.

Concurrently, IPPV also exerts deleterious effects on right ventricular afterload by increasing pulmonary vascular resistance. The elevated alveolar pressures generated during positive pressure inspiration can compress pulmonary capillaries and arterioles, thereby increasing resistance to blood flow within the pulmonary circulation. This elevation in pulmonary vascular resistance raises the afterload that the right ventricle must overcome to eject blood into the pulmonary artery. As the right ventricle faces increased resistance and mechanical impedance, its efficiency and output decline, further exacerbating the reduction in left ventricular filling and systemic blood pressure. Together, these alterations in preload and afterload constitute the principal pathophysiologic basis for IPPV-induced hypotension in anesthetized patients, particularly in those with marginal cardiovascular reserve or inadequate intravascular volume. The net result is a ventilation-associated decline in arterial pressure, which is often more pronounced in hypovolemic, vasodilated, or critically ill patients, or those under deep planes of anesthesia (Figure 7.11).

Mitigation Strategies for IPPV-Induced Hypotension

To attenuate the hemodynamic consequences of intermittent positive pressure ventilation (IPPV), the anesthetist must carefully balance the goals of adequate ventilation and oxygenation with the imperative to preserve cardiovascular stability. This requires a thoughtful and physiologically informed approach to ventilator settings and patient support. One of the most effective strategies involves minimizing the peak inspiratory pressure (PIP) by using the lowest value necessary to achieve adequate tidal volume—typically between 10 and 15 cm H_2O in small animals. Lower PIP reduces intrathoracic pressure fluctuations and minimizes the impedance of venous return. Additionally, minute ventilation should be precisely titrated by adjusting both respiratory rate and tidal volume to prevent alveolar overdistension and avoid respiratory alkalosis. Alkalemia shifts the oxyhemoglobin dissociation curve to the left, increasing hemoglobin's affinity for oxygen and thereby impairing peripheral oxygen unloading, especially in metabolically active tissues.

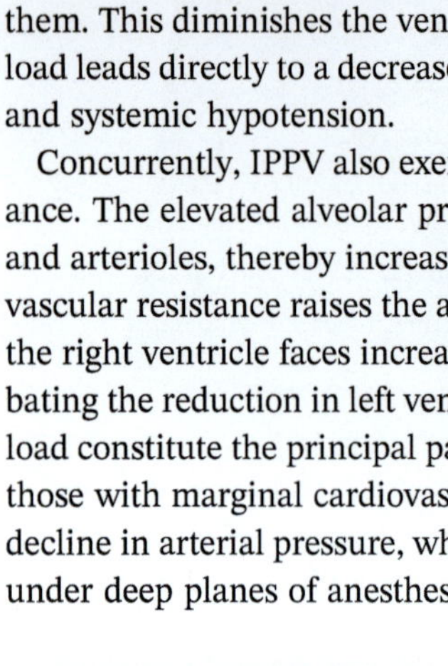

Figure 7.11 Hemodynamic effects of intermittent positive-pressure ventilation (IPPV), showing the cascade from increased intrathoracic pressure to reduced venous return, preload, stroke volume, and arterial blood pressure. *Source:* Image created by Schaeffer (2025).

Recruitment maneuvers, although occasionally necessary to improve ventilation-perfusion matching and reopen atelectatic alveoli, should be employed cautiously. Prolonged or excessive increases in airway pressure can significantly reduce preload and exacerbate hypotension. Close monitoring of arterial pressure during such maneuvers is essential. Ensuring adequate circulating volume is equally important. Patients should be evaluated for volume status preoperatively, and if hypovolemia is identified, fluid resuscitation should be initiated before the onset of controlled ventilation. IPPV should not be implemented in an unstable or volume-depleted patient without first optimizing preload.

Furthermore, positive end-expiratory pressure (PEEP), while useful for maintaining alveolar recruitment and preventing atelectasis, must be carefully titrated. Excessive PEEP can elevate mean intrathoracic pressure and thereby further diminish venous return and cardiac output. In patients who remain hypotensive despite optimal ventilator adjustments and fluid therapy, pharmacologic support may be required. The judicious use of vasopressors, such as dopamine or norepinephrine, can enhance systemic vascular resistance, while positive inotropes, such as dobutamine, may be employed to improve myocardial contractility and augment cardiac output.

Close coordination between ventilation management and cardiovascular monitoring is essential. In such cases, direct arterial pressure monitoring is ideal, as it provides continuous, beat-to-beat assessment of perfusion during respiratory cycles.

Monitoring Techniques and Interpretation

Direct arterial catheterization remains the gold standard for blood pressure measurement, particularly in patients requiring IPPV, where rapid shifts in intrathoracic pressure and hemodynamic load necessitate high-fidelity monitoring. The associated arterial pressure waveform can also reveal ventilation-associated changes such as pulsus paradoxus—a drop in systolic pressure during inspiration exceeding 10 mmHg—often seen in volume-responsive states or pericardial effusion (Haskins 2015; Duke-Novakovski et al. 2016). In situations where invasive monitoring is not available, Doppler sphygmomanometry is preferred over oscillometric methods, particularly in small (<5 kg), hypotensive, or vasoconstricted patients, and during IPPV, where oscillometric cycling may become unreliable due to motion artifact or low pulse amplitude.

The plethysmographic waveform from pulse oximetry can also support blood pressure interpretation. Respiratory variation in the amplitude of the pleth waveform during IPPV may indicate fluid responsiveness. Flattened pleth waveforms, concurrent with falling SpO_2 and MAP, should alert the anesthetist to deteriorating perfusion associated with ventilatory compromise. Perfusion assessment is incomplete without evaluating mucous membrane color, capillary refill time (CRT), and pulse quality, which reflect peripheral perfusion and vascular tone (Figure 7.12).

Oxygenation and Ventilation

Oxygenation is defined as the process by which oxygen molecules bind to hemoglobin in the pulmonary capillaries, forming oxyhemoglobin for systemic delivery to tissues. This process is fundamentally dependent on adequate alveolar ventilation, intact diffusion across the alveolar-capillary interface, sufficient hemoglobin concentration, and proper cardiovascular perfusion. Intraoperatively, the most widely used method for assessing a patient's oxygenation status is pulse oximetry (SpO_2)—a noninvasive, continuous monitoring tool that provides an estimate of arterial hemoglobin saturation. While not a

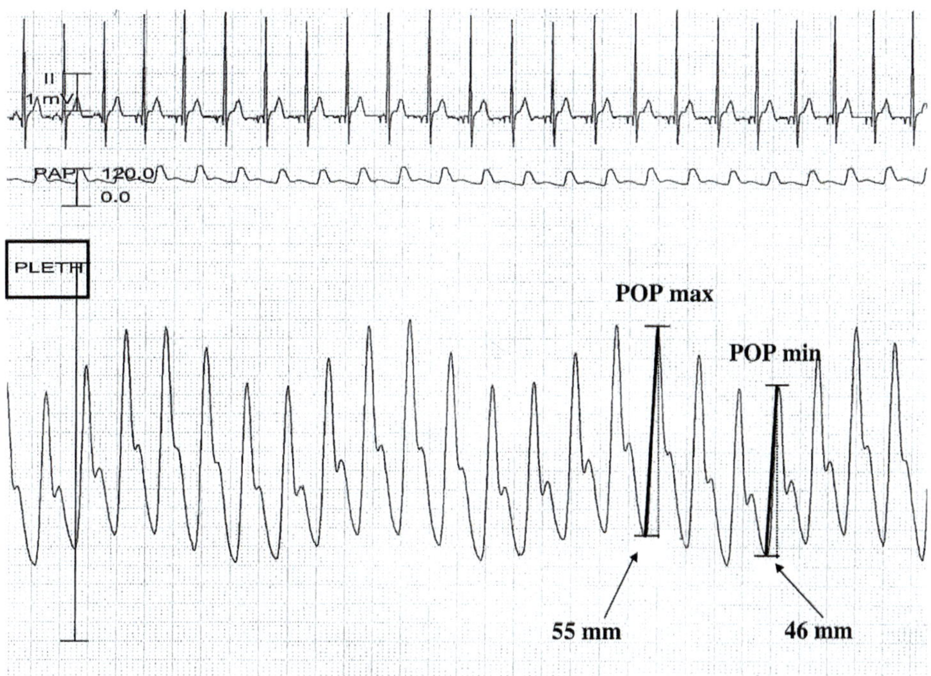

Figure 7.12 Simultaneous arterial pressure (AP) and pulse oximetry plethysmographic (PLETH) waveforms during intermittent positive-pressure ventilation (IPPV). Note the respiratory variation in pleth amplitude (ΔPOP), which can indicate fluid responsiveness. *Source:* Adapted from Cannesson et al. (2005).

substitute for arterial blood gas analysis (PaO_2), SpO_2 serves as a vital real-time indicator of pulmonary function and systemic oxygen delivery. A normal SpO_2 in anesthetized patients should remain above 95%, which corresponds to a PaO_2 greater than 80 mmHg on the oxyhemoglobin dissociation curve. Values below this threshold warrant immediate investigation and intervention, as declining saturation may precede critical hypoxemia.

The Plethysmographic Waveform (Pleth Form)

Modern pulse oximeters often display a plethysmographic waveform, commonly referred to as the "pleth." This waveform represents the pulsatile flow of arterial blood through the monitored tissue and serves as a graphical adjunct to the numerical SpO_2 reading. Beyond confirming probe placement, the pleth provides valuable insight into pulse quality, peripheral perfusion, and vascular tone.

A normal pleth waveform is characterized by a smooth, repeating upstroke and downstroke that corresponds with each cardiac cycle. A strong, well-defined pleth suggests robust peripheral perfusion and probe accuracy, whereas a weak, flattened, or erratic waveform may indicate hypovolemia, vasoconstriction, hypotension, or probe misalignment. The height of the waveform is influenced by stroke volume and vascular compliance, while the regularity may be altered by arrhythmias or patient motion.

Veterinary technicians trained to interpret pleth waveforms can detect peripheral vasoconstriction secondary to hypothermia or α2-agonist administration, recognize pulsus paradoxus in pleural effusion or pericardial tamponade, and identify periods of cardiovascular collapse before the loss of SpO_2 readings altogether. As such, waveform morphology should be continuously evaluated alongside the numerical saturation value.

Anatomical Sites and Probe Types

Pulse oximeters utilize two types of probes—transmission and reflectance—both of which rely on spectrophotometric detection of light absorption at two wavelengths (typically 660 and 940 nm) to differentiate between oxyhemoglobin and deoxyhemoglobin (Duke-Novakovski et al. 2016; Hofmeister and Brainard 2009). Transmission probes are the most common in veterinary practice and require the probe to be placed on thin, nonpigmented tissues with arterial blood flow between an emitter and a detector. Common anatomical sites include:

- **Tongue** (most reliable in anesthetized patients; highly vascular and centrally located)
- **Pinna** (ear flap; especially effective in cats and small dogs)
- **Toe web** (between digits; useful in recumbent patients)
- **Vulva or prepuce** (delicate mucosa with strong perfusion)
- **Tail tip** (especially in larger breeds when other sites are inaccessible) (Figure 7.13)

Reflectance probes, in contrast, measure light reflected back to the sensor and are often used on surfaces where transmission is not possible. These are suitable for placement on:

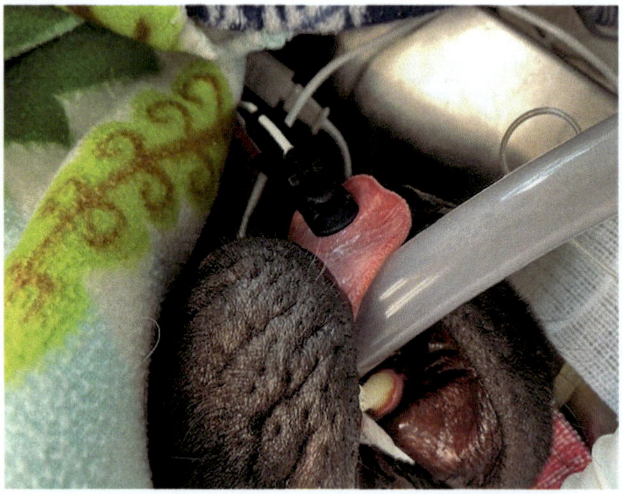

Figure 7.13 Veterinary pulse oximeter with a transmission probe applied for SpO_2 monitoring. *Source:* Courtesy of Schaeffer (2025).

- **Forehead or temporal region**
- **Base of the tail**
- **Thoracic or flank skin**, particularly in large animals

Proper placement is crucial. Probes should be secure but not constrictive, and the tissue should be pink, warm, and free of pigment or debris. Pigmented tissues or vasoconstriction can falsely depress SpO_2 readings, while ambient light or patient movement may cause signal dropout or artifact. When using reflectance probes, care must be taken to ensure stable contact and signal consistency, as these are more susceptible to motion artifact and low perfusion errors.

Oxyhemoglobin Dissociation Curve: Clinical Implications

The relationship between SpO_2 and PaO_2 is not linear, but sigmoidal, and is best visualized via the oxyhemoglobin dissociation curve. The curve illustrates how readily hemoglobin binds to or releases oxygen at varying partial pressures. In the upper flat portion of the curve, small changes in PaO_2 result in minimal changes in SpO_2. For example, PaO_2 values above 100 mmHg will still yield SpO_2 readings near 100%, offering limited insight into hyperoxia or impending hypoxia. However, as PaO_2 declines below 80 mmHg, the curve begins to steepen, and small decreases in PaO_2 produce rapid and clinically significant drops in SpO_2. When PaO_2 falls below 60 mmHg, the corresponding SpO_2 may drop below 90%, indicating critical hypoxemia with insufficient oxygen delivery to tissues.

Several factors can shift the curve and alter hemoglobin's affinity for oxygen:

- A rightward shift of the oxygen-hemoglobin dissociation curve (indicating reduced affinity) facilitates oxygen unloading to tissues and may occur with hypercapnia, acidosis (low pH), hyperthermia, or elevated 2,3-diphosphoglycerate (2,3-DPG) levels (Muir et al. 2000; Tilley and Smith 2015). This is beneficial during metabolic stress but results in lower SpO_2 values at any given PaO_2.
- A leftward shift (increased affinity) impairs oxygen release and is seen with hypocapnia, alkalosis, and hypothermia. This can lead to falsely reassuring SpO_2 values despite poor tissue oxygenation.

Understanding the physiologic and pathophysiologic implications of this curve is essential when interpreting SpO_2 values, especially in patients with altered acid-base balance, temperature regulation, or respiratory function. Pulse oximetry is a powerful tool, but only when interpreted in the full context with perfusion, ventilation, and underlying pathology.

Ventilation

Ventilation encompasses the exchange of carbon dioxide (CO_2) between alveoli and the atmosphere. It is influenced by minute ventilation, dead space ventilation, and alveolar compliance. Capnography, through measurement of end-tidal carbon dioxide ($EtCO_2$), offers real-time insight into ventilatory adequacy. Normal $EtCO_2$ values typically range between 35–45 mmHg. A rising $EtCO_2$ may indicate hypoventilation, decreased respiratory rate, or increased CO_2 production, while declining values may signal hyperventilation, reduce cardiac output, or impending cardiopulmonary arrest.

Capnography provides continuous, noninvasive monitoring of a patient's ventilatory status by measuring the concentration or partial pressure of carbon dioxide (CO_2) in the respiratory gases throughout the respiratory cycle. The terminal point of the exhalation phase—known as end-tidal CO_2 ($EtCO_2$)—is considered the best approximation of alveolar CO_2 and, under normal circumstances, closely reflects the partial pressure of arterial CO_2 ($PaCO_2$).

In anesthetized canines, normal $EtCO_2$ values range between 35 and 45 mmHg, corresponding to a normocapnic state and indicating adequate alveolar ventilation and systemic perfusion. Feline patients typically exhibit a slightly lower end-tidal CO_2 ($EtCO_2$), usually ranging between 32 and 38 mmHg, due to several species-specific physiological differences. Cats have a higher baseline respiratory rate and lower tidal volume compared to dogs. As a result, their minute ventilation per kilogram is elevated, enhancing CO_2 elimination. Additionally, feline pulmonary architecture, characterized by a relatively greater alveolar surface area and a thinner alveolar-capillary membrane, promotes more efficient CO_2 diffusion. This combination of increased ventilatory efficiency and reduced functional residual capacity contributes to consistently lower $EtCO_2$ readings in cats, even under anesthesia (Steffey and Mama 2007; Duke-Novakovski et al. 2016). Veterinary technicians must interpret these values in the context of species norms to avoid overventilation or unnecessary intervention.

Capnogram Interpretation and Waveform Recognition

The capnogram, a graphical representation of exhaled CO_2 over time, is divided into four distinct phases:

1) **Phase I (Baseline)**: This represents exhalation of dead space gas, which contains no CO_2 and appears as a flat baseline at 0 mmHg.
2) **Phase II (Ascending Limb)**: A sharp upward incline occurs as CO_2-rich alveolar gas begins to mix with dead space gas.
3) **Phase III (Alveolar Plateau)**: The waveform reaches a near-horizontal plateau, reflecting uniform alveolar emptying. The end of this phase represents the $EtCO_2$ value.
4) **Phase IV (Descending Limb)**: A rapid decline back to baseline as inhalation begins.

Veterinary technicians should become adept at recognizing both normal and pathological waveform patterns. The most common abnormal capnograms include:

- **Gradual upward drift of $EtCO_2$ with normal waveform**: Suggestive of hypoventilation or decreased minute ventilation. This may occur due to excessive anesthetic depth, opioid-induced respiratory depression, or CO_2 rebreathing. Mitigation includes lightening the plane of anesthesia, initiating manual or mechanical ventilation, and inspecting the anesthetic circuit for exhausted CO_2 absorbent or inadequate fresh gas flow.
- **Abrupt decrease in $EtCO_2$ to zero**: May indicate disconnection of the breathing circuit, esophageal intubation, or complete airway obstruction. Immediate action involves checking the integrity of the endotracheal tube (ETT), re-establishing airway patency, confirming placement via direct visualization or re-intubation, and assessing for ventilatory movement.
- **Shark-fin waveform (slanted Phase III)**: Characteristic of airway obstruction or bronchoconstriction, this is often observed in feline asthma or in cases of kinked or occluded ETTs. Troubleshooting includes verifying ETT patency, suctioning secretions, repositioning the tube, and administering bronchodilators or anticholinergics as prescribed.
- **Gradual downward drift in $EtCO_2$ with normal waveform**: May suggest hyperventilation, hypotension, or decreased cardiac output. A decline in pulmonary perfusion reduces alveolar CO_2 content. This pattern is common in early stages of hemorrhage, anesthetic overdose, or hypovolemia. Interventions include volume resuscitation, reduction in inhalant anesthesia concentration, and increasing perfusion via inotropes or fluid boluses under veterinary guidance.
- **Oscillating baseline or "bouncy" waveform**: Often a result of cardiac oscillations or spontaneous movement in light planes of anesthesia. This can occur due to the proximity of the heart to the airways. If perfusion is adequate and $EtCO_2$ values are stable, no intervention is necessary, but close monitoring is required to prevent anesthetic emergence without support (Figure 7.14).

Troubleshooting and Mitigation

To ensure accuracy of capnographic monitoring, veterinary technicians must routinely evaluate both the numeric $EtCO_2$ value and the waveform morphology in tandem. When irregularities are observed, a systematic troubleshooting approach should be employed:

1) **Verify airway integrity**: Check for ETT kinks, displacement, cuff leaks, or obstruction. Ensure proper placement within the trachea, especially in small or brachycephalic patients, where anatomical challenges may obscure visualization.
2) **Evaluate the capnograph sampling line**: Condensation, mucus, or patient secretions can occlude sidestream sampling lines. These should be cleared or replaced immediately.
3) **Assess patient ventilation**: Count the respiratory rate manually and compare it to the capnograph readings. Look for paradoxical breathing, decreased chest excursions, or abnormal breath patterns that may indicate ventilatory compromise.
4) **Inspect equipment**: Confirm that the anesthesia machine is functioning properly, that there is no CO_2 absorbent exhaustion, and that the fresh gas flow is appropriate for the rebreathing system in use.
5) **Interpret in context**: Consider the patient's ASA status, comorbid conditions (e.g., pulmonary fibrosis, diaphragmatic hernia, anemia), and anesthetic depth when evaluating $EtCO_2$ trends (Figure 7.15).

In animals under general anesthesia, hypoventilation is the rule, due to the depressive effects of inhalants, opioids, and neuromuscular interference. Controlled mechanical ventilation is often required in patients with high ASA scores, thoracic procedures, or obesity. Blood gas analysis, though invasive, remains the definitive method to evaluate $PaCO_2$, PaO_2, and acid-base status.

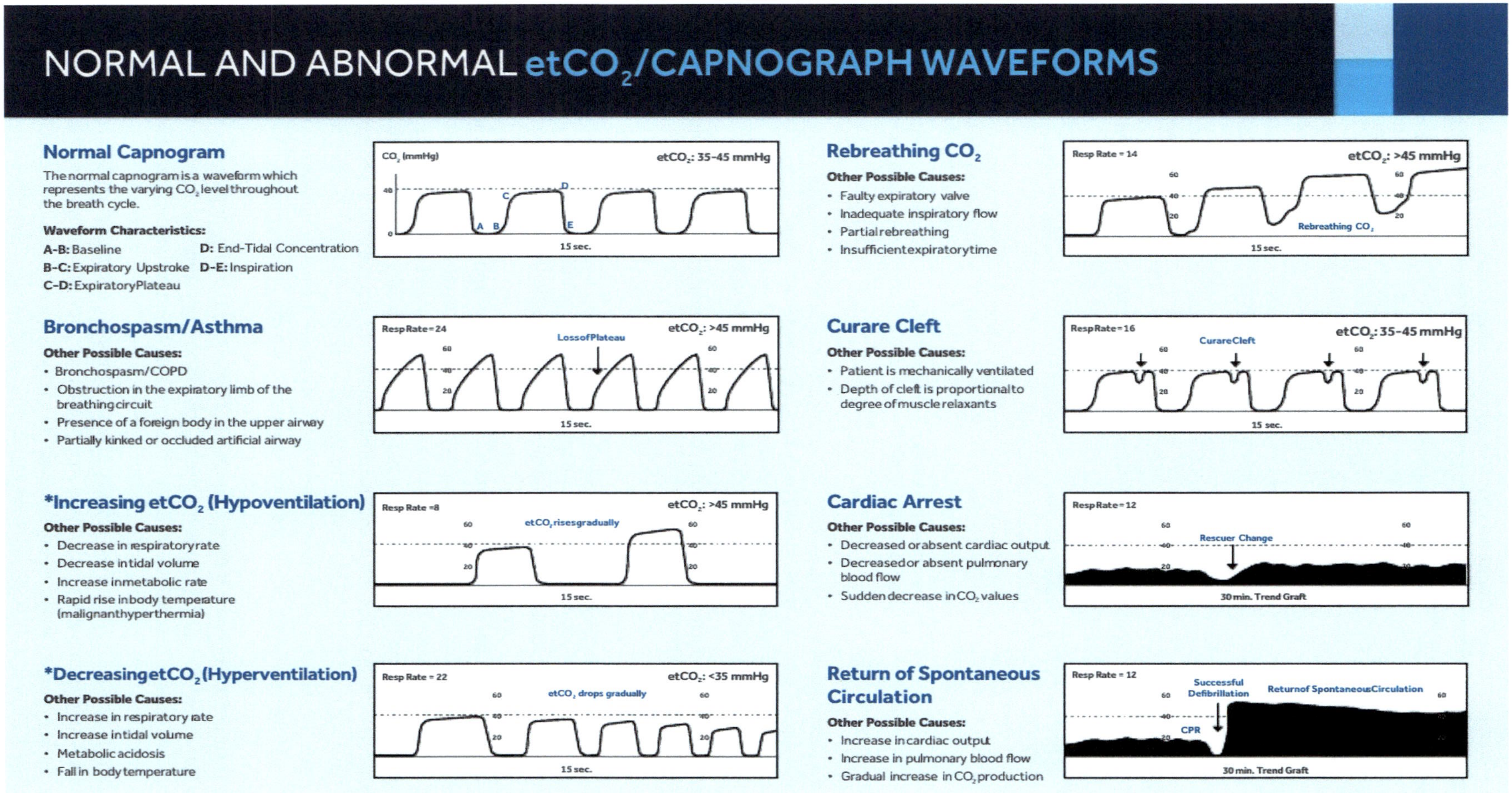

Figure 7.14 Examples of normal and abnormal capnography waveforms, including rebreathing, curare clefts, cardiac arrest, and return of spontaneous circulation (ROSC). *Source:* Image source: MDedge Emergency Medicine, 2025 / Frontline Medical Communications Inc.

Capnographic Troubleshooting Chart

Waveform Abnormality	Possible Cause(s)	Corrective Action(s)
Flat line (no CO_2 detected)	Disconnected circuit, apnea, airway obstruction, cardiac arrest, esophageal intubation	Check airway and breathing, confirm ET tube placement, reconnect circuit, begin CPR if indicated
Low $EtCO_2$ with normal shape	Hyperventilation, hypothermia, decreased metabolic rate, pulmonary embolism, poor perfusion/cardiac arrest	Reduce ventilation rate, correct underlying perfusion issue, assessfor embolism/shock
Elevated $EtCO_2$ with normal shape	Hypoventilation, rebreathing, increased metabolic rate (fever, sepsis, malignant hyperthermia)	Increase ventilation rate/tidal volume, check for CO_2 absorber exhaustion or faulty valves
'Shark-fin' waveform (slanted upstroke)	Bronchospasm, COPD, asthma, partial airway obstruction, kinking of ET tube	Administer bronchodilators, suction airway, reposition or replace ET tube
Curare cleft (dip in plateau)	Inadequate muscle relaxation, spontaneous breaths during mechanical ventilation	Increase anesthetic depth or administer neuromuscular blockade
Gradual rise in baseline	Rebreathing of CO_2, faulty expiratory valve, exhausted CO_2 absorber, inadequate fresh gas flow	Replace CO_2 absorbent, check circuit valves, increase fresh gas flow
Sudden drop in $EtCO_2$	Dislodged ET tube, circuit disconnection, massive pulmonary embolism, sudden cardiac arrest	Reconnect circuit, confirm tube placement, assess circulation, initiate resuscitation if needed
Oscillating base line	Cardiogenic oscillations (heart beating against lungs), patient movement	Typically benign; confirm diagnosis, minimize interference if needed

How to Use This Chart

1. First, always assess the patient before the monitor—look for breathing, pulse, and airway integrity.
2. Confirm the equipment setup: ET tube placement, circuit connections, and gas sampling line.
3. Apply corrective actions based on both clinical status and waveform appearance.
4. Use the waveform trends over time in conjunction with patient parameters to make clinical decisions.

Figure 7.15 Capnographic troubleshooting chart summarizing common waveform abnormalities, potential causes, and corrective actions. *Source:* Chart created by Schaeffer (2025).

Thermoregulation

Hypothermia is among the most common anesthetic complications in small animal practice, especially in pediatric, geriatric, or lean patients. Under general anesthesia, thermoregulatory mechanisms are blunted due to inhibition of hypothalamic function, peripheral vasodilation, and reduced metabolic rate. A decrease in core body temperature below 98 °F (36.7 °C) can reduce drug metabolism, impair coagulation, delay recovery, and exacerbate bradycardia and hypotension. Continuous temperature monitoring via esophageal or rectal probes is essential, with proactive warming measures—including circulating water blankets or forced-air warmers—applied throughout the procedure.

It is important to consider that core body temperature plays a critical role in anesthetic depth and cardiovascular performance. Hypothermia, a common complication in small animal anesthesia, particularly in pediatric or geriatric patients, can significantly deepen the anesthetic plane. This occurs through several mechanisms. As core temperature declines below approximately 97 °F (36.1 °C), hepatic metabolism of anesthetic agents—including inhalants and intravenous drugs such as propofol and opioids—slows markedly due to reduced enzymatic activity in cytochrome P450 pathways (Redondo et al. 2012; Grimm et al. 2015). Consequently, these drugs remain in circulation for longer periods and at higher plasma concentrations, potentiating their central nervous system depressant effects. Additionally, hypothermia reduces neuronal excitability, slows synaptic transmission, and depresses the medullary respiratory and vasomotor centers, which can mimic or augment the signs of excessive anesthetic depth, including bradycardia, hypotension, hypoventilation, and delayed recovery (Figure 7.16).

Compounding this challenge is the diminished efficacy of anticholinergic agents—such as atropine and glycopyrrolate—in hypothermic patients. These agents exert their chronotropic effects by competitively antagonizing muscarinic acetylcholine receptors (primarily M2 receptors) within the sinoatrial (SA) node, thereby reducing parasympathetic vagal tone and allowing the intrinsic pacemaker rate to increase. However, at core body temperatures below approximately 94 °F (34.4 °C), myocardial responsiveness to sympathetic and parasympathetic modulation is severely impaired. The sinoatrial (SA) node

Complications of Anesthetic-Induced Hypothermia in Dogs and Cats

Complication	Clinical Impact
Delayed drug metabolism	Slower breakdown of anesthetic agents leading to prolonged anesthetic depth
Prolonged recovery	Extended time to regain consciousness and ambulation
Bradycardia	Lower heart rate reducing cardiac output
Hypotension	Lower blood pressure decreasing tissue perfusion
Reduced immune function	Increased susceptibility to infection post-operatively
Impaired coagulation	Higher risk of bleedingdue to impaired clotting mechanisms
Decreased oxygen delivery	Left-shifted oxygen dissociation curve reducing oxygen availability to tissues
Shivering during recovery	Increased oxygen consumption and patient discomfort during recovery

Figure 7.16 Complications of anesthetic-induced hypothermia in dogs and cats. *Source:* Adapted from Brodbelt et al. (2008), Redondo et al. (2012), Dyson and Maxie (2017), and Grimm et al. (2015).

becomes refractory to pharmacologic stimulation due to reduced receptor-ligand binding kinetics, impaired ion channel function, and decreased cellular ATP availability, rendering the heart less responsive to both endogenous and exogenous chronotropes. As a result, administration of an anticholinergic in a hypothermic patient may produce little or no improvement in bradycardia until normothermia is restored (Grimm et al. 2015; Steffey and Mama 2007; Sessler 2008).

This blunted response underscores the importance of proactive thermal support during anesthesia. Passive warming measures (e.g., blankets and towels) are insufficient alone; active warming using circulating warm water blankets, forced-air systems, and warmed fluids is essential to maintain normothermia and ensure both anesthetic predictability and drug responsiveness. Core temperature should be monitored continuously using esophageal or rectal probes, with intervention initiated when body temperature drops below 98 °F (36.7 °C) and escalated aggressively when it falls below 95 °F (35 °C). Restoration of normothermia not only enhances drug metabolism and clearance but also re-establishes receptor sensitivity to autonomic pharmacologic agents, including anticholinergics.

Furthermore, hypothermia-induced bradycardia must be interpreted within the context of the anesthetic plane and perfusion status. A patient exhibiting profound bradycardia, accompanied by hypotension and hypoventilation, should not automatically be assumed to require pharmacologic stimulation. If hypothermia is present, the priority should be rewarming, as this may correct the cardiovascular depression without the need for additional drugs that may be ineffective or potentially detrimental under cold physiological conditions.

Ultimately, the integration of thermal regulation into the broader anesthetic management plan is not optional—it is imperative. Hypothermia distorts the anesthetic profile, alters drug pharmacokinetics and pharmacodynamics, deepens anesthetic depth, increases recovery time, impairs immune function, and may lead to serious perioperative complications such as coagulopathy or ventricular arrhythmias. In the setting of controlled ventilation and cardiovascular monitoring, a hypothermic patient presents a diagnostic challenge, as many of the expected physiologic parameters—such as heart rate, blood pressure, and responsiveness to intervention—are skewed or blunted. The veterinary technician must be equipped to identify these physiologic changes, understand the mechanisms behind them, and advocate for appropriate, evidence-based interventions aimed at preserving homeostasis and ensuring safe anesthetic outcomes.

Pain Assessment and Multimodal Analgesia

Pain is not only an ethical consideration but a physiological stressor that provokes neuroendocrine responses capable of destabilizing the anesthetized patient. Nociceptive stimulation results in activation of the hypothalamic-pituitary-adrenal (HPA) axis, catecholamine release, tachycardia, hypertension, increased metabolic demand, and in some cases, arrhythmogenesis or immunosuppression. Therefore, analgesia must be preemptive, multimodal, and titrated to both the procedure and patient response.

Pain scoring systems, such as the Colorado State University Acute Pain Scale or the Glasgow Composite Pain Scale, provide structured approaches to identifying and quantifying pain in companion animals. Parameters such as body posture, facial expression, vocalization, heart rate, respiratory rate, and response to palpation are used to assess pain severity and guide analgesic adjustments intraoperatively and postoperatively.

Multimodal analgesia refers to the simultaneous use of agents that act on different nociceptive pathways—thereby allowing for dose reduction, improved efficacy, and reduced adverse effects. This may include:

- **Opioids** (e.g., methadone, hydromorphone, fentanyl) acting at mu-opioid receptors in the CNS
- **NSAIDs** (e.g., meloxicam, carprofen) inhibiting peripheral cyclooxygenase enzymes
- **Local anesthetics** (e.g., lidocaine, bupivacaine) blocking sodium channels at the level of the nerve membrane
- **NMDA receptor antagonists** (e.g., ketamine) reducing central sensitization and wind-up phenomena
- **Alpha-2 adrenergic agonists** (e.g., dexmedetomidine) providing sedation and analgesia via presynaptic inhibition of norepinephrine release (Table 7.20)

Table 7.20 Perianesthetic agents in veterinary medicine and their effects on the nociceptive pathway.

Drug Class	Examples	Transduction(injury → nerve)	Transmission(nerve → spinal cord)	Modulation (spinal cord)and Perception (brain)
Opioids	Morphine, Hydromorphone, Methadone, Fentanyl	—	✓ inhibit afferent nerve firing	✓ dorsal horn inhibition; Methadone also blocks NMDA✓ alters brain's perception
NSAIDs	Carprofen, Meloxicam, Robenacoxib	✓ block prostaglandins, ↓ sensitization	—	—
Local Anesthetics	Lidocaine, Bupivacaine	✓ block sodium channels in nociceptors	✓ block conduction along nerves	—
Alpha-2 Agonists	Dexmedetomidine, Xylazine	—	—	✓ enhance inhibitory spinal pathways ✓ sedation, anxiolysis, ↓ perception
NMDA Antagonists	Ketamine, Methadone (partial)	—	—	✓ blocks wind-up, central sensitization ✓ dissociative/anesthetic effect
Gabapentinoids	Gabapentin, Pregabalin	—	✓ ↓ excitatory neurotransmitter release	✓ calcium channel modulation in spinal cord
Inhalant Anesthetics	Isoflurane, Sevoflurane	—	—	✓ global CNS depression → ↓ perception
Acetaminophen	Paracetamol (dogs only, toxic to cats)	✓ central COX inhibition	—	✓ central analgesic effect
Melatonin	Melatonin supplements	—	—	✓ anxiolytic, mild sedative; supports sleep–wake cycles
Maropitant	Cerenia (NK-1 receptor antagonist)	✓ blocks substance P at NK-1 receptors	—	✓ visceral pain modulation via NK-1 in dorsal horn
Trazodone	Trazodone	—	—	✓ serotonin antagonist/reuptake inhibitor; reduces anxiety/stress perception

Key Notes

- Methadone is unique among opioids with NMDA antagonist effects, reducing wind-up pain.
- Gabapentin targets neuropathic pain via calcium channel modulation.
- Maropitant, while primarily an antiemetic, also provides visceral analgesia by blocking substance P.
- Melatonin serves as an anxiolytic adjunct, supporting stress reduction and smoother recovery.
- Trazodone is a perianesthetic anxiolytic that improves patient compliance and decreases stress perception.

Source: Adapted from Lamont et al. (2020); Grimm et al. (2015); Robertson and Taylor (2004); Gaynor and Muir (2009).

The choice and timing of each agent must reflect the patient's comorbid status, cardiovascular stability, and procedure-specific requirements. In patients with renal compromise, NSAIDs may be contraindicated due to reduced renal prostaglandin synthesis and perfusion risk. In contrast, patients with neuropathic pain or central sensitization may benefit from low-dose ketamine infusions or gabapentinoids.

The safe and effective management of anesthesia requires not only technical proficiency but also a deep understanding of applied physiology, pharmacologic principles, and individualized patient care. Intraoperative anesthetic monitoring and analgesic techniques are not passive activities but deliberate, data-driven interventions that influence patient outcomes minute by minute. Veterinary technicians must be capable of interpreting trends in cardiovascular performance, oxygenation, ventilation, and thermoregulation with both urgency and nuance, while concurrently advocating for compassionate, multimodal pain management that respects the biological and emotional experience of the animal.

Anesthesia is not a static protocol; it is a dynamic and deeply layered discipline that demands continuous learning, critical evaluation, and reflective practice. As such, the author of this textbook strongly encourages readers to seek additional training and reference materials that extend beyond this foundational discussion. Anesthesia, by its nature, encompasses a vast and intricate body of knowledge. No single chapter can encompass its full depth or account for the variability introduced by patient species, comorbidities, procedural complexity, or evolving pharmacologic strategies.

Readers are urged to explore anesthesia-specific textbooks and to pursue continuing education (CE) opportunities through conferences, workshops, and online credentialing platforms. Active participation in CE not only sharpens technical skill and clinical reasoning but also fosters a network of professional support essential for those navigating advanced anesthetic care.

Veterinary anesthesia is as humbling as it is rewarding. Its mastery requires discipline, patience, and a lifelong commitment to growth. The veterinary technician who aspires to excellence in this area must remain a student of physiology, a steward of patient safety, and an advocate for pain-free medicine.

Neonatal Resuscitation in Veterinary Medicine

Neonatal resuscitation is a critical skill in veterinary practice, especially in species such as dogs and cats, where dystocia, large litter sizes, and unattended whelpings increase the risk of perinatal mortality. Neonates are physiologically distinct from adults; they possess immature thermoregulatory mechanisms, a limited hepatic glycogen reserve, and cardiopulmonary systems that transition abruptly at birth. Successful transition from fetal to neonatal life depends on the timely establishment of effective respiration, thermoregulation, and glucose homeostasis. Failure in any of these domains—namely oxygenation, temperature control, or nutrient delivery—may result in life-threatening compromise. The three most common causes of neonatal mortality in veterinary patients are hypoxia, hypothermia, and malnutrition (hypoglycemia) (Moon and Erb 1983; Root Kustritz 2006; Davidson 2019). Understanding their pathophysiology and developing intervention strategies to mitigate them are central to the resuscitation of newborn veterinary patients.

The Pathophysiology of Neonatal Compromise

Hypoxia is the primary cause of neonatal morbidity and mortality. In utero, the fetus is maintained in a relatively hypoxic environment ($PaO_2 \approx 25–30$ mmHg) but is protected by fetal hemoglobin, which has a higher oxygen affinity than adult hemoglobin (Silver and Buffenstein 1995; Root Kustritz 2006). Upon parturition, abrupt umbilical cord compression or placental separation terminates maternal oxygen supply, necessitating the immediate onset of pulmonary gas exchange. Failure to establish effective respiration results in persistent fetal circulation: pulmonary vascular resistance remains elevated, right-to-left shunting through the ductus arteriosus persists, and systemic hypoxemia ensues. Cellular hypoxia leads to anaerobic metabolism, lactic acidosis, cerebral hypoperfusion, and bradycardia. Mitigation requires rapid airway clearance, stimulation, and if necessary, assisted ventilation with supplemental oxygen.

Hypothermia in neonates occurs due to a high surface area-to-volume ratio, poor subcutaneous insulation, and limited brown adipose tissue reserves. Newborns are incapable of effective shivering thermogenesis, relying instead on nonshivering mechanisms that are oxygen and glucose-dependent. A drop in core temperature below 94 °F (34.5 °C) impairs surfactant production, decreases pulmonary compliance, depresses respiratory drive, and causes peripheral vasoconstriction, further impairing oxygen delivery (Davidson 2019; Sessler 2008; Root Kustritz 2006). Cold stress also increases metabolic demand, exacerbating hypoglycemia. Prevention includes immediate drying, use of warming devices, and close monitoring of core body temperature.

Table 7.21 Veterinary-modified neonatal APGAR score for dogs and cats.

Domain	Score 0	Score 1	Score 2
Mucous Membrane Color	Cyanotic/pale	Pink body, blue extremities	Completely pink
Heart Rate	Absent	<200 bpm	≥200 bpm
Reflex Irritability	No response	Weak grimace	Strong response (cough/sneeze)
Muscle Tone	Flaccid	Some flexion	Active motion
Respiratory Effort	Absent	Slow/irregular	Strong, regular

Interpretation

- Total score 7–10: Neonate requires routine observation.
- Total score 4–6: Moderate distress, requires supportive measures.
- Total score ≤3: Critical depression, immediate resuscitation required.

Source: Adapted from Veronesi et al. (2009) and Root Kustritz (2006).

Hypoglycemia results from the neonate's limited hepatic glycogen storage and immature gluconeogenic pathways. During the first hours post-birth, neonates transition from transplacental glucose supply to intermittent oral intake. If suckling is delayed or inadequate, blood glucose levels fall precipitously. Hypoglycemia impairs central nervous system function, blunts respiratory effort, and predisposes the myocardium to electrical instability. Clinical signs may include lethargy, tremors, seizures, and in severe cases, coma. Intervention consists of early and frequent feedings or supplementation with dextrose-containing fluids, either orally or parenterally in compromised patients.

Neonatal Assessment and APGAR Scoring

The neonatal APGAR score is a systematic tool used to assess viability at 1 and 5 minutes post-delivery. The veterinary-modified APGAR scale evaluates mucous membrane color, heart rate, reflex irritability, muscle tone, and respiratory effort (Veronesi et al. 2009; Root Kustritz 2006). Each domain is scored from 0 to 2, with a maximum score of 10. A total score of 7 to 10 indicates a neonate requiring routine observation; 4 to 6 suggests moderate distress requiring supportive measures; and ≤3 denotes critical depression necessitating immediate resuscitative intervention. APGAR scoring provides a reproducible metric for guiding the depth of required intervention and monitoring recovery (Table 7.21).

Tying of the Umbilicus

Tying of the umbilicus in a newborn is an essential step in neonatal care that aims to control hemorrhage and prevent ascending infection through the umbilical vessels. In most uncomplicated natural deliveries, the umbilical cord ruptures spontaneously due to the natural traction between the dam and the neonate. However, when delivery is assisted—such as during dystocia or cesarean section—or if the dam does not sever the cord, manual intervention becomes necessary to ensure safe cord management.

The umbilical cord should be ligated or clamped approximately one to two centimeters from the neonate's abdominal wall. This distance minimizes the risk of traction-related injury or herniation while preserving enough cord length for adequate handling and antiseptic treatment. A sterile absorbable suture material or tightly applied hemostatic clamp is typically used to tie off the cord. It is crucial to avoid excessive tension that might damage the surrounding skin or underlying structures, particularly in premature or compromised neonates. After securing the tie, the distal portion of the cord can be transected using sterile scissors or a scalpel blade.

Once the umbilicus has been tied and cut, attention must turn to cord antisepsis. Tincture of iodine, specifically 2% to 7% iodine solutions (often povidone-iodine or traditional iodine tincture), remains the gold standard for umbilical cord disinfection due to its broad-spectrum antimicrobial properties and effectiveness in preventing neonatal omphalitis (Davidson 2019; Root Kustritz 2006; Schaeffer and Dziuk 2002). The high iodine content provides broad-spectrum antimicrobial activity against both Gram-positive and Gram-negative organisms. The alcohol-based vehicle in tincture formulations enhances drying of the umbilical stump, creating an inhospitable environment for microbial colonization and accelerating necrosis and desiccation of the remaining cord tissue.

To apply, the tied umbilical stump should be dipped or generously painted with tincture of iodine, ensuring that the solution fully penetrates the base of the cord near the abdominal wall. This application should ideally occur immediately post-ligation and may be repeated once or twice daily for the first 24–48 hours in high-risk environments, such as barns, kennels, or surgical suites where sterility is not absolute. It is important to allow the iodine to air-dry thoroughly, as occlusion or wrapping of the stump can retain moisture and increase the risk of anaerobic infection.

Inappropriate or delayed umbilical care can result in complications such as omphalophlebitis, septicemia, and intra-abdominal abscessation. Therefore, diligent technique in ligation and antiseptic application is paramount. Observing the stump for signs of inflammation, discharge, or swelling in the first few days of life is essential to identify early signs of infection. Proper handling of the umbilicus immediately post-parturition plays a central role in neonatal survival and long-term health, particularly in high-risk or medically managed deliveries.

Airway Management and Initial Resuscitation

If a neonate is apneic, bradycardic, or cyanotic, immediate steps must be taken to establish a patent airway and initiate ventilation. The neonate should be suspended in a 45-degree head-down position to facilitate gravity-assisted drainage of fetal fluids from the oropharynx and nasopharynx. Gentle oropharyngeal suctioning with a bulb syringe or low-pressure suction device can clear meconium, blood, or mucus. Deep or aggressive suctioning, particularly in the posterior pharynx, may induce vagally mediated bradycardia or laryngospasm and should be avoided.

Tactile stimulation—such as vigorous rubbing of the thorax and back with a warmed towel—stimulates cutaneous afferent nerves, which activate the respiratory centers in the medulla oblongata. If spontaneous breathing does not commence within 15–20 seconds, positive pressure ventilation is indicated.

Oxygen Delivery and Ventilation Protocols

Oxygen supplementation is fundamental in neonatal resuscitation. Initially, room air may suffice, but if cyanosis or bradycardia persists, enriched oxygen (40–60%) should be delivered via a tight-fitting face mask. Neonates should be ventilated with a tidal volume of 10–15 mL/kg, using a neonatal anesthesia bag or mechanical ventilator. Positive inspiratory pressure (PIP) should not exceed 25 cm H_2O to avoid alveolar overdistention and barotrauma. Ventilation is delivered at a rate of 40–60 breaths per minute, with chest rise used as the primary indicator of effective ventilation.

Endotracheal intubation may be required in neonates with persistent apnea, ineffective mask ventilation, or airway obstruction. A properly sized uncuffed endotracheal tube (typically 2.0–3.0 mm ID in puppies and kittens) should be used. Proper placement must be confirmed via visualization of the tube tip between the arytenoid cartilages and observation of symmetric chest excursion. Continuous monitoring of heart rate and mucous membrane color is essential (Figure 7.17).

Cardiopulmonary Support and Contraindicated Medications

If, after at least thirty seconds of effective positive-pressure ventilation with oxygen, the neonate's heart rate remains critically low—RECOVER suggests a threshold of fewer than 50 beats per minute—chest compressions should be initiated without delay. The preferred method is the two-thumb encircling technique, with the thumbs placed directly over the heart and the fingers supporting the thorax. Compressions should depress the chest to approximately one-third to one-half of its width, or one-third of the anteroposterior diameter if the patient is positioned in sternal recumbency and should be delivered at a rate of 120–150 per minute with complete recoil between compressions. Ventilation must be coordinated according to airway status: when a cuffed endotracheal tube is not in place, compressions and ventilations should be synchronized at a 4:1 compression-to-ventilation ratio, whereas once the neonate has been intubated with a cuffed tube, ventilations can be delivered asynchronously, allowing compressions to remain uninterrupted. Throughout resuscitation, the administration of 100% oxygen is strongly recommended. Effective chest compressions are essential to generating coronary perfusion pressure, which is the critical determinant for achieving return of spontaneous circulation (RECOVER 2025).

Epinephrine at a dose of 0.01–0.1 mg/kg can be administered intravenously, intraosseously, or intratracheally in cases of asystole or pulseless electrical activity, consistent with the recommendations outlined in the RECOVER neonatal resuscitation guidelines. Its use is indicated when effective ventilation and compressions fail to restore adequate heart rate and circulation. However, several pharmacologic agents commonly used in adult resuscitation are specifically contraindicated in neonates. Atropine, for example, is not recommended; while it is a mainstay in treating adult bradycardia, the etiology of bradycardia in neonatal puppies and kittens is most often severe hypoxia rather than vagal stimulation. In these cases, blocking parasympathetic input without addressing the oxygen deficit can worsen myocardial ischemia and delay recovery (Davidson 2019; Moon and Erb 1983; Beasley and Dinn 2016; RECOVER 2025). Similarly, sodium bicarbonate should not be administered during the early phases of resuscitation unless profound metabolic acidosis is confirmed, since inadequate

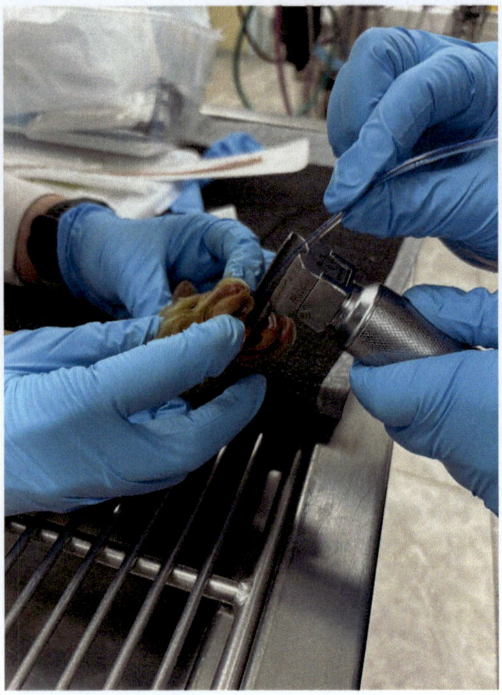

Figure 7.17 Newborn puppy undergoing endotracheal intubation with a 2.0 mm cuffless endotracheal tube. *Source:* Image from author's personal library.

ventilation can cause paradoxical intracellular acidosis and exacerbate CO_2 retention. The use of corticosteroids, vasopressin, and calcium solutions is also not supported in neonatal resuscitation due to their inconsistent efficacy and potential for disrupting the function of immature cardiomyocytes and other developing tissues (RECOVER 2025).

Post-Resuscitative Care

Post-resuscitation, neonates require vigilant supportive care to maintain homeostasis. Thermal support is critical; the target rectal temperature should be 96 °F–99 °F (35.5 °C–37.2 °C). Hypothermia depresses enzymatic function, slows gastric emptying, and suppresses immune response. Warmed incubators or heat lamps should be used, with careful avoidance of thermal burns or dehydration.

Nutritional support must be initiated early to avoid hypoglycemia. If suckling is inadequate or delayed, warmed colostrum or milk replacer should be administered orally or via orogastric tube at two to three hour intervals. Glucose levels should be monitored, and dextrose (5–10%) may be administered intravenously (0.5–1 mL/kg slowly) in compromised neonates. Passive transfer of maternal immunoglobulins via colostrum within the first eight hours of life is essential for immune competence. Neonates that fail to nurse may require serum supplementation (Figure 7.18).

Weight should be recorded daily; a failure to gain 5–10% of body weight daily is indicative of nutritional failure or underlying disease. Neonates should be monitored for persistent cyanosis, abdominal distension, regurgitation, or lethargy—early signs of aspiration, sepsis, or gastrointestinal dysfunction.

Neonatal resuscitation demands rapid identification of the pathophysiological cause of compromise and targeted, time-sensitive intervention. Hypoxia, hypothermia, and hypoglycemia are the predominant threats to neonatal viability, each exerting interrelated systemic effects that rapidly spiral into multisystem failure without intervention. A methodical approach encompassing airway clearance, ventilatory support, cardiovascular stabilization, and post-resuscitative care—grounded in the physiological principles of neonatal transition—is essential to reduce neonatal mortality and improve long-term health outcomes in veterinary patients.

Blood Product Administration in Canine and Feline Patients

Blood transfusion therapy is an essential component of emergency and critical care in small animal practice. It serves to restore oxygen-carrying capacity, address coagulopathies, expand plasma volume, and stabilize critically ill patients suffering from various hematologic and systemic conditions. Transfusion of whole blood or specific blood components must be conducted with precision, guided by evidence-based protocols and vigilant patient monitoring. We will discuss the clinical

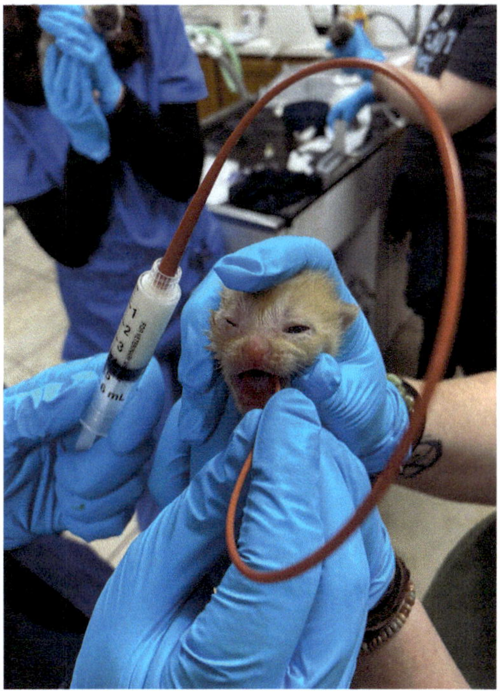

Figure 7.18 Neonatal kitten in an upright position receiving enteral nutrition via orogastric tube. *Source:* Image from the author's personal library.

indications for transfusion, blood collection and preparation techniques, nursing responsibilities during administration, and calculation of transfusion volumes and rates. It also outlines proper use of infusion equipment, including gravity systems and pulsatile pumps, and reviews recipient monitoring and post-transfusion assessment.

Clinical Indications for Transfusion

Blood products are indicated in numerous clinical scenarios where the patient's physiologic compensatory mechanisms are no longer sufficient to maintain tissue perfusion, oxygenation, or hemostatic function. Conditions that commonly warrant transfusion include acute or chronic anemia due to blood loss, immune-mediated hemolysis, or bone marrow suppression; hypovolemia with concurrent anemia; coagulopathies resulting from anticoagulant rodenticide ingestion, disseminated intravascular coagulation, hepatic insufficiency, or congenital factor deficiencies; and thrombocytopenia or thrombocytopathies causing active bleeding. Plasma transfusions may be used to address hypoproteinemia when oncotic pressure is compromised. In neonates, failure of passive transfer may necessitate administration of plasma or whole blood (Table 7.22).

Blood Component Therapy

Modern transfusion medicine emphasizes component therapy, in which specific elements of whole blood are administered to meet the individual needs of the patient. This approach improves safety, conserves donor resources, and minimizes the risk of volume overload. Packed red blood cells (pRBCs) are indicated when restoration of oxygen-carrying capacity is required without the need for plasma volume expansion. These are particularly beneficial in normovolemic anemia such as immune-mediated hemolytic anemia or nonregenerative anemia. The volume of pRBCs to administer is determined using the following equation:

$$\text{Volume (mL)} = [(\text{Desired PCV} - \text{Patient PCV}) \div \text{Donor PCV}] \times \text{Blood Volume (mL/kg)} \times \text{Body Weight (kg)}$$

In dogs, blood volume is approximately 90 mL/kg, and in cats, approximately 60 mL/kg. The donor PCV is typically assumed to be 70–80%.

Fresh frozen plasma (FFP) contains all coagulation factors, albumin, and antithrombin III, and is used to treat coagulopathies, liver dysfunction, or disseminated intravascular coagulation. It is not ideal for volume expansion unless given in large quantities. Cryoprecipitate, a fractionated product from FFP, contains concentrated fibrinogen, factor VIII, von

Table 7.22 Indications for blood component therapy in dogs and cats, including packed red blood cells, plasma products, cryoprecipitate, platelet products, whole blood, and albumin.

Component	Indications in Dogs	Indications in Cats	Clinical Notes
Packed Red Blood Cells (pRBCs)	Anemia due to hemorrhage, hemolysis, or decreased production; PCV <20%; clinical signs (tachycardia, weakness, collapse).	Anemia due to hemorrhage, hemolysis (FeLV, Mycoplasma haemofelis), or decreased production; PCV <15–20%.	Raises oxygen-carrying capacity without excessive volume; crossmatch required in cats, recommended in dogs with prior transfusion.
Fresh Frozen Plasma (FFP)	Coagulopathies (rodenticide toxicity, DIC, liver disease), hypoproteinemia with coagulopathy.	Coagulopathies (rodenticide toxicity, hepatic failure, DIC).	Provides clotting factors; must be used within one year of collection if frozen at −20 °C or −80 °C.
Cryoprecipitate	Hemophilia A (Factor VIII deficiency), von Willebrand disease.	Hemophilia A, von Willebrand disease (rare in cats).	Concentrated source of Factor VIII, vWF, and fibrinogen; small volume useful in patients that cannot tolerate large volumes.
Platelet-Rich Plasma (PRP)/ Platelet Concentrate	Thrombocytopenia or thrombocytopathia with active bleeding (IMT, DIC).	Severe thrombocytopenia with active bleeding (rarely performed due to poor availability).	Short shelf life; limited availability in veterinary medicine; risk of immune-mediated reactions.
Whole Blood	Acute hemorrhage with concurrent anemia and hypovolemia; trauma, surgery.	Acute hemorrhage with anemia and hypovolemia; trauma, surgery.	Contains RBCs, plasma proteins, clotting factors, and platelets; rarely ideal but sometimes necessary in acute emergencies.
Frozen Plasma (FP)	Rodenticide toxicity (Vitamin K antagonist) if factors II, VII, IX, X are required and FFP unavailable; coagulopathies without need for labile factors V and VIII.	Similar to dogs; rodenticide toxicity, hepatic insufficiency, coagulopathies without need for factors V and VIII.	Contains stable clotting factors (II, VII, IX, X) but lacks labile factors V and VIII; useful when FFP not available or expired beyond one year but stored up to five years.
Canine Albumin	Hypoalbuminemia due to protein-losing enteropathy, protein-losing nephropathy, severe hepatic insufficiency, or critical illness with oncotic support needs.	Use is controversial; canine-derived product may cause hypersensitivity or immune reactions; limited feline-specific formulations available.	Provides oncotic support and helps maintain colloid osmotic pressure; preferred over human albumin due to reduced risk of immune-mediated reactions, though cost and availability may limit use.

Source: Adapted from veterinary transfusion medicine guidelines and clinical literature (Davidow 2013; Holowaychuk 2016; Brooks 2017; Abrams-Ogg 2018; BSAVA 2020).

Willebrand factor, and fibronectin. It is the preferred treatment for von Willebrand disease, hemophilia A, and surgical bleeding in predisposed breeds. Cryosupernatant, or cryo-poor plasma, contains vitamin K–dependent factors (II, VII, IX, X) and is used in rodenticide toxicity or selective coagulopathies. Platelet-rich plasma and platelet concentrates may be prepared in specialized centers and are beneficial in treating life-threatening thrombocytopenia with active hemorrhage, though their availability and shelf-life limit routine use. Whole blood, which contains all cellular and plasma components, is typically reserved for patients suffering from acute hemorrhage who require both volume resuscitation and restoration of oxygen-carrying capacity.

Collection and Preparation of Blood Components

Donor selection is critical. All donors should be healthy, properly vaccinated, and screened for infectious diseases. Dogs should be typed for DEA 1.1 status, with DEA 1.1–negative dogs considered universal donors. Cats must always be blood typed (A, B, or AB) prior to donation, as they possess naturally occurring alloantibodies and are at high risk for transfusion reactions if mismatched. Cross-matching is required in previously transfused patients to avoid hemolytic reactions (Table 7.23).

Blood is collected using closed, sterile systems containing anticoagulant-preservative solutions such as CPDA-1. Once collected, whole blood may be processed by centrifugation to separate red cells, plasma, and platelets under aseptic

Table 7.23 Feline and canine blood donor requirements, including general eligibility criteria, blood typing, health and laboratory screening, infectious disease screening, donation frequency, and clinical considerations.

Species	General Requirements	Blood Typing	Health and Laboratory Screening	Infectious Disease Screening	Donation Frequency	Clinical Notes
Dog (Canine)	Healthy, good temperament; Age 1–8 years; Body weight >25 kg (55 lbs.); Current on vaccinations and parasite prevention; Not on medications other than preventatives; No previous transfusions.	DEA 1.1, DEA 1.2, DEA 7 typically tested; Ideal donors are DEA 1.1 negative; Crossmatch recommended after previous transfusion.	CBC, serum biochemistry, urinalysis performed at least annually; PCV/TP pre-donation; physical exam at each donation.	Ehrlichia canis, Anaplasma spp., Babesia spp., Borrelia burgdorferi (Lyme disease), Dirofilaria immitis (heartworm), Brucella canis (region-dependent), Leishmania spp. (in endemic areas).	Every 6–8 weeks; Blood volume collected ~15–20 mL/kg.	Sedation rarely required; Monitor for post-donation hypovolemia; Maintain donor health with good nutrition and regular veterinary exams.
Cat (Feline)	Healthy, good temperament; Age 1–8 years; Body weight >4–5 kg; Indoor-only preferred; Current on vaccinations and parasite prevention; Not on medications other than preventatives; No previous transfusions.	AB system (A, B, AB); Type A most common in DSH/DLH; Type B in certain purebreds (e.g., Devon Rex, British Shorthair); Crossmatch essential prior to each transfusion.	CBC, serum biochemistry, urinalysis performed at least annually; PCV/TP pre-donation; physical exam at each donation.	Feline Leukemia Virus (FeLV), Feline Immunodeficiency Virus (FIV), Mycoplasma haemofelis (hemotropic mycoplasmosis), Bartonella henselae, Cytauxzoon felis (in endemic areas).	Every 8–12 weeks; Blood volume collected ~10–12 mL/kg.	Sedation usually required; Smaller total volume collection; Donor cats at higher risk of stress and anemia, requiring careful monitoring.

Source: Adapted from transfusion medicine and donor screening guidelines (Davidow 2013; Wardrop et al. 2016; Brooks 2017; BSAVA 2020).

conditions. pRBCs are stored refrigerated at 1–6°C, while plasma components are frozen at −18°C or lower until use. All blood products should be inspected for discoloration, hemolysis, or contamination prior to administration.

Transfusion Preparation and Administration

Prior to administration, blood products must be prepared carefully. Plasma products are thawed with gentle agitation to avoid protein denaturation. Microwaving is contraindicated. Intravenous access is established using the largest appropriate catheter for the patient's size. For dogs, an 18–20 gauge catheter is typical; for cats, a 22–20 gauge is used. Inline filters (170–260 microns) must be employed to remove clots and microaggregates. Blood must never be administered concurrently through lines containing calcium-based fluids such as lactated Ringer's solution, as this may result in clot formation.

Initial transfusion should begin slowly at 0.25–0.5 mL/kg/h for the first 15–30 minutes while monitoring for signs of reaction. If no adverse effects are noted, the rate may be increased to a maximum of 5–10 mL/kg/h for packed red blood cells (pRBCs) or 6–10 mL/kg/h for plasma, with transfusion completed within four hours to reduce the risk of bacterial proliferation. Whole blood may be administered at 10–20 mL/kg over 2–4 hours, depending on cardiovascular status (Davidow 2013; Hackett and Mazzaferro 2015) (Figure 7.19).

When using gravity flow, veterinary technicians must calculate the required drip rate to ensure accurate delivery. The formula is:

$$\text{Drops/ min} = (\text{Volume to Infuse in mL}) \times (\text{Drip Factor in gtt/mL})/(\text{Time in minutes})$$

For example, to infuse 150 mL over three hours using a 20 drop/mL administration set:

$$(150 \times 20) \div 180 = 16.6 \approx 17 \text{ drops per minute or} \sim 3 \text{ drops/10 seconds}$$

When using pulsatile infusion pumps, it is essential to verify that the device is compatible with blood products. Peristaltic pumps that exert excessive shear forces may cause erythrocyte damage, leading to hemolysis and reduced viability of transfused cells (Davidow 2013; Wardrop et al. 2005). Infusion rates are entered in mL/h, and the pump should be set to deliver the volume evenly over the appropriate time frame, with inline filters in place.

Recipient Monitoring and Post-Transfusion Assessment

Prior to transfusion, baseline data including temperature, heart rate, respiratory rate, mucous membrane color, capillary refill time, and PCV/TS should be documented. Monitoring should occur every 15 minutes for the first hour, then every 30–60 minutes thereafter, with final assessment post-transfusion. Additional post-transfusion urinalysis may reveal hemoglobinuria indicative of hemolytic reactions.

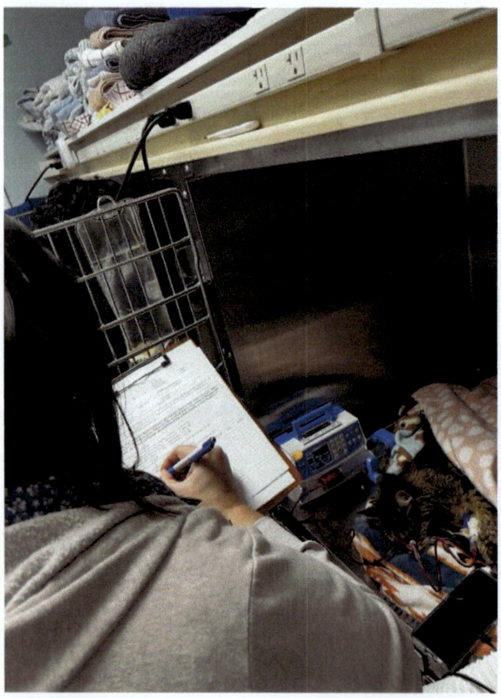

Figure 7.19 Cat receiving a whole blood transfusion via syringe pump, with a veterinary technician monitoring for adverse transfusion reactions. *Source:* Image from the author's personal library.

Clinical improvement following transfusion is expected to manifest as increased mentation, pinker mucous membranes, normalized heart rate, and improved capillary refill time. A follow-up PCV/TS should be obtained one to four hours post-transfusion. Each mL/kg of pRBCs administered is anticipated to raise the PCV by approximately 1% in dogs and 1.5% in cats, although this may vary based on ongoing losses or hemolysis.

Veterinary technicians must remain vigilant for transfusion reactions, which may be immunologic or nonimmunologic. Febrile nonhemolytic reactions are the most common and typically present with mild fever or vomiting. Acute hemolytic reactions can occur in mismatched or sensitized patients and are marked by hypotension, tachypnea, pigmenturia, and in severe cases, disseminated intravascular coagulation. Allergic reactions manifest as urticaria, pruritus, or facial swelling and are usually responsive to antihistamines. Volume overload is a concern, particularly in cats or patients with cardiac disease, and may be identified by tachypnea, pulmonary crackles, or nasal discharge.

The administration of blood products in dogs and cats is a complex but highly rewarding intervention that requires careful planning, precise nursing calculations, and diligent monitoring. Blood component therapy allows for targeted and efficient correction of anemia, coagulopathies, and hypoproteinemia, and has become a mainstay of modern veterinary critical care. By understanding the principles of donor selection, product preparation, transfusion technique, and recipient monitoring, veterinary professionals can optimize outcomes and improve survival in patients requiring transfusion support (Table 7.24).

Recognition and Management of Shock in Canine and Feline Patients

Shock is a life-threatening pathophysiologic condition characterized by inadequate tissue perfusion and oxygen delivery to meet cellular metabolic demands. If not promptly identified and treated, it results in cellular hypoxia, lactic acidosis, organ dysfunction, and ultimately death. In veterinary medicine, shock states are typically categorized into three primary mechanisms: hypovolemic, cardiogenic, and distributive. Each form of shock possesses distinct etiologies, physiologic manifestations, and therapeutic goals; however, all converge upon the same final common pathway of impaired perfusion and oxygenation.

Veterinary technicians serve a pivotal role in the recognition, triage, and initial stabilization of shock patients. A deep understanding of the pathophysiology underlying each type of shock state enhances the technician's ability to intervene promptly and appropriately.

Table 7.24 Clinical signs and onset timing of transfusion reactions during blood component therapy in dogs and cats.

Type of Reaction	Clinical Signs	Onset Timing
Acute Hemolytic Transfusion Reaction	Hemoglobinemia, hemoglobinuria, fever, tachycardia, hypotension, collapse, vomiting, pigmenturia, acute renal failure.	Within minutes to hours of transfusion.
Febrile Nonhemolytic Reaction	Fever, tachycardia, tachypnea, mild hypotension, restlessness, without hemolysis.	During or within 4 hours of transfusion.
Allergic/Hypersensitivity Reaction	Urticaria, pruritus, erythema, facial swelling, mild fever, usually within minutes of transfusion.	During or shortly after transfusion.
Anaphylactic Reaction	Severe dyspnea, hypotension, vomiting, diarrhea, collapse, cardiovascular shock, potentially fatal.	Immediate, within minutes of exposure.
Transfusion-Associated Circulatory Overload (TACO)	Dyspnea, tachypnea, coughing, pulmonary crackles, cyanosis, hypertension, evidence of volume overload.	During or within six hours of transfusion.
Transfusion-Related Acute Lung Injury (TRALI)	Acute hypoxemia, dyspnea, tachypnea, pulmonary edema not due to volume overload, onset within six hours of transfusion.	Within six hours of transfusion.
Delayed Hemolytic Reaction	Gradual fall in PCV/hematocrit days after transfusion, jaundice, bilirubinemia, persistent anemia, mild pyrexia.	Days to weeks post-transfusion.
Septic Reaction (bacterial contamination)	High fever, hypotension, tachycardia, shock, collapse, hemoglobinemia, hemoglobinuria, potentially fatal.	During or shortly after transfusion.

Source: Adapted from veterinary transfusion medicine guidelines and reference texts (Davidow 2013; Harvey 2012; Wardrop et al. 2016; BSAVA 2020).

Pathophysiology of Shock

In all forms of shock, the central feature is insufficient oxygen delivery (DO_2) to tissues, which leads to anaerobic metabolism, lactic acid accumulation, and cellular injury. Oxygen delivery is dependent upon both cardiac output (CO) and the oxygen content of arterial blood (PaO_2). Therefore, alterations in circulating blood volume, myocardial contractility, vascular tone, and oxygen-carrying capacity all influence shock dynamics.

Hypovolemic shock arises from a significant reduction in intravascular volume, commonly due to hemorrhage, severe dehydration, or third spacing (e.g., in gastrointestinal losses or peritonitis). The reduction in preload leads to diminished stroke volume and cardiac output. Despite intact myocardial function and vascular tone, the circulating volume is insufficient to perfuse tissues.

Cardiogenic shock results from intrinsic failure of the myocardium to generate adequate forward flow. Conditions such as dilated cardiomyopathy, arrhythmias, myocardial infarction, or severe valvular disease compromise cardiac output despite adequate volume status. This causes congestion, reduced stroke volume, and inadequate tissue perfusion.

Distributive shock, most associated with sepsis or anaphylaxis, is characterized by pathological vasodilation and increased vascular permeability. Despite adequate or even increased cardiac output in early phases, the loss of systemic vascular resistance and maldistribution of blood flow leads to impaired oxygen delivery. The most notable feature in distributive shock is relative hypovolemia, despite a normal intravascular volume.

Obstructive shock, as seen with conditions such as pericardial tamponade, pulmonary thromboembolism, or severe gastric dilatation-volvulus (GDV), is characterized by a physical impediment to cardiac filling or forward blood flow. Despite adequate myocardial contractility, mechanical obstruction reduces venous return or impedes ventricular outflow, leading to diminished stroke volume and cardiac output. The most notable feature in obstructive shock is impaired circulatory flow caused by an external or internal barrier, resulting in inadequate tissue perfusion despite normal intravascular volume and myocardial function.

Stages of Shock: Compensatory to Decompensatory Progression

All shock states progress through predictable clinical phases unless reversed. Understanding these stages allows veterinary technicians to detect subtle signs and initiate intervention before irreversible damage occurs.

In the compensatory phase, the body activates the sympathetic nervous system and the renin-angiotensin-aldosterone system (RAAS) in response to falling perfusion pressures. Heart rate increases (tachycardia), systemic vasoconstriction maintains blood pressure, and splenic contraction may transiently augment circulating volume. Mucous membranes may appear pink to slightly pale, with a brisk capillary refill time (CRT). Mentation is often still normal or only mildly subdued.

In early decompensatory shock, compensatory mechanisms begin to fail. Persistent hypoperfusion leads to anaerobic metabolism, resulting in metabolic acidosis and endothelial dysfunction. Clinical signs include pale to white mucous membranes, prolonged CRT, cold extremities, tachycardia or arrhythmias, hypothermia, and altered mentation. In this phase, lactate levels rise as tissues continue to operate in a hypoxic state.

Decompensatory or terminal shock is marked by profound cardiovascular collapse. Hypotension becomes refractory, bradycardia replaces earlier tachycardia due to myocardial hypoxia and vagal tone, and mentation deteriorates to stupor or coma. Pulselessness, severe hypothermia, and agonal breathing may precede cardiopulmonary arrest. Veterinary technicians must recognize that in cats, bradycardia and hypothermia—often observed in early decompensation—can be early indicators of serious pathology and should not be misinterpreted as benign.

Clinical Recognition of Shock by Veterinary Technicians

Veterinary technicians are often the first clinical personnel to assess a patient upon presentation. Early recognition of shock involves a thorough assessment of the animal's cardiovascular and neurologic status. Key parameters include heart rate, pulse quality (central and peripheral), mucous membrane color, CRT, rectal temperature, respiratory effort, and mentation. Rapid triage using a focused primary survey—airway, breathing, and circulation (ABC)—should be conducted immediately.

Dogs in compensatory hypovolemic shock may present with tachycardia, hyperdynamic pulses, and injected mucous membranes. As perfusion worsens, pulses weaken, mucous membranes become pale, and CRT lengthens. Cats are more insidious; they may be bradycardic, hypothermic, and hypotensive even in earlier phases, which may be mistaken for calmness or mild sedation.

Veterinary technicians must also be attuned to auscultable abnormalities such as muffled heart sounds (suggestive of pericardial effusion in cardiogenic shock), crackles or wheezes (indicative of pulmonary edema), and harsh lung sounds associated with distributive shock in septic patients (Table 7.25).

Immediate Interventions and Nursing Priorities

Upon identifying a potential shock patient, the veterinary technician must act with urgency. Oxygen supplementation should be provided immediately via flow-by, mask, oxygen cage, or nasal cannula, depending on the patient's tolerance and respiratory effort. Intravenous access must be obtained rapidly using the largest bore catheter feasible. In medium-to-large breed dogs, this often means a 16- to 18-gauge catheter in both cephalic veins to facilitate rapid volume resuscitation. For smaller patients or cats, 20- to 22-gauge catheters may be appropriate; however, placement in both forelimbs should still be attempted to allow for simultaneous administration of fluids, medications, or blood products.

In cases of hypovolemic or distributive shock, fluid resuscitation with isotonic crystalloids such as Lactated Ringer's or Normosol-R is initiated at a dose of 10–20 mL/kg boluses in dogs, and 5–10 mL/kg in cats, titrated to effect. Fluid responsiveness is evaluated through serial assessments of heart rate, blood pressure, pulse quality, CRT, mentation, and lactate levels. Caution must be exercised in cardiogenic shock, where fluid overload can exacerbate pulmonary edema. In such cases, vasodilators or positive inotropes may be prioritized over aggressive fluid therapy.

Veterinary technicians should concurrently collect a "Big Four" panel consisting of blood glucose (BG), lactate, packed cell volume (PCV), and total protein (TP). Each of these values provides critical insight:

- **Blood glucose** reflects perfusion and metabolic status. Hypoglycemia may be seen in sepsis, neonatal hypovolemia, or insulinoma, while stress-induced hyperglycemia is also common.
- **Lactate** is a key indicator of anaerobic metabolism. Elevated levels indicate inadequate oxygen delivery and can be used as a benchmark for resuscitative success.
- **PCV and TP** offer clues about blood loss or hemoconcentration. A normal PCV with low TP suggests protein loss (e.g., gastrointestinal or third spacing), while concurrent reductions may point to hemorrhage. Total protein also influences oncotic pressure and guides colloidal support.

Prompt placement of ECG leads and Doppler blood pressure monitoring should follow initial stabilization. Serial monitoring is essential to track the patient's response to therapy and guide further intervention. Central venous access, urinary catheterization for output monitoring, and continuous ECG are all procedures that veterinary technicians may assist with or perform under supervision as the patient's condition warrants.

Table 7.25 Clinical signs of compensatory, early decompensatory, and late decompensatory shock in dogs and cats, highlighting species-specific differences in pathophysiology and clinical presentation.

Stage of Shock	Pathophysiology	Clinical Signs in Dogs	Clinical Signs in Cats
Compensatory Shock	Sympathetic activation maintains cardiac output and perfusion via tachycardia, vasoconstriction, and splenic contraction.	Tachycardia, bounding pulses, injected/brick-red mucous membranes, rapid CRT (<1 second), bright mentation, mild hypertension or normotension.	Tachycardia may be less pronounced; normal to pale mucous membranes, rapid CRT or normal, mentation often subdued rather than bright.
Early Decompensatory Shock	Compensatory mechanisms fail; tissue hypoxia develops, anaerobic metabolism increases, leading to lactic acidosis.	Tachycardia, weak pulses, pale mucous membranes, prolonged CRT (>2 second), hypotension, hypothermia, dull mentation, tachypnea.	Bradycardia or normal heart rate (unlike dogs), weak pulses, pale mucous membranes, hypothermia common, hypotension, dull mentation, tachypnea.
Late Decompensatory Shock	Prolonged hypoperfusion results in cellular death, multi-organ dysfunction, and irreversible shock.	Severe hypotension, weak or absent pulses, pale or cyanotic mucous membranes, hypothermia, bradycardia (rare in dogs until terminal), stupor or coma, agonal respirations.	Marked bradycardia, severe hypothermia, hypotension, pale or cyanotic mucous membranes, weak or absent pulses, stupor or coma, agonal breathing.

Source: Adapted from veterinary internal medicine and critical care texts (Nelson and Couto 2019; Silverstein and Hopper 2015; King 2018; BSAVA 2020).

The veterinary technician's knowledge, clinical suspicion, and swift intervention are often the determining factors in the successful management of shock. Mastery of perfusion assessment, understanding of pathophysiologic principles, and competence in initiating stabilization are essential nursing skills. While veterinary medicine continues to advance, the timeless principles of early recognition, diligent monitoring, and appropriate resuscitative care remain cornerstones of successful shock management in dogs and cats (Table 7.26).

Oxygen Delivery Techniques and Respiratory Patient Support in Canine and Feline Nursing

The administration of supplemental oxygen is a foundation of emergency and critical care nursing. Hypoxemia, defined as a reduction in arterial oxygen tension, may occur due to pulmonary parenchymal disease, airway obstruction, hypoventilation, or circulatory failure. The role of the veterinary technician in recognizing early signs of respiratory distress, initiating oxygen therapy, and supporting both the physiological and psychological needs of the dyspneic patient is critical to successful intervention.

Veterinary patients rarely present with overt cyanosis unless hypoxemia is profound, making clinical recognition more reliant on subtler signs. Early indicators that a patient may require oxygen supplementation include increased respiratory rate, increased respiratory effort (notably abdominal effort or open-mouth breathing in cats), nasal flaring, orthopneic posturing, paradoxical abdominal motion, altered mentation, and audible respiratory noises such as stertor, stridor, or crackles. In some cases, tachycardia or bradycardia may be present depending on the underlying disease process and degree of systemic compromise. Veterinary technicians must also consider that stress, pain, and hyperthermia can all increase oxygen consumption, thus reducing available oxygen reserves. These signs should prompt immediate intervention before hypoxemia becomes life-threatening.

Table 7.26 Fluid restoration parameters in dogs and cats, including crystalloid and colloid shock doses, hypertonic saline administration, resuscitation endpoints, cautions, and recommended monitoring tools.

Parameter	Dogs	Cats	Clinical Notes	Monitoring Tools
Shock Dose (Crystalloids)	80–90 mL/kg IV (blood volume); given in ¼ dose increments (20–25 mL/kg), reassess after each bolus.	50–60 mL/kg IV (blood volume); given in ¼ dose increments (10–15 mL/kg), reassess after each bolus.	Use isotonic crystalloids (e.g., LRS, Norm-R, Plasma-Lyte).	Doppler BP monitoring, ECG for HR, lactate meter, capillary refill time assessment, urine output measurement.
Colloids (Synthetic)	10–20 mL/kg/day; use cautiously due to risk of coagulopathy, renal effects; can combine with crystalloids.	5–10 mL/kg/day; more sensitive to adverse effects; avoid overuse.	Small-volume resuscitation can reduce crystalloid load.	Same as crystalloids; monitor for coagulopathy (PT/PTT) if prolonged use.
Hypertonic Saline (7.2–7.5%)	3–5 mL/kg IV over 5–10 min; follow with crystalloids to restore interstitial volume.	2–4 mL/kg IV over 5–10 min; always follow with crystalloids.	Rapid intravascular expansion; transient effect without follow-up fluids.	Doppler BP monitoring, ECG, follow with fluids guided by perfusion parameters.
End Points of Resuscitation	HR: 80–120 bpm, CRT <2 second, pink mucous membranes, systolic BP ≥90 mmHg, MAP ≥60 mmHg, improved mentation, urine output ≥1 mL/kg/h, venous lactate <2.5 mmol/L or decreasing trend.	HR: 160–200 bpm (may normalize to 140–160), CRT <2 second, pink mucous membranes, systolic BP ≥90 mmHg, MAP ≥60 mmHg, improved mentation, urine output ≥1 mL/kg/h, venous lactate <2.5 mmol/L or decreasing trend.	Endpoints are clinical, not just numerical—tailor therapy to patient.	Doppler BP, SpO_2, lactate monitoring, urine output catheterization, mentation scoring, temperature monitoring.
Cautions	Avoid excessive crystalloids (risk: pulmonary edema, hemodilution). Frequent reassessment every 10–15 minutes.	Highly sensitive to volume overload; monitor closely for pulmonary edema/pleural effusion. Reassess frequently.	Cats especially at risk; use smaller boluses and monitor closely.	Monitor with thoracic auscultation, SpO_2, point-of-care ultrasound (lung ultrasound for B-lines), frequent perfusion reassessment.

Source: Adapted from veterinary emergency and critical care guidelines (Silverstein and Hopper 2015; Nelson and Couto 2019; DiBartola 2020; BSAVA 2020).

Oxygen delivery must be tailored to the patient's size, temperament, degree of respiratory compromise, and tolerance of handling. Several modalities are available in small animal practice, each with variable ability to deliver a fraction of inspired oxygen (FiO_2) and differing requirements for patient restraint and cooperation.

Flow-by oxygen is often the least invasive method and is typically the first technique employed during triage. This method involves holding oxygen tubing or an anesthesia circuit near the patient's nares, usually at a distance of 1–2 cm. Flow-by oxygen is typically delivered at flow rates of 2–5 L/min, achieving a fraction of inspired oxygen (FiO_2) of approximately 25–40%, depending on patient size, distance from the nares, and ambient airflow (Duke-Novakovski et al. 2016; Hofmeister and Brainard 2009). While simple and rapid, flow-by is inefficient and does not provide high FiO_2 unless the patient is extremely cooperative or sedated, which limits its utility in patients with moderate to severe hypoxemia.

Fitted oxygen masks provide a higher FiO_2 than flow-by, typically in the range of 50–60% when a tight seal is maintained and oxygen is delivered at flow rates of 5–10 L/min (Duke-Novakovski et al. 2016; Hofmeister and Brainard 2009). However, this technique can induce significant respiratory anxiety and may worsen dyspnea in uncooperative patients. Heat, CO_2 retention, and claustrophobia may contribute to stress, especially in brachycephalic breeds or patients with airway obstruction. Careful assessment of the patient's stress level must be weighed against the benefits of higher FiO_2.

Oxygen cages or chambers offer the advantage of hands-off oxygen delivery and are generally well-tolerated, particularly by cats. Oxygen enclosures, such as oxygen cages and hoods, can deliver an FiO_2 of 50–60% in standard designs, and up to 80% in high-efficiency units, depending on the seal integrity and flow rate, which typically ranges from 5 to 15 L/min (Duke-Novakovski et al. 2016; Hofmeister and Brainard 2009). The rise in FiO_2 is not instantaneous and may take several minutes to stabilize. One of the primary limitations is that opening the chamber door drastically reduces FiO_2, which must be considered during diagnostic staging. Humidity, temperature control, and carbon dioxide accumulation also become concerns with prolonged use, and close monitoring is essential.

Nasal cannulization is an efficient method of delivering supplemental oxygen while allowing ongoing diagnostics and nursing care. FiO_2 delivery ranges from 30% to 50%, depending on cannula placement and flow rate (typically 50–100 mL/kg/min) (Duke-Novakovski et al. 2016; Rudloff and Hopper 2004). Bilateral placement of cannulas, secured with tissue adhesive and sutures or tape across the nasal bridge and behind the head, provides greater FiO_2 than unilateral placement. This method is particularly useful in small-breed dogs or cats that are too dyspneic to tolerate masks or cages but are stable enough for minor restraint. Excessive flow rates can lead to nasal dryness, aerophagia, or discomfort, requiring humidification in long-term use (Table 7.27).

Veterinary technicians must understand that respiratory anxiety is both a psychological and physiological barrier to stabilization. Increased sympathetic tone, muscle tension, and struggling increase oxygen demand and can worsen hypoxemia. The prevention or mitigation of anxiety in respiratory patients is not optional—it is critical to patient survival. Common signs of respiratory anxiety include restlessness, panicked eyes, open-mouth breathing, exaggerated chest excursions, vocalization, and frantic behavior.

Mitigation strategies involve both environmental control and pharmacologic intervention. The patient should be placed in a quiet, dimly lit area with minimal auditory and visual stimuli. Handling must be minimal and should only occur when absolutely necessary. Veterinary technicians should advocate for rapid, hands-off oxygen delivery first, followed by diagnostic staging only once the patient is more stable. Sedation is often life-saving in the distressed respiratory patient. Butorphanol, a kappa-agonist and mu-antagonist opioid, provides both anxiolysis and mild respiratory depression. At doses of 0.1–0.4 mg/kg IV, IM, or intranasally, it can reduce oxygen demand and facilitate more effective oxygenation (Grimm et al. 2015; Plumb 2018). In patients with upper airway obstruction or severe distress, acepromazine or a short-acting benzodiazepine (e.g., midazolam) may be combined with butorphanol to further reduce anxiety and allow for procedures such as radiography or catheter placement.

Veterinary technicians must assess each patient's stress level and respiratory status before proceeding with any diagnostics. In unstable patients, oxygenation should be initiated prior to radiography or blood collection. Once the patient is more stable or lightly sedated, diagnostic staging may begin in a tiered fashion. Point-of-care ultrasound of the thorax and heart (TFAST/AFAST), pulse oximetry, thoracic radiography, and venous blood gas analysis may all contribute to diagnosis, but each step must be justified against the patient's ability to tolerate handling.

Restraint of respiratory patients must be approached with extreme caution. Physical restraint may lead to panic, worsening dyspnea, or collapse. In many cases, gentle support without direct pressure on the thorax is sufficient. Thoracic radiographs, when required, must be performed efficiently and with attention to the respiratory cycle. Dorsoventral (DV)

Table 7.27 Oxygen delivery techniques in dogs and cats, with approximate inspired oxygen fraction (FiO_2) values and associated clinical considerations.

Delivery Method	Approx. FiO_2 (%)	Clinical Notes
Flow-by Oxygen	25–40%	Simple, well tolerated, requires high flow rates (2–10 L/min). Inefficient as much oxygen is lost. Good for short-term stabilization.
Face Mask	35–55%	Provides moderate FiO_2. Can cause stress or rebreathing if low flow. Suitable for short-term use.
Nasal Cannula (Single)	30–40%	Flow rate 50–100 mL/kg/min. Requires tolerance and secure placement. Risk of nasal irritation.
Nasal Cannula (Double)	40–50%	Provides more consistent FiO_2 compared to single cannula. Higher risk of nasal irritation/epistaxis.
Oxygen Cage/Chamber	40–60% (up to 80% if sealed)	Stable FiO_2, minimal stress. Delayed access to patient. Risk of hyperthermia and CO_2 buildup without venting.
Flow-by in Elizabethan Collar with Oxygen Port	30–50%	Useful for cats or stressed patients. Oxygen accumulates in collar. FiO_2 less predictable.
Endotracheal Intubation with 100% Oxygen	Up to 100%	Maximal FiO_2 delivery. Used in anesthesia or resuscitation. Requires intubation and airway control.
Tracheostomy/ Transtracheal Catheter	40–100% depending on flow	Used for upper airway obstruction. Invasive; requires maintenance and monitoring.
High-Flow Nasal Oxygen (HFNO)	50–90%	Delivers warmed, humidified O_2 at high flow. Improves tolerance and FiO_2. Limited availability in veterinary practice.

Source: Adapted from veterinary emergency and critical care references (Silverstein and Hopper 2015; King 2018; BSAVA 2020; Nelson and Couto 2019).

projections are preferred over ventrodorsal (VD) in the respiratory patient because they reduce thoracic compression, require less manipulation, and allow for a more natural respiratory pattern during exposure. If lateral views are needed, patients should be handled gently with appropriate padding and support. Oxygen supplementation should continue uninterrupted when possible, during radiographic procedures.

Veterinary technicians must recognize their essential role in respiratory stabilization—both in technical skill and clinical judgment. Their actions and advocacy often determine the success of respiratory interventions. Oxygen delivery is not a singular act but a continuum of nursing care, requiring thoughtful assessment, careful restraint, pharmacologic support, and unwavering attention to the patient's response.

Cardiopulmonary Arrest and Cardiopulmonary Resuscitation in Small Animal Patients: Adherence to RECOVER 2.0 (2024) Guidelines

Cardiopulmonary arrest (CPA) is the abrupt cessation of spontaneous ventilation and effective circulation. In veterinary medicine, it is most commonly observed in patients with critical underlying pathology, such as trauma, sepsis, cardiac disease, or profound metabolic derangement. Cardiopulmonary resuscitation (CPR) aims to reestablish spontaneous circulation, ventilation, and tissue oxygen delivery through structured and timely interventions. The Reassessment Campaign on Veterinary Resuscitation (RECOVER) has served as the gold standard for veterinary cardiopulmonary resuscitation (CPR) since its first publication in 2012, and in 2024, RECOVER 2.0 introduced updated evidence-based guidelines reflecting the most current knowledge in resuscitative science (Fletcher et al. 2012; Boller et al. 2024). These updates emphasize algorithmic structure, early recognition of CPA, consistent team-based execution of CPR, and post-resuscitative care to optimize survival.

Veterinary technicians are often the first responders to a patient in CPA and are essential to effective resuscitation. Proficiency in recognizing CPA, initiating basic life support (BLS), coordinating team efforts, administering emergency drugs, and providing ongoing post-cardiac arrest nursing care is vital. This final discussion serves as both a comprehensive clinical guide and an ethical reminder of the technician's role in restoring life with skill and compassion.

Early Recognition of Cardiopulmonary Arrest

Immediate recognition of CPA remains the most significant determinant of survival. Veterinary technicians must maintain vigilance in monitoring critically ill patients, recognizing that CPA may present silently, particularly in cats or in patients under anesthesia. The hallmark indicators of arrest include sudden unresponsiveness, absence of spontaneous breathing, lack of palpable pulses, and absence of detectable heart sounds on auscultation. Agonal gasping—a reflexive, ineffective respiratory pattern—may be present in the initial seconds following CPA but should not be mistaken for functional respiration. Time is of the essence. If CPA is suspected, CPR must be initiated without delay. Pulse checks should never exceed ten seconds. An "assess less, act more" philosophy underpins the RECOVER 2.0 emphasis on early, decisive action.

Basic Life Support (BLS): Chest Compressions and Ventilation

The foundation of resuscitative efforts lies in BLS, which comprises chest compressions and ventilation. Chest compressions should begin immediately and continue uninterrupted, with a goal of 100–120 compressions per minute. The patient must be placed in lateral recumbency, and compressions should be performed over the widest portion of the thorax in most breeds. In keel-chested dogs or cats, compressions are more effective over the cardiac silhouette. Barrel-chested dogs such as bulldogs may benefit from a dorsal recumbent technique with compressions directly over the sternum.

Full chest recoil between compressions is critical to allow venous return. Hands must remain perpendicular to the thorax, and excessive leaning should be avoided. Compression depth should be one-third to one-half of the chest's width. Compressions should occur in two-minute uninterrupted cycles, with rescuers switching roles to reduce fatigue and maintain quality. Chest compression quality directly influences coronary and cerebral perfusion pressure, and as such, interruptions are minimized even during intubation or defibrillation.

Ventilation, while important, must not delay compressions. Patients should be intubated as soon as possible, with ventilation provided at 10 breaths per minute using 100% oxygen. The ventilation rate remains the same whether using manual ventilation with a rebreathing bag or a mechanical ventilator. Overzealous ventilation should be avoided, as hyperventilation can increase intrathoracic pressure, impair venous return, and reduce cardiac output.

Advanced Life Support (ALS): Rhythm Diagnosis, Drug Therapy, and Defibrillation

Advanced life support builds upon effective BLS and requires electrocardiographic (ECG) rhythm analysis, vascular access, and administration of resuscitative medications. Upon completing each two-minute cycle of compressions, a rapid (<5 seconds) rhythm assessment is performed. The RECOVER guidelines categorize arrest rhythms into two primary groups: shockable and nonshockable.

Shockable rhythms include ventricular fibrillation (VF) and pulseless ventricular tachycardia (VT). These patients require immediate defibrillation. A monophasic or biphasic defibrillator is used to deliver one shock at 4–6 joules/kg. After the shock is delivered, chest compressions resume immediately without delay for rhythm reassessment or pulse checks. Repeat shocks, if needed, are delivered every other cycle, with concurrent evaluation of antiarrhythmic therapy.

Nonshockable rhythms include asystole and pulseless electrical activity (PEA). These rhythms are managed through continued high-quality compressions, ventilation, and administration of vasopressors. Epinephrine is the cornerstone of drug therapy, administered at 0.01 mg/kg IV every 3–5 minutes. In cases of asystole or PEA, vasopressin (0.8 U/kg IV) may be used as an alternative or in combination. Atropine (0.04 mg/kg IV) is also indicated in cases of suspected high vagal tone or brady-asystolic rhythms.

Intravenous administration is preferred; however, intraosseous access may be used in small patients or when IV access is not immediately available. Intratracheal drug delivery is considered a last resort and requires a 2–3× dose dilution with sterile saline. The importance of rapid, effective drug administration cannot be overstated. Veterinary technicians must be fluent in dosage calculations, drug preparation, and communication with the resuscitation leader to avoid delays or dosing errors.

Capnography, when available, is an invaluable tool during CPR. End-tidal CO_2 ($EtCO_2$) values >18 mmHg suggest effective compressions, and a sudden increase in $EtCO_2$ is a reliable early indicator of return of spontaneous circulation (ROSC). Veterinary technicians should monitor capnography trends and report changes promptly to guide clinical decision-making.

Post-Resuscitative Care

Successful resuscitation does not end with ROSC. Veterinary technicians play a critical role in intensive monitoring and management that follows. The post-cardiac arrest period is characterized by global ischemia-reperfusion injury, myocardial dysfunction, and risk of re-arrest. Patients require oxygen supplementation, blood pressure support, temperature regulation, glucose monitoring, and seizure surveillance.

Oxygen should be titrated to maintain SpO_2 between 94–98% during post-cardiac arrest care, as recommended by the RECOVER 2.0 guidelines, to optimize tissue oxygen delivery while minimizing oxidative injury associated with hyperoxia (Boller et al. 2024). Hypoxia must be avoided, but emerging evidence also discourages prolonged hyperoxia. Intravenous fluids may be indicated for hypovolemia, but must be balanced against the risk of fluid overload in patients with compromised cardiac function. Positive inotropes or vasopressors may be required to maintain mean arterial pressure above 80 mmHg.

Neurologic support is paramount. Hypothermia may be beneficial in selected patients, though evidence in veterinary species remains inconclusive. Glucose should be monitored closely, as both hyperglycemia and hypoglycemia are associated with poor outcomes. Medical staff should ensure continuous ECG monitoring, accurate urine output measurement, and serial neurologic assessments to document recovery or deterioration.

Veterinary technicians also serve as the patient's advocate. Honest communication with the veterinary team and pet owners regarding prognosis, neurologic status, and expectations for recovery is vital. Many patients who experience ROSC require prolonged hospitalization and intensive care. When recovery is not achievable, technicians must support the team in providing palliative care with dignity and compassion.

Cardiopulmonary resuscitation is the ultimate test of clinical readiness, teamwork, and skill. The RECOVER guidelines offer a precise framework that empowers veterinary teams to act swiftly and decisively. However, the success of these interventions lies not in the algorithm alone, but in the preparedness, training, and clinical intuition of those who implement them.

Veterinary technicians stand at the heart of the resuscitation effort. Their hands deliver the compressions, their voices coordinate the rhythm, and their knowledge fuels the drive for survival. Through continued education, simulation training, and adherence to evidence-based protocols, veterinary technicians elevate CPR from a last hope to a structured, life-saving discipline. As this chapter concludes, let it be a reminder that the technician's role in CPR is not only mechanical, but profoundly human—rooted in competence, courage, and compassion.

Conclusion

Veterinary nursing is a profession defined by resilience, compassion, technical excellence, and an unwavering commitment to the patients who cannot speak for themselves. This chapter has explored the depth and breadth of knowledge required to stand at the forefront of patient care—from stabilizing the critically ill and recognizing the subtle signs of decline, to mastering advanced clinical skills and advocating for evidence-based practice. These pages serve not only as a resource, but as a reflection of the essential and irreplaceable role veterinary technicians play in every corner of the profession.

To be a veterinary technician is to be a healer, a thinker, a protector, and a voice. It is to meet suffering with science, fear with comfort, and uncertainty with skill. It is to hold the line in the moments that matter most, and to find fulfillment not in accolades, but in the quiet triumphs of lives saved, suffering eased, and dignity preserved.

Let this work affirm what you already know deep in your heart: that you are not "just" a veterinary technician. You are a critical thinker, a life-saver, an educator, and an advocate. You are a leader in your own right. May you carry the knowledge gained here with pride, continue to grow in confidence and competence, and never forget the power you hold in your hands—the power to make a difference, one patient at a time.

This is not the end of your learning journey. It is the foundation upon which you will continue to build. Celebrate how far you've come, embrace the challenges still ahead, and stand tall in the knowledge that veterinary nursing is a calling—one that chooses those strong enough to answer.

You are seen. You are valued. You are vital. Keep going. The profession is better because you are in it.

References

Abrams-Ogg, A.C.G. (2018). *Transfusion medicine in small animals*. In: *Textbook of Veterinary Internal Medicine*, 8e (ed. S.J. Ettinger, E.C. Feldman, and E. Côté), 1267–1283. St. Louis: Elsevier.

Acierno, M.J., Brown, S., Coleman, A.E. et al. (2018). ACVIM consensus statement: guidelines for the identification, evaluation, and management of systemic hypertension in dogs and cats. *Journal of Veterinary Internal Medicine*, pp.1803–1822 32 (6). https://doi.org/10.1111/jvim.15331 (accessed 27 June 2025).

American Animal Hospital Association (AAHA), 2010. AAHA nutritional assessment guidelines for dogs and cats. *Journal of the American Animal Hospital Association*, 46(4), pp.285–296. doi:https://doi.org/10.5326/0460285

American Society of Anesthesiologists (2014) *ASA physical status classification system*. https://www.asahq.org/standards-and-practice-parameters/asa-physical-status-classification-system

Bassert, J.M., Thomas, J.A., and McCurnin, D.M. (2021). *McCurnin's Clinical Textbook for Veterinary Technicians and Nurses*, 10e, 106–108. St. Louis: Elsevier.

Beasley, G.M. and Dinn, H.M. (2016). Cardiopulmonary resuscitation in neonatal and pediatric patients. In: *Small Animal Critical Care Medicine*, 2e (ed. D.F. Brobst and K.R. Tilley), 723–726. St. Louis, MO: Elsevier.

Boller, M., Fletcher, D.J., Brainard, B.M. et al. (2024). The RECOVER 2.0 clinical guidelines on veterinary cardiopulmonary resuscitation (CPR): Update and evidence synthesis. *Journal of Veterinary Emergency and Critical Care* 34 (S1): S1–S84.

Brodbelt, D.C., Blissitt, K.J., Hammond, R.A. et al. (2008). The risk of death: the confidential enquiry into perioperative small animal fatalities. *Veterinary Anaesthesia and Analgesia* 35 (5): 365–373.

Brondani, J.T., Luna, S.P.L., Minto, B.W., Santos, B.P., Beier, S.L. and Matsubara, L.M., 2013. Validation of the English version of the UNESP-Botucatu multidimensional composite pain scale for assessing postoperative pain in cats. *BMC Veterinary Research*, 9, p.143. doi:https://doi.org/10.1186/1746-6148-9-143

Brooks, M. (2017). Blood products and transfusion therapy. In: *Small Animal Critical Care Medicine*, 2e (ed. D.C. Silverstein and K. Hopper), 617–622. St. Louis: Elsevier.

Brown, D.C. and Kowalewich, N.J. (2012). Wound lavage: from bench science to clinical practice. *Compendium: Continuing Education for Veterinarians* 34 (3): E1–E10.

Cannesson, M., Besnard, C., Durand, P.G., Bohe, J. and Jacques, D. (2005). Relation between respiratory variations in pulse oximetry plethysmographic waveform amplitude and arterial pulse pressure in ventilated patients. Critical Care, 9(5), pp. R562–R568. https://doi.org/10.1186/cc3799.

Cammarota, G., Ianiro, G., Tilg, H. et al. (2017). European consensus conference on faecal microbiota transplantation in clinical practice. *Gut* 66 (4): 569–580. https://doi.org/10.1136/gutjnl-2016-313017.

CapnoAcademy (2018). *Normal and abnormal capnography waveforms infographic*. https://www.capnoacademy.com/2018/10/03/normal-and-abnormal-capnography-waveforms-infographic/

Chaitman, J., Jergens, A.E., Gaschen, F. et al. (2020). Commentary on fecal microbiota transplantation and its potential to modulate the gastrointestinal microbiome in dogs and cats. *Journal of Veterinary Internal Medicine* 34 (6): 2502–2507. https://doi.org/10.1111/jvim.15936.

Cooper, R.A. and Bowler, P.G. (2003). Wound antiseptics—do they work? *International Wound Journal* 1 (2): 63–70.

Davidow, E.B. (2013). Transfusion medicine. In: *Manual of Veterinary Transfusion Medicine and Blood Banking*, 1e (ed. D.J. Polzin and M.A. Oyama), 71–86. Wiley-Blackwell: Hoboken, NJ.

Davidson, A.P. (2019). Neonatal care. In: *Small Animal Pediatrics: The First 12 Months of Life*, 2e (ed. S.E. Peterson and M.A. Kutzler), 219–226. St. Louis, MO: Elsevier.

Davis, H. and Jensen, T. (2006). Arterial catheterization and blood pressure monitoring. *Clinical Techniques in Small Animal Practice* 21 (3): 122–130. https://doi.org/10.1053/j.ctsap.2006.06.003.

DiBartola, S.P. (2020). *Fluid, electrolyte, and acid–base disorders in small animal practice*, 5the. St. Louis, MO: Elsevier.

Digicare Animal Health (2025). *PocketSigns Reflectance Probe*. https://www.digi-vet.com/Accessories/Monitoring/Pulse-Oximetry/View-All/PocketSigns-Reflectance-Probe.html

Duke-Novakovski, T., de Vries, M., and Seymour, C. (2016). *Veterinary Anesthesia and Analgesia: The Fifth Edition of Lumb and Jones*, 5e, 484–486. Ames, IA: Wiley-Blackwell.

Dyson, D.H. and Maxie, M.G. (2017). Hypothermia in the anesthetized dog and cat: risk factors and treatment. *Veterinary Clinics of North America: Small Animal Practice* 47 (3): 437–448.

Fletcher, D.J., Boller, M., Brainard, B.M. et al. (2012). RECOVER evidence and knowledge gap analysis on veterinary CPR. Part 1: preparedness and prevention. *Journal of Veterinary Emergency and Critical Care* 22 (s1): S2–S13.

Frontiers in Cellular and Infection Microbiology (2023) *Dissecting the role of the gut microbiome and fecal microbiota transplantation in gastrointestinal health.* https://www.frontiersin.org/articles/10.3389/fcimb.2023.1298264/full

Gaynor, J.S. and Muir, W.W. (2009). *Handbook of Veterinary Pain Management*, 2e. St. Louis: Mosby Elsevier.

Grimm, K.A., Lamont, L.A., Tranquilli, W.J. et al. (2015). *Veterinary Anesthesia and Analgesia: The Fifth Edition of Lumb and Jones*, 5e, 160–163. Ames, IA: Wiley-Blackwell, 888–890.

Grimm, K.A., Lamont, L.A., Tranquilli, W.J. et al. (2017). *Veterinary Anesthesia and Analgesia: The Fifth Edition of Lumb and Jones*, 5the. Ames, IA: Wiley-Blackwell.

Grosenbaugh, D.A. and Muir, W.W. (1998). Evaluation of Doppler ultrasonography for measurement of arterial blood pressure in cats. *Journal of the American Veterinary Medical Association* 212 (4): 517–521.

Hackett, T.B. and Mazzaferro, E.M. (2015). Transfusion therapy. In: *Small Animal Critical Care Medicine*, 2e (ed. D.F. Brobst and K. R. Tilley), 697–702. St. Louis, MO: Elsevier.

Harvey, J.W. (2012). *Veterinary Hematology: A Diagnostic Guide and Color Atlas.* St. Louis: Elsevier Saunders.

Haskins, S.C. (2015). Monitoring the critically ill patient. In: *Small Animal Critical Care Medicine*, 2e (ed. D.F. Brobst and K.R. Tilley), 453–460. St. Louis, MO: Elsevier.

HealthManagement.org (n.d.) *A disposable, canister-free negative-pressure wound therapy device.* https://healthmanagement.org/c/icu/issuearticle/a-disposable-canister-free-negative-pressure-wound-therapy-device

Hewson, J. and McCready, M. (2019). Wound management. In: *Small Animal Surgical Nursing: Skills and Concepts*, 4e (ed. J. Heinrich and J.R. Neath), 247–263. St. Louis, MO: Elsevier.

Hofmeister, E.H. and Brainard, B.M. (2009). Monitoring anesthetized patients. In: *Lumb and Jones' Veterinary Anesthesia and Analgesia*, 4e (ed. W.J. Tranquilli, J.C. Thurmon, and K.A. Grimm), 483–486. Ames, IA: Blackwell Publishing; 492–494.

Holowaychuk, M.K. (2016). Blood component therapy in dogs and cats. *Compendium: Continuing Education for Veterinarians* 38 (5): E1–E8.

Hopper, K. and Haskins, S.C. (2015). Clinical blood gas analysis. In: *Small Animal Critical Care Medicine*, 2e (ed. D.L. Carlson and K. Hopper), 108–113. Elsevier Saunders: St. Louis.

Hosgood, G. (2006). Wound healing and management. In: *Kirk's Current Veterinary Therapy XIV: Small Animal Practice*, 14e (ed. J. D. Bonagura and D.C. Twedt), 1194–1199. Saunders Elsevier: St. Louis, MO.

Iizuka, R., Itami, T., Ishizuka, T. et al. (2019). Advantages of a novel device for arterial catheter securement in dogs. *Frontiers in Veterinary Science* 6: 171. https://doi.org/10.3389/fvets.2019.00171.

Kelly, C.R., Kahn, S., Kashyap, P. et al. (2015). Update on fecal microbiota transplantation 2015: indications, methodologies, mechanisms, and outlook. *Gastroenterology* 149 (1): 223–237. https://doi.org/10.1053/j.gastro.2015.05.008.

King, L.G. (2018). *Textbook of Respiratory Disease in Dogs and Cats.* St. Louis: Elsevier.

Lamont, L.A., Mathews, K.A., Carroll, G.L. et al. (2020). Analgesic drugs. In: *Veterinary Anesthesia and Analgesia: The Fifth Edition of Lumb and Jones* (ed. K.A. Grimm, W.J. Tranquilli, L.A. Lamont, et al.), 251–288. Wiley-Blackwell: Ames.

Mathews, K.A., Kronen, P.W., Lascelles, D., Nolan, A., Robertson, S., Steagall, P.V., Wright, B. and Yamashita, K., 2014. Guidelines for recognition, assessment and treatment of pain. *Journal of Small Animal Practice*, 55(6), pp.E10–E68. doi:https://doi.org/10.1111/jsap.12200

MDedge Emergency Medicine (2025). *End tidal capnography in the emergency department.* https://www.mdedge9-ma1.mdedge.com/ed-primarycare/article/88388/end-tidal-capnography-emergency-department

Moon, P.F. and Erb, H.N. (1983). Perinatal and neonatal mortality in the dog: retrospective studies. *Journal of the American Animal Hospital Association* 19 (6): 729–736.

Muir, W.W., Hubbell, J.A.E., Bednarski, R.M., and Skarda, R.T. (2000). *Handbook of Veterinary Anesthesia*, 3e, 39–41. St. Louis, MO: Mosby.

Nelson, R.W. and Couto, C.G. (2019). *Small Animal Internal Medicine*, 6e. St. Louis: Elsevier.

OpenAI (2025). *Cephalocaudal Veterinary Nursing Assessment [Infographic].* Generated using DALL·E, 29 August 2025.

Pavletic, M.M. (2010). *Atlas of Small Animal Wound Management and Reconstructive Surgery*, 3e, 42–45. Ames, IA: Wiley-Blackwell.

Pavletic, M.M. (2018). *Atlas of Small Animal Wound Management and Reconstructive Surgery*, 4the. Hoboken, NJ: Wiley-Blackwell.

Plumb, D.C. (2018). *Plumb's Veterinary Drug Handbook*, 9e, 166–169. Stockholm, WI: PharmaVet Inc.

Radlinsky, M.G. (2016). Negative pressure wound therapy. In: *Veterinary Surgery: Small Animal*, 2e (ed. K. Tobias and S.A. Johnston), 1040–1044. St. Louis, MO: Elsevier.

RECOVER (2025). RECOVER guidelines: newborn resuscitation in dogs and cats—clinical guidelines. *Journal of Veterinary Emergency and Critical Care* 35: S1–S59.

Redondo, J.I., Suesta, P., Serra, I., and Soler, C. (2012). Retrospective study of the prevalence of hypothermia in anesthetized dogs. *Veterinary Record* 171 (15): 374.

Reid, J., Scott, E.M., Calvo, G. and Nolan, A.M., 2017. Definitive Glasgow Composite Measure Pain Scale: Reliability and responsiveness to change in dogs with postoperative pain. *Journal of Small Animal Practice*, 58(6), pp.314–321. doi:https://doi.org/10.1111/jsap.12637.

Robertson, S.A. and Taylor, P.M. (2004). Pain management in dogs and cats. *In Practice* 26 (7): 370–379.

Root Kustritz, M.V. (2006). Clinical management of pregnancy, parturition, and dystocia in the bitch and queen. *Theriogenology* 66 (3): 575–584.

Rudloff, E. and Hopper, K. (2004). Critical care medicine. In: *Textbook of Veterinary Internal Medicine*, 6the (ed. S.J. Ettinger and E. C. Feldman), 501–518. Elsevier Saunders: St. Louis, MO.

Schaeffer, C. (2025). *Veterinary Nursing Strategy*. Hoboken, NJ: Wiley-Blackwell In press.

Schaeffer, D.J. and Dziuk, H.E. (2002). Evaluation of navel antisepsis protocols in newborn calves. *Journal of the American Veterinary Medical Association* 221 (4): 582–587.

Sessler, D.I. (2008). Temperature monitoring and perioperative thermoregulation. *Anesthesiology* 109 (2): 318–338.

Silver, I.A. and Buffenstein, R. (1995). Oxygen transport in fetal and neonatal mammals. *Comparative Biochemistry and Physiology Part A: Physiology* 111 (4): 619–627.

Silverstein, D.C. and Hopper, K. (2015). *Small Animal Critical Care Medicine*, 2e. St. Louis: Elsevier.

Steagall, P.V.M., Monteiro, B.P., Beauchamp, G. and Beauchamp, D., 2022. The Feline Grimace Scale: update and overview. *Journal of Feline Medicine and Surgery*, 24(3), pp.157–165. doi:https://doi.org/10.1177/1098612X221077462

Steffey, E.P. and Mama, K.R. (2007). Inhalation anesthetics. In: *Lumb and Jones' Veterinary Anesthesia and Analgesia*, 4e (ed. W.J. Tranquilli, J.C. Thurmon, and K.A. Grimm), 355–393. Ames, IA: Blackwell Publishing; 375–376.

Sugita, K., Yanuma, N., Ohmori, K., and Momoi, Y. (2019). Fecal microbiota transplantation in veterinary medicine. *Journal of Veterinary Medical Science* 81 (1): 2–8. https://doi.org/10.1292/jvms.18-0454.

Tilley, L.P. and Smith, F.W.K. (2015). *Blackwell's Five-Minute Veterinary Consult: Canine and Feline*, 6e, 992–994. Ames, IA: Wiley-Blackwell.

Thomovsky, E.J., Johnson, P.A., Moore, G.E., and Whitley, N.T. (2016). *Small Animal Emergency and Critical Care for Veterinary Technicians*. Ames, IA: Wiley-Blackwell.

Tobias, K.M. and Johnston, S.A. (2017). *Veterinary Surgery: Small Animal*, 2e. St. Louis, MO: Elsevier.

Tutorials, V. (2020). *How to Perform An Arterial Blood Draw [Video Still]*. YouTube. https://www.youtube.com/watch?v=abc123.

Veronesi, M.C., Panzani, S., Faustini, M., and Rota, A. (2009). An Apgar scoring system for routine assessment of newborn puppy viability and short-term survival prognosis. *Theriogenology* 72 (3): 401–407.

Wardrop, K.J., Reine, N.J., Birkenheuer, A.J. et al. (2005). Canine and feline blood donor screening for infectious disease. *Journal of Veterinary Internal Medicine* 19 (1): 135–142.

Wardrop, K.J., Weiss, D.J., and Thrall, M.A. (2016). *Schalm's veterinary hematology*, 7the. Ames, IA: Wiley-Blackwell.

Weese, J.S., Blondeau, J.M., Boothe, D. et al. (2011). Antimicrobial use in dogs and cats: antimicrobial guidelines from the International Society for Companion Animal Infectious Diseases. *Veterinary Medicine International*, 2011 1–9. https://doi.org/10.4061/2011/163140.

Zanghi, B.M., 2016. Comparison of rectal and auricular temperature measurements in dogs by veterinary practitioners and pet owners. *Journal of the American Veterinary Medical Association*, 249(5), pp.505–511. doi:https://doi.org/10.2460/javma.249.5.505

8

Holistic Veterinary Nursing Approaches

Introduction

Veterinary nursing is a discipline grounded in both technical proficiency and compassionate patient care. Yet, as the profession continues to evolve, there is an increasing recognition that true excellence in nursing extends beyond the mechanical execution of tasks. Holistic nursing approaches challenge veterinary technicians to rise above task-oriented thinking and embrace a model of care that considers the entirety of the patient's needs. This involves assessing not only the immediate medical concerns but also evaluating the patient's emotional state, environment, nutritional needs, pain management, and overall quality of life. In essence, holistic veterinary nursing is a mindset—a way of thinking and practicing that demands critical reflection, situational awareness, and the unwavering prioritization of the patient's well-being.

The modern veterinary technician plays a critical role in patient outcomes, particularly in high-stakes environments such as intensive care units. It is within these complex clinical scenarios that holistic nursing principles become most vital. A patient's survival may depend not only on the interventions performed but also on the attentive eyes, thoughtful observations, and compassionate advocacy provided by the nursing team. Holistic nursing asks the practitioner to think beyond checklists and protocols, continually asking, "What more can I do for this patient?" This chapter explores how holistic nursing can be applied in clinical settings, providing a foundation for whole-patient care that integrates physical health, emotional welfare, environmental considerations, and advocacy through the lens of critical thinking.

Understanding Holistic Nursing in Practice

Holistic nursing begins with the recognition that patients are more than their presenting conditions. While it is often tempting to focus solely on stabilizing vital signs or managing a specific diagnosis, such a narrow approach overlooks the complex interplay between physiological, emotional, and environmental factors that influence recovery. Every nursing action, from adjusting a patient's bedding to advocating for nutritional support, contributes to the broader goal of healing. When these actions are performed with intention and awareness, they become part of a comprehensive therapeutic plan rather than isolated tasks.

One of the foundational concepts in holistic nursing is the understanding that nothing within the patient's experience exists in isolation. This is particularly evident in critical care environments, where small physiological changes can have cascading effects on the patient's overall condition. A patient's altered mentation may not simply reflect fatigue but could indicate underlying hypoglycemia, hypoxia, or inadequate perfusion. Holistic nursing requires the practitioner to observe these subtle changes, connect them to broader clinical patterns, and advocate for timely interventions before the patient reaches a point of crisis (Monroe 2020).

This interconnected thinking also applies to the patient's environment. Environmental stressors such as excessive noise, poor lighting, or inadequate bedding can negatively impact recovery by elevating stress hormones, impairing immune function, and prolonging hospitalization (McMillan 2017). Holistic nursing calls upon the veterinary technician to proactively create an environment conducive to healing, recognizing that comfort measures are not luxuries but essential components of patient care.

Nutrition is another critical element in holistic nursing that is often underestimated in its impact on recovery. Malnutrition and food aversion can delay wound healing, weaken the immune system, and contribute to poor outcomes in critical patients (Brown et al. 2019). The veterinary technician must view nutrition not as an afterthought but as a central therapeutic tool. This includes exploring creative solutions to encourage intake, preventing food aversion through positive feeding experiences, and collaborating with the medical team to ensure appropriate nutritional plans are implemented based on the patient's specific metabolic demands.

Pain management is also integral to the holistic nursing model. Pain is not only a physical experience but also a profound emotional and psychological burden. Patients in pain often experience increased stress, decreased mobility, and diminished will to recover. Veterinary technicians must advocate for appropriate analgesia, using validated pain scoring systems and clinical observations to ensure that patients are not silently suffering. In this role, the technician becomes the voice for those who cannot express their discomfort, ensuring that every effort is made to provide comfort alongside medical care (Mathews et al. 2014).

Holistic Nursing vs. Task-oriented Nursing

This table compares key characteristics of holistic nursing and task-oriented nursing approaches. While task-oriented nursing focuses on completing procedures, holistic nursing emphasizes the patient's entire experience, including physical, emotional, and environmental factors. Understanding the differences between these two models highlights the evolving role of the veterinary technician as both a clinical provider and patient advocate.

The shift from task-oriented care to holistic nursing represents a transformation in how veterinary technicians approach patient care. Rather than focusing solely on procedures, holistic nursing integrates emotional, physical, and environmental awareness into every clinical decision. The table below contrasts the two approaches, highlighting how holistic nursing elevates the technician's role from task completer to proactive patient advocate (Table 8.1).

Historical Development of Holistic Nursing in Veterinary Medicine

The concept of holistic nursing, while often viewed as a modern advancement, has roots that trace back to the very origins of nursing itself. In human medicine, early pioneers such as Florence Nightingale emphasized the importance of environmental factors on patient recovery, recognizing that cleanliness, nutrition, and emotional well-being played critical roles in health outcomes (Dossey et al. 2015). Nightingale's environmental theory, which focused on creating conditions that supported the natural healing process, laid the groundwork for a more holistic understanding of nursing care. Over time, this evolved into broader nursing theories such as Jean Watson's Theory of Human Caring, which underscored the importance of compassion, emotional presence, and the recognition of the patient as a whole being (Watson 2008).

Although veterinary medicine historically focused primarily on physical health and disease management, the increasing recognition of the emotional bonds between humans and their animals has transformed expectations surrounding veterinary care. By the late 20th century, pet owners began to view animals not just as property but as family members, leading to heightened concern for their emotional and psychological well-being (Rollin 2011). This societal shift prompted veterinary

Table 8.1 Holistic patient assessment checklist for comprehensive veterinary nursing care.

Aspect	Task-oriented Nursing	Holistic Nursing
Focus	Specific tasks and procedures	Whole-patient care including physical, emotional, and environmental needs
Mindset	Checklist-driven	Reflective and patient-centered
Assessment	Vital signs and presenting complaint only	Includes behavior, environment, nutrition, and emotional state
Interventions	Administer treatment as directed	Advocate for changes based on nuanced observations
Communication	Minimal, often one-way	Collaborate with clients and the interdisciplinary team
Patient Experience	May overlook stress or discomfort	Actively seeks to improve comfort and reduce stress
Success Measures	Completion of tasks or procedures	Improvement in patient well-being and quality of life

Source: Jennings, M. (2025). Author's own compilation.

professionals to reexamine their approach to patient care, integrating practices that addressed not only physical health but also environmental comfort, emotional stability, and quality of life.

Veterinary nursing developed alongside this cultural change, moving from a largely task-oriented role focused on technical skills to one that emphasizes patient advocacy and whole-patient care. As the veterinary profession became more specialized, particularly in fields like emergency and critical care, it became evident that survival alone was not a sufficient measure of success. Patient outcomes had to be assessed in terms of overall well-being, comfort, and the ability to return to an acceptable quality of life posttreatment (Fowler 2021). This realization paved the way for the widespread adoption of holistic nursing principles in modern veterinary practice.

Holistic nursing today stands as a natural progression of this historical evolution, challenging technicians to think beyond the narrow confines of disease management. By applying concepts originally developed in human nursing and adapting them to the unique challenges of veterinary care, veterinary technicians have redefined their professional identity as caregivers who address the full spectrum of patient needs.

The Role of Critical Thinking in Holistic Nursing

Holistic nursing relies heavily on the application of critical thinking skills. This extends beyond recognizing clinical signs and administering treatments to engaging in active problem-solving and situational awareness. In a holistic framework, the veterinary technician continuously evaluates the patient's evolving condition, interpreting subtle changes in behavior, posture, mentation, and physiological parameters to anticipate needs before they become critical. This form of thinking demands a high level of attentiveness and the ability to integrate diverse information sources into a cohesive clinical picture (Benner et al. 2010). For example, a patient recovering from major abdominal surgery may exhibit restlessness and tachycardia during a postoperative check. A task-oriented technician might simply document the vital signs and administer the next scheduled medication without further consideration. In contrast, a holistic technician will pause to question the underlying cause of these changes. Is the patient experiencing unrecognized pain despite the current analgesic plan? Could hypovolemia or an emerging septic process be contributing factors? Is the patient's environment exacerbating stress levels, thereby influencing physiologic responses? Through critical thinking, holistic technicians move from observation to intervention taking steps to assess perfusion, advocate for a reassessment of the pain management plan, or modify the environment to reduce stress stimuli.

The following flowchart illustrates a critical thinking pathway used by holistic veterinary technicians when evaluating a postoperative patient exhibiting signs of restlessness and tachycardia. Rather than attributing these symptoms to a single cause, the holistic approach prompts the technician to assess pain control, investigate underlying physiological imbalances, evaluate environmental stressors, and communicate observations to the medical team. This structured process highlights how holistic nursing moves beyond task completion to embrace comprehensive, patient-centered problem-solving that supports timely, effective interventions and improved clinical outcomes (Figure 8.1).

Holistic nursing also involves recognizing patterns and trends over time. Rather than viewing a single abnormal laboratory value or vital sign in isolation, the technician assesses the trajectory of the patient's condition. Is the patient's lactate level trending upward despite fluid therapy? Has the respiratory rate steadily increased over the past four hours? Identifying these trends allows the technician to foresee potential deterioration and initiate appropriate communication with the medical team before the patient reaches a crisis point. This proactive approach not only improves patient outcomes but also reinforces the technician's critical role as a frontline advocate for patient well-being (Fowler 2021).

Emotional Intelligence and Its Impact on Patient Care

In addition to critical thinking, emotional intelligence is a vital component of holistic nursing. Emotional intelligence encompasses self-awareness, self-regulation, empathy, and effective interpersonal communication. Veterinary technicians with high emotional intelligence are better equipped to manage the emotional demands of patient care, respond appropriately to client concerns, and maintain positive working relationships with colleagues (Goleman 1995).

Holistic nursing requires the ability to recognize and manage one's emotional responses in high-stress situations. Caring for critically ill patients, particularly those with uncertain prognoses, can elicit feelings of frustration, sadness, or helplessness. Rather than suppressing these emotions, holistic technicians acknowledge and process them, allowing for sustained emotional resilience. This emotional regulation prevents burnout and compassion fatigue, ensuring that the technician remains present and engaged in delivering high-quality patient care (Figley 2002).

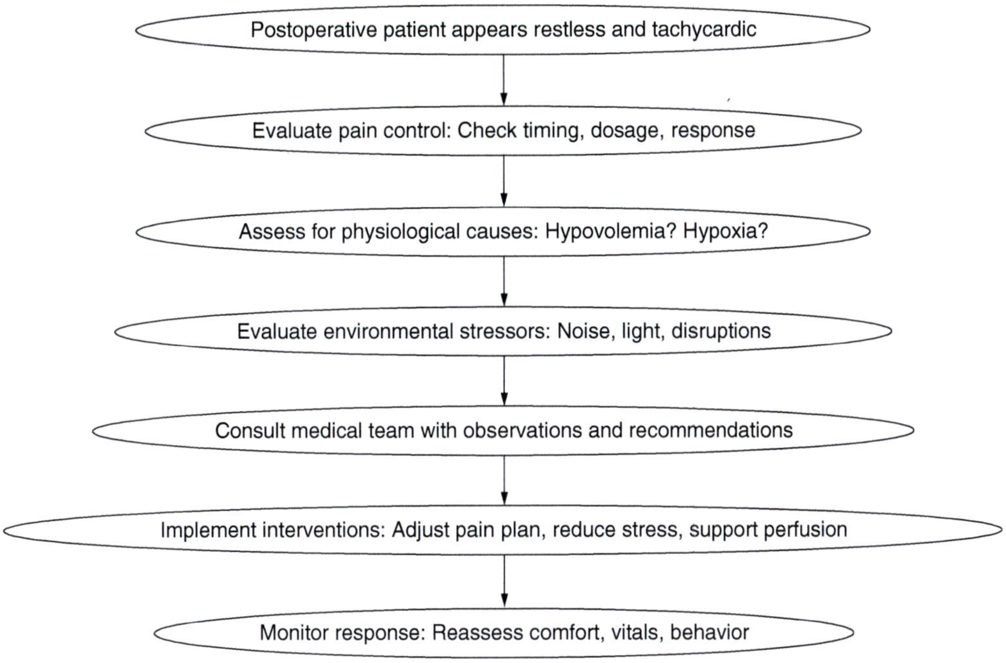

Figure 8.1 Holistic critical-thinking pathway. *Source:* Jennings, M. (2025) Author's own illustration.

Empathy is another critical aspect of emotional intelligence in holistic nursing. Veterinary patients cannot verbally express their discomfort, fears, or emotional distress. It is the responsibility of the technician to interpret nonverbal cues and advocate for interventions that improve not only physical comfort but also emotional well-being. For instance, a hospitalized patient who consistently turns away from caregivers or refuses food may be experiencing emotional withdrawal due to prolonged stress. Recognizing this, the holistic technician might suggest introducing familiar scents, playing calming music, or encouraging short periods of human interaction to alleviate anxiety and promote a sense of safety (McMillan 2017).

Emotional intelligence also plays a pivotal role in client interactions. Veterinary technicians must frequently navigate difficult conversations regarding prognosis, treatment limitations, and end-of-life decisions. Approaching these discussions with empathy and emotional sensitivity fosters trust and facilitates more effective communication. By acknowledging the emotional weight of these decisions for pet owners, technicians create a supportive environment that empowers clients to make informed and compassionate choices for their pets (Johnson 2021).

Applying Holistic Nursing in Clinical Practice

The practical application of holistic nursing requires veterinary technicians to view every interaction with a patient as an opportunity to influence their recovery and comfort. This involves intentional consideration of the patient's immediate surroundings, emotional state, physiological needs, and the broader context of their care plan. Rather than approaching nursing tasks as isolated duties to be completed, holistic technicians understand that every action has a ripple effect on the patient's well-being. Small adjustments to the patient's environment, thoughtful handling, and vigilant monitoring contribute to meaningful improvements in both physiological stability and emotional resilience (Monroe 2020).

One of the most immediate and impactful areas where holistic nursing is applied is in environmental management. The clinical environment can significantly influence a patient's stress levels, which in turn affects immune function, cardiovascular health, and recovery times. Excessive noise, bright lighting, and constant activity can create a state of chronic sympathetic arousal, elevating cortisol levels and impairing healing processes (McMillan 2017). A holistic technician actively works to mitigate these stressors by creating a calmer, more predictable environment. This may include placing a towel over a cat's kennel to provide visual security, ensuring that canine patients receive regular opportunities for quiet rest away from high-traffic areas, and using species-specific calming aids such as synthetic pheromones.

Attention to recumbency care is another critical aspect of holistic nursing. Patients who are unable or unwilling to reposition themselves are at increased risk for pressure sores, compromised circulation, and respiratory difficulties. Rather than waiting for pressure injuries to develop, a holistic technician takes proactive steps to reposition patients regularly, assess for early signs of skin compromise, and implement supportive bedding solutions that reduce pressure points. This level of care requires more than simply following a rotation schedule; it demands careful assessment of the patient's comfort and an individualized plan that supports their physical limitations while promoting optimal circulation and oxygenation (Brown et al. 2019).

Holistic nursing also emphasizes the importance of building positive emotional connections with patients. While it is easy to overlook the value of gentle touch and reassuring presence amidst the clinical demands of critical care, these small moments contribute significantly to patient well-being. A dog recovering from trauma may initially resist interaction, but with patient, gentle handling and positive reinforcement, the technician can help rebuild trust and reduce anxiety. These interactions not only improve the patient's emotional state but also foster cooperation with necessary medical procedures, reducing the need for chemical restraint and minimizing additional stress (Monroe 2020).

Nutrition remains a cornerstone of holistic patient care, particularly for hospitalized patients whose appetite and intake may be compromised. The holistic technician recognizes that food aversion is a common complication of hospitalization, often resulting from negative associations with feeding experiences during periods of illness or discomfort. Preventing food aversion requires creativity and sensitivity to the patient's preferences and emotional state. This may involve offering highly palatable foods, warm meals to enhance aroma, and providing quiet, low-stress environments during feeding times. The goal is to associate eating with comfort and safety, ultimately supporting the patient's recovery through improved nutritional intake (Brown et al. 2019).

Pain management continues to be a critical area of advocacy in holistic nursing. Veterinary technicians are often the first to recognize subtle signs of pain that may go unnoticed during brief medical rounds. A change in posture, reluctance to move, or decreased engagement with caregivers may indicate inadequate analgesia. Holistic technicians use validated pain scales in combination with their own clinical observations to advocate for adjustments to pain management protocols. This advocacy is particularly important in cases where patients may have normalized their pain or become too withdrawn to outwardly display discomfort. By ensuring that every patient receives appropriate pain control, holistic technicians uphold the highest standards of compassionate, ethical care (Mathews et al. 2014).

Holistic Assessment Tools and Nursing Models

The effective application of holistic nursing requires not only a compassionate mindset but also structured tools and models that support comprehensive patient evaluation. These tools guide veterinary technicians in systematically assessing the full spectrum of patient needs, ensuring that critical elements of care—physical, emotional, environmental, and social—are not overlooked. By integrating formal assessment models into daily practice, veterinary technicians enhance both the quality and consistency of care provided across diverse clinical settings.

Holistic Patient Assessment Checklist

In addition to formal models and scales, veterinary technicians can benefit from using structured checklists during daily care. This checklist was developed by the author to operationalize a holistic nursing approach during patient interaction. It is designed to standardize observations and handoffs so no essential aspect of the patient's experience is overlooked. It supports consistent evaluation of physical health, emotional well-being, and environmental conditions throughout hospitalization. The categories were selected because they map to modifiable drivers of patient outcomes (pain, nutrition, mobility, environment, psychosocial state) and align with day-to-day nursing responsibilities, making them practical for shift-based reassessment and team communication (Table 8.2).

One widely used tool in veterinary medicine is the HHHHHMM Quality of Life Scale, which evaluates seven key factors: Hurt, Hunger, Hydration, Hygiene, Happiness, Mobility, and More Good Days Than Bad (Villalobos and Kaplan 2007). Although originally developed to assist pet owners and veterinarians in making end-of-life decisions, this tool also serves as a valuable framework for holistic patient assessments in general and critical care environments. Veterinary technicians can use the scale to monitor hospitalized patients, identify areas where comfort measures need improvement, and advocate for adjustments to care plans when quality-of-life indicators decline.

Table 8.2 Holistic patient assessment checklist (author-developed).

Assessment Category	Key Considerations
Physical Health	Vital signs, pain level, hydration status, appetite, mobility, and presence of wounds or pressure sores
Emotional State	Signs of fear, anxiety, depression, withdrawal, or stress; response to handling and interaction
Environment	Noise levels, lighting, cleanliness, comfort items (bedding, toys), and kennel location
Nutrition	Current intake, food preferences, feeding method, signs of nausea or food aversion
Pain Management	Use of pain scoring tools, behavioral indicators of discomfort, and medication effectiveness
Hygiene	Cleanliness of patient, bedding, and surrounding area; evidence of urine/fecal soiling
Mobility Support	Ability to change position, need for physical therapy or assistance, risk of pressure sores
Behavioral Trends	Changes in behavior over time; tracking patterns such as activity level, sleep, and alertness
Social Interaction	Engagement with staff, interest in surroundings, response to familiar voices or people
Quality of Life	Overall condition and trajectory, signs of decline or improvement, use of QOL tools

Source: Jennings, M. (2025). Author's own compilation.

HHHHHMM Quality of Life Scale

This table outlines the components of the HHHHHMM Quality of Life Scale developed by Villalobos and Kaplan (2007). It is a helpful tool for evaluating the comfort and well-being of veterinary patients, especially those approaching end-of-life care. Each category should be assessed individually to provide an objective understanding of the patient's quality of life (Table 8.3).

In addition to quality-of-life assessments, structured nursing models adapted from human healthcare, such as the Roy Adaptation Model, offer a framework for understanding how patients respond to illness and environmental changes. This model emphasizes the patient's ability to adapt to internal and external stimuli, highlighting the importance of nursing interventions that support physiological stability, emotional resilience, and environmental comfort (Roy and Andrews 1999). Veterinary technicians applying this model assess how well patients are coping with hospitalization and treatment interventions, then tailor care strategies to support adaptive responses. For example, providing familiar bedding, minimizing environmental stressors, and supporting mobility through gentle physical therapy all contribute to positive adaptive outcomes.

Another practical tool is the use of nursing care plans, which provide a structured approach to individualized patient management. Care plans incorporate subjective and objective assessments, identify nursing diagnoses, establish measurable

Table 8.3 Quality-of-life assessment framework for evaluating patient comfort and well-being.

Category	Description/Indicators
Hurt	Is pain adequately managed? Evaluate for signs of discomfort, including vocalization, restlessness, or posture changes.
Hunger	Is the pet eating willingly? Monitor appetite, food interest, and potential weight loss.
Hydration	Are hydration needs being met? Assess mucous membranes, skin turgor, and intake/output.
Hygiene	Can the pet maintain grooming and cleanliness, or is help required? Look for soiling, unkempt coat, and pressure sores.
Happiness	Does the pet express joy or interest in interaction? Consider playfulness, tail wagging, purring, and engagement.
Mobility	Is the pet able to move around comfortably? Assess gait, willingness to walk, and any signs of stiffness or lameness.
More Good Days Than Bad	Are there more good days than bad? Track trends in daily behavior and overall well-being.

Source: Jennings, M. (2025). Author's own compilation.

goals, and outline specific interventions. In a holistic framework, these plans extend beyond addressing medical conditions to include strategies for emotional support, pain management, environmental enrichment, and client education. The consistent use of nursing care plans ensures that each patient receives thoughtful, personalized attention throughout their hospitalization, with clearly documented evaluations and adjustments based on the patient's evolving needs (Monroe 2020).

Holistic assessment also involves the use of pain scoring systems tailored to veterinary patients. Tools such as the Glasgow Composite Pain Scale for dogs and the Feline Grimace Scale for cats provide objective measures of pain that guide analgesic interventions (Reid et al. 2007; Evangelista et al. 2019). These tools empower veterinary technicians to identify and address pain promptly, reinforcing the role of the technician as an advocate for patient comfort.

By integrating these tools and models into daily nursing practice, veterinary technicians reinforce their role as critical thinkers and patient advocates. Structured assessments help transform subjective observations into actionable clinical information, ensuring that the holistic needs of each patient are consistently met and that care remains dynamic and responsive throughout the treatment process (Table 8.4).

The Holistic Patient Radar

The Holistic Patient Radar turns your shift observations into a single, glanceable picture that guides advocacy and handoffs. Eight domains—pain, hydration, nutrition, mobility, hygiene, environment, emotional comfort, and engagement—are scored on a simple 0–5 scale and plotted at two time points (e.g., 08:00 and 16:00). The overlay shows improvement, plateau, or decline, helping the team prioritize action (Figure 8.2).

Good practice means the team uses **consistent anchors** so scores mean the same thing for everyone—here, "3" explicitly signals "needs attention" and "5" indicates "high concern/urgent." With those anchors, a morning Pain = 4 triggers an analgesia review, while an Engagement = 2 prompts low-effort enrichment and environmental adjustments. It is **action-linked**: every low score drives a concrete change (e.g., Pain 4 → titrate analgesia and recheck in 60 minutes; Engagement 2 → quiet-zone signage, dimmed task lighting, and two scheduled interactions), and these actions are documented next to the radar so the plan is visible at handoff. It is also **comparative over time**: two outlines tell the story—AM → PM improvement (Pain 4 → 2; Engagement 2 → 3) suggests the plan is helping but engagement remains a focus; if any domain worsens (e.g., Hydration 2 → 4), the team escalates promptly and adjusts the plan before the next round (Figure 8.3).

Holistic Ethics

Holistic nursing inherently intersects with ethical decision-making, requiring veterinary technicians to navigate complex situations that involve patient welfare, client expectations, and the limitations of available resources. As advocates for patients who cannot voice their own needs, veterinary technicians often find themselves in the center of morally challenging

Table 8.4 Pain scoring tools for holistic assessment: comparison of the Glasgow Composite Pain Scale (dogs) and the Feline Grimace Scale (cats).

Criteria	Glasgow Composite Pain Scale (Canine)	Feline Grimace Scale (Feline)
Purpose	Assess acute pain in dogs using behavioral and physiological signs	Assess acute pain in cats using facial expressions
Scoring system	Numerical score from behavioral categories; higher scores = more pain	Five facial action units scored 0–2; higher score = more pain
Categories/ indicators	Vocalization, posture, mobility, attention to wound, demeanor, appetite	Ear position, orbital tightening, muzzle tension, whisker change, head position
Ease of use	Requires observation and handling; moderate time investment	Quick visual assessment; noninvasive and efficient
Clinical utility	Guides when to initiate or escalate analgesia; validated for post-op use	Useful for monitoring hospitalized cats; sensitive to subtle signs of discomfort
Limitations	Less effective for highly anxious or stoic dogs	May be impacted by sedation, facial structure, or fear responses

Source: Author's synthesis based on Reid et al. (2007) and Evangelista et al. (2019). Jennings, M. (2025). Author's own.

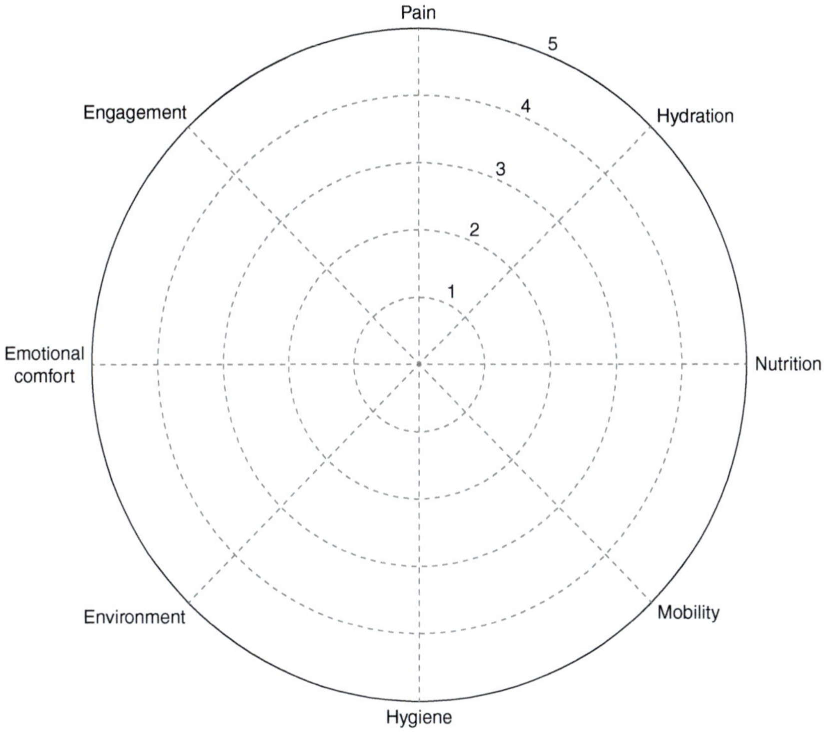

Template: plot two traces (e.g., 08:00 and 16:00). Scale 0–5 across eight domains.
CC0 (public domain)

Figure 8.2 Holistic patient radar template (author-developed). *Source:* Jennings, M. (2025). Author's own illustration.

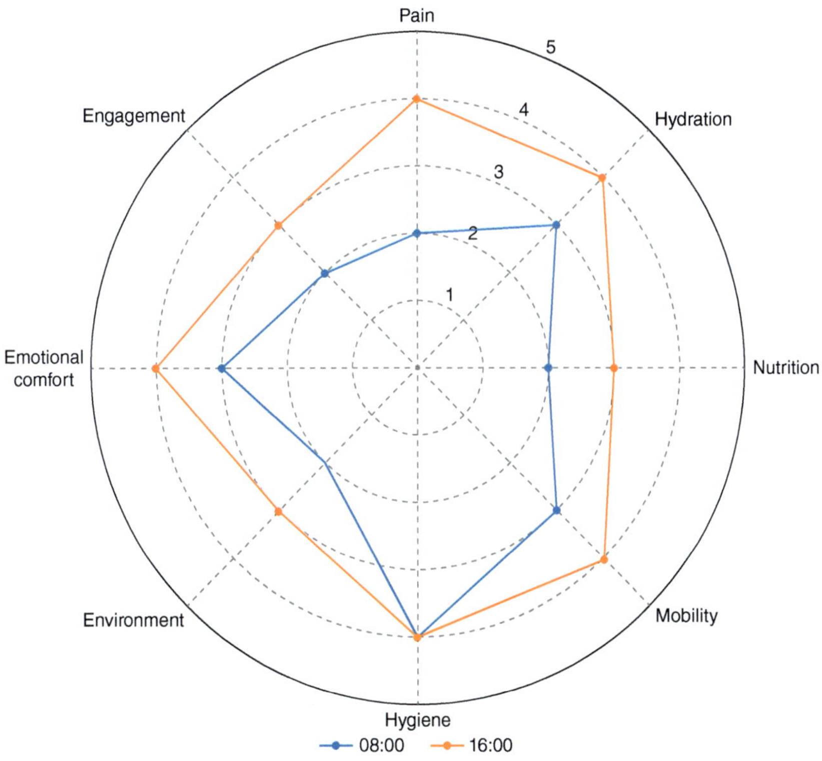

Illustrative values only. CC0 (public domain).

Figure 8.3 Holistic patient radar—shift-comparison template across eight nursing domains (author-developed). *Source:* Jennings, M. (2025). Author's own illustration.

scenarios. These moments demand not only clinical knowledge and emotional intelligence but also a clear understanding of ethical principles such as beneficence, non-maleficence, autonomy, and justice (Beauchamp and Childress 2019).

One of the most frequent ethical dilemmas encountered in holistic nursing involves the tension between pursuing aggressive treatment and preserving a patient's quality of life. While medical interventions may offer a chance at prolonged survival, they do not always guarantee comfort or a return to meaningful function. Veterinary technicians must weigh the benefits and burdens of continued treatment, advocating for decisions that prioritize the patient's well-being even when this means confronting difficult conversations about transitioning to palliative care or euthanasia. The use of quality-of-life assessment tools, such as the HHHHHMM Scale, supports objective evaluations in these emotionally charged situations, providing a framework for guiding clients toward humane, patient-centered decisions.

Financial limitations often add another layer of ethical complexity. Veterinary technicians may encounter cases where the optimal course of treatment is financially out of reach for the client. In these moments, the technician must balance respect for the client's autonomy with the ethical duty to advocate for the patient's welfare. Holistic nursing does not dismiss the realities of financial constraints but seeks creative solutions within those boundaries. This may involve proposing alternative care plans that prioritize comfort, exploring financial assistance programs, or coordinating with charitable organizations to secure support for critical interventions (Rollin 2011).

Veterinary technicians often find that the greatest ethical challenges do not stem from a lack of knowledge or willingness to advocate but from the difficulty of having their concerns acknowledged and acted upon by the veterinary team. Despite being the individuals most closely engaged with patient care, technicians frequently encounter situations where their observations and recommendations are dismissed, particularly in hierarchical environments where the voices of technicians are undervalued. This dismissal can lead to significant moral distress, especially when the technician believes that inaction or inappropriate medical decisions are compromising patient welfare (Fowler 2021). The experience of being unheard is particularly painful when a technician repeatedly advocates for improved pain management, adjustments to treatment plans, or consideration of a patient's declining quality of life, only to be met with resistance or indifference. In some cases, the attending veterinarian may be focused solely on clinical outcomes or procedural goals, neglecting the broader perspective of patient comfort and emotional well-being that the technician brings to the case. This creates a dissonance between the technician's professional responsibility to advocate for the patient and their limited authority to enact meaningful change (Rollin 2011). The emotional toll of this disconnect cannot be overstated. Technicians may internalize feelings of guilt and helplessness when they are unable to prevent suffering despite recognizing clear indicators that a patient is in distress (Rollin 2011). Over time, this persistent moral distress can erode professional satisfaction, contribute to burnout, and even lead some technicians to question their role within the veterinary team. Addressing these challenges requires not only personal resilience but also institutional cultural change that fosters respect for nursing perspectives and encourages collaborative, interdisciplinary decision-making (Monroe 2020).

Ethical dilemmas also arise when clients request treatments that the veterinary team believes are not in the patient's best interest. For example, a client may insist on pursuing aggressive therapies for a terminally ill patient despite significant suffering and poor prognosis. In these situations, holistic technicians must employ empathetic communication strategies to help clients understand the implications of their choices while respecting their right to make informed decisions. Technicians play a vital role in presenting clear, honest information about the patient's condition and likely outcomes, supporting clients as they navigate these emotionally difficult decisions (Johnson 2021).

Workplace ethics further complicate the holistic nursing role, particularly when institutional policies or cultural practices conflict with patient-centered care. Technicians may encounter situations where staffing shortages compromise the ability to provide optimal nursing care or where financial pressures lead to recommendations for unnecessary diagnostics and treatments. In these cases, holistic technicians must advocate not only for individual patients but also for systemic changes that promote ethical, compassionate care across the organization. This may involve participating in ethics committees, providing feedback to leadership, and modeling ethical behavior for colleagues and new team members (Monroe 2020).

Veterinary technicians must develop strong, assertive communication skills to navigate these situations while maintaining professionalism. Using structured frameworks such as SBAR can help technicians present their concerns clearly and objectively, framing observations in clinical terms that resonate with the medical team. When advocacy efforts continue to be dismissed, it may be necessary to escalate concerns through appropriate leadership channels or ethics committees to ensure that the patient's welfare remains the primary focus of care (Benner et al. 2010). Despite these challenges, the commitment to patient advocacy remains a defining characteristic of holistic nursing. Even when their voices are not immediately heard, technicians who consistently advocate for their patients lay the groundwork for long-term cultural shifts toward more collaborative and compassionate veterinary care.

Holistic Approaches in End-of-Life and Palliative Care

Holistic nursing becomes especially vital in the context of end-of-life and palliative care, where the focus of treatment shifts from curative efforts to ensuring comfort, dignity, and emotional peace for both the patient and their caregivers. In these scenarios, veterinary technicians take on a central role in managing the physical symptoms of decline, advocating for compassionate care plans, and guiding clients through some of the most difficult decisions they will make regarding their pets.

A key component of holistic palliative care is the management of physical comfort. Veterinary technicians assess and address pain through frequent evaluations using validated pain scales. They advocate for adjustments in analgesic protocols and introduce non-pharmacological comfort measures such as environmental modifications, gentle handling, and supportive bedding to minimize discomfort. Effective symptom management extends beyond pain control and includes addressing nausea, respiratory distress, mobility challenges, and inappetence, all of which significantly impact a patient's final days (Mathews et al. 2014).

Equally important is the emotional and psychological support provided to both patients and their caregivers. Animals at the end of life are highly sensitive to the emotional states of their human companions and the energy of their environment. Veterinary technicians practicing holistic care strive to create a peaceful, low-stress atmosphere that honors the patient's need for security and comfort. This may include providing quiet spaces, using calming pheromones, incorporating familiar objects from home, and ensuring the presence of trusted caregivers during the final stages of life (McMillan 2017).

For pet owners, the end-of-life phase is an emotionally overwhelming time marked by grief, uncertainty, and often guilt. Holistic nursing includes preparing clients for what to expect as their pet approaches death, explaining the natural processes involved, and offering reassurance that their decisions are being made in the patient's best interest. Technicians provide guidance on creating meaningful moments during this time, such as taking final walks, offering favorite treats, or simply sitting quietly with their pet to provide comfort. These actions help families create cherished final memories and promote emotional healing (Johnson 2021). When the decision for euthanasia is reached, holistic nursing focuses on making the experience as peaceful and dignified as possible. Technicians play an essential role in preparing the environment, ensuring that the setting is calm and private, and that the patient is physically comfortable and free of anxiety. They assist in managing the technical aspects of the procedure while also providing compassionate presence to the family, offering words of comfort, and facilitating time for goodbyes (Villalobos and Kaplan 2007).

After the loss of a patient, holistic care does not end. Veterinary technicians often follow up with grieving families, offering condolences, resources for grief support, and reassurance that their loved one's passing was handled with kindness and respect. This ongoing support helps foster long-term trust between the veterinary team and the community, demonstrating that holistic nursing is not limited to the clinical setting but extends into the emotional lives of those who have experienced loss. In embracing holistic approaches to end-of-life and palliative care, veterinary technicians honor their highest calling: to provide comfort in the face of suffering, advocate for dignity in death, and support the human-animal bond through its most profound transitions.

Fostering Emotional Resilience in Holistic Nursing

Holistic nursing demands a high level of emotional investment in patient care. While this deep engagement contributes to improved outcomes and more compassionate care, it also exposes veterinary technicians to the emotional toll of frequent exposure to suffering, ethical dilemmas, and patient loss. Without intentional strategies to foster emotional resilience, veterinary technicians are at risk for compassion fatigue, burnout, and moral distress, all of which can undermine their ability to provide the very level of care they strive to maintain (Figley 2002).

Emotional resilience is not an innate quality but a skill that can be developed and strengthened over time. It begins with self-awareness, the ability to recognize personal limits, identify signs of emotional exhaustion, and acknowledge the impact that challenging cases have on mental well-being. Veterinary technicians practicing holistic care must prioritize self-reflection, regularly assess their emotional state and seek support when needed. Journaling, peer discussions, and debriefings after particularly difficult cases provide valuable opportunities for processing emotions and maintaining a balanced perspective (Goleman 1995).

Developing healthy emotional boundaries is another critical component of resilience. Holistic technicians often feel a profound sense of responsibility for their patients, which can lead to overextension and emotional depletion if not carefully managed. Recognizing the difference between professional empathy and personal emotional involvement allows technicians to maintain compassionate care without becoming overwhelmed by the emotional weight of every case. This balance enables technicians to remain present and effective in their roles while protecting their own mental health (Monroe 2020).

Mindfulness practices are increasingly recognized as effective tools for cultivating emotional resilience in healthcare settings. Techniques such as deep breathing, meditation, and focused attention exercises help technicians stay grounded during high-stress situations and recover more quickly from emotional setbacks. Even brief moments of mindfulness during a shift—such as taking a few deep breaths before entering a patient's room or practicing gratitude during a lunch break—can reset emotional equilibrium and improve overall well-being (Brown et al. 2019).

Professional support networks also play a vital role in building resilience. Veterinary technicians benefit from connecting with colleagues who understand the unique emotional demands of the profession. Regular participation in team debriefings, peer support groups, and mentorship programs creates a safe space for sharing experiences, validating emotions, and learning coping strategies. These professional relationships foster a sense of camaraderie and remind technicians that they are not alone in facing the challenges of holistic, emotionally intensive care (Fowler 2021).

Finally, maintaining a sense of purpose is central to sustaining long-term emotional resilience. Holistic nursing is a demanding but meaningful practice. When veterinary technicians remain connected to their core values—the desire to alleviate suffering, advocate for vulnerable patients, and contribute to meaningful moments in the human-animal bond—they strengthen their emotional endurance. Reflecting on personal successes, celebrating even small patient improvements, and remembering the positive impact of their work reinforces the intrinsic rewards of the profession and helps mitigate the effects of ongoing emotional strain (Mathews et al. 2014).

The Role of Leadership and Mentorship in Promoting Holistic Nursing

Holistic nursing practices flourish in environments where leadership actively fosters a culture of patient-centered care, critical thinking, and professional growth. Veterinary technicians often look to their supervisors, experienced colleagues, and hospital leadership to model the behaviors and attitudes that prioritize the well-being of both patients and staff. When leadership emphasizes the importance of holistic approaches, it creates a supportive environment where technicians feel empowered to fully advocate for their patients and practice their skills.

Effective leaders understand that holistic nursing is not simply a clinical framework but also a cultural value that must be intentionally cultivated. This involves creating policies and protocols that support comprehensive patient assessments, encourage interdisciplinary collaboration, and recognize the importance of addressing both physical and emotional aspects of patient care. Leaders can promote this culture by ensuring that nursing staff have the time and resources necessary to implement holistic care strategies, including adequate staffing levels, continuing education opportunities, and access to tools that support environmental enrichment and comfort-focused interventions (Monroe 2020).

Mentorship plays a critical role in shaping the next generation of veterinary technicians to embrace holistic thinking. Experienced technicians who have developed expertise in whole-patient care are uniquely positioned to guide less experienced colleagues in moving beyond task-oriented mindsets. Through mentorship, novice technicians learn how to critically evaluate complex cases, advocate confidently for patient welfare, and communicate effectively with both clients and the veterinary team. Mentors serve as role models, demonstrating how to integrate compassion, clinical knowledge, and ethical reasoning in daily nursing practice (Benner et al. 2010).

Structured mentorship programs can help formalize this process, pairing new technicians with experienced technicians who provide ongoing support, feedback, and encouragement. These relationships foster professional growth and help technicians navigate the emotional challenges associated with holistic care, including moral distress and compassion fatigue. By providing a safe space for reflection and discussion, mentors help their colleagues build emotional resilience and maintain a sense of purpose in their work (Figley 2002).

Leadership and mentorship also play a vital role in promoting open communication within veterinary teams. When leaders and mentors model respectful dialogue and active listening, they create a culture where nursing perspectives are valued and considered in clinical decision-making. This collaborative approach strengthens patient care by ensuring that the insights of those most closely involved in daily nursing tasks inform treatment plans and care strategies (Fowler 2021). Ultimately, the promotion of holistic nursing through strong leadership and mentorship ensures that veterinary teams provide not only excellent medical care but also compassionate, patient-centered support that honors the dignity and well-being of every patient. By fostering these values within their organizations, veterinary leaders contribute to a more sustainable, fulfilling, and ethically grounded profession.

Introduction to Case Studies

The application of holistic nursing principles is best understood through real-world examples that illustrate how theoretical concepts translate into clinical practice. Case studies provide a valuable lens for exploring the challenges, successes, and ethical considerations that veterinary technicians encounter when delivering whole-patient care. These examples highlight the critical role of nursing advocacy, creative problem-solving, and interdisciplinary collaboration in improving patient outcomes and ensuring emotional support for both patients and their caregivers. Through these cases, veterinary professionals can visualize the profound impact of holistic nursing approaches across a range of clinical scenarios, from critical care to palliative support.

Case Studies in Holistic Nursing Practice

Case Study 1: Preventing Food Aversion in a Postoperative Feline Patient

A five-year-old, FS, domestic short-haired cat named Luna presented for an exploratory laparotomy following a foreign body obstruction. Post-surgery, Luna exhibited reluctance to eat despite stabilization of her gastrointestinal tract. Recognizing the risk of developing a long-term food aversion, the holistic nursing team implemented a proactive nutritional plan. The nursing staff ensured that feeding times occurred in a quiet, low-stress environment, away from the sounds and smells of the treatment area. They offered highly palatable, warmed foods to stimulate appetite and avoided forcing syringe feeding, which could create negative associations. In addition, a pheromone diffuser was placed near Luna's recovery area to reduce anxiety. When Luna still failed to show interest in food, the nursing team collaborated with the veterinarian to explore appetite stimulants. Over the next 48 hours, Luna began accepting small meals voluntarily. This case highlights the importance of addressing emotional and environmental factors alongside medical interventions to prevent a common postoperative complication that could have led to prolonged hospitalization and poor recovery outcomes (Brown et al. 2019).

Case Study 2: Advocating for Effective Pain Management in a Critical Care Patient

Max, a 12-year-old, MN, Labrador Retriever, was hospitalized following a hit-by-car incident that resulted in multiple fractures and significant soft tissue injury. Despite being prescribed standard analgesics, Max exhibited signs of discomfort, including restlessness, shallow breathing, and reluctance to engage with caregivers. The attending veterinarian was initially reluctant to adjust the pain protocol due to concerns about sedation. The holistic nursing team utilized a validated pain assessment tool, documenting clear behavioral and physiological indicators of inadequate pain control. Armed with this data, the technician advocated for an adjustment to Max's analgesia plan, suggesting a multimodal approach that included both opioid and nonopioid analgesics, as well as local nerve blocks. Following these changes, Max's comfort improved, and his willingness to engage in physical therapy sessions increased, contributing to a smoother recovery. This case demonstrates the critical role of the veterinary technician in recognizing unaddressed pain and advocating effectively for the patient's comfort (Mathews et al. 2014).

Case Study 3: Environmental Modification for a Shelter Dog with Severe Anxiety

Bella, a three-year-old, F, Border Collie mix, was admitted to a rescue shelter exhibiting severe anxiety and fear-based aggression. Her history included prior neglect, and she spent much of her time cowering in the back of her kennel. Recognizing the detrimental effects of chronic stress, the holistic nursing team implemented environmental modifications designed to reduce anxiety and promote positive behavioral change. Bella's kennel was relocated to a quieter section of the shelter, and visual barriers were installed to provide her with a sense of security. Calming classical music was introduced during high-stress times of the day, and synthetic dog-appeasing pheromone diffusers were placed near her resting area. The nursing staff also initiated a structured desensitization program, slowly introducing positive human interactions paired with high-value treats. Over the following weeks, Bella's anxiety behaviors diminished, allowing her to become a candidate for adoption. This case exemplifies the power of environmental enrichment and behavioral support in holistic nursing practice (McMillan 2017).

Case Study 4: Balancing Aggressive Treatment with Quality of Life in End-Stage Disease

Charlie, a 10-year-old, MN, Golden Retriever, was diagnosed with metastatic hemangiosarcoma. His owners initially requested aggressive chemotherapy protocols in the hope of extending his life. Over time, however, Charlie's quality of life began to decline despite ongoing treatments. He experienced anorexia, persistent nausea, and significant lethargy. The holistic nursing team initiated a candid and compassionate conversation with the family, using a quality-of-life scale to objectively assess Charlie's condition. By focusing on Charlie's comfort and dignity, the technician helped the owners understand that continued aggressive treatment was unlikely to provide meaningful improvement. The family ultimately chose to transition Charlie to palliative care, prioritizing his comfort through pain management, environmental modifications, and supportive nursing care until the time of a peaceful euthanasia at home. This case highlights the importance of holistic nursing in guiding end-of-life decisions with empathy, compassion, and a focus on patient-centered outcomes (Fowler 2021).

Holistic Nursing Case Study Summary Table

This table summarizes key elements from the holistic nursing case studies presented in the chapter. It offers a comparative view of clinical situations, holistic interventions, and resulting outcomes to illustrate the practical application of whole-patient care principles (Table 8.5).

Conclusion

Holistic nursing in veterinary medicine is not defined by the mere addition of alternative therapies or wellness strategies; it is a fundamental shift in mindset that challenges veterinary technicians to embrace the full complexity of each patient's experience. This approach moves beyond the mechanical completion of tasks and instead demands an active, thoughtful, and compassionate engagement with every aspect of patient care. From critical thinking and environmental management to emotional intelligence and patient advocacy, holistic nursing empowers veterinary professionals to become true stewards of their patients' well-being.

In clinical practice, this model of care transforms the way veterinary technicians approach each case. Every interaction becomes an opportunity to influence not only the patient's physiological health but also their emotional comfort and dignity. Whether through advocating for improved pain management, recognizing subtle signs of emotional distress, or ensuring that hospitalized patients experience environments conducive to healing, holistic technicians embody a standard of care that elevates the profession and enhances patient outcomes.

The path to holistic nursing requires continuous self-reflection, professional growth, and emotional resilience. It challenges technicians to think critically, act decisively, and communicate effectively across interdisciplinary teams. Just as

Table 8.5 Clinical examples illustrating holistic nursing interventions and patient-centered outcomes.

Patient	Primary Issue	Holistic Interventions	Outcome
Luna (Feline)	Postoperative food aversion risk	Low-stress feeding, palatable warmed food, pheromones, and appetite stimulant	Voluntary eating resumed, no long-term aversion
Max (Canine)	Post-trauma pain under-managed	Pain scoring, technician advocacy, multimodal analgesia, nerve blocks	Pain controlled, improved comfort, and cooperation
Bella (Shelter Dog)	Severe anxiety and fear-based behavior	Environmental relocation, calming music, pheromones, desensitization	Reduced anxiety, became adoptable
Charlie (Canine)	Declining QOL from metastatic cancer	QOL scale assessment, client education, palliative shift	Peaceful euthanasia, family supported and informed

Source: Jennings, M. (2025). Author's own compilation.

importantly, it calls for the preservation of the technicians' own well-being through healthy boundaries, mindful self-care, and connection to a strong professional support network.

As veterinary medicine continues to evolve, the role of the veterinary technician must evolve with it. By embracing holistic nursing approaches, veterinary technicians not only advance their own professional competencies but also play a pivotal role in transforming veterinary care into a more compassionate, patient-centered, and ethically grounded practice. In doing so, they fulfill their highest calling—not simply as caregivers, but as advocates, educators, and champions for the animals entrusted to their care.

References

Beauchamp, T.L. and Childress, J.F. (2019). *Principles of Biomedical Ethics*, 8e. Oxford University Press.

Benner, P., Tanner, C.A., and Chesla, C.A. (2010). *Expertise in Nursing Practice: Caring, Clinical Judgment, and Ethics*, 2e. Springer Publishing Company.

Brown, W.Y., McNeill, C.J., and Young, A. (2019). Nutrition and the hospitalized veterinary patient. *Veterinary Clinics of North America: Small Animal Practice* 49 (2): 307–321. https://doi.org/10.1016/j.cvsm.2018.10.003.

Dossey, B.M., Luck, S., and Schaub, B.G. (2015). *Florence Nightingale: Mystic, Visionary, Healer*, 2e. F. A. Davis Company.

Evangelista, M.C., Benito, J., Monteiro, B.P. et al. (2019). Development of the Feline Grimace Scale: A new tool for acute pain assessment in cats. *Scientific Reports* 9: 19128. https://doi.org/10.1038/s41598-019-55693-8.

Figley, C.R. (2002). Compassion fatigue: Psychotherapists' chronic lack of self-care. *Journal of Clinical Psychology* 58 (11): 1433–1441. https://doi.org/10.1002/jclp.10090.

Fowler, H. (2021). *Veterinary Nursing Care: Theory and Practice*. CRC Press.

Goleman, D. (1995). *Emotional Intelligence: Why It Can Matter More than IQ*. Bantam Books.

Johnson, A. (2021). Communicating with clients during emotional decision-making in veterinary practice. *Veterinary Nursing Journal* 36 (4): 98–104. https://doi.org/10.1080/17415349.2021.1910002.

Mathews, K., Kronen, P.W., Lascelles, D. et al. (2014). Guidelines for recognition, assessment and treatment of pain. *Journal of Small Animal Practice* 55 (6): E10–E68. https://doi.org/10.1111/jsap.12200.

McMillan, F.D. (2017). *Mental Health and Well-Being in Animals*. CABI.

Monroe, J. (2020). Holistic veterinary nursing: Practical approaches for patient care. *Veterinary Nursing Journal* 35 (1): 12–19. https://doi.org/10.1080/17415349.2020.1712371.

Reid, J., Nolan, A.M., Hughes, J.M.L. et al. (2007). Development of the short-form Glasgow Composite Measure Pain Scale (CMPS-SF) and derivation of an analgesic intervention score. *Animal Welfare* 16 (S): 97–104.

Rollin, B.E. (2011). *Practical Ethics for Veterinarians: Animal Welfare in Practice*, 2e. Wiley-Blackwell.

Roy, C. and Andrews, H.A. (1999). *The Roy Adaptation Model*, 2e. Prentice Hall.

Villalobos, A.E. and Kaplan, L. (2007). *Canine and Feline Geriatric Oncology: Honoring the Human-Animal Bond*. Wiley-Blackwell.

Watson, J. (2008). *Nursing: The Philosophy and Science of Caring*, Reve. University Press of Colorado.

9

Patient Advocacy

Introduction

In veterinary medicine, where patients cannot express their needs, fears, or discomfort, the role of the veterinary technician as a patient advocate is both a profound responsibility and a critical component of quality care. Advocacy transcends the performance of technical tasks, requiring the veterinary technician to act as the voice, protector, and champion for each patient's welfare. This role demands not only clinical expertise but also the courage to stand firm in the face of adversity, the emotional intelligence to navigate complex interpersonal dynamics, and the ethical grounding to ensure that every patient receives care that prioritizes dignity, comfort, and well-being.

Veterinary technicians are uniquely positioned to fulfill this role because of their constant proximity to patients and their deep involvement in daily care. While veterinarians often focus on diagnostic processes and treatment plans, it is the technician who spends the most time observing patients, recognizing subtle changes in behavior, and interpreting nonverbal signs of distress or improvement. These close interactions create a bond that positions the technician as the patient's most dedicated guardian, charged with ensuring that care decisions reflect not only medical necessity but also the individual patient's comfort and emotional state (Fowler 2021).

Patient advocacy in veterinary medicine extends beyond direct patient care to encompass communication with clients, collaboration with the veterinary team, and the ethical management of complex medical decisions. It is a dynamic, multifaceted role that requires the veterinary technician to maintain vigilance, speak up when something is amiss, and consistently push for the highest standards of compassionate, patient-centered care. This chapter will explore the depth and breadth of patient advocacy, outlining the essential strategies veterinary technicians must develop to fulfill this role effectively and ethically. Through an examination of real-world case studies, practical communication frameworks, and ethical considerations, this chapter will provide a comprehensive guide for veterinary technicians seeking to enhance their advocacy skills and improve patient outcomes.

The Role of the Veterinary Technician as an Advocate

The veterinary technician's role as an advocate is rooted in the recognition that animals are vulnerable beings who rely entirely on their caregivers for their well-being. In the clinical setting, this dependence extends to the veterinary team, and within that team, the technician often stands closest to the patient's side. Veterinary technicians possess a unique perspective that combines clinical knowledge with intimate familiarity of the patient's daily experiences, making them ideally positioned to speak on behalf of the animal's needs, preferences, and comfort (Rollin 2011).

Patient advocacy encompasses several core responsibilities: ensuring effective pain management, promoting humane handling and stress reduction, identifying unmet physiological and emotional needs, and acting as a liaison between the veterinary team and the client. These responsibilities are not isolated; they exist in a continuous feedback loop that shapes every aspect of patient care. When a veterinary technician commits to the role of advocate, each observation, interaction, and intervention becomes an opportunity to influence outcomes in a way that prioritizes the patient's welfare (Monroe 2020).

One of the most critical aspects of advocacy is the technician's responsibility to ensure that pain and discomfort are properly addressed. Pain in animals is often under-recognized and undertreated due to their inability to communicate directly. Veterinary technicians are trained to interpret subtle behavioral cues that indicate pain, such as changes in posture, vocalization, withdrawal from interaction, and alterations in normal activity patterns (Mathews et al. 2014). Recognizing these signs is only the first step; the true act of advocacy lies in ensuring that these observations lead to timely and effective interventions. This may involve recommending additional analgesic support to the attending veterinarian or suggesting alternative pain management strategies, such as the use of multimodal analgesia or nonpharmacological methods like cold therapy or massage.

Beyond physical pain, veterinary technicians also advocate for the emotional well-being of their patients. Hospitalization, especially in high-stress environments like critical care units, is inherently distressing for many animals. The veterinary technician plays a pivotal role in creating environments that reduce fear and anxiety. This includes thoughtful kennel placement, minimizing exposure to stressful stimuli, incorporating familiar items from home, and ensuring that patient interactions are approached with gentle handling and calm, reassuring communication. The technician's ongoing assessment of a patient's emotional state, and their willingness to speak up when environmental factors are contributing to distress, is a powerful form of advocacy that often goes unrecognized but has a profound impact on recovery outcomes (McMillan 2017). In addition to direct patient care, veterinary technicians serve as advocates during medical decision-making processes. This requires clear, professional communication with both the veterinary team and the client. In cases where proposed treatment plans may not align with the patient's best interest, whether due to poor prognosis, financial constraints, or potential for suffering, the technician must have the courage to raise concerns. Advocacy is not about confrontation but about collaboration. By presenting objective clinical observations and ethical considerations, the veterinary technician supports the team in making balanced, humane decisions that reflect both medical realities and patient-centered care goals (Beauchamp and Childress 2019).

The technician's advocacy role also extends to educating clients. Pet owners often struggle to make informed decisions due to emotional distress, lack of understanding of medical terminology, or unrealistic expectations about outcomes. Veterinary technicians bridge this gap by providing clear, compassionate explanations of the patient's condition, available treatment options, and the potential impact of each choice. In doing so, they empower clients to make decisions that honor their pet's quality of life, often helping to ease the guilt and uncertainty that accompany difficult choices like palliative care or euthanasia (Johnson 2021).

Finally, veterinary technicians act as advocates for systemic improvements within the veterinary profession. By modeling holistic, patient-centered care and participating in quality improvement initiatives, technicians help shape hospital policies that support better patient outcomes. This may involve advocating for standardized pain assessment protocols, the implementation of low-stress handling guidelines, or the development of continuing education programs focused on patient advocacy. In this way, the role of the advocate extends beyond individual cases to foster lasting cultural change within veterinary institutions (Fowler 2021).

Advocacy for Pain Management

Pain management is a cornerstone of compassionate and ethical veterinary care, yet it remains one of the most challenging areas for consistent advocacy. Veterinary technicians stand at the front lines of this effort, acting as the patient's voice to ensure that discomfort does not go unnoticed or untreated. Advocacy for pain management is not a passive role; it requires vigilance, assertiveness, and a deep understanding of both the science of pain and the barriers that exist within veterinary medicine that contribute to its undertreatment.

Recognizing the Complexity of Pain

Understanding the multidimensional nature of pain is the first step toward effective advocacy. Pain is not merely a physiological response to injury; it is a complex experience that includes sensory, emotional, and cognitive components (Mathews et al. 2014). Acute pain, if not adequately managed, can transition into chronic pain syndromes, which are more difficult to treat and severely impact an animal's quality of life. Veterinary technicians must educate themselves on the mechanisms of both acute and chronic pain to effectively advocate for interventions that address the full scope of the patient's discomfort.

Subtle behavioral changes are often the first, and sometimes only, indicators of pain. Species like cats and rabbits, pain behaviors may manifest as immobility, hiding, changes in grooming habits, or flattened ears rather than vocalization or overt limping. Canine patients might exhibit restlessness, pacing, or altered posture. Critically ill patients may become withdrawn, showing minimal engagement with their environment. Veterinary technicians must develop an acute sensitivity to these behaviors, understanding that even minor deviations from a patient's baseline behavior warrant further investigation (Evangelista et al. 2019).

The Ethical Responsibility of Advocacy

Veterinary technicians have an ethical obligation to speak up when they observe signs of unmanaged pain. This is not always easy, especially in hierarchical environments where the technician's voice may be undervalued. However, remaining silent in the face of a patient's suffering violates the foundational ethical principles of beneficence and non-maleficence (Beauchamp and Childress 2019). Advocacy means taking the sometimes uncomfortable step of initiating conversations with attending veterinarians, even when those discussions involve questioning or challenging current pain management protocols. Technicians can strengthen their advocacy efforts by presenting objective data alongside their clinical observations. Utilizing validated pain scoring tools such as the Glasgow Composite Pain Scale for dogs and the Feline Grimace Scale provides concrete evidence to support their concerns (Reid et al. 2007). Documenting trends in behavior, appetite, mobility, and physiological parameters such as heart rate and respiratory rate creates a comprehensive clinical picture that reinforces the need for intervention.

Multimodal Pain Management Strategies

Effective advocacy also requires an in-depth understanding of available pain management options. Veterinary technicians should familiarize themselves with the concept of multimodal analgesia, which involves using multiple classes of medications and nonpharmacologic interventions to manage pain from different physiological angles. This approach typically yields better results than relying on a single medication class and can minimize adverse effects. For instance, a patient recovering from orthopedic surgery might benefit from the combined use of opioids for acute pain relief, NSAIDs to reduce inflammation, local anesthetics for targeted nerve blocks, and adjunctive therapies such as gabapentin or amantadine for managing neuropathic pain. Understanding the pharmacology behind these treatments enables technicians to make informed suggestions when advocating for changes to pain management protocols (Mathews et al. 2014).

Incorporating Non-Pharmacologic Therapies

Holistic pain management extends beyond pharmaceuticals. Veterinary technicians play a crucial role in implementing non-pharmacologic interventions that contribute to patient comfort. Techniques such as cold and heat therapy, massage, therapeutic laser treatments, and gentle physical rehabilitation can significantly reduce pain and improve mobility. The use of comfortable, pressure-relieving bedding and regular repositioning of recumbent patients also prevents the development of secondary pain sources such as pressure sores (Monroe 2020). Environmental considerations are equally important. Reducing sensory stressors in the hospital environment, such as loud noises, bright lights, and constant human traffic, can decrease sympathetic nervous system activation, which in turn can lower pain perception. Nursing staff should advocate for calm, quiet spaces for recovery and limit unnecessary handling of painful patients to avoid exacerbating discomfort (McMillan 2017).

Case Example: Advocacy in Action

Consider the case of Bella, a 10-year-old, Labrador Retriever recovering from a complex orthopedic surgery. Despite having a standard postoperative analgesic plan in place, Bella displayed signs of distress including rapid breathing, reluctance to lie down, and decreased appetite. The nursing staff carefully documented Bella's behaviors and utilized the Glasgow Composite Pain Scale to objectively quantify her discomfort.

Presenting this data to the attending veterinarian, the nursing team recommended a reassessment of Bella's pain management plan. They suggested the addition of a constant rate infusion (CRI) of analgesics combined with local lidocaine patches applied near the surgical site. They also recommend implementing passive range-of-motion exercises and providing padded bedding to reduce pressure on sensitive areas. Within 24 hours of implementing these changes, Bella's behavior improved noticeably. She began resting comfortably, her respiratory rate normalized, and her appetite returned. This case demonstrates the critical impact of nursing advocacy and the importance of a comprehensive, patient-centered approach to pain management.

Advocacy for Emotional Well-Being

While physical health remains a primary focus in veterinary medicine, the emotional and psychological well-being of patients is equally critical to achieving successful outcomes. Animals experience fear, anxiety, and stress in ways that profoundly impact their physiology, recovery rates, and quality of life. Veterinary technicians, through their close daily interactions with patients, are uniquely positioned to assess and advocate for the emotional health of the animals in their care. Recognizing emotional distress and implementing interventions to reduce it is a hallmark of holistic, compassionate nursing practice (McMillan 2017).

Understanding the Impact of Emotional Distress on Recovery

The physiological effects of chronic stress are well documented across species. Prolonged activation of the sympathetic nervous system leads to elevated cortisol levels, which suppress immune function, impair wound healing, increase susceptibility to infection, and contribute to gastrointestinal disturbances such as inappetence and vomiting (Koolhaas et al. 2011). In hospitalized patients, particularly those in critical care settings, this state of constant physiological arousal can delay recovery and worsen prognoses.

Veterinary technicians must understand that emotional distress is not a secondary concern but a critical factor that directly affects medical outcomes. Animals that experience unrelieved fear and anxiety often resist handling, refuse to eat, and show signs of learned helplessness, where they disengage from their environment entirely. Left unaddressed, these emotional responses can create a negative feedback loop that complicates treatment and prolongs suffering.

Identifying Signs of Emotional Distress

Advocating for emotional well-being begins with the ability to accurately assess and recognize when a patient is experiencing distress. Behavioral cues vary by species but often include trembling, panting, lip licking, avoidance behaviors, hypervigilance, and vocalizations such as whining or growling. In more extreme cases, patients may exhibit aggression as a fear response or become completely withdrawn, refusing food or social interaction (Overall 2013). Subtle signs should not be dismissed. A cat that hides at the back of the kennel, a dog that continuously paces or pants despite normal vitals, or a rabbit that sits motionless in a hunched position are all exhibiting classic signs of emotional discomfort. Veterinary technicians must advocate for these patients by ensuring that their emotional states are taken into account during daily rounds and treatment planning.

Creating Emotionally Supportive Environments

Environmental management is a primary tool for supporting emotional well-being. Veterinary technicians can significantly influence the recovery environment by advocating for quiet, low-stress spaces that minimize exposure to loud noises, harsh lighting, and frequent disturbances. Simple measures such as covering kennels to provide visual security, separating prey and predator species within the hospital, and limiting unnecessary handling can dramatically reduce stress responses (Mills et al. 2014). The use of pheromone therapies, such as Feliway for cats and Adaptil for dogs, provides species-specific calming signals that help patients feel more secure. These interventions, while sometimes viewed as supplemental, are critical components of a comprehensive emotional care plan and should be routinely recommended by veterinary technicians when stress-related behaviors are observed (Frank et al. 2010). Comfort items from home, such as familiar bedding or a piece of clothing with the owner's scent, can also reduce anxiety in hospitalized patients. When possible, technicians should advocate for these personal items to be included in the patient's recovery area, particularly for long-term hospitalizations or patients struggling with separation anxiety.

The Environmental Stress Audit translates kennel conditions into a simple 1–5 score across noise, light, traffic, odors/air, temperature, kennel placement, and comfort items. A score of 1 reflects optimal conditions, 3 signals "needs attention," and five indicates high stress requiring prompt intervention. Tallying the domains helps technicians prioritize quick fixes (e.g., quiet-zone signage, dimmed task lighting, relocating kennels, immediate cleanup/ventilation) and bring concrete, environment-focused recommendations to rounds (Figure 9.1).

Environment Stress Audit — 1 to 5 Scale (Author Developed)

Domain	1 (Ideal)	3 (Needs Attention)	5 (High Stress)	Notes/Quick Fixes
Noise	Consistently quiet, minimal alarms	Intermittent noise; occasional alarms	Frequent barking/alarms/ voices	Close doors: alarm etiquette: soft-close bins: sound-dampening
Light	Dimmed at rest; day-night cues	Mixed lighting, some glare	Bright/harsh, lights on overnight	Use task lights, dimmers, cover bright indicators
Traffic	Low traffic: minimal disruptions	Moderate traffic near kennels	High traffic: constant disruptions	Re-route paths: 'quiet zone' signs: cluster tasks
Odors/Air	Nautral; good ventilation	Occasional odors	Persistent odor, stake air	Immediate clean-up; increase ventilation, charcoal/HEPA as appropriate
Temperature	Thermally comfortable	Occasional hot/cold spots	The hot/cold: drafts	Adjust HVAC: add fans/warmers/blankets as indicated
Kennel Placement	Away from noise/doorways	Near occasional stressors	Next to door/ICU hub/loud area	Relocate kennel; add visual/sound barriers
Comfort Items	Bedding/toys as appropriate	Limited comfort items	No comfort items present	Add padding: familiar items if sale

Scoring: 1 = optimal/low stress, 3 = needs attention, 5 = high stress (urgent). Tally total to prioritize fixes.

Figure 9.1 Environment stress audit–1–5 scoring with quick fixes (author-developed).

Gentle Handling and the Power of Positive Associations

Handling practices have a significant impact on a patient's emotional state. Veterinary technicians must advocate for low-stress handling techniques and ensure that all staff members are trained in gentle, respectful restraint methods. The goal is to reduce fear during necessary procedures by using methods such as cooperative care training, minimal restraint, and the strategic use of anxiolytic medications when appropriate (Yin 2009). Positive reinforcement during handling and treatment can help create new, positive associations with the clinical environment. Veterinary technicians play a critical role in delivering treats, verbal praise, and comforting touch during and after procedures, reinforcing the idea that not all interactions within the hospital are negative. Over time, these small gestures contribute to a patient's sense of safety and can reduce overall stress levels.

Case Example: Emotional Advocacy in Action

Consider the case of Jasper, a seven-year-old, MN, mixed-breed dog admitted for treatment of acute pancreatitis. Upon admission, Jasper was anxious but cooperative. Over the course of his hospitalization, however, he became increasingly withdrawn, refused food despite medical stabilization, and began to growl defensively when approached. The veterinary nursing team recognized that Jasper's emotional state was deteriorating and took immediate action. They advocated for moving him to a quieter ward away from the busy treatment area and introduced a calming pheromone diffuser near his kennel. A familiar blanket from home was placed in his bedding area, and handling was limited to essential care only, performed by the same familiar staff members whenever possible to reduce anxiety from unfamiliar interactions. The technicians also implemented a positive reinforcement plan, offering high-value treats and soothing verbal praise during treatments. After two days of this adjusted care plan, Jasper's demeanor improved. He began accepting small meals, his defensive behaviors decreased, and his recovery progressed more rapidly. This case demonstrates how proactive emotional advocacy, led by the veterinary nursing team, can dramatically improve both the emotional well-being and clinical outcomes of hospitalized patients.

Advocacy During Medical Decision-Making

One of the most complex and demanding aspects of patient advocacy is the veterinary technician's role in influencing medical decision-making. While the veterinarian holds the legal and ultimate authority over treatment plans, the technician often has the most continuous and detailed knowledge of the patient's day-to-day condition. This intimate understanding of patient progress, comfort, and response to treatment places the veterinary technician in a critical position to provide meaningful input that shapes decisions affecting the patient's well-being (Fowler 2021).

Understanding the Barriers to Effective Advocacy

Despite their valuable insights, veterinary technicians frequently encounter barriers when attempting to participate in clinical decision-making. Hierarchical structures within veterinary practice often result in a dynamic where technicians feel their observations and recommendations are undervalued or dismissed. Some veterinarians may focus primarily on clinical metrics such as laboratory values or diagnostic imaging results, overlooking the importance of behavioral observations and quality-of-life assessments that technicians are uniquely qualified to provide (Rollin 2011). Additionally, cultural factors within the profession can discourage assertiveness among nursing staff, leading to situations where critical information about a patient's declining condition is not effectively communicated to decision-makers. Overcoming these challenges requires not only a strong commitment to advocacy but also the development of advanced communication skills and confidence in the value of the nursing perspective (Goleman 1995).

The Ethical Responsibility to Speak Up

Veterinary technicians have an ethical obligation to advocate for their patients when they believe that current treatment plans are not aligned with the patient's best interests. This may involve raising concerns about ineffective pain management, prolonged suffering without meaningful recovery, or the need to shift the focus of care from aggressive treatment to palliative support. These conversations can be difficult, particularly when they involve questioning the decisions of senior clinicians. However, remaining silent in these moments undermines the technician's professional duty to act as the patient's voice (Beauchamp and Childress 2019).

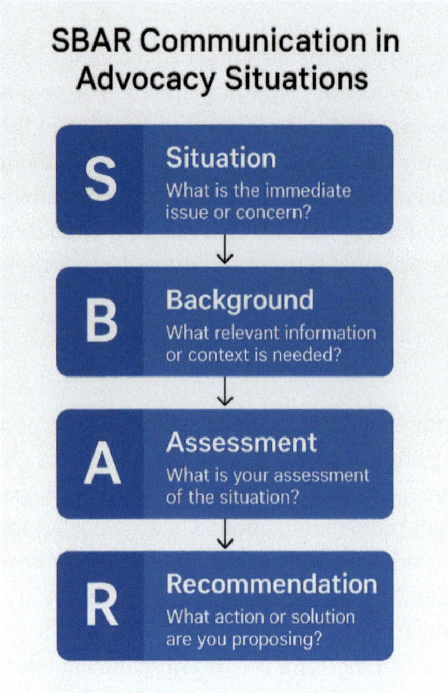

Figure 9.2 SBAR communication in advocacy situations (author-developed). *Source:* Jennings (2025). Author's own illustration.

Technicians must approach these conversations with professionalism, compassion, and clinical evidence. Using structured communication frameworks such as SBAR (Situation, Background, Assessment, Recommendation) helps organize information clearly and objectively, increasing the likelihood that recommendations will be received respectfully and acted upon. This approach allows the technician to present the current situation, provide relevant background details, offer their clinical assessment, and clearly state their recommendation for the patient's care moving forward (Benner et al. 2010) (Figure 9.2).

Advocating Within Legal and Professional Boundaries

While patient advocacy is a core responsibility of the veterinary technician, it must be practiced within the legal and ethical boundaries of the profession. Veterinary technicians cannot independently diagnose, prescribe treatment, or alter medical plans. However, this does not diminish the critical role they play in influencing care decisions. Understanding and respecting these boundaries ensures that advocacy remains collaborative and effective rather than confrontational or inappropriate.

Advocacy within scope involves gathering clinical observations, using validated assessment tools, and clearly communicating patient concerns to the veterinary team. For example, a technician may not adjust a pain medication dose without a doctor's order, but they can, and should, document behavioral indicators of discomfort and recommend a reassessment using pain scoring tools. By framing concerns around objective data and patient welfare, veterinary technicians support better outcomes while honoring the legal authority of the veterinarian. Navigating these boundaries with professionalism is key to maintaining trust and teamwork. When technicians consistently present their concerns respectfully and back them with clinical evidence, they become valued contributors to the decision-making process. Advocacy is most impactful when it is grounded in collaboration, clinical insight, and a clear understanding of the technician's role as both caregiver and communicator (Figure 9.3).

To make advocacy actionable and team-safe, Table 9.1 maps who does the work (R), who is ultimately accountable (A), who is consulted (C), and who is informed (I) across common scenarios—from pain-score triggers and SBAR escalation to discharge teaching and follow-up. Use this matrix to align expectations during rounds, avoid scope creep, and ensure that every low-score or concern raised by the technician links to a clear owner and next step.

Advocating for Balanced and Realistic Treatment Goals

One of the most challenging advocacy situations arises when treatment plans become increasingly aggressive despite a poor prognosis or declining quality of life. Veterinary technicians may observe that a patient is no longer benefiting from medical interventions, yet decisions continue to favor life-extending treatments at the expense of comfort. In these situations, technicians must balance respect for the veterinarian's authority and the client's wishes with their obligation to prioritize the patient's welfare. Advocacy in this context often involves introducing conversations about quality-of-life assessments, using objective tools like the HHHHHMM Scale to support recommendations for palliative care or humane euthanasia (Villalobos and Kaplan 2007). Technicians can play a pivotal role in reframing the conversation around treatment success, not in terms of survival at any cost, but in achieving a life free of suffering and distress. This patient-centered approach ensures that care decisions are grounded in compassion and ethical responsibility rather than solely in clinical outcomes.

Case Example: Influencing Medical Decisions through Advocacy

Consider the case of Luna, a 15-year-old, FS, domestic shorthair cat hospitalized for complications related to chronic renal failure. Despite aggressive interventions, including intravenous fluids, multiple medications, and nutritional support, Luna showed progressive deterioration. She was no longer grooming herself, refused to eat, and remained in a hunched posture, avoiding interaction. Laboratory values continued to worsen despite aggressive treatment. The veterinary technician caring for Luna carefully documented her declining physical condition and emotional withdrawal. During rounds, the technician respectfully raised concerns using the SBAR framework. She presented Luna's current situation, provided a summary of her clinical history and declining laboratory values, assessed that Luna was experiencing significant distress with minimal likelihood of meaningful recovery, and recommended a conversation with the client about transitioning to palliative care.

By presenting clear, objective data and framing the conversation around Luna's quality of life rather than medical failure, the technician facilitated a compassionate discussion between the veterinarian and the client. Ultimately, the family elected for humane euthanasia, grateful for the honest, empathetic guidance they received. The technician's advocacy ensured that Luna's final moments were peaceful and free from unnecessary suffering.

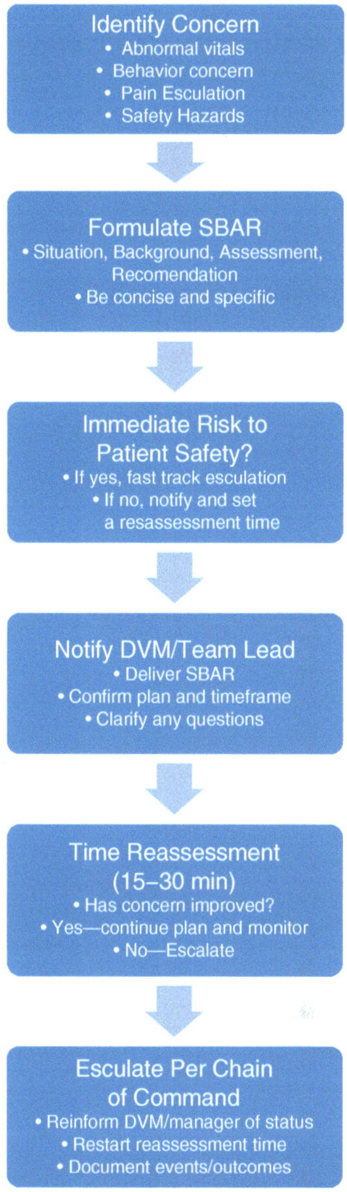

Figure 9.3 Escalation pathway for technician advocacy and patient safety (author-developed). *Source:* Jennings (2025). Author's own illustration.

Advocacy for Supportive and Adjunctive Medical Interventions

While advocacy is often associated with major clinical decisions or ethical dilemmas, some of the most impactful nursing advocacy occurs through the recognition and recommendation of supportive and adjunctive medical interventions. These are interventions that may not directly address the primary disease process but are essential in supporting the patient's comfort, physiological stability, and recovery. Veterinary technicians, due to their close observation of patients throughout hospitalization, are uniquely positioned to identify when these interventions are needed and advocate for their timely implementation (Brown et al. 2019).

Recognizing the Need for Supportive Interventions

Supportive care addresses the secondary challenges that often arise during illness and recovery. These include inappetence, dehydration, hypothermia, nausea, anxiety, and reduced mobility, which can hinder recovery if left unaddressed. Veterinary technicians must remain vigilant in monitoring for these conditions and be prepared to initiate conversations with the medical team when they recognize signs that a patient would benefit from additional supportive measures.

One of the most common scenarios requiring nursing advocacy is inappetence. Prolonged refusal of food leads to a cascade of negative health effects, including delayed healing, immune suppression, and the development of hepatic lipidosis in feline patients. Technicians frequently observe the earliest signs of inappetence, such as turning away from food, lip licking, and restlessness during feeding times. While these behaviors might be overlooked during brief veterinary assessments, the technician's ongoing interaction with the patient provides critical insight into emerging nutritional deficits (Evangelista et al. 2019).

Advocacy in this scenario includes recommending the use of antiemetics to alleviate nausea, suggesting appetite stimulants, and proposing alternative feeding methods such as syringe feeding or the placement of a feeding tube when voluntary intake does not improve. Presenting clear documentation of intake patterns, weight trends, and behavioral indicators supports the case for implementing these interventions early, before the patient experiences severe metabolic consequences (Mathews et al. 2014).

Proactive Intervention for Comfort and Stability

Beyond nutritional support, veterinary technicians must also advocate for adjunctive measures that promote patient comfort and physiological stability. These include maintaining normothermia in hypothermic patients through external warming devices, recommending supplemental oxygen for patients exhibiting signs of respiratory distress, and initiating mobility support plans for patients at risk of developing pressure sores or muscle atrophy due to prolonged recumbency.

Table 9.1 Roles and responsibilities matrix (RACI) for advocacy tasks (author-developed).

Task	Technician	Veterinarian (DVM)	Assistant	CSR/Client Liaison	Lead/Manager
Pain-score threshold reached → analgesia review	**R** (measure, report; propose timings)	**A** (orders/changes) • C	C (observe/ report)	I	C (policy/stock)
Escalation using SBAR/chain-of-command	**R** (prepare and deliver SBAR)	**A** (clinical decisions) • C	I	I	C (escalation pathway)
Environmental modification (noise/light/kennel)	**R** (implement changes)	C	C (set up, relocate)	I	**A** (resources/ approval)
Nutrition plan and owner education	**R** (teach-back; tools)	**A** (diagnose/ prescribe) • C	C	**R** (materials, scheduling)	I
Discharge instructions & demonstration	**R** (demo, verify teach-back)	**A** (final plan) • C	C	**R** (documents, appointments)	I
Rounds handoff (IPASS/SBAR)	**R** (prepare/lead nursing summary)	**A** (approve/modify plan) • C	I	I	C
Holistic Patient Radar (AM/PM trend + action points)	**R** (score and plot; propose actions)	C	C	I	I
HHHHHMM quality-of-life scoring and discussion	**R** (score; communicate trends)	**A** (treatment decisions) • C	I	I	I
EMR documentation (nursing note & care plan updates)	**R** (chart findings/ actions)	**A** (medical orders) • C	I	I	I
Safety event reporting & debrief	**R** (file report; participate)	C	C	I	**A** (investigate/ close loop)
Post-discharge follow-up/ telecheck	**R** (within scope; reinforce plan)	**A** (medical advice as needed) • C	I	**R** (schedule/ confirm)	I
Records transfer/continuity paperwork	I	**A** (clinical sign-off)	I	**R** (send/confirm)	C

Key: R = Responsible (does the work) • A = Accountable (final authority) • C = Consulted • I = Informed.
Note: Adjust to local laws and hospital policy (e.g., prescribing/diagnosing remain DVM accountabilities). If your team prefers one "R" per row, set the CSR as **C** (not **R**) on "Nutrition" or "Discharge" rows and keep the technician as the sole **R**.
Source: Jennings (2025). Author's own illustration.

For example, a recumbent patient recovering from trauma may show signs of discomfort or increased respiratory effort when lying flat. The technician observing these changes should advocate for postural adjustments, the use of supportive slings or bedding to relieve pressure points, and passive range-of-motion exercises to preserve joint mobility and circulation. These supportive measures, while seemingly minor, have a profound impact on both comfort and recovery outcomes (Monroe 2020).

Case Example: Addressing Inappetence Through Advocacy

Teddy, a five-year-old, M, Golden Retriever hospitalized for acute pancreatitis, had not eaten voluntarily for over 36 hours despite stabilization of his primary condition. The veterinary team focused on fluid therapy and pain control but had not yet addressed his ongoing nausea and inappetence. Observing Teddy's repeated refusal of food, lip licking, and restlessness, the nursing staff documented his behavioral cues and presented their concerns during medical rounds. The veterinary technician recommended the administration of an antiemetic such as maropitant and suggested that if no improvement occurred within 24 hours, a feeding tube should be considered to prevent further nutritional decline. After receiving maropitant, Teddy began accepting small meals later that day, and his recovery progressed more smoothly. This example highlights how timely nursing advocacy for supportive interventions can prevent secondary complications and improve patient outcomes.

Advocacy Through Client Education

An essential but often underrecognized aspect of patient advocacy is the veterinary technician's role in educating clients. While the clinician focuses on diagnostics and treatment planning, it is frequently the veterinary technician who spends the most time communicating with pet owners, guiding them through complex decisions, and ensuring they fully understand their pet's medical condition and care options. Effective client education is not simply about relaying information; it is about empowering clients to make informed, compassionate decisions that prioritize the well-being of their pets (Johnson 2021).

Cultural Competency in Advocacy

Veterinary technicians must recognize that patient advocacy also involves cultural competency, understanding, and respecting the diverse beliefs, backgrounds, and communication styles of the clients they serve. Clients come from a wide range of cultural and religious traditions, each of which may influence how they perceive animal care, treatment decisions, and end-of-life considerations. A culturally competent approach helps build trust, reduce misunderstandings, and support decision-making that honors both the patient's welfare and the client's values. For example, some clients may hold beliefs that restrict certain types of medical intervention, such as blood transfusions or euthanasia. Others may prioritize spiritual or holistic approaches to treatment. Language barriers, literacy levels, and previous experiences with veterinary care can also influence how clients interact with the veterinary team. In these situations, the veterinary technician serves as a bridge, ensuring that the patient's needs remain central while respecting the client's worldview.

Advocacy in these cases may include slowing down to clarify information, using visual aids, involving interpreters when needed, or gently reframing treatment goals in a way that aligns with the client's cultural context. It also requires self-awareness, acknowledging personal biases, and avoiding assumptions. By approaching each interaction with openness and empathy, veterinary technicians can provide inclusive, respectful care that supports both the patient and the client in meaningful ways.

Understanding the Emotional State of Clients

Veterinary technicians must approach client education with a deep understanding of the emotional turmoil that accompanies pet illness and hospitalization. Clients often experience feelings of fear, guilt, confusion, and helplessness. These emotions can cloud judgment and make it difficult for pet owners to process information, especially when faced with unfamiliar medical terminology and stressful decisions about their pet's care (Goleman 1995).

Recognizing this, the veterinary technician must employ active listening skills and demonstrate empathy during every client interaction. This involves giving the client space to express concerns and emotions, validating those feelings, and responding with compassion. By creating a trusting, supportive environment, technicians encourage open communication and help clients feel safe in asking questions or expressing uncertainty about recommended treatment plans (Fowler 2021).

Simplifying Complex Medical Information

Clients frequently struggle to comprehend complex medical explanations, particularly during emotionally charged situations. Veterinary technicians serve as interpreters of medical language, breaking down technical information into clear, concise, and relatable explanations. This includes explaining diagnoses, treatment options, prognoses, and potential outcomes using terms that are free from jargon and accessible to individuals without a medical background (Johnson 2021).

Visual aids such as diagrams, handouts, and treatment schedules can further enhance understanding. Demonstrating how to administer medications or perform basic nursing care at home empowers clients and increases compliance. Veterinary technicians should also assess a client's preferred learning style, whether visual, auditory, or hands-on, and tailor education strategies accordingly to ensure information is retained effectively.

Guiding Clients Through Difficult Decisions

One of the most emotionally challenging aspects of client education is assisting pet owners in making difficult decisions regarding their pet's care, especially in cases involving poor prognoses, chronic illnesses, or end-of-life considerations. Veterinary technicians must approach these discussions with both honesty and sensitivity, ensuring that clients have all the necessary information to make decisions grounded in compassion and informed consent (Beauchamp and Childress 2019). In these moments, it is helpful to introduce objective tools, such as quality-of-life scales, to guide discussions and help clients assess their pet's current state. Veterinary technicians play a key role in reframing treatment success away from purely survival-focused metrics and toward considerations of comfort, dignity, and meaningful quality of life. These discussions, while difficult, are often the most impactful moments of advocacy in a patient's journey.

Case Example: Advocating Through Client Education

Milo, a 12-year-old, MN, domestic short-haired cat, was diagnosed with chronic kidney disease and presented to the clinic with severe weight loss, dehydration, and inappetence. The attending veterinarian outlined treatment options, including subcutaneous fluid therapy, prescription diets, and appetite stimulants. However, Milo's owner appeared overwhelmed and struggled to ask questions during the appointment. The veterinary technician took additional time after the consultation to sit with the owner, explaining the condition in simpler terms and demonstrating how to administer subcutaneous fluids at home. She provided a written care plan and used a feline body condition scoring chart to help the owner monitor Milo's progress. Recognizing the owner's anxiety about performing home treatments, the technician offered a follow-up demonstration during a scheduled technician appointment.

By providing ongoing education, reassurance, and resources, the technician empowered the client to confidently manage Milo's care at home, improving his quality of life and reducing the need for frequent hospital visits. This case illustrates the transformative power of client education as a form of advocacy, ensuring that pet owners are not only informed but also capable of providing effective and compassionate care.

Advocacy in Preventive and Wellness Care

While patient advocacy is often discussed in the context of critical illness, hospitalization, or end-of-life care, it is equally vital in preventive medicine and wellness appointments. In fact, some of the most impactful moments of veterinary technician advocacy occur when patients are outwardly healthy. Preventive care offers a unique opportunity to promote long-term health, detect early signs of disease, and protect animals from preventable conditions. By embracing their role in wellness care, veterinary technicians help shift the focus of veterinary medicine from reactive to proactive, and ensure that advocacy becomes a daily, integrated practice.

Championing Preventive Care

Veterinary technicians are often the first to engage with clients during wellness visits, making them ideally positioned to promote the value of routine preventive care. Preventive measures like vaccination schedules, parasite control, dental health, weight and nutritional assessments, and early screenings for breed-specific conditions are foundational to maintaining patient health. During these appointments, veterinary technicians advocate by not only administering care but also educating clients about the importance of these interventions. For instance, when discussing parasite prevention, technicians explain how consistent heartworm prevention not only avoids the disease itself but also mitigates the risks and costs involved in its treatment. Similarly, dental prophylaxis, when implemented early, can prevent oral health problems and systemic infections, contributing to overall well-being. Veterinary technicians should emphasize how these practices prevent pain, improve quality of life, and save owners from unexpected, expensive treatments in the future. By linking the benefits of preventive care to the animal's comfort and long-term health, technicians play a pivotal role in changing how clients view routine veterinary visits.

Technicians also need to foster a relationship where clients feel comfortable asking questions. For instance, clients may have concerns about the cost of preventive treatments or be unaware of their pet's need for certain interventions. By proactively addressing these concerns and offering information in a way that aligns with the pet owner's values, technicians can advocate for long-term health while supporting the client's ability to make informed choices.

Identifying Early Warning Signs

Wellness visits provide the perfect setting for technicians to notice and act upon subtle changes that may indicate underlying health issues. While these signs may seem minor, they can be crucial in catching diseases early, when they are most treatable. For example, changes in weight, behavior, or eating habits could be the first indication of conditions such as diabetes, thyroid imbalances, or kidney disease. Although these changes might not be severe enough for an owner to notice, technicians, who are accustomed to observing patients closely, may detect them.

For example, a technician might notice a dog that has gained weight over the past year and suggest adjusting the diet or discussing exercise plans with the owner. They may observe a cat that is grooming less frequently, which could be an early sign of arthritis or dental pain, prompting a conversation about further diagnostics or pain management options. When these observations are raised with the veterinarian, they not only show the technician's keen eye but also demonstrate their role in keeping the patient's best interest at heart. Early intervention often prevents a small problem from turning into a significant medical issue, reinforcing the importance of regular wellness visits.

Advocating for Behavior and Mental Wellness

Advocacy in preventive care extends to emotional well-being as well. Veterinary technicians are in a unique position to observe behavior that may otherwise go unnoticed, such as anxiety, house soiling, or aggression. Clients may not always bring up behavioral issues unless prompted, so technicians must feel empowered to initiate these conversations. A pet's mental and emotional health is just as important as their physical health, and technicians must advocate for addressing any concerns. For example, when a dog presents for a wellness checkup and shows signs of anxiety, such as excessive panting, pacing, or destructive behavior, the technician should ask the client open-ended questions to gauge the severity. "Have you noticed any changes in your pet's behavior recently, especially at home?" This inquiry can uncover emotional distress that could be linked to environmental changes, new household members, or health issues like pain. When these problems are recognized early, the technician can suggest strategies to manage them, such as anxiety-reducing products, behavior consultations, or changes in the pet's routine. By initiating these conversations, veterinary technicians advocate for the pet's mental health, helping to create an emotionally supportive environment that supports recovery, prevents future behavior problems, and improves the pet's quality of life.

Promoting Client Education and Health Literacy

Clients cannot advocate for their pets if they don't fully understand their needs. Veterinary technicians play a critical role in simplifying complex medical information and correcting misconceptions about preventive care. Educating clients effectively involves breaking down complicated topics like vaccination schedules, parasite prevention, and early screenings into digestible, actionable pieces. Use the Client Understanding Ladder to match teaching to readiness: begin at Functional (plain language and show-and-do with teach-back), move to Communicative (co-planning that fits the home routine and constraints), and, when appropriate, step into Critical (framing options, risks/benefits, and agreeing on next steps). For example, clients may be unaware that indoor pets still require parasite protection or that their pet's weight is a critical factor in overall health; start with a clear explanation, then co-design how and when they'll give preventives or measure food, and finally compare options to align with their goals.

This ladder is an author-developed application of Nutbeam's functional–communicative–critical model of health literacy, using AHRQ's teach-back method and veterinary health-literacy guidance (Figure 9.4).

For clients who may be overwhelmed with medical terminology, the veterinary technician serves as the translator, explaining treatment options, potential side effects, and the benefits of specific interventions. At the Functional rung, avoid jargon and confirm understanding with teach-back ("Can you show me how you'll give this?"). As understanding grows, shift to the Communicative rung by tailoring dosing times, reminder tools, and handling tips to the client's context; when the client is ready, use the Critical rung to weigh alternatives and define what "success" will look like at home. By making sure clients are well-informed, technicians empower them

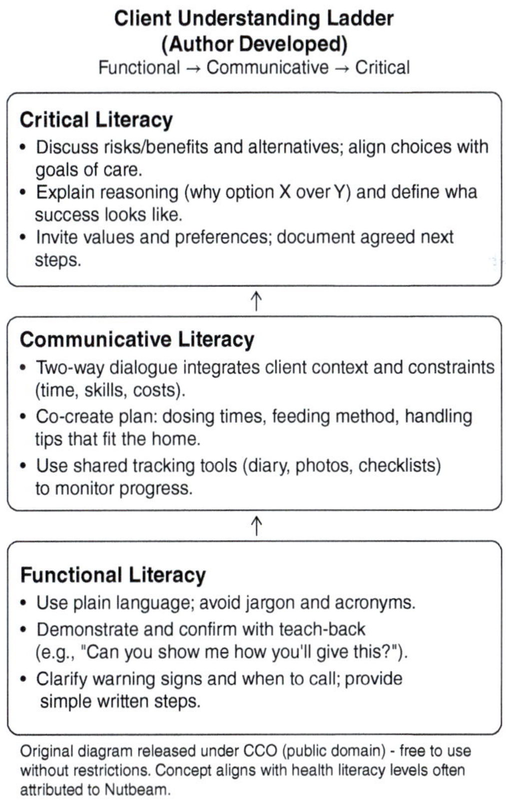

Figure 9.4 Client Understanding Ladder—functional, communicative, and critical literacy prompts for veterinary technicians (author-developed). *Source:* Jennings (2025). Author's own illustration; aligns with Nutbeam's health literacy levels.

to make choices that are not only medically sound but also aligned with their values. Using clear, concise language is key, ensuring clients feel heard and understood. When explaining the importance of early screenings, such as for heart disease or cancer, the technician can gently emphasize how routine diagnostics can catch potential problems before they progress, making treatment more effective and less expensive. For example, recommending an annual blood panel or dental examination can give both technician and client peace of mind, knowing they're staying ahead of any developing health issues. Document the ladder step you used (Functional/Communicative/Critical), the client's teach-back, one barrier identified, and the adaptation made; this keeps advocacy visible in the record and guides the next visit.

Supporting Patients Through Life Stages

Each stage of a pet's life requires tailored preventive care, and the technician's role in advocating for the patient evolves accordingly. During early life stages, advocacy includes ensuring that puppies and kittens receive their full vaccine series, are socialized appropriately, and are given the proper care to ensure healthy growth and development. Technicians advocate for these young patients by educating owners about early care requirements and helping them set up a strong foundation for lifelong health.

For adult pets, advocacy shifts to maintaining wellness through proper nutrition, weight management, and behavioral monitoring. Weight and diet can impact a pet's health far more than most owners realize, and technicians should routinely discuss these factors during wellness visits. In particular, technicians can offer support in addressing challenges such as obesity, poor dental hygiene, or behavior issues, all of which can affect long-term health.

For senior pets, preventive care becomes even more critical. Advocacy for geriatric patients often involves monitoring for signs of age-related conditions, including arthritis, kidney disease, and cancer. Technicians can advocate for early intervention by ensuring that owners are aware of the need for semi-annual exams, adjusted dietary plans, and screenings for common geriatric diseases. By advocating for these proactive measures, technicians help seniors live longer, more comfortable lives.

Preventive Advocacy for the Veterinary Team

Veterinary technicians are often the first line of defense in spotting potential problems in patients, but they should also be vigilant about fostering wellness within their team. Preventive care doesn't just apply to patients; it also applies to the team. Advocating for a healthy work environment, reducing stress, and preventing burnout are equally important for maintaining high standards of patient care. Technicians can advocate for their colleagues by encouraging breaks, checking in with overwhelmed team members, and creating a supportive atmosphere where open communication is prioritized. By ensuring their own well-being and supporting each other, the veterinary team can work together to provide the best possible care for patients.

Advocacy in preventive and wellness care is just as critical as advocacy during acute illness or end-of-life situations. It requires foresight, communication skills, and a proactive mindset. When veterinary technicians embrace this role fully, they help clients understand their pet's needs, prevent suffering before it begins, and foster lifelong bonds built on trust and education. In doing so, technicians affirm that their advocacy is not just reactive, it is anticipatory, intentional, and foundational to every aspect of patient care.

Preventative Care Case Studies

Case Study 1: Preventing Disease in a Young Adult Dog

PATIENT: *"Wally," a three-year-old, MN, Labrador Retriever*
PRESENTING FOR: Annual wellness exam and vaccines

Wally presented for his routine check-up and appeared happy and energetic. During the technician's pre-exam assessment, Wally's owner mentioned he had gained a few pounds over the winter, and they laughed it off as "winter fluff." The technician performed a body condition score and noted that Wally had moved from a 5/9 to a 7/9 since his last visit. His weight had increased by nine pounds over the past year.

The technician took the opportunity to advocate for early intervention in weight management. Instead of simply documenting the weight gain, she explained how even modest weight increases in young dogs can lead to joint strain, reduced stamina, and early onset of arthritis. She used clear, client-friendly terms and offered to create a feeding and exercise plan tailored to Wally's routine. She also recommended baseline bloodwork to check for any underlying metabolic causes.

The client admitted that Wally's portions had crept up and that long walks had been replaced by quick backyard time. With encouragement and a collaborative tone, the technician helped the client understand that this was a perfect time to adjust course, before the excess weight led to more serious health consequences. This preventive advocacy empowered the owner to take action and preserved Wally's long-term health through simple lifestyle changes.

Case Study 2: Addressing Dental Disease in a Middle-Aged Cat

PATIENT: *"Mittens," an eight-year-old, FS, domestic shorthair cat*
PRESENTING FOR: Semiannual wellness exam

Mittens was presented for a routine visit with no complaints from the owner. During the physical exam, the technician noticed mild dental tartar, gingivitis, and a faint but distinct odor from the mouth. When asked about Mittens' eating habits, the owner said she was still eating "just fine" and hadn't shown any signs of discomfort. The technician explained that cats are skilled at hiding pain and that eating normally does not rule out oral discomfort. She discussed how chronic dental inflammation can contribute to systemic inflammation, heart and kidney strain, and progressive pain. The client had never considered a dental cleaning for Mittens, believing that indoor cats had minimal dental risk. Using an educational dental chart, the technician demonstrated the progression of periodontal disease and offered a detailed explanation of what a prophylactic cleaning would entail. The technician also brought up the long-term benefits of treating dental disease early, before extractions would be necessary. She advocated for a treatment plan not because of obvious distress, but to **prevent** future discomfort. Her clinical observations and calm, educational approach reassured the owner, who ultimately agreed to schedule a dental procedure for the following month.

Case Study 3: Supporting a Senior Dog Through Wellness Transitions

PATIENT: *"Toby," a 12-year-old, MN, Border Collie mix*
PRESENTING FOR: Annual exam and medication refill

Toby had been a long-time patient at the clinic. His owner requested a refill for Toby's arthritis medication during his yearly exam. The technician conducting the intake noticed that Toby was slower to rise than in past visits and had difficulty stepping onto the scale. The owner said, "He's just getting older, nothing to be done." Rather than accept this as normal aging, the technician gently pointed out Toby's mobility changes and advocated for a quality-of-life assessment. She explained that while aging is inevitable, suffering is not. There were several noninvasive tools the team could use to assess pain more thoroughly, and additional options like laser therapy, joint supplements, or adjustments to his current medication protocol that could improve comfort. The owner seemed hesitant at first, fearing the conversation was headed toward end-of-life care. The technician clarified that the goal was to enhance Toby's golden years, not shorten them. Her advocacy shifted the tone of the appointment from resignation to empowerment. The client agreed to additional diagnostics and left with a new care plan aimed at improving comfort, not just managing decline.

Building Confidence as a Patient Advocate

Confidence is an essential trait for effective patient advocacy, yet many veterinary technicians struggle with self-doubt when attempting to assert their observations and recommendations. This hesitation often stems from imposter syndrome, a psychological pattern where individuals doubt their skills and fear being exposed as inadequate despite their competence (Clance and Imes 1978). In the hierarchical structure of veterinary medicine, where technicians may feel subordinate to veterinarians and practice managers, it becomes even more challenging to voice concerns, particularly when those concerns challenge existing treatment plans.

Building confidence as a patient advocate begins with acknowledging the value and validity of the nursing perspective. Veterinary technicians are uniquely positioned to observe behavioral, physiological, and emotional changes in patients that may not be evident during brief veterinary examinations. Recognizing this proximity as a form of clinical expertise helps technicians understand that their insights are not only valuable but critical to patient welfare (Fowler 2021).

Mentorship is a powerful tool for developing advocacy confidence. Experienced technicians can provide guidance, share strategies for effective communication, and model assertive behavior in clinical settings. Through mentorship, newer technicians can gain the courage to voice their observations, knowing they have the support of more seasoned colleagues. Structured mentorship programs also create opportunities for case discussions and role-playing exercises, which help technicians practice presenting their recommendations with clarity and professionalism (Benner et al. 2010).

Developing assertive communication skills is another key component of building confidence. Veterinary technicians should practice using structured communication tools such as SBAR (Situation, Background, Assessment, Recommendation) to clearly articulate their concerns and proposed solutions. This framework enables technicians to present clinical observations objectively and professionally, reducing the fear of being dismissed or disregarded (Beauchamp and Childress 2019).

Finally, small victories in advocacy efforts should be celebrated. Each successful intervention, no matter how minor, reinforces a technician's belief in their ability to make a meaningful impact. Over time, these experiences build a foundation of confidence that empowers veterinary technicians to become strong, unwavering voices for their patients.

Navigating Conflict in Advocacy

Advocacy often requires veterinary technicians to navigate conflict, whether it arises from disagreement with a veterinarian, differing opinions among nursing staff, or a client's resistance to recommended care. Conflict is a natural part of the advocacy process, but when handled skillfully, it can lead to better patient outcomes and stronger professional relationships. The first step in managing conflict is recognizing that disagreement does not equate to disrespect. Differing perspectives often stem from unique professional experiences, varying ethical frameworks, or differing interpretations of clinical data. Veterinary technicians should approach conflicts with curiosity rather than confrontation, seeking to understand the other party's viewpoint before presenting their own (Goleman 1995).

Using emotional intelligence is critical when navigating conflict. This involves self-regulation to prevent defensive or emotional reactions, empathy to understand the motivations and concerns of others, and social skills to facilitate open, respectful dialogue. Veterinary technicians must remain calm and focused on the patient's welfare, using objective data and clinical observations to support their advocacy efforts (Goleman 1995). When conflict arises with clients, technicians should employ compassionate communication strategies. This includes active listening, validating the client's emotions, and gently guiding them toward informed decisions through education and reassurance. Offering clear explanations of the patient's condition and the potential consequences of various choices helps clients feel empowered rather than pressured, reducing the likelihood of confrontation (Johnson 2021). In cases where conflict persists despite these efforts, veterinary technicians should seek support from practice managers or hospital leadership. Escalating concerns through appropriate channels ensures that patient advocacy remains a priority while maintaining professional decorum and team cohesion.

Ethical Considerations in Patient Advocacy

Patient advocacy is deeply rooted in ethical responsibility. Veterinary technicians must constantly navigate situations where competing interests, such as the client's wishes, financial limitations, and the patient's best interests, create ethical dilemmas. Effective advocacy requires a thorough understanding of ethical principles and the courage to act in alignment with them, even when doing so is challenging (Beauchamp and Childress 2019).

Utilitarianism, deontology, and virtue ethics provide frameworks for ethical decision-making in advocacy. Utilitarianism focuses on achieving the greatest good for the greatest number, often guiding decisions around resource allocation in shelters or critical care settings. Deontology emphasizes adherence to professional duties and ethical codes, requiring technicians to advocate for humane treatment regardless of potential conflicts. Virtue ethics centers on the character of the technician, promoting honesty, compassion, and integrity in all interactions (Rollin 2011).

Moral distress frequently arises when technicians recognize the ethically appropriate course of action but are constrained by external factors, such as client finances or hospital policies. Left unaddressed, moral distress can lead to burnout and reduced job satisfaction. Veterinary technicians must develop strategies to manage moral distress, including seeking mentorship, participating in ethics discussions, and engaging with hospital leadership to advocate for systemic changes that support ethical patient care (Figley 2002). By grounding their advocacy efforts in well-established ethical frameworks, veterinary technicians can navigate even the most difficult situations with confidence and clarity, ensuring that their actions remain focused on the patient's welfare above all else.

Advocating for Vulnerable Patient Populations

Certain patient populations require heightened levels of advocacy due to their increased vulnerability. Geriatric patients, neonates, exotic species, and shelter animals face unique challenges that demand specialized nursing interventions and a proactive approach to ensuring their welfare. Geriatric patients often suffer from multiple chronic conditions and may experience cognitive decline, reduced mobility, and chronic pain. Advocacy for these patients involves ensuring that pain management protocols are consistently applied, promoting environmental modifications to support mobility, and initiating discussions about quality-of-life considerations when aggressive treatments may no longer be appropriate (Mathews et al. 2014).

Neonates require vigilant monitoring and immediate intervention when signs of distress appear. Veterinary technicians must advocate for appropriate environmental support, including thermoregulation, nutritional supplementation, and careful monitoring for early signs of failure to thrive. Advocacy also includes ensuring that nursing protocols for neonates are clearly documented and followed consistently by all members of the veterinary team (Brown et al. 2019). Shelter animals often enter veterinary care with a history of neglect, malnutrition, and emotional trauma. These patients benefit greatly from environmental enrichment, gentle handling, and a structured approach to behavior modification. Advocacy in shelter medicine also involves working with rescue organizations to secure funding for necessary treatments and ensuring that resources are distributed equitably among high-need cases (Rollin 2011).

The Future of Patient Advocacy in Veterinary Medicine

The role of the veterinary technician as a patient advocate will continue to expand as the profession evolves. Advances in telemedicine, pain management, and integrative therapies are reshaping how care is delivered, providing new opportunities for technicians to influence treatment plans and improve patient outcomes (Fowler 2021).

Telemedicine platforms offer expanded access to veterinary care, particularly for underserved communities. Veterinary technicians can play a critical role in telehealth consultations by educating clients, performing virtual patient assessments, and ensuring that remote care plans address both the medical and emotional needs of patients. As technology becomes more integrated into veterinary practice, technicians will need to develop new competencies in virtual communication and remote patient monitoring.

Pain management continues to advance, with new medications and therapies emerging to address chronic pain and improve quality of life for aging and critically ill patients. Veterinary technicians must stay informed about these advancements to advocate effectively for modern, evidence-based pain control protocols (Mathews et al. 2014).

The integration of veterinary social work into clinical practice offers another exciting avenue for expanding patient advocacy. By collaborating with social workers, veterinary technicians can better support clients facing emotional, financial, or logistical barriers to providing optimal care for their pets. This interdisciplinary approach enhances patient outcomes and reinforces the veterinary technician's role as a holistic caregiver and advocate (Johnson 2021). As the profession continues to embrace patient-centered care models, veterinary technicians will remain at the forefront of this cultural shift, ensuring that every patient receives compassionate, dignified, and ethically grounded care.

Advocacy Within the Support Staff Team

While much of patient advocacy focuses on interactions with veterinarians and clients, veterinary technicians must also be prepared to advocate within their own team. Technician-to-technician advocacy involves supporting colleagues, speaking up about unsafe practices, and fostering a workplace culture where every technician feels empowered to act in the patient's best interest. These internal dynamics are essential to maintaining consistent, high-quality care across the veterinary team.

Veterinary technicians often work in fast-paced, emotionally intense environments where stress, fatigue, and burnout can impair clinical judgment or lead to oversights. In these situations, technicians must look out for one another, whether that means offering help during a busy shift, checking in on a colleague's emotional well-being, or tactfully addressing a missed

Am I Advocating for My Patient?

This reflective tool helps veterinary technicians assess whether they are fully supporting their patients in both medical and non-medical dimensions.

- ☐ Have I identified any unmet needs (e.g., pain, nutrition, emotional comfort)?
- ☐ Have I clearly communicated concerns to the veterinary team using an organized format (e.g. SBAR)?
- ☐ Have I educated the client about the patient's needs in clear, compassionate language?
- ☐ Have I checked for signs of discomfort or stress that may not be outwardly visible?
- ☐ Have I advocated for diagnostic testing or interventions when early disease is suspected?
- ☐ Have I provided reassurance and clarification to the client when uncertainty arises?
- ☐ Have I acted with empathy while maintaining clinical objectivity?
- ☐ Have I supported my fellow veterinary technicians to ensure team-wide patient advocacy?

Figure 9.5 "Am I Advocating for My Patient?"—reflective checklist (author-developed). *Source:* Jennings (2025). Author's own illustration.

protocol that could impact patient safety. Effective technician-to-technician advocacy is grounded in mutual respect and shared responsibility.

Supporting less experienced technicians is another vital form of advocacy. New graduates or junior team members may hesitate to voice concerns or make recommendations, even when they notice something clinically significant. Senior technicians can advocate for their colleagues by encouraging open dialogue, validating their observations, and mentoring them in confident communication strategies. When technicians advocate for each other, the result is a stronger, more cohesive team and better patient outcomes.

Advocacy Tool

As you finish this chapter, use the following self-reflection checklist to assess how well you are incorporating advocacy into your daily practice. This tool is designed to help you translate the concepts discussed into actionable habits (Figure 9.5).

Conclusion

The role of the veterinary technician as a patient advocate is both a privilege and a profound responsibility. As frontline caregivers, technicians have the unique opportunity to observe, assess, and respond to the physical and emotional needs of their patients with a level of attentiveness and compassion unmatched by any other member of the veterinary team. Through confident communication, ethical clarity, and unwavering commitment to patient welfare, veterinary technicians ensure that each patient receives not only effective medical treatment but also care grounded in dignity, comfort, and respect.

Building advocacy skills requires intentional practice and the courage to speak up even in challenging environments. Whether advocating for improved pain management, supporting emotionally distressed patients, or guiding clients through difficult decisions, veterinary technicians play a critical role in influencing both individual outcomes and the broader culture of veterinary medicine. By embracing this role with confidence and integrity, technicians contribute to a future where patient-centered, compassionate care remains the foundation of veterinary practice.

As veterinary medicine continues to evolve, the voice of the veterinary technician will remain a powerful force for change. With each act of advocacy, whether in the hospital ward, during a client consultation, or through systemic improvements in care, technicians reaffirm their essential place in the healing journey of every patient they serve.

References

Beauchamp, T.L. and Childress, J.F. (2019). *Principles of Biomedical Ethics*, 8e. Oxford University Press.

Benner, P., Sutphen, M., Leonard, V., and Day, L. (2010). *Educating Nurses: A Call for Radical Transformation*. Jossey-Bass.

Brown, D.C., Agnello, K., Iadarola, M.J., and Lascelles, B.D.X. (2019). Pain in companion animals: Beyond physiology. *Veterinary Clinics of North America: Small Animal Practice* 49 (6): 1043–1056.

Clance, P.R. and Imes, S.A. (1978). The imposter phenomenon in high achieving women: Dynamics and therapeutic intervention. *Psychotherapy: Theory, Research & Practice* 15 (3): 241–247.

Evangelista, M.C., Benito, J., Monteiro, B.P. et al. (2019). Clinical applicability of the Feline Grimace Scale: Real-time versus image scoring and the influence of sedation and surgery. *PeerJ* 7: e6791.

Figley, C.R. (2002). Compassion fatigue: Psychotherapists' chronic lack of self care. *Journal of Clinical Psychology* 58 (11): 1433–1441.

Fowler, H. (2021). *Veterinary Nursing: A Systems Approach*, 2e. Wiley-Blackwell.

Frank, D., Beauchamp, G., Palestrini, C., and Gauthier, M. (2010). Systematic review of the use of pheromones for treatment of undesirable behavior in cats and dogs. *Journal of the American Veterinary Medical Association* 236 (12): 1308–1316.

Goleman, D. (1995). *Emotional Intelligence: Why It Can Matter More Than IQ*. Bantam Books.

Johnson, C. (2021). *Client Communication and Education for Veterinary Technicians*. Elsevier.

Koolhaas, J.M., Bartolomucci, A., Buwalda, B. et al. (2011). Stress revisited: A critical evaluation of the stress concept. *Neuroscience & Biobehavioral Reviews* 35 (5): 1291–1301.

Mathews, K.A., Kronen, P.W., Lascelles, D. et al. (2014). Guidelines for recognition, assessment and treatment of pain. *Journal of Small Animal Practice* 55 (6): E10–E68.

McMillan, F.D. (2017). *Mental Health and Well-Being in Animals*. CABI.

Mills, D.S., Karagiannis, C.I., and Zulch, H. (2014). Stress, Its effects on health and behavior: A guide for practitioners. *Veterinary Clinics of North America: Small Animal Practice* 44 (3): 525–541.

Monroe, T. (2020). *Veterinary Technician's Guide to Pain Management*. CRC Press.

Overall, K.L. (2013). *Manual of Clinical Behavioral Medicine for Dogs and Cats*. Elsevier Health Sciences.

Reid, J., Nolan, A.M., Hughes, J.M.L. et al. (2007). Development of the short-form Glasgow Composite Measure Pain Scale (CMPS-SF) and derivation of an analgesic intervention score. *Animal Welfare* 16 (S1): 97–104.

Rollin, B.E. (2011). *An Introduction to Veterinary Medical Ethics: Theory and Cases*, 2e. Wiley-Blackwell.

Villalobos, A.E. and Kaplan, L. (2007). *Canine and Feline Geriatric Oncology: Honoring the Human-Animal Bond*. Wiley-Blackwell.

Yin, S. (2009). *Low Stress Handling, Restraint and Behavior Modification of Dogs and Cats: Techniques for Developing Patients Who Love Their Visits*. CattleDog Publishing.

10

Communication in Veterinary Nursing

Introduction

Communication lies at the heart of veterinary nursing. It is the thread that connects patients to their caregivers, unites clinical teams in shared goals, and enables pet owners to participate meaningfully in their animal's care. While clinical knowledge and technical skills are critical to the practice of veterinary nursing, the ability to communicate clearly, compassionately, and effectively is equally vital. Veterinary technicians must be able to explain complex medical information to clients, collaborate with diverse team members, advocate for their patients, and navigate emotionally sensitive situations with confidence and empathy.

In a profession where patients cannot speak for themselves, the veterinary technician becomes the essential bridge between patient needs and human understanding. Every interaction, whether it involves providing discharge instructions, discussing a treatment plan, or voicing a concern during rounds, is an opportunity to influence outcomes and build trust. Poor communication can result in misunderstanding, reduced compliance, conflict among colleagues, and even compromised patient care. In contrast, strong communication skills promote team cohesion, client satisfaction, and improved clinical results (Fossum 2020).

This chapter explores the fundamental role of communication in veterinary nursing. It will examine the qualities that make communication effective, discuss strategies for client and colleague interactions, and address common challenges such as handling conflict and delivering difficult news. Through clinical examples and evidence-based techniques, veterinary technicians will learn how to refine their communication style, strengthen relationships within the veterinary team, and provide exceptional support to pet owners throughout the continuum of care.

The Importance of Communication Skills in Veterinary Nursing

The ability to communicate effectively is as critical to the role of the veterinary technician as any technical competency. While mastery of clinical skills allows technicians to perform procedures and support medical treatments, communication skills are what enable them to work collaboratively within a healthcare team and ensure that pet owners understand and follow through with care instructions. Without clear, compassionate, and confident communication, even the most advanced medical interventions may fail to produce successful outcomes (Fossum 2020).

Enhancing Patient Outcomes Through Communication

Communication directly impacts patient outcomes by improving client compliance and fostering a clearer understanding of treatment plans. Studies in human healthcare have shown that when medical professionals communicate effectively, patients experience better recovery outcomes, improved medication adherence, and higher satisfaction with care (Street et al., 2009). The same principles apply to veterinary medicine. When clients fully understand their pet's medical condition and the reasons behind specific treatment recommendations, they are more likely to follow through with home care instructions and return for necessary follow-up visits.

Veterinary technicians serve as the primary educators for clients regarding medication administration, dietary management, wound care, and ongoing monitoring. Explaining these tasks requires more than simply relaying information, it demands the ability to assess the client's emotional state, gauge their level of understanding, and adapt the communication approach accordingly. For example, a technician discharging a diabetic pet must not only explain how to administer insulin but also provide reassurance, demonstrate the technique, and offer written materials for later reference. These strategies ensure that the client leaves the hospital feeling prepared and confident, which directly influences the pet's health and safety at home.

Communication Across the Patient Life Cycle

Veterinary technicians serve as the constant presence throughout a patient's life, from early wellness visits to end-of-life care. Each stage of life presents unique medical, emotional, and educational needs, not only for the patient but also for the client. Adapting communication strategies to match these evolving needs is a hallmark of holistic nursing. By tailoring their approach to each phase of the patient's journey, veterinary technicians ensure that clients are supported, informed, and empowered at every turn.

Pediatric Communication focuses heavily on education and reassurance. Clients with new puppies or kittens are often overwhelmed by the volume of care information. Vaccination schedules, diet transitions, behavior expectations, parasite prevention, and socialization information in the allotted visit time create a barrier to digestible information amounts. Veterinary technicians must use clear, structured explanations and repeat key points throughout multiple visits. It is also essential to normalize the learning curve, affirming that client questions are welcome and expected. Holistic communication at this stage involves checking the emotional temperature of the client, ensuring they feel capable and supported rather than judged or rushed. Imploring written tools that can be handed or mailed to clients can be a useful way to ensure clients are receiving information in a digestible manner.

Adult Wellness Communication shifts toward partnership and preventive care. This is the stage where clients may begin to disengage if they feel visits are routine or unimportant. Veterinary technicians can maintain engagement by helping clients understand the "why" behind recommendations, connecting wellness bloodwork, nutrition choices, or behavior interventions to long-term quality of life. Building rapport during this stage means avoiding script-like delivery and instead asking open-ended questions about lifestyle changes, concerns, or observed trends. Communication becomes a tool for proactive partnership, not just compliance.

Geriatric and Chronic Care Communication requires a more emotionally attuned approach. Older pets often have multiple conditions and fluctuating quality of life. Clients may experience anticipatory grief or guilt, especially when facing difficult decisions. Veterinary technicians must balance clarity with compassion, helping clients interpret lab results, recognize subtle signs of pain or cognitive decline, and feel confident managing medications or mobility aids. Discussions should include frequent check-ins: "How are you feeling about what we just covered?" or "Would you like me to go over this again in writing?" These interactions build trust and reinforce the technician's role as a nonjudgmental guide through uncertainty.

Palliative and End-of-Life Communication demands the highest level of emotional intelligence (EI) and presence. Clients are often in distress, vacillating between hope and grief. Veterinary technicians must be able to read the room, offering empathy without presumption, and clarity without detachment. This stage of communication is not just about explaining options, it's about holding space for the family's emotional experience. Tone, pace, silence, and body language carry as much weight as words. Providing a warm blanket, pausing before responding, or simply sitting quietly for a moment can offer comfort beyond any spoken explanation. Clear and gentle language, such as "We want to help you make choices that feel right for your family," helps clients feel seen, not pushed.

By adapting communication styles to each life stage, veterinary technicians fulfill their holistic responsibility to treat the patient as more than a clinical case. They become educators, counselors, and advocates, assuring that every interaction honors the patient's experience and the client's role in their care. This life-stage approach deepens client relationships and reinforces the technician's critical position as a lifelong care partner (Figure 10.1).

Strengthening Team Dynamics and Clinical Efficiency

Effective communication also enhances collaboration within the veterinary healthcare team. Veterinary technicians work alongside veterinarians, fellow technicians, assistants, and administrative staff in a dynamic and often high-pressure environment. Miscommunication can lead to errors, duplicated tasks, and tension among colleagues. In contrast, clear, respectful, and timely communication fosters teamwork, increases efficiency, and reduces the risk of mistakes in patient care (Goleman 1995).

A well-communicated patient handoff during shift changes, for example, ensures continuity of care and prevents critical details from being overlooked. Utilizing structured communication tools such as the SBAR (Situation, Background,

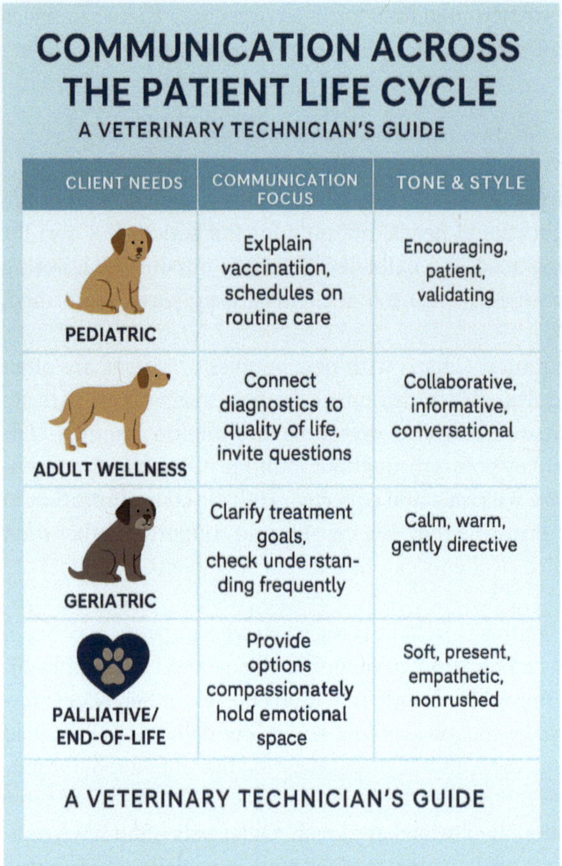

Figure 10.1 Communication across the patient life cycle. Jennings (2025). Author's own illustration.

Assessment, Recommendation) model supports this process by providing a clear framework for conveying patient status and care priorities. When all team members are informed and working from the same information, patient safety improves, and the hospital environment becomes more cohesive and supportive.

Building Trust and Reducing Client Anxiety

Veterinary medicine is emotionally charged, often involving highly stressful situations for pet owners. Fear, grief, and financial concerns can overwhelm clients, making it difficult for them to process medical information or make rational decisions. Veterinary technicians play a vital role in alleviating client anxiety by providing clear explanations, offering emotional support, and demonstrating empathy during every interaction (Johnson 2021). Building trust through effective communication starts with active listening, giving clients the space to express their concerns without interruption, and validating their emotions. When technicians demonstrate genuine care and take time to answer questions patiently, they foster a trusting relationship that encourages clients to be honest about their challenges, including financial limitations or emotional distress. This transparency allows the veterinary team to develop realistic, compassionate treatment plans that are both medically sound and aligned with the client's capabilities.

Communicating Through Uncertainty and Diagnostic Ambiguity

One of the most challenging and emotionally charged moments in veterinary nursing occurs when a patient's condition is unclear. Veterinary technicians are often tasked with supporting clients during these in-between spaces, before a diagnosis is confirmed, while waiting on lab results, or when differentials are still broad. These moments can create anxiety for clients, who may expect definitive answers and become frustrated or fearful when uncertainty remains. Holistic veterinary technicians must be equipped not only to convey what is known but to hold space for what is not yet known, guiding clients with clarity, compassion, and emotional steadiness.

Uncertainty is not failure, it is part of medicine. But to the client, it may feel like something is being missed, delayed, or mishandled. Technicians serve a crucial role in helping clients reframe this uncertainty as a natural step in the diagnostic process. Communicating that ambiguity is expected, and that the team is actively working through it, can alleviate fear and restore trust. For example, if a pet presents with lethargy, vomiting, and mild dehydration, the technician might say: *"Right now, your pet's symptoms could be caused by a few different things, some mild, some more serious. Our first step is to gather more information through bloodwork and imaging so the doctor can narrow down the possibilities. I know it's hard not to have a definite answer yet, but we'll keep you updated as we learn more today."* This approach is both honest and grounding. It avoids false reassurance while offering the client a clear picture of the plan ahead.

Technicians must also tune in to the emotional undercurrent. Clients may respond to uncertainty with fear, impatience, guilt, or even anger. Some may seek frequent updates, while others withdraw or shut down. Recognizing these emotional patterns allows the technician to adapt their approach. A highly anxious client may benefit from more frequent touchpoints: *"The doctor is still reviewing the ultrasound, but I wanted to check in and see how you're holding up while we wait."* This simple outreach acknowledges the client's emotional experience and reinforces that they are not being forgotten, even when definitive information isn't yet available.

The following chart outlines key principles for effective communication during uncertain clinical situations, with examples of language that fosters clarity, reassurance, and confidence (Table 10.1).

Table 10.1 Communication principles for navigating diagnostic uncertainty in veterinary nursing.

Communication Principle	Explanation	Example Statement
State What is Known	Clearly share confirmed findings using straightforward language.	"We know their temperature is elevated and they're a bit dehydrated. That tells us there's likely an inflammatory process at play."
Explain What is Being Investigated	Describe the rationale behind diagnostics or next steps.	"The bloodwork will show us whether there's an infection, anemia, or organ involvement, which will help us narrow this down."
Avoid Overpromising or Speculation	Don't make assumptions—balance optimism with transparency.	"We're hopeful this is something simple, but we're being thorough, so we don't miss anything."
Validate Emotional Responses	Acknowledge and normalize the client's feelings.	"It's completely understandable to feel anxious when we don't have all the answers yet. We're going to keep communicating with you."
Use Bridge Statements	Offer interim steps or reassurances to connect uncertainty with action.	"While we wait on results, let's make sure your pet is comfortable and hydrated—that gives them the best support as we learn more."

Source: Jennings (2025). Author's own compilation.

In cases of ongoing ambiguity, such as chronic, waxing-and-waning symptoms or suspected autoimmune disease, clients may feel exhausted by the lack of resolution. Veterinary technicians can provide continuity of communication, offering emotional support even when answers remain elusive. Holistic nursing in these cases means shifting focus to what *can* be controlled, comfort, quality of life, daily observations, and empowering the client to remain engaged in the patient's journey, even without a definitive label. Ultimately, clear and compassionate communication during uncertain moments prevents panic, builds client resilience, and reinforces the veterinary technician's role as a stabilizing presence. Holding space for diagnostic ambiguity is a powerful expression of holistic care, it acknowledges the clinical complexity of veterinary medicine while centering the client's emotional experience as an integral part of the healing process.

Case Example: The Power of Effective Communication

Consider the case of Daisy, a three-year-old French Bulldog hospitalized for a foreign body obstruction. Daisy's owner was visibly distressed and overwhelmed by the financial implications of surgery. The veterinary technician recognized the client's anxiety and took the time to sit down and thoroughly explain the surgical procedure, possible outcomes, and the importance of postoperative care. Using simple language and visual aids, the technician walked through the discharge instructions and demonstrated how to monitor Daisy's surgical site and administer medications at home. In addition to technical explanations, the technician acknowledged the owner's emotional distress, offering reassurance and providing contact information for follow-up questions. As a result, the client left feeling more confident in managing Daisy's recovery. Daisy returned for her postoperative check-up with excellent wound healing and no complications, a direct outcome of the technician's effective communication and the client's improved compliance.

Basic Communication Techniques in Veterinary Nursing

Mastering basic communication techniques is fundamental to building trust, reducing misunderstandings, and promoting effective collaboration within the veterinary healthcare team and with clients. These foundational skills serve as the bedrock upon which more complex communication strategies, such as conflict resolution or delivering difficult news, are built. Without a strong grasp of these techniques, even the most well-intentioned messages can fail to achieve their desired outcomes.

The Foundation of Effective Communication: Clarity and Simplicity

One of the most critical aspects of effective communication is clarity. Veterinary nursing often involves explaining complex medical information, treatment protocols, and care instructions to individuals who may have no background in animal health. Using clear, straightforward language ensures that information is understood and retained. This means avoiding technical jargon whenever possible. For example, instead of saying, "We'll need to administer subcutaneous fluids to support hydration," a technician might say, "We'll give fluids under the skin to help keep your pet hydrated." This simple reframing makes the information accessible and less intimidating to clients, improving compliance and confidence. When communicating with colleagues, clarity also involves providing complete and relevant information during handoffs and updates. Technicians should practice delivering concise summaries that include the key facts necessary for continued patient care, avoiding vague or incomplete statements that can lead to errors.

The Power of Active Listening

Communication is as much about listening as it is about speaking. Active listening involves fully engaging with the person speaking, demonstrating attentiveness through verbal and nonverbal cues, and responding appropriately to show understanding. In practice, this means making eye contact, nodding, and using affirming phrases such as "I understand" or "That makes sense." It also involves resisting the urge to interrupt or immediately offer solutions. By allowing clients and colleagues to fully express their thoughts and concerns before responding, veterinary technicians foster trust and demonstrate respect for the other person's perspective (Goleman 1995). Active listening also includes paraphrasing or summarizing what was said to confirm understanding. For example, after a client expresses worry about medication administration, the technician might respond, "So what I'm hearing is that you're feeling unsure about giving the insulin at home. Is that correct?" This technique not only confirms clarity but also shows empathy.

Nonverbal Communication: Saying More Without Words

Nonverbal communication often speaks louder than words. Body language, facial expressions, posture, and tone of voice all contribute to how messages are received. Veterinary technicians should be conscious of their nonverbal cues, ensuring they convey openness, confidence, and empathy. For example, crossing arms, avoiding eye contact, or using a harsh tone can unintentionally communicate disinterest or impatience, even if the words spoken are supportive. In contrast, open body language, relaxed posture, and a calm, reassuring tone foster trust and reduce anxiety, particularly in emotionally charged situations.

In team environments, nonverbal cues are equally important. Acknowledging a colleague's contributions with a smile or nod during discussions can promote a sense of teamwork and respect. Positive body language enhances collaboration and encourages open dialogue within clinical teams.

Timing and Environment: Setting the Stage for Effective Communication

The timing and environment in which communication takes place greatly influence how messages are received. Veterinary technicians should be mindful of when and where conversations occur, particularly those involving complex instructions or sensitive topics. Delivering discharge instructions in a busy, noisy treatment area may leave clients distracted and unable to focus. Instead, choosing a quiet, private space allows for uninterrupted, thoughtful conversation. Similarly, addressing performance concerns with a colleague should be done privately rather than in front of other team members, fostering a culture of mutual respect.

Timing also plays a critical role. Attempting to discuss detailed instructions with a client who is visibly upset or overwhelmed may not be productive. In such cases, it is often better to address immediate emotional needs first, then return to the necessary information once the client is more receptive.

Case Example: Applying Basic Communication in Practice

Consider the case of Rocky, a young Labrador Retriever recently diagnosed with a severe food allergy. His owners, confused and frustrated after weeks of unsuccessful treatments, expressed skepticism about trying yet another diet change. The veterinary technician practiced active listening, allowing the clients to fully explain their previous experiences without interruption. She summarized their concerns by saying, "It sounds like you've tried a lot of changes already, and you're feeling frustrated that nothing has helped." This simple statement validated their experience and created a foundation for trust.

Using clear, jargon-free language, the technician explained how the proposed prescription diet differed from previous attempts and why it was important to give it a fair trial. She provided written feeding guidelines and offered to schedule a follow-up call to check on Rocky's progress. Her calm demeanor, open body language, and clear explanations reassured the clients, and they agreed to try the new plan. At the follow-up visit, the owners reported significant improvements and expressed gratitude for the supportive communication they received.

Advanced Communication in Veterinary Nursing

As veterinary technicians refine their foundational communication skills, they must also develop the ability to navigate more complex interpersonal dynamics, particularly when dealing with heightened emotions, stress, and varying communication preferences. Advanced communication is not only about conveying information effectively but also about reading subtle cues, adjusting one's approach to match the emotional and cognitive state of others, and maintaining clarity and compassion even under pressure. Mastery of these skills allows veterinary technicians to strengthen relationships with clients and colleagues, prevent conflict, and ensure that critical information is delivered and received accurately in emotionally charged situations.

Recognizing Different Communication Styles and Preferences

Every individual processes and expresses information differently. Understanding and adapting to these differences is a hallmark of advanced communication. Broadly, communication styles can be categorized into four primary types: analytical, driver, amiable, and expressive (Merrill and Reid 1981). While few people fit perfectly into a single category, recognizing the dominant tendencies in others helps veterinary technicians tailor their communication strategies for maximum effectiveness.

Analytical Communicators are logical, data-driven, and highly focused on accuracy. They tend to be cautious decision-makers and may need time to process information before arriving at a conclusion. Veterinary technicians interacting with analytical clients or colleagues should provide detailed, fact-based explanations and offer supporting materials like printed discharge instructions, laboratory results, or research articles. Emotional appeals are less effective with this group; instead, focus on evidence and logical reasoning to build trust and compliance.

Driver Communicators are highly goal-oriented, assertive, and focused on results. They prefer direct, concise communication and become frustrated with what they perceive as unnecessary details or emotional discussions. When dealing with drivers, veterinary technicians should quickly outline the problem, present actionable solutions, and emphasize outcomes. Time efficiency is key. These individuals respect competence and clarity but may view overly cautious or uncertain language as weakness.

Amiable Communicators prioritize harmony, relationships, and emotional well-being. They are often highly empathetic but may struggle with making difficult decisions, particularly when those decisions involve negative outcomes. Veterinary technicians should create a supportive and non-confrontational environment, using gentle language and offering emotional validation. Allowing extra time for decision-making and providing ongoing reassurance helps amiable communicators feel more confident and less overwhelmed.

Expressive Communicators are enthusiastic, optimistic, and future-focused. They enjoy storytelling and often rely on personal experiences to make decisions. While they can be highly engaged, they may lose interest in overly detailed or technical explanations. Veterinary technicians should highlight the big-picture benefits of treatment plans, engage clients with relatable anecdotes, and maintain a positive, energetic tone during conversations. Visual aids and forward-thinking discussions about quality of life resonate well with this style.

Recognizing these communication styles requires ongoing observation of verbal and nonverbal cues, including tone of voice, preferred pacing of conversations, and how decisions are approached. Veterinary technicians should remain flexible and willing to adjust their communication style in real-time based on these observations (Figure 10.2).

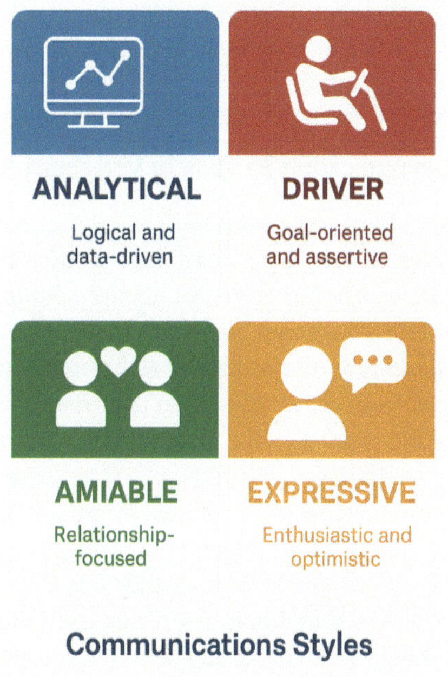
ANALYTICAL
Logical and data-driven
DRIVER
Goal-oriented and assertive
AMIABLE
Relationship-focused
EXPRESSIVE
Enthusiastic and optimistic
Communications Styles

Figure 10.2 Common communication styles and their core characteristics in clinical interactions. Jennings (2025). Author's own illustration.

How Communication Styles Are Heightened During Stress

Stress amplifies existing communication tendencies, often pushing individuals toward extreme manifestations of their preferred style. Under these heightened emotional states, clients and colleagues may become less receptive to information and more focused on meeting their immediate emotional or cognitive needs. Recognizing and addressing these stress-induced shifts is a critical skill for veterinary technicians.

Analytical Communicators Under Stress: These individuals may become paralyzed by indecision, insisting on more data before making even urgent choices. They may ask repetitive questions or fixate on small, often irrelevant details. Veterinary technicians can support stressed analytical communicators by gently guiding them toward timely decisions, offering the most critical information upfront, and reassuring them that further details can be provided after initial steps are taken.

Driver Communicators Under Stress: Drivers under stress often become more controlling, demanding immediate answers and quick decisions. Their tone may become abrupt or even aggressive as they attempt to regain a sense of control over a chaotic situation. Veterinary technicians should remain calm and assertive, provide direct and confident recommendations, and avoid overly lengthy explanations. Meeting their need for control by offering clear options restores their sense of agency and helps de-escalate tension.

Amiable Communicators Under Stress: Stress can cause amiable communicators to retreat emotionally, avoid decisions altogether, or become tearful and overwhelmed. They may defer decisions to others out of fear of making the wrong choice. Veterinary technicians should offer emotional support, validate the client's feelings, and help break decisions into smaller, manageable steps. Providing written resources and following up after discussions can further reduce their anxiety.

Expressive Communicators Under Stress: When stressed, expressive communicators may oscillate between overly optimistic views and emotional outbursts. They may focus on unrealistic outcomes and struggle to process negative information. Veterinary technicians can help ground expressive communicators by acknowledging their emotions while gently bringing conversations back to realistic expectations. Visual aids, timelines for treatment progress, and focusing on small, positive milestones can help these individuals stay engaged and hopeful without becoming disconnected from reality.

Understanding these patterns allows veterinary technicians to remain composed during difficult conversations and guide both clients and colleagues toward constructive outcomes. This adaptability is essential not only for reducing stress in others but also for protecting the technician's own emotional resilience during challenging situations.

Communication Barriers in Veterinary Nursing

One of the most common challenges in achieving effective communication is the presence of barriers that hinder clear understanding. These barriers may be verbal, emotional, environmental, or cultural. Veterinary technicians must be aware of how such obstacles can disrupt communication and develop strategies to overcome them.

Medical jargon is one of the most frequent barriers encountered when communicating with clients. While technical terms are necessary for professional dialogue, they often confuse or intimidate clients. For example, in a busy emergency room, a technician once told a client that their dog was in "hypovolemic shock," which only increased the client's panic. Recognizing the confusion, the technician calmly rephrased the statement: "Your dog's blood pressure is very low, and we are working quickly to stabilize them." This clearer explanation allowed the client to better understand the severity of the situation without feeling overwhelmed by unfamiliar language. Technicians should consciously translate medical language into plain terms and check frequently for understanding, using open-ended questions like, "Does that make sense?" or "Would you like me to explain that another way?"

Cultural differences also create communication challenges. Beliefs about animal care, euthanasia, and financial decision-making vary significantly between cultures. For instance, a client from a culture that prioritizes the sanctity of life may resist discussions about euthanasia, even in cases of severe suffering. In one case, a veterinary technician recognized the client's discomfort and shifted the conversation from the concept of euthanasia to focusing on the pet's quality of life, using gentle, compassionate language. By asking open-ended questions and actively listening to the client's values, the technician helped guide the family toward a decision that honored both their beliefs and the pet's well-being. Demonstrating respect for cultural differences fosters trust and helps guide conversations toward mutually acceptable solutions.

Emotional barriers arise when clients are overwhelmed with fear, grief, or guilt. These intense emotions can prevent them from fully processing information or making rational decisions. For example, when discussing an expensive treatment plan with a grieving client, a veterinary technician noticed that the client had stopped asking questions and appeared withdrawn. Recognizing this as emotional overload, the technician paused the conversation, offered tissues and a quiet space to sit, and suggested returning to the discussion after the client had a moment to gather themselves. Providing written instructions and contact information for follow-up questions also alleviates emotional barriers, allowing clients to review information when they are more emotionally prepared.

Environmental factors, such as noisy treatment areas or rushed consultations, impede effective communication. For example, in a busy surgical ward, a technician attempted to review complex home-care instructions with a client amidst loud equipment and constant interruptions. The client left confused and called back later, having misunderstood critical medication instructions. Learning from this experience, the hospital created a dedicated discharge room for quiet, focused conversations, which significantly improved client satisfaction and compliance. Veterinary technicians should advocate for appropriate environments when discussing complex treatment plans or delivering difficult news, ensuring clients have the physical and emotional space to process important information effectively. By recognizing these barriers and implementing strategies to overcome them, veterinary technicians can dramatically improve their communication effectiveness, strengthen relationships with clients, and ensure that every patient receives the highest standard of care.

Nonverbal Communication in Clinical Settings

Nonverbal communication is a powerful tool in clinical practice, often speaking louder than words. While verbal communication conveys factual information, nonverbal cues express emotional intent, build rapport, and provide insight into the unspoken feelings of clients and colleagues. Veterinary technicians must develop strong observational skills to interpret these cues and adjust their communication strategies accordingly, ensuring that both emotional and informational needs are met.

Positive nonverbal behaviors include maintaining open body language, making appropriate eye contact, and using a calm, reassuring vocal tone. For example, when delivering discharge instructions to a nervous client, standing at eye level, smiling gently, and speaking softly can reduce anxiety and help the client focus on absorbing the information. Leaning slightly forward during conversations shows interest and engagement, while nodding affirmatively communicates understanding and encouragement for the client to continue expressing their concerns. Conversely, negative nonverbal cues such as crossed arms, avoiding eye contact, hurried movements, or fidgeting can unintentionally signal disinterest, impatience, or discomfort. Veterinary technicians should remain mindful of their body language, especially during emotionally sensitive discussions. Even small adjustments, like sitting down rather than standing over a seated client during end-of-life conversations, demonstrate respect and compassion, creating a more supportive environment for difficult decisions.

Interpreting nonverbal cues also involves closely observing clients for signs of confusion, discomfort, or distress. A client who avoids eye contact, shifts uncomfortably, or tightly grips their belongings may be overwhelmed or anxious, even if they verbally agree to a treatment plan. Veterinary technicians should recognize these indicators and gently check in by asking, "Do you have any questions about what we've discussed?" or "Would you like me to go over that again?" This approach encourages clients to voice unspoken concerns and ensures their full understanding.

Nonverbal cues are equally critical when interacting with colleagues. In a busy treatment area, a colleague's hurried movements or clipped responses may indicate stress or overwhelm. Veterinary technicians can offer assistance or check in with a simple, "Do you need a hand with anything?" Recognizing and responding to these nonverbal signals strengthens teamwork and reduces the likelihood of conflict. Advanced interpretation of nonverbal communication also involves cultural sensitivity. In some cultures, direct eye contact may be considered disrespectful, while in others it is a sign of honesty and engagement. Veterinary technicians should be aware of these cultural nuances and adapt their body language accordingly to avoid unintentionally offending or alienating clients.

Case Example: A client arrives to discuss treatment options for their elderly cat, recently diagnosed with kidney failure. Though verbally agreeing to the proposed plan, the client avoids eye contact, wrings their hands, and has a tense posture. Recognizing these signs of emotional distress, the veterinary technician pauses and says, "I know this is a lot of information. How are you feeling about everything we've discussed so far?" The client visibly relaxes and admits feeling overwhelmed and unsure about the financial commitment. This opens the door for a compassionate conversation about alternative care options and financial support resources, ultimately leading to a plan that the client feels comfortable with and can follow through on. By developing a keen awareness of both their own nonverbal behaviors and those of others, veterinary technicians create more meaningful and supportive interactions. This attentiveness fosters trust, improves client satisfaction, and strengthens collaboration within the veterinary team, ultimately contributing to better patient outcomes.

Navigating Digital Communication in Veterinary Practice

In today's veterinary environment, communication extends far beyond the exam room. Text messages, emails, mobile apps, client portals, and even social media messaging have become routine channels through which veterinary technicians engage with pet owners. While these platforms offer convenience and immediacy, they also introduce new challenges. Tone, clarity, timeliness, and emotional nuance can be easily lost, or misunderstood, when communication happens without vocal inflection or body language.

Holistic veterinary technicians recognize that digital messages are not just administrative tasks, they are clinical interactions that influence how clients perceive care, respond to instructions, and remain connected to the veterinary team. Even a short email or a prescription refill message has the potential to reinforce trust, reduce anxiety, or accidentally create confusion. As such, digital communication must be approached with the same intention and emotional awareness as face-to-face conversations.

Tone matters more when tone is all you have. A message like, *"Your refill is ready,"* may sound brisk or impersonal without context. By adding a friendly and professional tone, *"Hi Amanda, I wanted to let you know Bailey's refill is ready and waiting at the front desk. Let us know if you have any questions!"*, the message becomes both functional and relational. Small adjustments to language soften the interaction and ensure the client feels supported, not dismissed (Figure 10.3).

Clarity is essential in written instructions. Clients may refer to digital messages when administering medications, preparing for surgery, or reviewing follow-up care. Technicians must write with precision, avoiding abbreviations, minimizing medical jargon, and organizing information clearly. For example: *"Give 1 tablet by mouth twice daily"* is far clearer than *"1 tab PO BID."* Lists, line breaks, or bullet formatting can make multistep instructions easier to follow in digital text.

Timeliness and responsiveness shape client trust. If a client messages with a question and receives no reply for several hours, or worse, days, they may feel neglected, regardless of the clinic's workload. While technicians may not always be able to respond immediately, setting expectations helps. An auto-response like, *"Thank you for reaching out! Our team will review your message and respond within the next 24 hours,"* provides reassurance and outlines a clear timeframe.

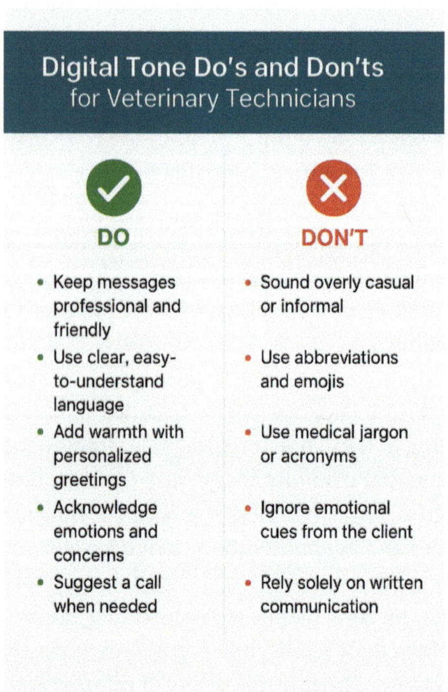

Figure 10.3 Guidelines for professional digital communication in veterinary nursing. *Source:* Jennings (2025). Author's own illustration.

In more emotionally sensitive cases, such as postoperative recovery, hospice care, or ongoing illness, clients may reach out digitally with nuanced concerns. Messages like, *"He seems a little off today"* or *"She didn't eat much and is just sleeping"* may not sound urgent, but often reflect anxiety or uncertainty. Holistic technicians learn to read between the lines and respond with empathy:

> *"Thank you for the update, I know it can be stressful when she's not acting like herself. Would you be open to a quick call so we can talk it through together?"*

Knowing when to transition a digital conversation to a phone call or in-person visit is a key clinical judgment. Written communication has limitations. When clients are expressing emotional distress, confusion about treatment, or frustration with the care process, a technician's voice, calm, compassionate, and real, can bridge the gap in ways text never will.

Privacy and professionalism must also be preserved. Even when texting from a work device or responding through a clinic app, veterinary technicians must avoid casual tone drift. Using abbreviations, emojis, or overly informal phrases can unintentionally diminish the credibility of the message. Likewise, digital platforms must comply with legal and ethical standards of recordkeeping. Any recommendations, updates, or clinical observations provided digitally should be documented in the medical record.

Finally, digital communication can extend holistic care beyond the walls of the hospital. Sending a follow-up message after an emotionally difficult visit, a thank-you note after euthanasia, or a reminder about an upcoming recheck shows the client they remain cared for. These small touches build lasting relationships and demonstrate that veterinary care is not a transaction, it's a partnership. In the hands of a mindful veterinary technician, digital communication becomes a tool not just for efficiency, but for connection. When approached with intention, empathy, and clarity, even the simplest message can convey the same core truth: *we see you, we care, and we are here for your pet's journey, every step of the way.*

The Role of Emotional Intelligence in Communication

Emotional intelligence (EI) is the ability to recognize, understand, and manage one's own emotions while effectively navigating the emotions of others. High EI is a critical trait for veterinary technicians, as it directly influences their ability to connect with clients, collaborate with colleagues, and manage the emotional demands of veterinary practice.

The four core components of EI are self-awareness, self-regulation, empathy, and social skills (Goleman 1995). Self-awareness allows technicians to recognize their own emotional triggers and avoid reacting impulsively. Self-regulation enables them to remain calm and composed during stressful situations. Empathy involves recognizing and validating the emotions of clients and colleagues, while strong social skills foster effective teamwork and conflict resolution.

Self-awareness involves understanding one's own emotional state and recognizing how it impacts behavior and communication. In clinical practice, this means being aware of personal stressors and emotional triggers that may affect interactions with clients and team members. For instance, a technician who notices feelings of frustration during a particularly busy shift can take a moment to pause and reset before engaging with a distressed client. This awareness prevents negative emotions from influencing conversations and ensures that communication remains compassionate and professional.

Self-regulation is the ability to control emotional reactions and respond thoughtfully rather than impulsively. Veterinary nursing is a high-stress environment where emotions can run high, especially when dealing with critical cases or challenging clients. A technician practicing self-regulation remains calm and composed even when confronted with an angry client or a difficult situation. For example, if a client becomes confrontational about treatment costs, a technician with strong self-regulation skills will avoid responding defensively and instead calmly redirect the conversation toward constructive solutions, maintaining a focus on the patient's best interest.

Empathy is the capacity to understand and share the feelings of others. In veterinary practice, this involves recognizing the emotional struggles that clients face when their pets are ill and acknowledging those feelings without judgment. Practical applications of empathy include actively listening to clients' concerns, using validating language such as "I can see how difficult this is for you," and adjusting communication styles to meet the emotional needs of each client. For example, when discussing euthanasia, a technician who practices empathy might sit with the client in a private room, offer tissues, and provide gentle reassurance that their decision is compassionate and humane.

Social skills encompass the ability to build and maintain positive relationships, navigate social complexities, and work collaboratively with others. In a veterinary setting, this means fostering open communication within the healthcare team, offering support to colleagues under stress, and participating actively in case discussions. Technicians with strong social skills help create a cohesive team environment by encouraging teamwork, offering assistance without being asked, and addressing conflicts diplomatically. For instance, during a busy day when tensions are high, a technician might notice a colleague struggling and offer to share the workload, promoting a spirit of collaboration and mutual support.

By consciously applying these four components of EI in daily practice, veterinary technicians can improve client satisfaction, enhance team dynamics, and contribute to a more positive and effective workplace culture. EI not only benefits interpersonal relationships but also plays a critical role in reducing compassion fatigue and promoting personal resilience, ensuring that technicians can continue to provide high-quality care for their patients over the long term. For example, when a client becomes visibly upset after learning about a terminal diagnosis, a technician with high EI will recognize the client's grief, respond with appropriate empathy, and avoid overwhelming them with excessive medical details. Instead, they will offer comfort, provide space for the client to process their emotions, and schedule a follow-up conversation to discuss treatment options once the client is ready.

Delivering Difficult News: Structured Approaches

Delivering bad news is one of the most challenging responsibilities in veterinary nursing. Whether discussing a poor prognosis, euthanasia options, or financial limitations, these conversations require sensitivity, clarity, and compassion. Structured approaches, such as the SPIKES protocol, help veterinary technicians navigate these discussions effectively (Baile et al. 2000).

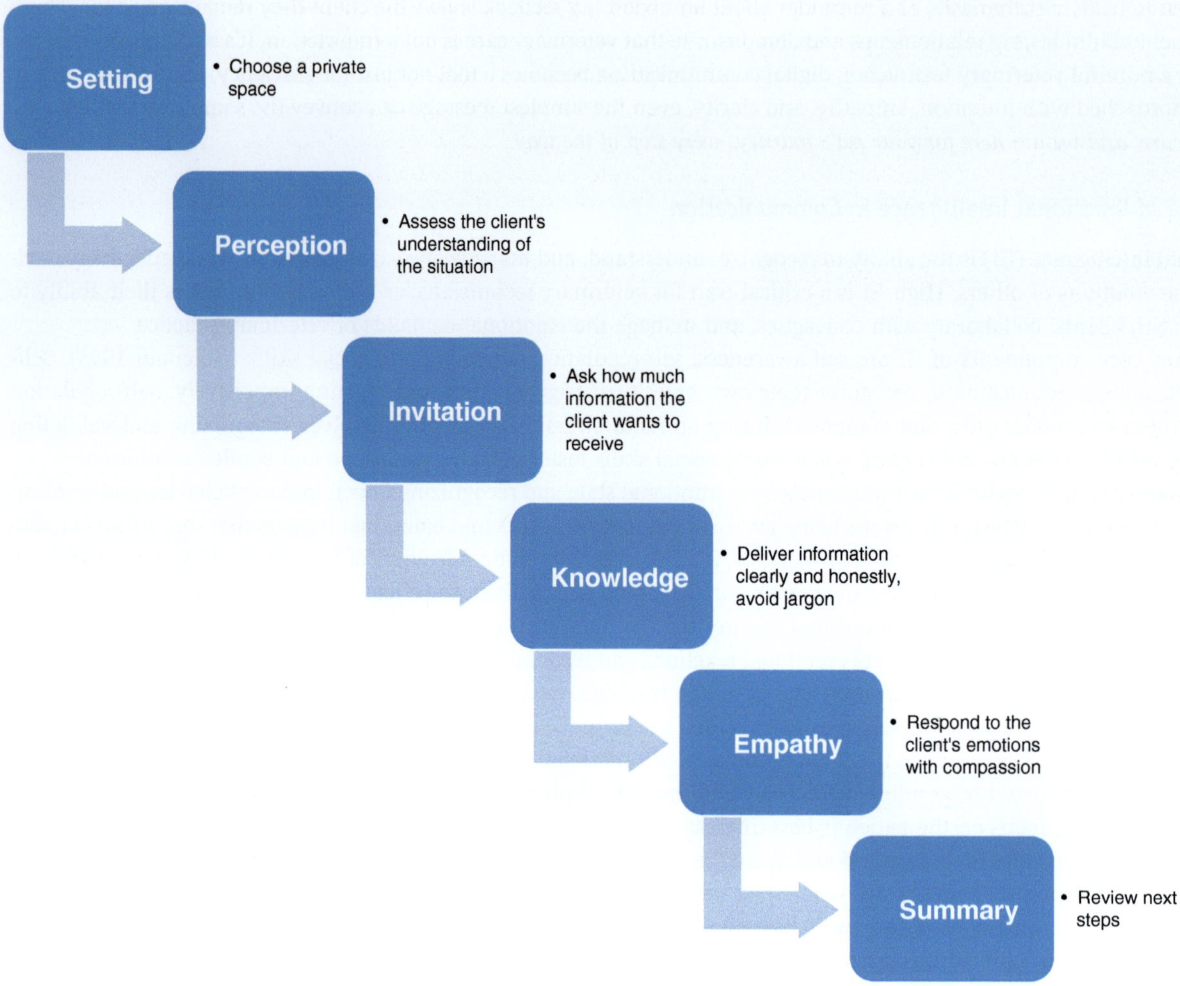

Figure 10.4 The SPIKES communication framework adapted for veterinary client interactions. *Source:* Jennings (2025). Author's own illustration; adapted from SPIKES model.

The SPIKES protocol involves setting, perception, invitation, knowledge, empathy, and summary (Figure 10.4).

Using this approach ensures that clients feel supported throughout difficult conversations and have the information they need to make informed decisions about their pet's care.

Case Study: Applying the SPIKES Protocol

Bella, a 13-year-old, FS, Labrador Retriever, was presented to the veterinary hospital for progressive hindlimb weakness. After a thorough neurological evaluation and advanced imaging, the diagnosis of a spinal tumor was made. The prognosis was guarded to poor, and the recommended options were either referral for radiation therapy or palliative care with euthanasia as a likely outcome in the near future. The veterinary technician prepared to deliver this difficult news using the SPIKES protocol.

Setting: She invited the owners into a private consultation room, ensured tissues were available, and closed the door to minimize distractions. She positioned herself at eye level, sitting down across from the couple to create a supportive and respectful atmosphere.

Perception: She began by asking, "Can you tell me what you've understood so far about Bella's condition?" This allowed the owners to express their expectations and understanding before she added more details.

Invitation: She then asked, "Would it be okay if I share what the tests have shown and what it means for Bella's health moving forward?" Gaining permission ensured the clients were emotionally ready to hear the information.

Knowledge: Using clear, nontechnical language, the technician explained, "The results show that Bella has a mass pressing on her spinal cord. It's affecting her ability to use her legs and unfortunately, it's not something we can cure with surgery. There are some options to help her be more comfortable, but we want to talk through what feels right for your family."

Empathy: As the owners began to cry, the technician paused, offered tissues, and said, "I can see how much you love her and how hard this is. It's okay to feel overwhelmed right now." She allowed silence to let the owners process the information.

Summary: She then gently outlined the available options, emphasizing that there was no pressure to decide immediately. She handed them a written summary of the discussion and let them know the team would be available for any follow-up questions.

In this case, the SPIKES protocol helped guide a complex and emotional conversation with clarity and compassion. The owners later expressed appreciation for how the news was delivered and felt supported throughout their decision-making process. This structured yet empathetic approach ensured that Bella's needs were honored, and her family was treated with the dignity and understanding they deserved.

Conflict Resolution and De-Escalation Techniques

Conflict is an inevitable reality in the fast-paced, emotionally charged environment of veterinary medicine. Whether it arises between colleagues over patient care decisions or with clients distressed by difficult news, the ability to navigate and resolve conflict is a critical skill for veterinary technicians. More importantly, advanced conflict resolution and de-escalation techniques not only restore harmony but also preserve relationships and support the emotional well-being of all parties involved.

Understanding the Psychological Principles Behind Conflict

To effectively manage conflict, veterinary technicians must first understand the underlying psychological processes that contribute to it. Conflict often stems from perceived threats to an individual's needs, values, or control over a situation. When people feel unheard, disrespected, or powerless, their brains trigger a physiological stress response, often referred to as the fight, flight, or freeze response (Cannon 1932). In these moments, rational thinking diminishes, and emotional reactions dominate. Recognizing these stress responses is the first step in de-escalating conflict. Veterinary technicians must remain calm and centered to help guide clients or colleagues back to a state of cognitive clarity. This begins with self-awareness and self-regulation, recognizing one's own emotional reactions and consciously choosing to respond rather than react impulsively.

Effective de-escalation starts with maintaining a calm, neutral demeanor: speak in a low, even voice, avoid raising your volume or mirroring someone's agitation, and use your steady presence to signal that the situation is manageable. Pair this with reflective listening to show understanding and reduce defensiveness, paraphrase the person's concerns, and check for accuracy (e.g., "It sounds like you're feeling overwhelmed by the treatment plan and worried about managing it at home, does that sound right?"). Before moving to solutions, acknowledge emotions to lower intensity and build rapport; statements such as "I can see this is very stressful" or "It's understandable to feel frustrated" validate feelings without implying agreement. Throughout, keep your body language open and nonthreatening: uncross your arms, keep your hands visible, stay at eye level with appropriate eye contact, and avoid looming over seated clients or adopting closed, defensive postures.

Using the LEAPS Model to Navigate Challenging Conversations in Veterinary Medicine

The LEAPS model offers a structured, empathetic approach to de-escalation and resolution. It helps veterinary professionals maintain control of difficult conversations while ensuring the client feels heard and supported. Each component of the LEAPS model plays a role in transforming conflict into collaboration:

L—Listen Actively

Active listening goes beyond hearing words; it involves full attention, open body language, and acknowledgment of the client's concerns. Avoid interrupting and show that you're present by nodding, making eye contact, and using minimal encouragers like "I see" or "Go on."

E—Empathize with Emotion

Recognize and validate the client's emotional state, even if the facts are still unclear. For example, "I can see this is really upsetting for you" signals compassion and calms defensive responses.

A—Ask Clarifying Questions

Gently guide the conversation with open-ended questions that help uncover the root of the concern. For example, "Can you tell me more about what's been worrying you since your pet's last visit?"

P—Paraphrase Understanding

Restate the client's concern in your own words to confirm you've understood accurately. This might sound like, "So what I'm hearing is that you're concerned the medication may be causing side effects?"

S—Summarize and Strategize

End with a concise summary of what was discussed and outline clear next steps. This provides closure and reassures the client that a plan is in place: "We'll go ahead and recheck Luna's lab work today, and I'll have the doctor speak with you about adjusting her medication."

By practicing LEAPS, veterinary technicians can remain grounded in moments of tension, reduce emotional escalation, and restore trust (Figure 10.5).

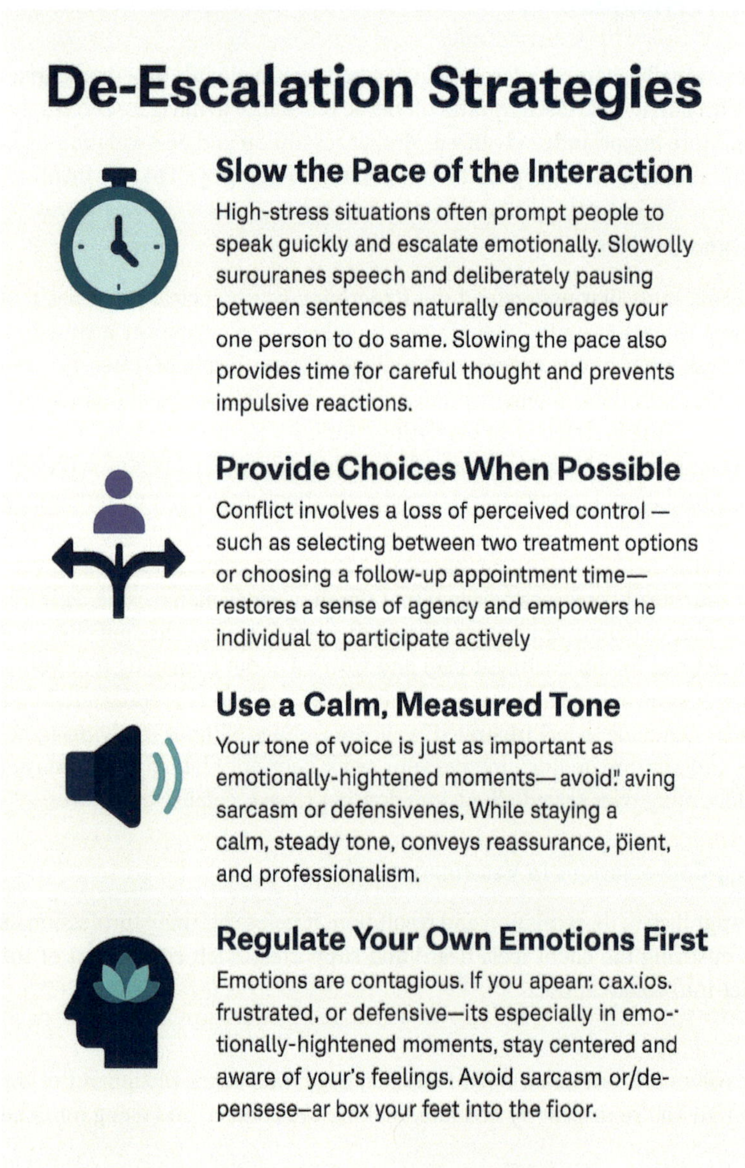
De-Escalation Strategies
Slow the Pace of the Interaction
High-stress situations often prompt people to speak guickly and escalate emotionally. Slowolly surouranes speech and deliberately pausing between sentences naturally encourages your one person to do same. Slowing the pace also provides time for careful thought and prevents impulsive reactions.
Provide Choices When Possible
Conflict involves a loss of perceived control — such as selecting between two treatment options or choosing a follow-up appointment time— restores a sense of agency and empowers he individual to participate actively
Use a Calm, Measured Tone
Your tone of voice is just as important as emotionally-hightened moments— avoid:' aving sarcasm or defensivenes, While staying a calm, steady tone, conveys reassurance, ṗient, and professionalism.
Regulate Your Own Emotions First
Emotions are contagious. If you apean: cax.ios. frustrated, or defensive—its especially in emo-tionally-hightened moments, stay centered and aware of your's feelings. Avoid sarcasm or/de-pensese—ar box your feet into the fioor.

Figure 10.5 Practical de-escalation strategies for maintaining professionalism and emotional safety in client interactions.

Case Example: De-Escalating a High-Stress Client Interaction

During an emergency visit, a client whose dog had ingested a foreign object became highly agitated upon learning that surgery would be expensive and immediate. The client raised their voice and began accusing the staff of only caring about money. The veterinary technician calmly acknowledged the client's emotional distress by saying, "I can see how scary and overwhelming this situation feels right now." She maintained a calm tone and open posture while using reflective listening to clarify the client's financial concerns. Employing the LEAPS model, she asked clarifying questions, summarized the medical urgency, and offered realistic payment options. By remaining composed and empathetic, the technician successfully de-escalated the situation, and the client agreed to proceed with the surgery after exploring financial solutions.

Communication with Colleagues in Clinical Practice

Veterinary medicine is inherently collaborative. From patient handoffs to surgical procedures, every aspect of care requires coordination among veterinary technicians, veterinarians, assistants, client service representatives, and hospital leadership. Effective communication among colleagues is therefore not only a professional courtesy but a clinical necessity. Poor communication can lead to misunderstandings, missed treatments, interpersonal tension, and ultimately diminished patient care. In contrast, well-developed interprofessional communication skills help veterinary technicians navigate high-stakes situations, advocate for patients, and foster a team environment rooted in mutual respect and shared purpose.

One of the key components of strong communication with colleagues is clarity. Veterinary technicians often serve as the communication bridge between multiple parties: doctors, support staff, and clients. When relaying critical patient updates, such as changes in mentation or vital signs, the technician must provide information that is succinct, accurate, and free from ambiguity. Tools like SBAR (Situation, Background, Assessment, Recommendation) help structure this information in a way that promotes efficient and informed decision-making. For example, when transitioning a patient at shift change, a technician might say, "Situation: Rocky is a postop foreign body. Background: surgery was three hours ago, and he's on a fentanyl CRI. Assessment: his heart rate has increased, and he's whining more. Recommendation: consider increasing his pain management or reassessing his comfort level."

Another vital element is respectful dialogue, particularly in situations of disagreement. In a busy hospital, it is common for team members to have different opinions about treatment approaches, case priorities, or workflow protocols. Veterinary technicians may observe a patient deteriorating and feel urgency to act, while a veterinarian is balancing multiple cases. In these moments, assertive yet respectful communication allows technicians to advocate without undermining team cohesion. Rather than saying, "You're not listening to me, this patient is crashing," a technician might say, "I've noticed some changes in our patient's respiratory rate and gum color, and I'm concerned we need to intervene quickly. Can we reassess together?"

Peer support and EI also play essential roles in interprofessional communication. Veterinary technicians work under significant emotional pressure and are often the first to recognize when a colleague is overwhelmed, burned out, or at risk for compassion fatigue. Offering to assist without being asked, checking in with a simple, "Are you okay?" or validating a colleague's concerns with, "That was a tough case, we did everything we could," reinforces team solidarity. These small gestures build trust and psychological safety, creating a workplace culture where team members feel valued and supported.

Conflicts will arise, but the key is in how they are managed. If a technician feels a colleague has acted unfairly, such as assigning tasks unequally or offering harsh criticism, addressing the issue directly and privately is far more effective than allowing resentment to fester. A veterinary technician might say, "I noticed I've been handling the ICU patients the past few shifts, and I'm feeling a bit stretched. Can we talk about how we're dividing responsibilities?" This approach focuses on behavior and solutions rather than blame, preserving professional relationships.

Lastly, transparency and accountability are crucial. Mistakes happen in any clinical setting, and when they do, owning them openly rather than deflecting blame fosters a culture of trust. If a technician administers the wrong medication dose but immediately reports it, explains the error, and helps develop a corrective plan, they model integrity and professionalism. This openness also encourages others to speak up without fear of reprisal, ultimately improving patient safety.

In summary, strong communication with colleagues is a blend of structured clarity, respectful assertion, EI, and shared responsibility. Veterinary technicians who prioritize these values help foster a cohesive, resilient team capable of delivering high-quality patient care in even the most demanding clinical environments.

Communicating Across Interdisciplinary Boundaries

In many clinical cases, veterinary technicians act as the connective tissue not only within the hospital but across the broader veterinary care network. Patients may receive care from multiple providers over time, general practitioners, specialists, emergency teams, physical rehabilitation therapists, and even external partners like shelters or referring veterinarians. Communication in these interdisciplinary settings requires not only clarity and professionalism but also consistency, respect, and proactive collaboration. Veterinary technicians are often the ones summarizing and relaying key information between these intersecting teams. Whether preparing a patient referral for an internal medicine consult, relaying updates to a shelter partner, or interpreting a specialist's recommendations for the general practice team, technicians must ensure that messages are accurate, thorough, and clearly understood. The stakes are high: any lapse in communication can lead to gaps in care, conflicting instructions, or client confusion.

A holistic approach to interdisciplinary communication includes the following elements:

Consistency in Messaging: When care is shared between teams, clients can feel overwhelmed or misinformed if the language and expectations shift from provider to provider. Veterinary technicians should strive to deliver messages that echo the same priorities and goals as the larger care team. If a specialist has outlined a treatment plan, it is the technician's responsibility to reinforce, not reinterpret, that plan when reviewing it with the client or primary care team. This consistency builds trust and prevents contradictory advice from derailing treatment.

Clarity in Summarizing: Writing a discharge summary or patient transfer note is not simply a clerical task, it is a clinical skill. Technicians must highlight relevant medical history, diagnostics performed, treatments administered, and the current status of the patient in a way that is easy for another clinician to understand. Omitting crucial context, such as response to previous medications or owner-specific limitations, can significantly impair continuity of care.

Respectful Collaboration: Interdisciplinary work requires humility and mutual respect. Different teams may have varied perspectives, resources, and philosophies of care. A holistic technician listens openly, seeks clarification when needed, and presents their own insights diplomatically. For example, if a referring veterinarian's history doesn't match the current clinical findings, the technician might say, *"The referring notes mention recent GI upset, though we haven't seen signs here. We'll keep it on our radar. Do you think we should run additional diagnostics?"* This honors the contributions of the previous team while staying grounded in the current assessment.

Client Advocacy Across Teams: Clients navigating multiple providers may feel like their pet's story is fractured. Veterinary technicians serve as the throughline. When clients are confused by conflicting recommendations, technicians can help clarify by rephrasing medical language and identifying where misunderstandings may have occurred. They can also help advocate for realistic expectations when specialists recommend advanced diagnostics or therapies that exceed the client's financial or emotional bandwidth. A holistic technician does not pass the client off, they walk beside them throughout the referral process.

Timely Follow-Up and Documentation: When interdisciplinary communication is delayed, the patient suffers. Veterinary technicians should ensure that communications, such as emailed summaries, case notes, or client callbacks, are completed promptly. When sending or receiving external medical records, it is critical to confirm that all necessary documentation is included. Creating a culture of reliable follow-through shows respect not only for colleagues but for the patient's whole journey through the healthcare system.

In an increasingly collaborative veterinary landscape, the technician's voice is not ancillary, it is central. Holistic nursing means not only seeing the whole patient but also understanding the whole system that supports their care. Interdisciplinary communication, when done with clarity and compassion, elevates patient outcomes, smooths transitions between teams, and reinforces the technician's role as a vital clinical partner.

When Communication Breaks Down: Strategies for Rebuilding and Repair

Despite the best intentions and training, there will be times when communication fails. Messages are misunderstood, emotions escalate, and conversations may leave veterinary technicians or their clients and colleagues feeling frustrated, dismissed, or even disrespected. Recognizing when communication has broken down, and knowing how to respond effectively is a vital part of advanced communication in veterinary nursing.

Veterinary technicians may find that even after employing active listening and empathy, the other party remains closed off or defensive. Alternatively, a technician may realize that their own attempts to convey information are falling flat or being misinterpreted. In these moments, it is essential not to double down on the same approach, but to pause, reassess, and apply strategies that can reset the conversation.

The first step is acknowledging the breakdown without blame. Phrases like, "I feel like we may not be on the same page right now, can we take a moment to reset?" or "I may not have explained that as clearly as I could have, can I try again?" shift the focus away from fault and toward resolution. This vulnerability models humility and opens the door for collaborative repair.

In cases where technicians are being communicated with poorly, such as being spoken to dismissively, shouted at, or disrespected, professional boundaries must be maintained. In the moment, technicians should remain calm and assertive. For example, a technician might respond, "I want to help, but I need us to have a respectful conversation so we can work together on this." If the behavior persists or escalates, it may be appropriate to disengage and seek support from a supervisor or another team member. Ensuring personal safety and maintaining professionalism are top priorities.

Sometimes communication difficulties stem from emotional overwhelm. A veterinary technician trying to explain euthanasia options to a grieving client may notice the client zoning out or becoming agitated. In this scenario, it is wise to pause and ask, "Would it help if we took a short break? I can come back in a few minutes and we can talk more when you're ready." Offering space can allow the emotional temperature to cool, making room for clarity and compassion to return.

In longer-term situations, such as ongoing tension between team members, poor communication must be addressed proactively. Scheduling a private, structured conversation to discuss communication concerns, perhaps facilitated by a manager, can prevent resentment from growing. Using "I" statements helps keep these discussions constructive: "I feel dismissed when my patient updates are not acknowledged," or "I've noticed our conversations sometimes feel tense, and I'd like to work on improving that."

When appropriate, utilizing feedback loops, asking for clarification, or inviting feedback can also preempt misunderstandings. A veterinary technician might say, "I just want to make sure I explained that well, what questions do you have?" or "I'd love your feedback on how I handled that conversation, anything you'd suggest I do differently next time?"

Finally, veterinary hospitals should support a culture that encourages reflection, conflict resolution, and emotional support. Role-playing scenarios during team meetings, debriefing after high-stress cases, and promoting psychological safety all reinforce the message that communication is a skill to be nurtured, not a performance to be perfected. By recognizing when communication is faltering and knowing how to address it without blame or defensiveness, veterinary technicians uphold their commitment to patient advocacy, client trust, and team collaboration. These moments of rupture, when handled with skill and EI, often lead to greater connection and mutual respect.

Building Psychological Safety in Team Communication

Psychological safety refers to a workplace culture in which team members feel safe expressing ideas, admitting mistakes, and offering constructive feedback without fear of embarrassment or punishment (Edmondson 1999). Creating psychologically safe environments leads to more effective communication, improved patient outcomes, and stronger teamwork.

Veterinary technicians play a vital role in fostering psychological safety by modeling respectful communication, encouraging team participation during rounds and case discussions, and validating the contributions of all team members. When mistakes occur, focusing on solutions rather than blame promotes learning and growth. For example, if a medication error occurs, a psychologically safe team environment encourages open reporting and collaborative problem-solving to prevent future incidents. Veterinary technicians should advocate for regular team meetings focused on open communication, continuous improvement, and shared learning. By mastering advanced communication techniques, veterinary technicians elevate their role within the healthcare team, foster stronger client relationships, and ensure that every patient receives compassionate, informed, and dignified care.

Communication as a Tool for Technician Empowerment

For veterinary technicians, communication is not only a skill but also a source of power. In the fast-paced and hierarchical world of veterinary medicine, technicians often find themselves balancing clinical responsibilities with emotional labor, all while navigating complex team dynamics and client expectations. Communication, when mastered and used intentionally, becomes a tool that elevates the technician's role, reinforces their clinical authority, and ensures their voice is heard in decisions that affect patient care.

Empowered communication begins with clinical confidence. Technicians who can articulate patient changes, advocate for interventions, or explain diagnostic rationales are more likely to influence outcomes and gain the respect of their colleagues. Saying, *"This patient's heart rate has increased significantly since morning rounds, and I believe they may be painful,"* carries more weight than *"I think something might be wrong."* Precise, evidence-based communication not only supports better medicine but also repositions the technician as a decision-making contributor, not just a task executor. It also serves as a foundation for professional visibility. In hospitals where technicians struggle to gain recognition for their efforts, clear and consistent communication becomes a vehicle for visibility. Participating actively in rounds, contributing to treatment plans, and updating the team on patient progress shows initiative and reinforces professional value. Communication empowers technicians to say, *"I've been monitoring this patient closely, here's what I've noticed and what I recommend,"* rather than passively waiting to be asked.

In interactions with clients, strong communication builds credibility and trust. When technicians are able to explain medications, discharge instructions, or diagnostic reasoning clearly and compassionately, clients view them as knowledgeable, reliable, and approachable. This deepens the technician-client relationship and fosters long-term loyalty to the hospital. A technician who can say, *"I'll walk you through this step-by-step so you feel confident at home,"* becomes not only a caregiver, but an educator and advocate.

Beyond client and patient care, communication also strengthens a technician's leadership potential. Peer mentorship, conflict navigation, team debriefing, and cross-department collaboration all hinge on strong interpersonal skills. Technicians who lead with calm, clear communication can de-escalate stress, unify fractured teams, and promote a healthier workplace culture. This kind of leadership is often quiet but deeply influential, it fosters psychological safety and encourages others to rise to the same standard.

Empowered communication also includes knowing how to set boundaries. Technicians are often expected to absorb high volumes of emotional labor without being given space to express their own needs. Knowing how to say, *"I'd like to support this conversation, but I need a short break to regulate myself,"* or *"Can we schedule a time to revisit this when we're both less rushed?"* is a form of self-advocacy. It models professionalism while protecting the technician's own well-being.

Finally, communication is the foundation of career advancement. Whether applying for a leadership role, giving a case presentation, mentoring a junior technician, or pursuing a specialty credential, technicians must be able to communicate their insights, their value, and their vision. Those who practice clear, assertive, and emotionally intelligent communication stand out, not only to clients and teammates but also to hospital leadership, educators, and industry partners. Holistic nursing is not just about tending to the needs of the patient, it is about honoring the full identity and capacity of the veterinary technician. Communication is how that identity takes shape in the world. It is how the technician advocates, collaborates, teaches, learns, leads, and grows. In the hands of a thoughtful veterinary professional, communication is far more than a tool, it is a reflection of empowerment, integrity, and purpose.

Reflection Exercise: *Finding Your Voice, A Communication Empowerment Journal*

Purpose: This journaling activity is designed to help veterinary technicians reflect on how they currently use communication in their clinical work, and how they can grow to become more empowered, visible, and confident in their role. Holistic nursing begins with self-awareness, and this reflection supports that inward understanding (Figure 10.6).

Empowerment doesn't come from knowing all the answers, it comes from choosing to engage, even when it feels uncomfortable. Every time you use your voice in service of a patient, a teammate, or yourself, you are practicing the heart of holistic nursing: presence, purpose, and courage.

Conclusion

Mastering advanced communication is not simply a desirable skill for veterinary technicians, it is a fundamental requirement for delivering compassionate, effective, and patient-centered care. Throughout this chapter, we explored the diverse challenges veterinary technicians face in both client and colleague interactions, from managing communication barriers and interpreting nonverbal cues to employing EI and delivering difficult news with grace. Each of these components plays a crucial role in ensuring that critical information is not only conveyed but truly understood and acted upon.

Veterinary nursing is a profession rooted in advocacy, empathy, and clinical excellence. In no area is this more apparent than in the way technicians communicate. Whether calming a distressed pet owner, guiding a family through the final

Step 1: Where Are You Now?	
Take a quiet moment to consider your current communication habits in the workplace. Reflect on the following prompts and jot down your thoughts When was the last time I clearly advocated for a patient? What did I say? How was it received? Do I feel Confident speaking up during rounds or team meetings? If not, what holds me back? When clients ask me questions, do I feel prepared to answer them clearly? Have I ever stayed silent about a concern because I was unsure how to say it "the right way"?	
Step 2: Identifying Strengths and Blind Spots	
Divide a page into two columns:	
My Strengths	My Growth Areas
Where do I already excel in communication? Think about tone, empathy, clarity, teamwork, or client education.	Where do I feel stuck, silenced, or unsure? Be honest and gentle—these are opportunities for growth.
Step 3: Empowered Reframing	
Choose one scenario where you wish you had communicated differently. Without judgment, write down: • What you did say • What you wish you had said • How you would say it now if you had the chance again This helps shift passive reflection into actionable insight. It also builds a mental "library" of language you can use in the future.	
Step 4: Intentions for Empowered Communication	
Complete the following statements to set communication goals rooted in empowerment: This week, I will speak up when ______________________________. I will practice confidence by using phrases like ______________________. I will remind myself that my voice matters because ____________________. When I feel unsure, I will ground myself by __________________________. Post your answers somewhere visible or revisit them weekly to build accountability.	

Figure 10.6 Structured reflection prompts to support growth in professional communication and advocacy.

moments of their beloved companion's life, or collaborating with colleagues to make swift, informed decisions in the ICU, communication remains at the heart of every meaningful interaction.

Importantly, communication is not a static skill but one that must be continuously developed and refined. By embracing self-awareness and self-regulation, veterinary technicians can manage their own emotional responses even in the most stressful moments. By practicing empathy and honing their social skills, they create stronger, more supportive relationships with both clients and team members. And by learning to recognize when communication falters, and having the courage to repair it, technicians demonstrate leadership and integrity that inspire trust and respect. In an environment as emotionally charged and fast-paced as veterinary medicine, the ability to communicate clearly, compassionately, and effectively is nothing short of transformative. These advanced communication strategies not only enhance patient outcomes and client satisfaction but also foster healthier workplace dynamics, reduce compassion fatigue, and elevate the role of veterinary technicians as essential advocates within the healthcare team. Through thoughtful, intentional communication, veterinary technicians truly become the voice for those who cannot speak and the steady presence for those who need it most.

References

Baile, W.F., Buckman, R., Lenzi, R. et al. (2000). SPIKES, A six-step protocol for delivering bad news: Application to the patient with cancer. *The Oncologist* 5 (4): 302–311.

Cannon, W.B. (1932). *The Wisdom of the Body*. W.W. Norton & Company.

Edmondson, A. (1999). Psychological safety and learning behavior in work teams. *Administrative Science Quarterly* 44 (2): 350–383.

Fossum, T.W. (2020). *Small Animal Surgery*, 5e. Elsevier.

Goleman, D. (1995). *Emotional Intelligence: Why It Can Matter More Than IQ*. Bantam Books.

Johnson, C. (2021). *Client Communication and Professional Relationships in Veterinary Practice*, 2e. CRC Press.

Merrill, D. and Reid, R. (1981). *Personal Styles and Effective Performance*. Chilton Book Company.

Street, R.L., Makoul, G., Arora, N.K., and Epstein, R.M. (2009). How does communication heal? Pathways linking clinician–patient communication to health outcomes. *Patient Education and Counseling* 74 (3): 295–301.

Part IV

Specialized Topics

11

Mental Health and Well-being

Introduction: Caring for the Caregivers

Veterinary technology is intimate work with high cognitive load. The day can move from calm routine to crisis within minutes; there may be little control over caseload, frequent interruptions, and intense interpersonal encounters with colleagues and clients. The emotional labor is continuous: one conversation requires transparent cost-of-care discussion; the next demands calm boundary-setting in the face of anger or grief; the third asks a technician to support a teammate who is quietly spiraling after a difficult shift. In environments where scheduling is tight, staffing fluctuates, and the inbox never ends, people begin to borrow from sleep, shorten meals into snacks taken standing, and carry unresolved conflict home. The result is not a failure of character but a predictable human response to chronic strain. A holistic perspective reframes well-being as a shared competency and a system property rather than an individual perk. The aim of this chapter is to give technicians and leaders common language for the problems they face, practical tools that fit the tempo of real clinics, and a credible path to workplaces where people can do demanding work without sacrificing their health or identity (Maslach and Leiter 2016).

Well-being in this chapter is organized across three interlocking levels: individual skills that steady attention and emotion, team practices that make candor and learning routine, and organizational design that restores time, predictability, and clarity. Figure 11.1 summarizes this framework and previews the practices explored in the sections that follow. Readers may use the inner ring to locate personal techniques, the middle ring to find team routines, and the outer ring to identify structural levers that prevent chronic overload.

The Landscape: Burnout, Compassion Fatigue, Moral Distress, and Moral Injury

Burnout is best understood not as a personal weakness but as a syndrome arising from persistent imbalance between job demands and available resources. It typically manifests as emotional exhaustion, depersonalization or cynical distancing, and a reduced sense of accomplishment. In practice, a burned-out technician may feel dread before shifts, annoyance toward clients or coworkers that would not have bothered them months earlier, and hollow relief at clock-out that never restores energy. Compassion fatigue describes the erosion of empathic capacity after repeated exposure to others' distress; it can travel with secondary traumatic stress, where images or moments replay uninvited. Moral distress occurs when a person knows or believes a particular action would be ethically preferable yet cannot enact it due to institutional constraints, interpersonal dynamics, legal limits, or financial reality. When moral distress is repeated and unresolved, it risks consolidating into moral injury, which is not simply "feeling bad" but a violation of the person's core moral expectations of themselves or their system. A technician who believes "we do right by people" may experience deep disorientation when outcomes depend on wallet size or when safety corners are cut. Naming these phenomena precisely matters because different problems require different remedies. Rest days do not repair moral injury; yoga does not fix structural understaffing; more effort does not offset contrary incentives. Teams must therefore pair individual skill-building with organizational change and ethical repair to see durable gains (Table 11.1) (Maslach and Leiter 2016; Litz et al. 2009).

Psychological Safety and Just Culture

Psychological safety is the shared belief that the group is safe for interpersonal risk-taking. In a psychologically safe team, people can ask naïve questions, challenge a plan respectfully, admit uncertainty, or disclose a mistake without fear of humiliation or retribution. This is not softness; it is a performance multiplier. When safety is high, concerns surface early rather than fester, and course corrections happen before harm. Just culture complements psychological safety by distinguishing

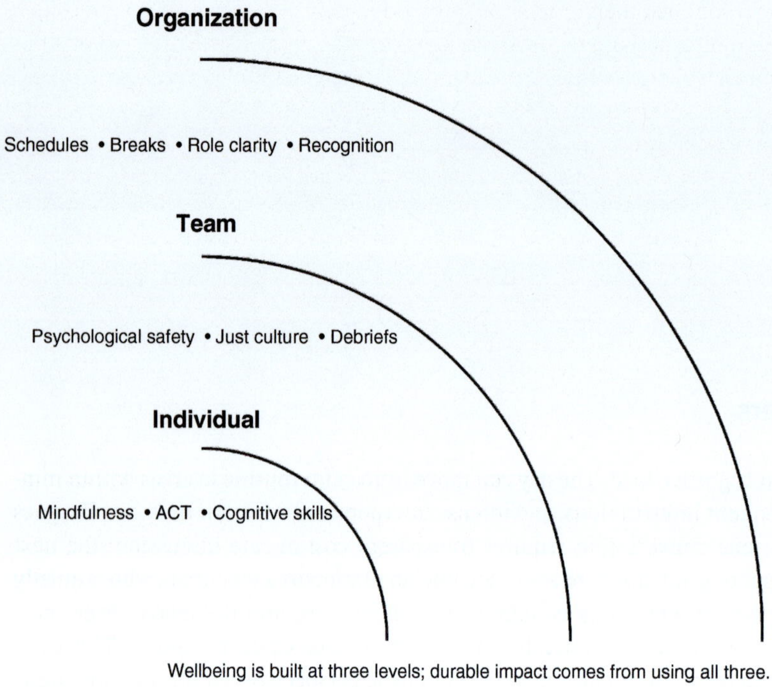

Figure 11.1 Concentric three-level framework: inner = individual skills (mindfulness, ACT, cognitive); middle = team practices (psychological safety, just culture, debriefs); outer = organizational design (schedules, breaks, role clarity, recognition). *Source:* Jennings (2025). Owner's own illustration.

Table 11.1 Concept comparison table—mental health constructs.

Concept	Definition	Common Triggers	Early Signs	Helpful Responses	When to Escalate
Burnout	Chronic demand–resource mismatch.	Overload; low control; quick turns.	Exhaustion; cynicism; inefficacy.	Predictable schedules; protected breaks; role clarity; targeted recognition.	Function impaired >2 weeks or risky coping → supervisor + EAP.
Compassion fatigue	Empathic depletion from repeated distress.	High emotional caseload; poor recovery.	Numbness; irritability; low patience.	Boundaries; rotation; brief debriefs; self-compassion routines.	Ongoing withdrawal or sleep loss → EAP/ clinician.
Secondary traumatic stress	Indirect trauma symptoms.	Exposure to traumatic events/ accounts.	Intrusions; hyperarousal; avoidance; nightmares.	CISM debriefs; second-victim support; grounding; short duty mods.	Symptoms >1–2 weeks or safety risk → licensed care.
Moral distress	Knows right action but blocked.	Cost limits; understaffing; conflicting directives.	Rumination; anger/ shame; avoidance.	Name strain; ethics huddle; tiered options; standard scripts.	Recurrent with impairment → leadership + counseling support.
Moral injury	Enduring value/identity violation.	Repeated unresolved distress; perceived betrayal.	Profound guilt; meaning collapse; bitterness; withdrawal.	Moral repair: acknowledge, change, facilitated processing.	Despair or self-harm thoughts → emergency care immediately.

among human error, at-risk behavior, and reckless conduct, then responding proportionately. Human error invites consoling and system fixes; at-risk behavior calls for coaching and risk awareness; reckless conduct has consequences. In practice, consider two contrasting incident conversations. In the first, a technician documents a near-miss and is met with silence or sarcasm; they learn to keep quiet. In the second, the supervisor thanks them, asks what made the slip likely, and removes the trap for others; the technician learns that speaking up improves the system. Over time, a just culture shifts people from self-protection to shared problem-solving and reduces the shame that feeds burnout. Leaders operationalize this by closing the loop on raised concerns, visibly sharing "what changed," modeling their own fallibility, and embedding nonpunitive postevent reviews that include human factors. When a senior technician says in a huddle, "I missed something yesterday; here's how the environment contributed and what I'm trying today," the team receives permission to be honest and curious rather than fearful (Edmondson 1999).

Mental Health First Aid and Second-Victim Support

Mental Health First Aid (MHFA) adapts the logic of basic life support to psychological crises: notice early warning signs, approach with care, listen nonjudgmentally, encourage professional support, and ensure safety. In veterinary workplaces, peers often notice the first indicators: a colleague who has become unusually irritable, markedly withdrawn, or suddenly reckless with breaks and boundaries. A trained teammate can say privately, "I'm noticing you're carrying a lot; would you be open to talking and planning support?" and then actually walk with them to an Employee Assistance Program (EAP) number, a private office, or a manager who knows how to respond. After adverse events, the "second-victim" experience is common: intrusive memories, shame, hypervigilance, avoidance of similar cases, and even insomnia. The solution is not to command resilience but to supply a prepared response pathway. A simple three-step protocol helps: a same-day check-in by a trained peer to ensure immediate safety and normalize reactions; a scheduled follow-up within seventy-two hours to assess sleep, appetite, and functional impairment; and a menu of supports from modified duties and buddy shifts to counseling referrals. The phrase "second-victim" is imperfect and sometimes contested, but the need it highlights is real: clinicians deserve structured care when care goes badly for any reason, including systems failures or interpersonal conflict (Mental Health First Aid USA n.d.).

Key steps in MHFA include:

1) **Recognize the Signs of Distress:** Veterinary technicians must develop the observational skills to recognize behavioral and emotional changes in their colleagues. Warning signs include noticeable shifts in mood, withdrawal from social interactions, increased irritability, decreased job performance, unexplained absenteeism, and expressions of hopelessness or overwhelm. A colleague who was once enthusiastic and engaged may become quiet, detached, or visibly fatigued. Recognizing these shifts early allows for timely intervention before the situation escalates.
2) **Approach with Compassion and Nonjudgment:** Approaching a colleague about mental health concerns requires sensitivity and genuine care. Choose a private, quiet space to have the conversation, and start with open-ended, nonconfrontational language. For example, say, "I've noticed you seem a bit down lately, and I'm really concerned. Is there anything you'd like to talk about or anything I can do to help?" This gentle approach signals empathy and creates a safe space for the person to open up without feeling judged or embarrassed.
3) **Listen Without Trying to Fix the Problem Immediately:** One of the most powerful tools in MHFA is active listening. Often, individuals experiencing emotional distress need to feel heard before they are ready to seek solutions. Avoid offering immediate advice or dismissive reassurances like, "You'll be fine" or "Just try to stay positive." Instead, practice reflective listening by repeating back what the person shares and acknowledging their emotions. Phrases such as "That sounds incredibly difficult" or "I can't imagine how heavy that feels for you" validate their experience and demonstrate understanding.
4) **Encourage Professional Help and Resource Utilization:** While peer support is invaluable, it is not a substitute for professional mental health care. Encourage colleagues to access available resources, such as EAPs, counseling services, or mental health hotlines. If a colleague is reluctant to seek help, gently emphasize that mental health is just as important as physical health and that professional support is a sign of strength, not weakness.
5) **Know How to Respond in Crisis Situations:** In cases where a colleague expresses thoughts of self-harm or suicide, immediate action is required. Veterinary technicians should familiarize themselves with crisis intervention protocols and know when and how to involve supervisors, HR personnel, or emergency services. Remaining calm, ensuring the person is not left alone, and connecting them with immediate support can be lifesaving.

Emotional Debriefing and Critical Incident Stress Management

Critical Incident Stress Management (CISM) offers structured, time-limited processes to metabolize emotional load after difficult events. Effective debriefs are optional, confidential, facilitated by someone trained, and focused on human experience rather than technical critique. They are not therapy and should not become blame sessions. A 20-minute debrief at the end of a brutal day might begin with a brief grounding exercise, invite each person to name what hit hardest and what helped, validate normal stress responses, and end with concrete next steps, such as schedule adjustments or outreach to those most affected. Every day, "micro-debriefs" matter too. When a tense client interaction ends, two colleagues can take three minutes to acknowledge adrenaline, identify one skill that worked, and decide how to document and escalate if needed. This short circuit prevents people from carrying unresolved activation into the next room and lays the groundwork for a culture where feelings are not treated as private defects but as data that inform safer practice (Figure 11.2).

Boundaries, Empathy, and Sustainable Compassion

Boundaries, empathy, and sustainable compassion are presented as interlocking skills that keep care steady rather than sacrificial. The first section examines boundaries in clinical reality, clear definitions, early warning signs of erosion in body, mood, and schedule, and precise language and micro-habits that make limits visible and repairable, supported by team coverage and predictable breaks. The second section deepens empathy by distinguishing cognitive perspective-taking from affective resonance, outlining methods to prevent empathic distress, and offering practical routines such as precontact perspective checks, concise in-the-moment reflection lines, and postinteraction resets that protect energy while improving connection. The final section develops sustainable compassion, integrating daily self-compassion practices, compassionate limit-setting that pairs warmth with clarity, closure rituals that help leave work at work, and unit-level scaffolds, brief debriefs, and buddy coverage, so difficult moments are not carried alone. Each section provides recognition cues for when skills are slipping, ready-to-use scripts, short practice drills, and leadership actions that embed these capacities as durable team norms (Neff 2011).

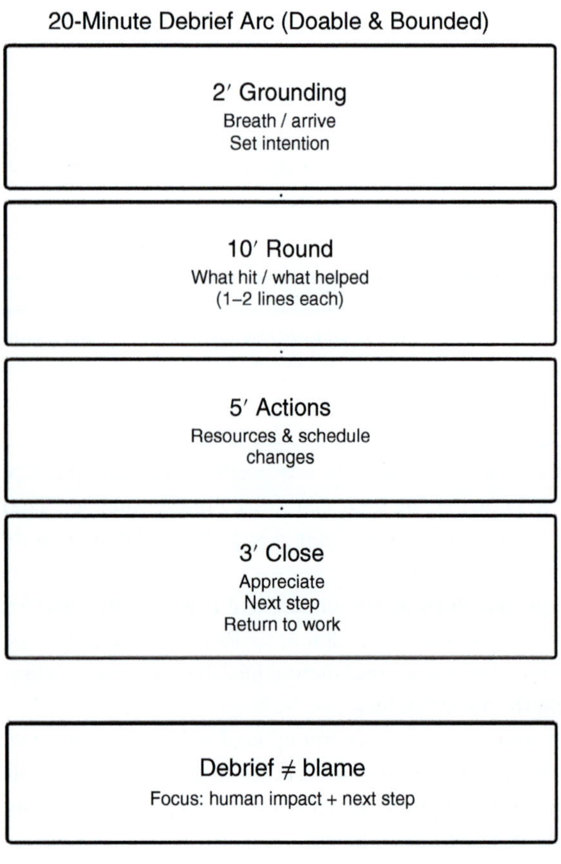

Figure 11.2 2′ grounding → 10′ "what hit/what helped" round → 5′ resources and schedule actions → 3′ close. *Source:* Jennings (2025). Author's own illustration.

Boundaries

Boundaries are the rules by which you protect finite human capacities, time, attention, emotion, privacy, and recovery, so your care remains steady rather than sacrificial. In busy hospitals, boundary erosion rarely announces itself dramatically; it creeps in through calendar "quick favors," skipped breaks, after-hours messages answered out of guilt, and the quiet belief that being dependable means being always available. Early signs that your boundaries are slipping include resentment at reasonable requests, irritability that lingers after small interactions, a sense that you are performing friendliness while feeling empty, and difficulty transitioning to nonwork roles after a shift. Some people notice boundary trouble somatically before they see the pattern, jaw clenching, headaches, shallow breathing, or cognitively through rumination about work while doing ordinary home tasks. The corrective begins by externalizing boundaries from private willpower to visible agreements. Drafting a one-paragraph "personal practice policy" is a practical start: specify when you take breaks and who can interrupt, how you handle after-hours communication, and what you do when you feel flooded. Share this with your lead or manager and anchor it in team norms so it is not merely a personal preference but a safety practice. Build small environmental cues that support the agreement: a "step-out" card you can hand a colleague when you need two minutes to reset, a five-minute block on your schedule after emotionally intense calls to complete notes and breathe, and a door-frame reminder that says "arrive-home ritual" to prevent carrying the last case into your evening.

Language makes boundaries practicable. Prerehearsed sentences prevent over-explaining in the heat of the moment. In client conversations, you might say, "I want to give you a clear update. I'll gather the details and call you by 2 p.m. so I can be thorough rather than rushed." In colleague requests that exceed current capacity: "I can do the medication reconciliation now or the discharge call in 15 minutes; which keeps us safest?" When emotions run high, pairing empathy with limit-setting keeps both intact: "I hear how worried you are, and I'm going to step out to get support so I can respond well. I'll return in two minutes." Repair matters when boundaries are crossed. If you say yes and realize it was a mistake, close the loop: "I overcommitted and can't complete this safely today. Here's what I can own, and here's what needs to shift." At the team level, leaders reinforce boundaries by scheduling predictable breaks, discouraging "quick turns," publishing coverage plans for protected time, and modeling their own limits so staff see that saying no appropriately is a mark of professionalism, not defiance (Maslach and Leiter 2016). Individually, track "boundary drift" for one week by jotting down each time you worked through a break, answered messages after hours, or said yes with resentment. Reviewing this list with a peer or supervisor converts vague overwhelm into a specific redesign. Boundaries are not barriers to caring; they are the frame that makes durable caring possible (Table 11.2).

Empathy

Empathy is the capacity to understand and resonate with another person's experience; in practice, it has two parts that need different care. Cognitive empathy is perspective-taking, grasping what the other person believes and values. Affective empathy is feeling with, recognizing, and, to a degree, sharing their emotion. When untrained, affective empathy can tip into empathic distress, where we absorb another's feelings without regulation and become overwhelmed ourselves. Trained empathy uses the information of feeling to guide skillful action, not to drown the clinician. Signs that your empathy is struggling include fast judgments about "difficult clients," sarcasm as a default relief valve, narrative shortcuts that assume bad faith, and dread at the thought of specific conversations. On the other end of the spectrum, over-identification shows up as taking responsibility for outcomes you do not control, staying late reflexively without strategic benefit, and feeling personally rejected when plans change. The practical work is to widen the gap between perception and reaction just enough to choose a response. A simple sequence helps: notice what you feel ("tight chest, heat in face"), name what the other might feel using plain words before content ("this sounds frightening and frustrating"), reflect concisely ("you were expecting X and got Y"), and then ask one clarifying question that moves the problem forward ("so that I don't miss what matters most, what is the smallest helpful next step right now?"). This pattern reduces adrenaline for everyone and keeps you anchored to purpose rather than to your own discomfort.

Structured empathy exercises can be woven into daily work without special sessions. Before a charged phone call, spend 30 seconds writing the client's likely story from their vantage point; then revise it once with the most generous plausible interpretation. After the call, note which parts of your guess were accurate and which were not; this trains calibration over time. In huddles, practice "looped listening" in pairs: one person speaks for 30 seconds about a recent tough interaction; the other reflects content and emotion in two sentences and asks one genuine question. Switching roles reveals how concise reflections can feel surprisingly validating. When you sense empathic distress rising mid-conversation, a brief internal cue

Table 11.2 Boundary language bank.

Empathy + Limit—sentence stems	Repair after over-commit
• "I can hear how important this is. To give a reliable answer, I will check the chart and call by [time]." • "I want to help. I can do [task A] now or [task B] in 15 minutes—which keeps us safest?" • "I hear the urgency, and I need two minutes to get support so I respond well. I will be right back." • "I am not able to [request] right now. I can [alternative] by [time] or tomorrow at [time]." • "Let's keep our language respectful so we can solve this. If it continues, I will pause and bring in a lead." • "I can stay on this for five minutes, then I need to return to my assignment."	• "I overcommitted earlier and cannot finish [task] safely today. Here is what I can complete now: [scope]. Let's adjust [plan/owner]." • "I said yes too quickly. To maintain quality, I need to move this to [time] or ask [name] to take lead." • "Thanks for your flexibility while I correct this."

One-Week Boundary Drift Tracker (review on Day 7)

Day	Break taken	After-hours OFF	Said NO/deferral	1-line note
Mon	[ ]	[ ]	[ ]	
Tue	[ ]	[ ]	[ ]	
Wed	[ ]	[ ]	[ ]	
Thu	[ ]	[ ]	[ ]	
Fri	[ ]	[ ]	[ ]	
Sat	[ ]	[ ]	[ ]	
Sun	[ ]	[ ]	[ ]	

Replace over-explaining with clean scripts. Pair empathy with a clear limit; repair quickly if you over-commit; track boundary drift for one week. How to use: check a box each day. If boxes stay unchecked → boundaries are holding. If checks cluster, review with a peer/lead and adjust schedule, scripts, or coverage.
Source: Jennings (2025). Author's own illustration.

such as "soften belly, slow voice" paired with a single present-moment breath interrupts escalation and restores choice (Kabat-Zinn 1994). Team culture amplifies or extinguishes empathy. Psychological safety, permission to speak honestly without humiliation, enables technicians to ask for help when they feel flooded and to debrief without fear afterward (Edmondson 1999). Leaders can protect empathy by centralizing responses to online criticism so individuals do not carry digital blast radius on their own time and by explicitly teaching staff that empathic accuracy plus clear boundaries, not emotional fusion, is the target. Empathy becomes sustainable when it is precise, time-bound, and linked to action rather than to self-sacrifice (Table 11.3).

Sustainable Compassion

Sustainable compassion converts empathic understanding into balanced, values-guided action while maintaining the caregiver's humanity. It is the felt stance of "I am with you and I will help in the ways that are mine to give," combined with a clear recognition of limits. The opposite poles, numb detachment on one side, martyrdom on the other, are both signs that compassion has slipped out of balance. Warning lights for depletion include a flatness that persists across interactions, cynicism that masquerades as humor, compulsive fixing that overrides consent, and exhaustion wildly disproportionate to the actual time spent helping. The antidote is not to care less but to care differently. Self-compassion is the keystone skill: responding to one's own moments of suffering with kindness, awareness of shared humanity, and mindful presence rather than self-criticism. Practiced regularly, it reduces shame after inevitable mistakes, increases willingness to seek help, and stabilizes mood under strain (Neff 2011). A workable daily routine might begin with a two-minute compassion practice before shift, silently acknowledging that the day will include limits, wishing yourself steadiness, and setting one value you will try to embody in your tone. During the day, use "compassionate limit-setting" language that keeps warmth and boundary together: "I hear that you need an immediate answer; the safest way to give you that is to review the chart

Table 11.3 Empathy micro-sequence—quick reference chart.

Step	Purpose	Micro-actions (body cue/reset)	Example language	Pitfall to avoid
1) Notice (body cue)	Widen attention and interrupt autopilot.	• Feet on floor • Longer exhale (4–6 second) • Name the cue (e.g., "tight chest").	—	Jumping straight to fixing or defending.
2) Name emotion first	Validate affect before facts to lower arousal.	• Softer tone • First words label feeling (not cause).	"This sounds worrying." "This is upsetting and frustrating."	Explaining policy before acknowledging emotion.
3) Reflect content	Show you heard the core mismatch/need.	• Mirror one sentence, neutral • Avoid blame words.	"You expected X and received Y." "You needed a clear cost and got mixed messages."	Arguing details or adding justifications.
4) Clarifying question	Focus the next helpful step and share control.	• One question only • Offer a small next action.	"What would help most right now?" "Would two options help?"	Multiple questions or shifting back to policy talk.

Under pressure: Notice → Name emotion → Reflect content → Clarifying question.
Jennings (2025). Author's own Illustration.

and call you by three. I'm putting that on my list now." End the day with a closure ritual that marks completion: write down three small moments of effectiveness, name one hard thing you are not taking home, and perform a brief physical reset like a shoulder roll and slow exhale. These micro-practices, repeated, train the nervous system to move out of threat and into engagement.

Teams can scaffold sustainable compassion by normalizing "compassion budgets" on intense services, short recovery windows built into flow, a designated quiet space, and buddy coverage for five-minute resets after charged encounters. Leaders should model compassionate self-talk publicly after hard moments, "That was rough; I'm going to take two minutes to settle so my next call gets my best," so staff see that care for self is part of care for others. Debriefs that ask "what was hardest" and "what helped" metabolize acute activation before it calcifies into avoidance. When moral distress is involved, sustainable compassion includes moral repair: candid acknowledgment of constraint, shared problem-solving to reduce recurrence, and explicit statements of professional identity that are not outcome-contingent ("we tell the truth kindly, we act within our scope, and we stand with each other even when we cannot change the facts"). Organizations contribute by designing schedules that protect sleep and breaks, rewarding relational skills in evaluations, and providing access to timely counseling so people can process accumulated stress rather than white-knuckling through it (Maslach and Leiter 2016). Over time, sustainable compassion feels like grounded warmth rather than glow or drain: present enough to connect, steady enough to think, clear enough to stop when the work of the moment is done. It is not a personality trait some have and others lack; it is a trainable stance supported by individual habits, team practices, and humane work design (Figure 11.3).

Evidence-Based Coping: Mindfulness, Acceptance, and Cognitive Skills

This section presents mindfulness, acceptance-based skills, and cognitive strategies as an integrated toolkit for protecting attention and flexibility under stress. It begins by clarifying what each skill set is and is not, then outlines recognition cues that signal trouble, mindfulness lapses marked by rumination and reactivity, acceptance pitfalls such as experiential avoidance or value-drift, and cognitive traps like catastrophizing and mind-reading. The mindfulness subsection focuses on brief, workflow-friendly drills, a one-minute precall reset, between-task body scans, and a consistent "arrive-home" ritual, paired with examples from common clinical moments to demonstrate transfer. The acceptance (ACT) subsection develops diffusion phrases, values clarification, and a simple "choice point" map to guide behavior when emotions surge, with sample self-talk that re-anchors steadiness or kindness. The cognitive subsection trains distortion spotting, reality-testing questions, and if-then coping plans that keep thinking accurate under pressure. Each subsection provides concrete scripts, short practice

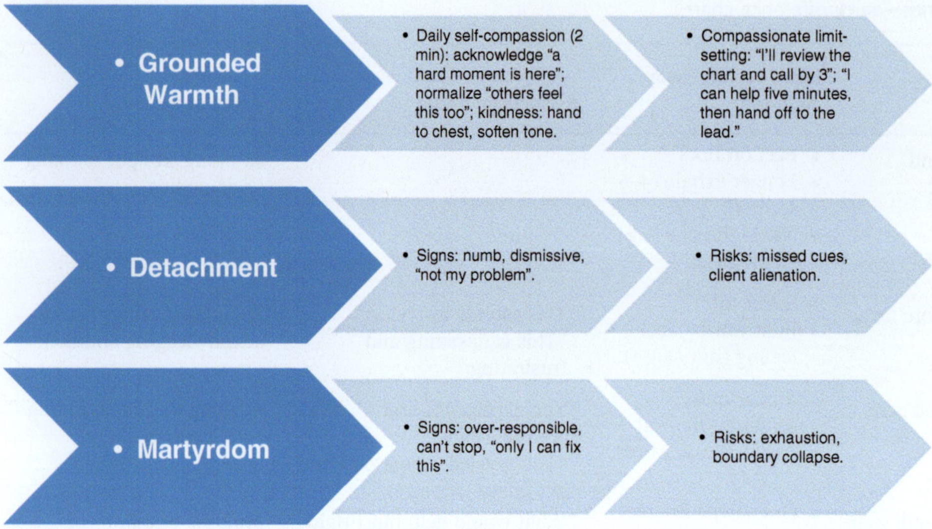

Figure 11.3 Sustainable compassion outline with "Grounded Warmth" practices. *Source:* Jennings (2025). Author's own Illustration.

progressions, and leader actions, embedding skills in huddles, posting visual prompts, protecting micro-practice windows, and knowing when to route someone to professional support, so these methods function as job tools rather than private wellness hobbies.

Mindfulness

Mindfulness refers to training attention to return, on purpose and without judgment, to present-moment experience. In clinical reality, this means noticing sensory cues, thoughts, and emotions as they arise and recovering steadiness quickly enough to choose the next helpful action. The aim is not blankness or passivity; it is an agile attention that can widen or narrow on demand. Early signals that mindfulness is slipping include automatic reactions to tone or facial expression, rumination that replays conversations long after they end, and abrupt swings in pace, rushing when deliberate speed would be safer or stalling when decisive movement is required. Many clinicians first detect lapses somatically: clenched jaw, shallow breathing, or a sense of tunnel vision during difficult calls. Treating these signals as prompts rather than failures allows a return to skill: a short breath reset before speaking, a deliberate label of the emotion that is present, and a single clear intention for the next minute.

Micro-practices make mindfulness feasible in busy hospitals. A one-minute precontact reset, taken before a charged phone call or conversation, stabilizes tone and word choice; it can be as simple as feeling the feet on the floor, letting the breath lengthen naturally, and setting a quiet intention such as steadiness or clarity. Between tasks, a brief body scan, relaxing the brow, softening the shoulders, and releasing the tongue from the roof of the mouth interrupts cumulative tension that otherwise masquerades as irritability. After emotionally dense encounters, a "note-and-name" check converts vague activation into information: identify one emotion in plain language, identify one fact that is still true, and identify one next step that honors both. At day's end, an "arrive-home" ritual tells the nervous system the shift is over: put keys down in the same place, wash hands slowly while recounting three competent moments, and take one deliberate breath at the threshold before entering home roles. None of these practices requires special equipment or long sessions, but repetition creates accessible grooves the mind can fall back into when stress spikes (Kabat-Zinn 1994).

Mindfulness scales from individual habit to team norm. When prehuddle includes a 60-second shared breath before complex days, teams begin on the same cadence. When leaders narrate their own resets, "that conversation activated me; I am taking one minute to settle so the next client gets my best," permission to pause becomes part of professionalism rather than a private indulgence. Visual cues placed thoughtfully, small "breathe before you brief" cards near phones, or "arrive-home" notes at exits, keep skills in the environment rather than in memory alone. Over time, clinics that protect these micro-windows see fewer verbal escalations, clearer documentation, and a steadier emotional climate, not because people care less but because attention is trained to return where it is most useful (Kabat-Zinn 1994).

Acceptance and Commitment Skills (ACT)

Acceptance and Commitment Therapy skills translate well to healthcare because they assume that internal experiences, thoughts, emotions, images, and urges are often uncontrollable in the moment, while behavior can still be guided by chosen values. Acceptance in this context is not resignation; it is a willingness to make room for inevitable discomfort so that actions can align with what matters. The common breakdowns are experiential avoidance and value drift. Avoidance shows up as chronic email refreshing to delay a difficult call, detouring into low-leverage tasks, or over-explaining to dampen anxiety. Value drift appears as tone and choices that no longer match professional identity, such as sarcasm with colleagues despite a commitment to kindness, or rushed discharges that contradict a value of clarity. Recognition of these patterns is the first intervention; naming them restores discretion.

Defusion techniques help unhook from sticky thoughts without arguing with them. A simple internal phrasing, "I am having the thought that this client will attack me online," creates a few centimeters of distance between the thinker and the thought. Noticing the mind's habit of catastrophizing and labeling it as a habit rather than as a prophecy makes room for values to steer the next step. Values clarification then provides the compass. When steadiness and honesty are the chosen anchors, the next sentence can be shaped accordingly: "Here is what is known, here is what is uncertain, and here is what happens next." A practical "choice-point" sketch on scrap paper can be done in under a minute: current trigger in the center, helpful moves that bring behavior toward values on one side, unhelpful moves that pull away on the other. Having named both paths, even a single value-consistent move, lowering the voice, pausing to verify a fact, or inviting a colleague to join, shifts the interaction's trajectory. After high-arousal moments, a brief postevent note that connects action to value, "today's steady tone in triage matched the value of safety," reinforces identity and makes it more likely that the same move will be available next time (Hayes et al. 2012).

Teams can embed ACT skills without formal therapy by normalizing language that reflects defusion and values. Leaders who say in debrief, "a story showed up in my head that I was failing; the helpful move was to return to accuracy," model process, not just outcome. Unit posters that quietly ask, "What value is needed in these next five minutes?" cue behavior without shaming emotion. Supervisors can include a two-question check in one-to-ones: what thoughts or feelings have been loud this week, and what value would guide the next call or case, so that staff practice mapping discomfort to action. This approach does not minimize distress; it gives it a place while insisting that behavior remains aligned with professional purpose (Hayes et al. 2012).

Cognitive Skills

Cognitive skills target the accuracy of thinking under pressure. The cognitive model proposes that emotions and behaviors are influenced by how situations are interpreted; when interpretations skew negative or absolute, decisions and tone suffer. In practice, a technician might jump from a delayed callback to a conclusion that the client is hostile, or from a single documentation oversight to a global judgment of incompetence. The first task is detection. Common distortions include catastrophizing, mind-reading, all-or-nothing evaluations, and confirmation seeking that ignores disconfirming facts. Somatic cues again assist recognition: a rising heart rate and narrowed attention often accompany stories that are racing ahead of evidence. Once noticed, interpretations can be tested rather than obeyed.

Reality-testing questions keep cognition tethered to data. Useful prompts include: what facts are known now; what equally plausible, less threatening explanations exist; what evidence would I accept as sufficient to change my mind; and what small experiment could gather that evidence quickly. Translating these into action might mean calling a client with a neutral, structured opener rather than composing a defensive script, or asking a colleague to read a note before sending rather than assuming it will be misinterpreted. If-then plans convert insight into reliability: if a review or email triggers dread, then read it once aloud in a neutral voice and list three verifiable points before deciding how to respond; if an error is discovered, then notify the appropriate person using a standard template that separates emotion from facts. When cognitive skills are paired with mindfulness and acceptance, accuracy improves without sliding into toxic positivity; the target is not cheerful reinterpretation but usable, testable understanding (Beck 2011).

Leaders can cultivate cognitive accuracy at the team level by modeling thoughtful reappraisal in real time. During huddle, a supervisor might say, "The schedule looks stacked; the story that shows up is 'today will be chaos'. A more accurate frame is that the morning is dense and the afternoon has flex; the plan is to redistribute two appointments and assign a float for triage." Incident reviews can be run through a thinking-accuracy lens that asks, "What assumptions did we make, which were right, which were wrong, and how will we test the next one?" Over time, teams that practice noticing and testing interpretations become faster at distinguishing signal from noise. People waste less energy on imagined attacks, apologize sooner when wrong, and choose communication that reflects reality rather than reflex.

Shift Work, Sleep, and the Physiology of Recovery

Shift and rotating schedules misalign circadian timing with required wakefulness, degrading mood regulation, attention, and executive function; in practice, this shows up as irritability, slowed processing, memory slips, and a higher likelihood of error. Framing sleep as clinical equipment rather than a personal luxury aligns with the burnout literature's central claim that performance and well-being deteriorate when demands chronically exceed resources, and that restoring fundamental resources (time, recovery, staffing) is a systems responsibility rather than an individual fix (Maslach and Leiter 2016).

Physiology-informed routines make recovery more reliable after nights and rotations. A consistent wind-down and daytime-sleep protocol, cool, dark, quiet, helps consolidate sleep, while simple attentional resets reduce carryover arousal: a one-minute breath before leaving work, a brief body-scan on arriving home, and a deliberate "arrive-home" ritual that marks the end of role demands. These micro-practices do not aim for blankness but for steadier awareness under stress, a goal supported by foundational mindfulness work showing that short, repeatable practices can improve regulation and reduce reactivity (Kabat-Zinn 1994). Caffeine used early in a shift with a firm cutoff, strategic short naps on prolonged nights, and minimized bright-light exposure before daytime sleep further protect alertness and rest without requiring long training blocks.

Whether recovery actually happens depends on design. "Quick turns" that compress rest windows, unpredictable rosters, and unprotected meal and restroom breaks cumulatively erode capacity; the antidote is schedule architecture that preserves recovery time after nights, publishes assignments early, and treats breaks as safety practices, not perks. When supervisors routinely ask in huddle, "Who is coming off nights, and what assignments protect their bandwidth?" they model the psychologically safe behavior of naming human limits without stigma, which in turn makes it easier for staff to surface fatigue risks before they become mistakes (Edmondson 1999). In clinics that consistently align work structure with human physiology, the predictable result is fewer lapses and steadier morale, not because people try harder, but because the system returns essential resources to the people doing the work (Maslach and Leiter 2016).

Communication Pressures, Client Incivility, and Digital Well-being

In many hospitals, the hardest moments come not from clinical complexity but from conversations under pressure. Cost-of-care discussions, boundary enforcement, and emotionally charged feedback can trigger adrenaline surges, narrow attention, and leave lingering rumination long after a shift ends. Three domains determine whether communication drains or sustains teams: the skill to de-escalate in real time, the policy backbone that defines how incivility and abuse are handled, and digital habits that prevent online interactions from invading rest and recovery. When these domains work together, skill, policy, and digital boundaries, staff remain warm and clear, risk decreases, and difficult exchanges become manageable rather than corrosive.

Communication Pressures

Communication under load is a physiologic event as much as a linguistic one. Heart rate rises, breath shortens, and the mind begins to predict threat, which pushes tone toward speed or sharpness. Recognizing this pattern early allows a return to choice. A brief, internal reset before high-stakes contact, feeling both feet, letting the exhale lengthen, naming a single intention such as steadiness, widens attention enough to hear the other person rather than only reacting to their tone. From there, three practices make a measurable difference: visible listening, emotion-first reflection, and structured clarity. Visible listening means silence long enough to let the other person finish a sentence without interruption, eye contact that is steady but relaxed, and nods or short verbal acknowledgments that show tracking. Emotion-first reflection places feelings before content: "this has been frustrating and worrying," so nervous systems settle enough to process information. Structured clarity then offers brief, ordered steps: "here is what is known, here is what is uncertain, and here is what happens next," so the conversation has a direction rather than a swirl.

Scripts help under pressure because they reduce decision load in the moment. In a cost-of-care call, a technician might say, "I want to make sure nothing important is missed. I'll summarize what has been discussed, name what is still uncertain, and then outline options so you can decide the next step." When emotions rise, pairing empathy with limits preserves both: "I can hear how urgent this feels, and the safest way to give you a reliable answer is to check the chart and call you by two o'clock." After a tense exchange, a short closure helps prevent rumination: one sentence acknowledging difficulty, one sentence naming an effective action taken, and one sentence committing to the next step. Practiced regularly, these tiny rituals reduce spillover into subsequent conversations and shorten the emotional tail of a hard day. Team culture reinforces skill when shared language is adopted across roles. If everyone uses the same phrases to reflect emotion and to set next steps, clients experience consistency, and staff can hand off seamlessly. Leaders signal expectations by modeling resets aloud, "that was charged; taking one minute to settle so the next call gets my best," and by scheduling brief debrief windows after predictable pressure points so learning is captured while the experience is fresh. Over time, communication becomes less about personality and more about repeatable patterns that hold up under stress.

Client Incivility

Not all difficult communication is equal. Incivility includes discourtesy, sarcasm, raised voices, and dismissive comments; abuse includes threats, slurs, persistent harassment, and any behavior that compromises safety. Treating every sharp edge as abuse dilutes credibility; treating any abuse as "part of the job" erodes morale and retention. A clear, rehearsed policy draws the line and explains the response. Staff need to know the exact language that constitutes a warning, how that warning is delivered, what happens if it is ignored, and who steps in. A technician might say, in a steady tone, "I want to help and can continue once we keep our language respectful. If the language continues, I will pause this conversation and involve my supervisor." If the boundary is crossed again, the follow-through should be immediate and calm: "We are pausing now. My supervisor will join us to determine next steps." Consistency matters more than volume. When policies are enforced predictably across clients and the time of day, staff learn that their well-being is not negotiable, and clients learn that anger will not buy access to exceptions.

Preparation reduces escalation. Posting a brief, plainly worded code of conduct at entrances and on invoices sets expectations before problems arise. Training should include role clarity about who issues warnings, who terminates conversations or visits, and how documentation occurs so that follow-up is grounded in facts. After any abusive episode, support for the staff member involved should be automatic rather than requested, private check-in on the same day, a short follow-up within 72 hours to assess impact and sleep, and modest scheduling adjustments if needed. This is not about dramatizing routine friction; it is about acknowledging that the body remembers threat and benefits from a structured return to baseline. Leaders contribute by closing the loop publicly, without naming clients, on what changed because staff spoke up, such as adding a second person to certain conversations or revising front-desk scripts that reliably triggered conflict. When accountability sits with policy and leadership rather than with individual willpower, people stop grinding through hostility alone and start engaging boundaries as a shared safety practice (Figure 11.4).

Digital Well-being

Online spaces amplify both praise and harm, and the timing is rarely humane. A scathing review read at midnight lingers into the next morning; a group-chat debate during a day off converts recovery time into unpaid labor; a flurry of after-hours messages teaches staff that availability is a measure of loyalty. Digital well-being reframes technology usage so it supports care rather than colonizes private life. The first shift is structural: route public-facing complaints to a single point of contact, such as a manager or small communications team, and remove the expectation that individual technicians monitor or respond to reviews on personal time. Standard responses should be calm, brief, and oriented to offline resolution, acknowledging concern, avoiding clinical specifics, and inviting a direct conversation with leadership. This keeps reputational management professional and prevents staff from becoming targets in back-and-forth threads that rarely help anyone.

Internal communication deserves similar boundary setting. Clear expectations about response times, quiet hours, and the difference between urgent and nonurgent messages prevent constant low-level vigilance. If the culture expects unread badges to be cleared immediately, attention never fully returns to rest; if the culture expects batch responses during set windows and reserves true emergencies for phone calls, bodies relearn that off time is safe. Leaders set the tone by adhering to the norms themselves and by scheduling messages to send during work hours when possible. Staff can support themselves with small habits: disabling push notifications during sleep windows, moving social apps off the home screen, and choosing a personal ritual that marks the end of online clinic time each day. Privacy and professionalism guide the final layer. Declining to engage with clients on personal accounts, avoiding case details online, and routing disputes into documented, secure channels protect both staff and the organization. When digital boundaries, centralized responses, and humane messaging norms are in place, online noise stops dictating mood and availability, and recovery becomes possible again.

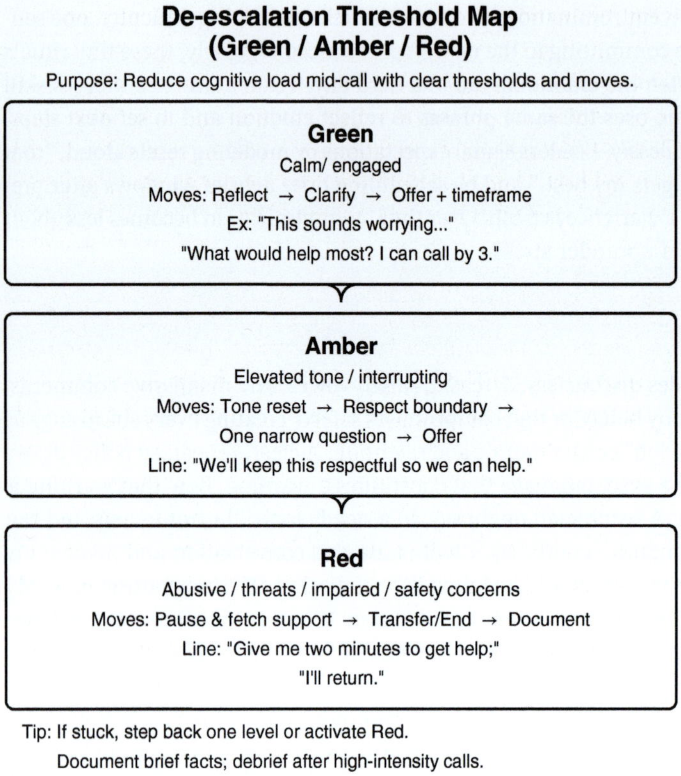

Figure 11.4 De-escalation threshold map. *Source:* Jennings (2025). Author's own illustration.

Economic Realities, Moral Distress, and Meaning

Financial constraints are powerful generators of moral distress because they collide with professional identity and purpose. Many in helping professions hold a core belief, "we help," and experience a particular kind of injury when help appears contingent on money or when staffing limits force corners to be cut. This is not ordinary sadness; repeated exposure to value-conflict can erode meaning and, if unresolved, consolidate into moral injury, a wound to conscience and identity that persists beyond the immediate event (Litz et al. 2009). In veterinary settings, cost-of-care pressures and resource scarcity are frequent sources of ethical conflict, making moral distress a predictable occupational hazard rather than a rare exception (Moses et al. 2018).

Recognition is the first repair step. Moral distress often presents as lingering anger or shame after encounters, ruminative replay of conversations, avoidance of similar situations, or a sense of contamination, "this isn't who I am at work." It may also appear somatically as tightness in the chest, restless sleep, or an uncharacteristically short fuse. These signals differ from ordinary fatigue because they are tied to perceived violations of values rather than to workload alone. Naming the injury, "this was an ethical strain, not a simple bad day," helps move from self-blame to shared problem-solving and prevents the accumulation of unresolved "moral residue" that amplifies the next event (Litz et al. 2009).

Conversation design can reduce harm even when resources cannot be changed. Tiered options prepared in advance allow technicians to describe paths clearly without implying false guarantees; uncertainty should be labeled in plain language and paired with a next step so families and teams are not cornered at peak emotion. Phrases that hold honesty and kindness together are protective: "Here is what is known, here is what remains uncertain, and here are two feasible next steps." Inviting pauses is equally protective: "This is a lot to take in; it is reasonable to be hesitant, and we can revisit in a few minutes." After charged exchanges, brief closures prevent rumination: one sentence to acknowledge difficulty, one sentence to note an effective action taken, and one to define the immediate follow-up. These small, repeatable moves do not erase constraints, but they preserve integrity under constraint. Team response should treat moral distress as an expected human reaction, not a private failing. Short, nonpunitive debriefs, 10–20 minutes, optional, facilitated, help metabolize acute moral strain. Three questions are sufficient: what felt worst, what was within the team's control, and what will change next time. Leaders strengthen trust by closing the loop on those answers, even when the change is incremental. Psychological safety is crucial at this stage; when staff can name ethical tension without fear of humiliation or reprisal, distress is shared and addressed rather than silently carried (Maslach and Leiter 2016).

Organizational design turns isolated coping into durable protection. Standardized payment pathways and transparent scripts reduce ad hoc bargaining that feels arbitrary. Where feasible, compassionate-care funds provide a structured, accountable way to assist without relying on individual exceptions; when funds are limited, clear criteria prevent moral injury from case-by-case improvisation. Regular ethics huddles or brief consult channels give staff a place to surface dilemmas early and distribute responsibility for decisions. Workload and staffing policies remain foundational: chronic overload magnifies ethical strain and accelerates burnout, whereas restoring time, recovery, and role clarity returns essential resources to the people doing the work (Maslach and Leiter 2016).

This debriefing outline is designed for veterinary technicians and frontline teams, including those stepping into lead or supervisory roles. It is used after moments that carry moral stress, value conflicts, cost-of-care constraints, adverse outcomes, near misses, or incidents of disrespect, not during an active crisis. The goal is quick, nonpunitive sense-making: a 10–20 minute, optional huddle with a named facilitator (any trained peer, shift lead, or manager) that turns distress into one or two concrete changes. Psychological safety is the ground rule, no blame, one-mic, permission to pass, so experiences can be named without fear. The expected outputs are small but visible: a script tweak, a micro-policy adjustment, a clear owner and timeframe, and a "close the loop" update to the team. Scheduled at the end of a shift or within 24–72 hours, this outline normalizes moral emotions as an occupational signal and builds trust across roles; if risk remains high or questions exceed the team's scope, the discussion escalates to a formal review while preserving the same humane tone (Table 11.4).

Moral repair is a deliberate process: candid acknowledgment of the constraint and its impact, affirmation of shared values that were threatened, concrete steps to prevent recurrence when possible, and visible support for those most affected. A simple institutional statement, "This decision conflicted with our values; here is what we are changing, and here is the support available this week," signals that the organization sees and shares the weight. Over time, consistently naming tension and aligning language and policy reduce isolation and blunt the frequency and intensity of injury. The work does

Table 11.4 Moral stress debrief.

Step	Timebox	Purpose	Facilitator prompts (examples)	Output/owner
1) Set the frame	One minute	Signal safety; set scope and time.	"This is optional and timeboxed (10–20 minutes). This is for learning—not a performance review."	Shared aim and time agreement
2) Ground	Two minutes	Regulate; align on facts.	"Two slow breaths. One-line summary of the event."	Shared one-line facts
3) Round 1—What felt worst?	Three to five minutes	Name the human impact without blame.	"One sentence each; OK to pass. No cross-talk."	Themes captured
4) Round 2—What was in our control?	Three to five minutes	Distinguish controllables vs. constraints.	"What was within our control? What were the constraints?"	List of controllables
5) Round 3—What changes next time?	Three to five minutes	Identify a smallest helpful change.	"One tweak: script/micro-policy/handoff/coverage."	Shortlist of micro-changes
6) Capture actions	Two minutes	Convert ideas to owned tasks.	"Who owns which action? By when? Any support needed?"	Owner + timeframe; supports routed
7) Close the loop	One minute	State what will be escalated and when updates come back.	"Here's what we'll escalate and when you'll hear back. Thank you for speaking up."	Comms plan/follow-up date
8) Document for learning	30 seconds	Record brief, nonpunitive notes.	"Theme, actions, owners, review date."	Brief note filed

Moral Stress Debrief—Quick Reference Chart (10–20 minutes)
Optional, nonpunitive, facilitated; focus on human impact and the next step.
Jennings (2025). Author's own illustration.

not eliminate moral distress; it transforms it from a private wound into a shared signal that guides ethical improvement (Litz et al. 2009; Moses et al. 2018).

Measuring What Matters, and Routing to Care

Lightweight measurement earns trust only when it leads to visible change. The purpose is not surveillance but guidance: brief, voluntary pulse check-ins identify pressure points (energy, belonging, psychological safety), while periodic use of a validated tool such as the ProQOL tracks compassion satisfaction and fatigue over time (Stamm 2010). Data must be handled with care, aggregated to protect individuals, discussed in protected time, and explicitly tied to next steps, so that speaking up actually improves work design. Closing the loop ("here's what we heard; here's what will change, and why") converts disclosure into learning and strengthens the conditions that make candid reporting possible in the first place (Edmondson 1999). When teams see results, adding a float role on peak days, revising a triage script that reliably triggers conflict, and carving out a quiet space for short recovery breaks, measurement begins to function as a lever rather than a vent. This linkage matters because burnout is a systems problem: sustained mismatches between demands and resources predict exhaustion and depersonalization, which are mitigated when organizations restore time, staffing, and clarity (Maslach and Leiter 2016).

Signals must also route to support. Peers are often the first to notice changes, withdrawal, irritability, risk-taking, or rumination, and should be equipped to approach early, listen without judgment, and guide colleagues to appropriate help. MHFA offers a practical template: notice, approach, listen, encourage professional support, and ensure safety, while staying within the limits of a nonclinical role (Mental Health First Aid USA n.d.). A simple, well-published pathway keeps roles clear: peers invite conversation and share concerns; supervisors coordinate immediate practical supports (breaks, coverage, modified assignments); EAP or external clinicians provide care; human resources manages accommodations; leadership addresses recurrent causes through policy and design. Making this pathway visible, posting EAP contacts in break areas, listing local providers familiar with healthcare, outlining when and how to escalate a safety check, reduces barriers to care and normalizes mental health as part of occupational health.

Integrating sensing with support completes the loop. A quarterly ProQOL pulse might reveal rising secondary traumatic stress in a unit; leaders acknowledge the finding, pilot brief end-of-shift debriefs, and adjust staffing on predictable surge days. A monthly psychological-safety item might show reluctance to report near-misses; supervisors model fallibility, thank reporters, and publicly share "what changed because someone spoke up," reinforcing a climate where candor is safe (Edmondson 1999). Individual check-ins during one-to-ones can mirror the same structure: what has taken energy, what restored it, what one change would help next week, so small course corrections happen before crises. Framing help-seeking as professional strength ("using the right resource at the right time") further shifts identity away from stoicism and toward practiced competence. Over time, the organization behaves like a learning system: it senses lightly, responds concretely, and routes distress to care, reducing burnout risk by returning essential resources to the people doing the work (Maslach and Leiter 2016; Stamm 2010).

Work Design: Schedules, Breaks, Role Clarity, and Recognition

Work design is the structural antidote to chronic overload. When schedules are predictable, breaks are protected, roles are unambiguous, and recognition is specific and values-linked, demands and resources come back into balance, reducing burnout and stabilizing performance (Maslach and Leiter 2016). The following sections translate these four levers, schedules, breaks, role clarity, and recognition, into concrete practices that convert good intentions into daily norms.

Schedules

Predictable scheduling is the foundation on which every other well-being practice rests. Publishing rosters early, minimizing quick turns, and distributing high-intensity shifts equitably allow people to plan sleep, family obligations, and recovery. Effective teams treat the schedule as a living safety document rather than a static spreadsheet: surge hours have planned float coverage; known pinch points (first hour after open, last hour before close) are deliberately staffed; and on-call expectations are explicit so availability is not extracted informally through guilt. Self-scheduling within guardrails can increase perceived control without sacrificing coverage. Staff bid on shifts in waves, with the final pass ensuring equity and service needs. When a week turns volatile, leaders narrate the plan: which appointments will be redistributed, which nonurgent tasks will be deferred, and which roles will absorb triage so patient-facing staff are not simultaneously juggling phones and procedures. A simple end-of-day huddle that scans tomorrow's roster for gaps and assigns a named problem-solver prevents overnight anxiety from landing on individuals. Over time, predictable schedules signal that the organization respects human physiology and planning, which is a core resource in the burnout equation (Maslach and Leiter 2016).

Breaks

Breaks are not perks; they are safety equipment. Without protected pauses, cognitive speed, empathy, and decision quality degrade, and near-misses climb. Clinics that succeed make breaks operational, not optional. Coverage maps identify exactly who steps in when a technician taps out for 10 minutes; a visible "break board" or shared chat thread tracks who is out and who is up next; and "no-fault" language removes the need to justify stepping away. Microbreaks, two to three minutes between intense interactions, reset tone and reduce rumination when longer pauses are impossible. A quiet, uncluttered space matters as much as the minutes themselves; moving recovery out of hallways prevents constant interruption. Leaders reinforce the norm by asking at mid-shift, "Who has not had a meal or restroom break, what needs to shift so that happens by the next hour?" and by adjusting assignments in real time rather than applauding endurance. When breaks are built into flow and backed by coverage, the result is steadier attention and fewer errors for reasons grounded in basic human limits (Maslach and Leiter 2016).

Role Clarity

Ambiguity is an invisible drain on attention. Clear, shared maps of who decides, who executes, and who must be consulted reduce friction, rework, and postshift rumination. RACI-style responsibility matrices can be kept lightweight and practical: for triage, one role owns the decision to escalate, another owns documentation, and a third is consulted for complex calls; for discharges, one role verifies medications, another confirms client understanding, and a lead resolves disputes. When roles are clear, cross-training becomes a strength rather than a source of identity blur: people can flex to cover each other without losing a stable sense of mastery. Clarity also supports psychological safety because it makes speaking up easier; staff know whom to approach and how decisions are made, which lowers the interpersonal risk of asking questions or flagging concerns (Edmondson 1999). Leaders should make role expectations visible at the point of use, laminated one-pagers at phones, brief run-books at treatment stations, and revisit them after near-misses to see whether uncertainty, not effort, was the root cause. The aim is a calm, predictable handoff from task to task in which everyone understands their lane and the merge points.

Recognition

Recognition converts invisible effort into identity, mastery, and growth. Generic praise, "great job today," lands lightly and disappears; specific, values-linked feedback boosts learning and belonging (Maslach and Leiter 2016). Effective recognition names the behavior, ties it to a value, notes the impact, and, when appropriate, links to the next opportunity. A lead might say, "Your calm coaching during that tense call kept the room steady and aligned with our value of clarity; please pair with the next two new hires on phone skills." This framing helps the recipient understand exactly what to repeat and why it mattered. Recognition should not be reserved for heroics; routine excellence, thorough discharges, clean handoffs, and precise documentation deserve the same clarity. Public moments (end-of-shift huddles, weekly emails) build shared standards, while private notes convey care during hard weeks. Recognition also works upward and sideways; peers and supervisors benefit from hearing what they did that helped the team. When feedback is frequent, specific, and values-anchored, it counters depersonalization and strengthens the resources known to protect against burnout, efficacy, meaning, and connection (Maslach and Leiter 2016).

Implementation Roadmap: Converting Ideas into Norms

Culture shifts when everyday behavior changes, not when slogans appear on walls. The roadmap below translates well-being principles into repeatable routines, assigning ownership and staging work so progress is visible early and reinforced over time. Two anchor ideas guide the approach: first, burnout risk falls when organizations restore core resources, time, predictability, clarity, and belonging, rather than asking individuals to "cope harder" (Maslach and Leiter 2016); second, people speak up and learn together only when psychological safety is actively created, modeled, and protected by leaders (Edmondson 1999). The steps that follow turn those claims into practice.

Foundations and Ownership (Weeks 0–2)

The work begins by naming well-being as a safety and retention priority in a brief charter and assigning explicit owners: an executive sponsor for air cover, a site lead at each hospital for day-to-day execution, and a data/learning point person who tracks what is tried and what changes. The charter ties every action to two outcomes: fewer errors and steadier retention, so the program is seen as operational, not ornamental (Maslach and Leiter 2016). Leaders then make psychological safety a stated norm for meetings and huddles, modeling fallibility ("here's where I struggled; here's what I'm changing") and thanking people who raise concerns to signal that candor is welcome and useful (Edmondson 1999). This foundation prevents later steps from feeling like isolated wellness activities.

First 30 Days: Visible, Skill-Bearing Wins

Early actions should give staff something they can feel and use immediately. Train a small cross-shift cohort in MHFA, so every schedule has at least one person equipped to notice, approach, and route a colleague to appropriate help; publish their names where staff can find them (Mental Health First Aid USA n.d.). Identify two or three debrief facilitators per site and give them protected time; start with short, optional debriefs after predictably difficult days using a simple script focused on human impact and next steps rather than blame (Mitchell 1983). Publish a concise second-victim pathway and rehearse it like a code: same-day check-in, a 72-hour follow-up, and a menu of supports such as modified duties, peer buddying, and counseling referral (Litz et al. 2009). Adjust scheduling guardrails to minimize quick turns and guarantee recovery windows after nights so the system, not individual willpower, protects sleep. Embed a one-minute mindfulness or ACT micro-skill at the start of every shift, feet on the floor, longer exhale, one shared intention, such as steadiness, so regulation becomes part of standard work rather than a private hobby (Kabat-Zinn 1994). Each of these steps is small by design but collectively signals that the organization is changing how days actually run.

Days 31–90: Standardize and Scale

Once early habits take hold, convert them into standard work. Establish a monthly learning huddle that reviews near-misses through a just-culture lens, explicitly discussing human factors and system contributors; leaders close each review by naming what will change, who owns it, and when the team will hear back (Edmondson 1999). Build a simple routing pathway for distress into everyday operations: peers notice and invite conversation, supervisors coordinate immediate practical supports and coverage, EAP or external clinicians provide care, human resources manages accommodations, and leadership addresses recurrent causes through policy or design. Post-EAP and local clinical contacts in break areas and add them to onboarding packets so access does not depend on memory (Mental Health First Aid USA n.d.). Normalize manager one-to-ones that ask three questions: what took energy, what restored it, and what one change would help next week, so small adjustments occur before crises. Maintain schedule hygiene by publishing rosters earlier and assigning a daily "problem solver" to rebalance work in real time, keeping the link between staffing design and burnout risk explicit (Maslach and Leiter 2016).

Three to Twelve Months: Bake Into Systems and Measure Lightly

Sustained change requires embedding practices where people already work. Add debrief skills, the second-victim pathway, and micro-regulation drills to orientation and annual refreshers so new hires learn the same playbook. Update policy documents to include a short code of conduct for clients, a clear incivility/abuse response ladder, break protection as a safety norm, and a schedule standard that preserves recovery after nights. This shifts boundaries from personal preference to organizational expectation. Introduce light-touch sensing that always triggers action: a quarterly, voluntary ProQOL to watch compassion satisfaction and fatigue trends, discussed in protected time and followed by visible changes such as float coverage on surge hours or revisions to scripts that reliably trigger conflict (Stamm 2010). Each time staff provide input, leaders publicly close the loop with "what we heard" and "what changes now or later and why," reinforcing psychological safety and the credibility of measurement (Edmondson 1999). Recognition completes the cycle: supervisors and peers name specific behaviors tied to values and impact, converting invisible effort into identity and growth, an antidote to depersonalization (Maslach and Leiter 2016).

Keeping trust when constraints persist. Some requests will be delayed due to budgets or staffing. Credibility is preserved by stating constraints plainly, naming interim protections, and setting a date to revisit the decision. Saying "not now" paired with a concrete mitigation plan and a calendar reminder maintains psychological safety more effectively than silence, and it honors the core idea that burnout is a design problem to be worked on, not a character flaw to be pushed through (Maslach and Leiter 2016; Edmondson 1999). Over quarters, these micro-habits, training, rehearsal, schedule hygiene, learning huddles, light sensing with visible action, and values-linked recognition, accumulate into trust. People speak earlier, help each other sooner, and carry less home, and the organization becomes known as a place where demanding work is sustainably done.

Conclusion

Mental health is not ancillary to veterinary technology; it is a primary driver of safety, quality, retention, and the capacity to care over time. The strains named in this chapter, burnout, compassion fatigue, secondary traumatic stress, moral distress, and moral injury, are understandable human responses to conditions, not personal failings. The remedy is systemic and layered: evidence-informed personal skills that steady attention and emotion; psychologically safe teamwork with just-culture accountability that converts error into learning; and humane work design. When technicians and leaders commit to this whole-system approach, they create workplaces where empathy does not become exhaustion, accountability does not become shame, and skill can deepen across a full career. For support beyond the clinic, see Table 11.5 below.

Table 11.5 External mental health and well-being resources for veterinary technicians (U.S.).

Category	Resource	What it offers	How to access	Cost	Notes/eligibility
Crisis now	988 Suicide & Crisis Lifeline (n.d.)	24/7 confidential support by phone, text, or chat (suicidal thoughts, emotional distress).	Call or text 988; chat at 988lifeline.org	Free	U.S. only; bilingual support; TTY and ASL options available.
Crisis now	Crisis Text Line (n.d.)	24/7 confidential crisis support via text with trained counselors.	Text HOME to 741741	Free	U.S. only; also supports WhatsApp/Facebook in some regions—see site.
Crisis now	SAMHSA Disaster Distress Helpline (n.d.)	24/7 crisis counseling for disaster-related distress (natural or human caused).	Call or text 1-800-985-5990	Free	U.S. and territories; Spanish press "2"; 100+ languages via interpreters.
Information and referral	SAMHSA National Helpline (n.d.)	24/7 information and treatment referrals for mental health and substance use.	Call 1-800-662-HELP (4357)	Free	Information/referral; not ongoing counseling.
Information and referral	FindTreatment.gov (SAMHSA n.d.)	Search confidentially for local mental health and substance use treatment.	findtreatment.gov	Free directory	Filter by location, payment/insurance, levels of care.
Information and referral	NAMI n.d. HelpLine (noncrisis)	Peer-supported information and resources; not a crisis line.	Call 800-950-NAMI (6264) or text NAMI to 62640 (M–F, 10 a.m.–10 p.m. ET)	Free	Education and referral; for crisis use 988.
Information and referral	United Way n.d. 211	Local navigation for mental health, basic needs, financial help, etc.	Dial 211; 211.org for chat/text options	Free	Available in most of the U.S.; 180+ languages via interpretation.

(Continued)

Table 11.5 (Continued)

Category	Resource	What it offers	How to access	Cost	Notes/eligibility
Veterinary-specific	NOMV (Not One More Vet n.d.)—Peer Support	Peer support for veterinary teams (including support staff); moderated forums; info and education.	nomv.org → Peer Support/Support Staff forum	Free	Peer support (not therapy or crisis). Verification required to join forums.
Veterinary-specific	NOMV—Support Grants	Micro-grants to help eligible individuals with essentials (e. g., mental health, housing, transport).	nomv.org → Apply for a Grant	Free grants	Eligibility applies; amounts and programs vary.
Veterinary-specific	Shanti Project n. d.—Veterinary Mental Health Initiative (VMHI)	Evidence-based counseling and clinician-facilitated groups for veterinary professionals (availability varies).	See shanti.org → Veterinary Mental Health Initiative	Often free/ low-cost	Confirm current eligibility and offerings; not a crisis line.
Veterinary-specific	AVMA n.d. Wellbeing Resources	Well-being tools, education, and links for veterinary professionals.	avma.org → Resources → Wellbeing	Many free	Some materials are public; others may require membership.
Workplace/ insurance	Employee Assistance Program (EAP)	Short-term counseling, referrals, financial/legal consults (varies by employer).	Ask HR or your benefits portal	Usually free to employees	Confidential within legal limits; clarify session counts.
Workplace/ insurance	Your health plan's mental health benefits	In-network therapy lists, virtual care, and crisis coverage.	Number on back of insurance card; plan website/app	Copay or coverage varies	Ask about wait times, telehealth, and out-of-network options.
Global directories	Find A Helpline (ThroughLine n.d.)	Verified helpline locator for 130+ countries.	findahelpline.com	Free directory	Use if traveling or based outside the U.S.
Global directories	Befrienders Worldwide (n.d.)	International network providing emotional support and suicide prevention.	befrienders.org	Free directory	Find local centers outside the U.S.

Notes: If anyone is in immediate danger, call 911 (U.S.) or local emergency services. Availability and eligibility can change; check each site for current details.
Jennings (2025). Author's own illustration.

References

988 Suicide & Crisis Lifeline (n.d.). *988 Suicide & Crisis Lifeline.* https://988lifeline.org

American Veterinary Medical Association (n.d.). *Wellbeing resources.* https://www.avma.org/resources-tools/wellbeing

Beck, J.S. (2011). *Cognitive Behavior Therapy: Basics and Beyond*, 2e. Guilford Press.

Befrienders Worldwide (n.d.). *Befrienders Worldwide.* https://www.befrienders.org

Crisis Text Line (n.d.). *Crisis Text Line.* https://www.crisistextline.org

Edmondson, A. (1999). Psychological safety and learning behavior in work teams. *Administrative Science Quarterly* 44 (2): 350–383.

Hayes, S.C., Strosahl, K.D., and Wilson, K.G. (2012). *Acceptance and Commitment Therapy: The Process and Practice of Mindful Change*, 2e. Guilford Press.

Kabat-Zinn, J. (1994). *Wherever You Go, There You are: Mindfulness Meditation in Everyday Life.* Hyperion.

Litz, B.T., Stein, N., Delaney, E. et al. (2009). Moral injury and moral repair in war veterans: A preliminary model and intervention strategy. *Clinical Psychology Review* 29 (8): 695–706.

Maslach, C. and Leiter, M.P. (2016). *Burnout: A Multidimensional Perspective (Updated Discussions in Burnout at Work: A Psychological Perspective).* Psychology Press.

Mental Health First Aid USA (n.d.). *Mental Health First Aid.* National Council for Mental Wellbeing. https://www.mentalhealthfirstaid.org/.

Moses, L., Malowney, M.J., and Boyd, J.W. (2018). Ethical conflict and moral distress in veterinary practice: A survey of North American veterinarians. *Journal of Veterinary Internal Medicine* 32 (6): 2115–2122.

National Alliance on Mental Illness (n.d.). *NAMI HelpLine.* https://www.nami.org/help

Neff, K. (2011). *Self-Compassion: The Proven Power of Being Kind to Yourself.* William Morrow.

Not One More Vet (n.d.). *Peer support and support grants.* https://www.nomv.org

Shanti Project (n.d.). *Veterinary Mental Health Initiative (VMHI).* https://www.shanti.org

Stamm, B.H. (2010). *The concise ProQOL manual*, 2nde. ProQOL.org.

Substance Abuse and Mental Health Services Administration (n.d.). *Disaster Distress Helpline.* https://www.samhsa.gov/find-help/disaster-distress-helpline

Substance Abuse and Mental Health Services Administration (n.d.). *FindTreatment.gov.* https://findtreatment.gov

Substance Abuse and Mental Health Services Administration (n.d.). *National Helpline.* https://www.samhsa.gov/find-help/national-helpline

ThroughLine (n.d.). *Find a Helpline.* https://findahelpline.com

United Way Worldwide (n.d.). *211.* https://www.211.org

12

Professionalism

Introduction

Professionalism is a foundational pillar of veterinary nursing, shaping not only how individuals conduct themselves in clinical settings but also how the profession is perceived by colleagues, clients, and the broader community. In a field that combines scientific expertise with compassionate caregiving, professionalism serves as the bridge between technical competence and human connection. It influences every interaction, from client communication and patient advocacy to collaboration with veterinary teams and engagement in continuing education. Professionalism extends beyond outward appearance and behavior; it reflects a deep commitment to ethical practice, accountability, and personal growth.

In the fast-paced and emotionally charged environment of veterinary medicine, maintaining professionalism is both a challenge and a necessity. Veterinary technicians must navigate complex clinical situations, manage difficult client conversations, and work collaboratively within multidisciplinary teams while upholding rigorous standards of conduct and integrity. The demands of the profession require not only technical skill but also emotional intelligence, resilience, and a powerful sense of personal responsibility (Goleman 1995).

This chapter explores the multifaceted nature of professionalism in veterinary nursing, providing a comprehensive examination of what it means to be a professional, how to maintain professional standards under pressure, and the steps veterinary technicians can take to develop and strengthen their professional identity. By understanding and embodying these principles, veterinary technicians can elevate the quality of patient care, enhance client trust, and contribute to the advancement of their profession.

The Importance of Professionalism in Veterinary Nursing

Professionalism in veterinary nursing is not a superficial concept limited to appearance or polite behavior; it is a comprehensive standard that encompasses ethics, competence, accountability, and the ongoing commitment to personal and professional growth. The importance of professionalism extends far beyond the confines of individual careers, it directly impacts patient outcomes, the client experience, team dynamics, and the public perception of the veterinary nursing profession as a whole.

At its core, professionalism fosters trust. Clients place immense trust in veterinary teams, often entrusting them with beloved companions during times of crisis and uncertainty. Veterinary technicians who consistently demonstrate professionalism through clear communication, ethical behavior, and clinical competence reinforce this trust, leading to stronger client relationships and greater compliance with medical recommendations. When clients perceive veterinary technicians as knowledgeable, composed, and compassionate, they are more likely to follow through with care plans, which directly benefit patients' health outcomes.

Within the clinical environment, professionalism contributes to effective teamwork. Veterinary hospitals rely on collaboration among technicians, veterinarians, assistants, and administrative staff to deliver high-quality care. A professional veterinary technician understands the importance of respectful communication, reliability, and emotional regulation, even in stressful or fast-paced situations. These behaviors reduce conflict, promote efficient workflow, and create a positive, supportive atmosphere that benefits both the team and the patients under their care.

Professionalism also upholds the integrity of the veterinary nursing profession itself. As the field continues to advocate for greater recognition, credentialing, and autonomy, the collective behavior of veterinary technicians becomes a defining factor in how the profession is perceived by the broader healthcare community and society at large. Technicians who embody professionalism contribute to advancing the field, demonstrating that veterinary nursing is a vital and highly skilled healthcare discipline deserving of respect and acknowledgment.

Ethical behavior is another critical aspect of professionalism. Veterinary technicians are frequently confronted with challenging decisions involving patient advocacy, client finances, and treatment limitations. Upholding ethical standards, even when those decisions are difficult, ensures that patient welfare remains the central focus of care. This includes maintaining confidentiality, advocating for humane treatment, and refusing to participate in practices that compromise patient well-being or violate professional ethics.

In the context of holistic nursing, professionalism takes on an even broader role. It involves recognizing the interconnectedness of physical, emotional, and environmental factors that influence both patient care and team well-being. A professional veterinary technician not only provides technically competent care but also considers the emotional needs of patients and clients, fosters a supportive work environment, and contributes to a culture of compassion and respect.

The long-term success of veterinary technicians is also deeply tied to their professional conduct. Career advancement opportunities, mentorship roles, and leadership positions often arise for individuals who consistently demonstrate professionalism. Supervisors and colleagues are more likely to recommend and support professionals who exhibit strong interpersonal skills, accountability, and dedication to continued learning.

In sum, professionalism is not merely a standard to aspire to, it is a daily practice that shapes the culture of veterinary medicine, influences patient outcomes, and contributes to personal career fulfillment. By consistently upholding professional standards, veterinary technicians reinforce their value within the healthcare team, build stronger client relationships, and advocate for the continued growth and recognition of their profession.

Maintaining Professional Standards

Maintaining professional standards in veterinary nursing is a continuous, deliberate process that extends beyond basic job performance. It requires an unwavering commitment to ethical conduct, clinical competence, personal accountability, and the ongoing pursuit of knowledge. These standards serve as the foundation for high-quality patient care, effective teamwork, and the advancement of the veterinary nursing profession.

One of the core components of maintaining professional standards is a strong ethical framework. Veterinary technicians operate in a field where the line between what *can* be done and what *should* be done is often blurred by complex clinical situations, financial limitations, and emotional client interactions. A well-developed ethical framework acts as a moral compass, guiding decisions in ways that prioritize patient welfare, uphold professional integrity, and support humane treatment practices.

Ethical frameworks are informed by established guidelines, such as the codes of conduct provided by the National Association of Veterinary Technicians in America (NAVTA) and the American Veterinary Medical Association (AVMA). Table 12.1 distills the overlapping and distinct emphases of the NAVTA Code of Ethics and the AVMA *Principles of Veterinary Medical Ethics* (PVME) into practical themes for veterinary medicine. The table should be used as a quick reference guide, not a substitute for the full documents.

However, maintaining an ethical framework requires more than simply knowing these standards; it demands the ability to apply them in real-world scenarios where conflicting interests often arise. For example, when financial limitations prevent clients from pursuing the ideal treatment plan, an ethical veterinary technician must skillfully balance patient advocacy with respect for the client's autonomy. They must also recognize when to advocate for alternative solutions that minimize suffering while staying within the client's means.

Ethics in veterinary nursing also extends to honesty in communication. This includes providing clients with accurate, unbiased information, even when it is difficult to deliver, or resisting the temptation to present a more optimistic prognosis to avoid emotional discomfort. Upholding these values, even in challenging moments, demonstrates an elevated level of professionalism and ensures that clients can make informed decisions based on factual information rather than emotional reassurance.

Competence is another critical pillar of professionalism, encompassing not only the mastery of technical skills but also the ability to apply knowledge effectively and appropriately in varied clinical contexts. Veterinary technicians are responsible for a vast range of technical tasks, including medication administration, anesthesia monitoring, sample collection, wound care, and critical patient assessments. Competence ensures these tasks are performed with precision, minimizing the risk of medical errors and enhancing patient outcomes.

Table 12.1 Ethical responsibilities of veterinary technicians and veterinarians within the veterinary healthcare team.

Theme	NAVTA Code of Ethics (Technicians)	AVMA PVME (Veterinarians)
Primary Obligation	Serve society and animals through excellent care; prevent/relieve suffering; uphold laws; maintain the profession's dignity.	Provide competent, compassionate care within a valid VCPR; act with stewardship, integrity, and respect; prioritize animal welfare.
Professional Conduct and Integrity	Be accountable for professional actions; guard against incompetence and unethical practice; model ethical behavior.	Uphold professional integrity; avoid fraud/deceit; comply with law; maintain honesty in all professional communications.
Competence and Lifelong Learning	Maintain and advance competence through ongoing education; contribute to advancing the profession (ideal).	Maintain/advance knowledge and skills; seek consultation or referral when indicated; practice within areas of competence.
Client Relations and Confidentiality	Protect client confidentiality; educate the public (e.g., zoonoses) when appropriate.	Respect confidentiality; ensure clear, accurate communication and informed decision-making; maintain complete, accurate medical records.
Animal Welfare	Prevent and relieve suffering; promote animal health and well-being.	Place patient needs first; minimize pain, fear, anxiety, and stress; follow AVMA guidance on humane euthanasia and related policies.
Delegation, Scope, and Supervision	Work within legal scope of practice; collaborate with veterinarians; support standards and legislation that promote quality care.	Delegate appropriately within the VCPR; ensure supervision and accept responsibility for delegated tasks; follow state/federal requirements.
Interprofessional Relationships	Collaborate respectfully with veterinarians and team members to deliver quality care.	Treat colleagues with respect; avoid disparagement; foster appropriate team supervision, delegation, and consultation.
Public Health and Society	Promote public health and safety as part of professional responsibility.	Balance responsibilities to patients, clients, public, and environment; support continuity of care and emergency responsibilities.
Records, Continuity, and Transfers	— (implied via collaboration/standards)	Maintain accurate records; facilitate record transfers and continuity of care when appropriate.
Conflicts, Advertising, and Fees	— (not emphasized)	Manage conflicts of interest; ensure truthful advertising and fees; maintain transparency in business practices.
Accountability and Reporting	Be accountable; protect the public and the profession from incompetence or unethical conduct.	Report illegal or unethical practices to appropriate authorities; adhere to the code's conduct across clinical and business spheres.

However, competence is not static. Veterinary medicine is a rapidly advancing field, and maintaining clinical competence requires a commitment to ongoing education. Veterinary technicians must stay informed about new treatments, diagnostic technologies, pharmacological advancements, and best practices in patient care. This can be achieved through formal continuing education courses, attending professional conferences, participating in hospital in-service training, and reading current veterinary literature.

Equally important to technical competence is the development of critical thinking and clinical judgment. Veterinary technicians frequently make real-time decisions about patient monitoring, adjustments to treatment protocols, and emergency interventions. High professional standards require technicians to assess situations holistically, considering not only the immediate medical needs of the patient but also long-term implications for recovery, quality of life, and emotional well-being. Technicians must be confident in their knowledge while remaining open to seeking clarification or guidance when faced with unfamiliar or complex cases.

Accountability is the third major component of maintaining professional standards and is often the most difficult to master. True accountability involves taking full ownership of one's actions and their outcomes, regardless of whether they lead to success or failure. In a clinical setting, this means accepting responsibility for both the quality of patient care delivered and any mistakes that occur. When errors happen, which are inevitable in any medical field, professional veterinary technicians must promptly acknowledge the mistake, report it through the appropriate channels, and participate fully in corrective actions to prevent future occurrences. Accountability also means upholding commitments to colleagues and patients alike. This includes arriving at work prepared and on time, completing assigned tasks to the highest standard, and following through on promised actions. Reliable team members contribute to a workplace culture of trust and collaboration, while those who fail to meet their responsibilities create tension and compromise patient care. Importantly, accountability must be practiced without fear of undue punishment. Veterinary leaders play a critical role in creating a culture where accountability is encouraged through constructive feedback rather than blame. In such environments, veterinary technicians feel empowered to admit mistakes and learn from them, fostering continuous improvement rather than fear-driven concealment of errors.

Case Study: Accountability in Action

At a busy emergency hospital, a veterinary technician noticed that a patient had not received pain medication as ordered. Although it was a colleague's oversight, the technician chose to report the error and document the incident to ensure the patient received appropriate care. She later followed up with the team during rounds to discuss workflow improvements. This act of accountability not only protected the patient but fostered a culture of safety and transparency.

Professional appearance and demeanor also play a key role in maintaining standards. While appearance alone does not define professionalism, it does contribute to how veterinary technicians are perceived by clients, colleagues, and the public. Clean, well-maintained uniforms, appropriate personal hygiene, and a calm, confident presence demonstrate respect for the workplace and help instill confidence in clients. Body language, tone of voice, and verbal communication should consistently reflect courtesy, empathy, and professionalism.

Another critical aspect of maintaining professional standards is fostering effective communication. Veterinary technicians are often the primary point of contact between clients and the veterinary healthcare team. Clear, compassionate, and professional communication ensures that clients understand their pet's condition, treatment options, and care instructions. Within the healthcare team, open and respectful communication supports collaborative decision-making and reduces misunderstandings that can compromise patient care.

Time management and organizational skills also support professional standards. Veterinary technicians are responsible for managing multiple patients, treatments, and client interactions throughout the day. Maintaining professional standards means being efficient, prioritizing tasks appropriately, and ensuring that patient care is never compromised due to poor planning or disorganization. It also means respecting appointment schedules, meeting deadlines for documentation, and preparing adequately for procedures.

Professional boundaries are a lesser-discussed but equally essential element of maintaining standards. While empathy and compassion are critical to the nursing role, veterinary technicians must also maintain appropriate boundaries to protect their emotional health and maintain objectivity in clinical decision-making. Over-involvement in client relationships or taking on emotional burdens beyond one's control can lead to compassion fatigue and impaired judgment. Recognizing the line between professional support and personal involvement ensures that technicians can continue to provide high-quality care without compromising their well-being.

Finally, maintaining professional standards requires an ongoing commitment to self-reflection and growth. Veterinary technicians should regularly assess their performance, seek feedback from supervisors and colleagues, and identify areas for improvement. Participation in continuing education courses, professional conferences, and credentialing programs reinforces a dedication to lifelong learning and ensures that skills and knowledge remain current in an ever-evolving field.

Maintaining professional standards is not a singular event or a box to check, it is a continuous, active process that requires dedication, humility, and the pursuit of excellence. Through ethical conduct, clinical competence, accountability, and commitment to growth, veterinary technicians not only uphold the standards of their profession but also elevate the quality of care for the patients and clients they serve.

What Makes a Professional

Professionalism in veterinary nursing transcends simple job performance; it embodies a set of core values, behaviors, and attitudes that elevate the role from a technical position to a respected healthcare profession. While technical skills are undoubtedly important, it is the consistent application of integrity, accountability, empathy, and a commitment to continuous growth that truly defines a professional. Understanding what makes a professional helps veterinary technicians not only develop their own careers but also contribute to the advancement of the veterinary nursing profession as a whole.

To understand how professionalism operates in veterinary nursing, it's helpful to visualize the interconnected components that form its foundation. The framework below outlines the key pillars that uphold professional conduct in both clinical and interpersonal settings (Figure 12.1).

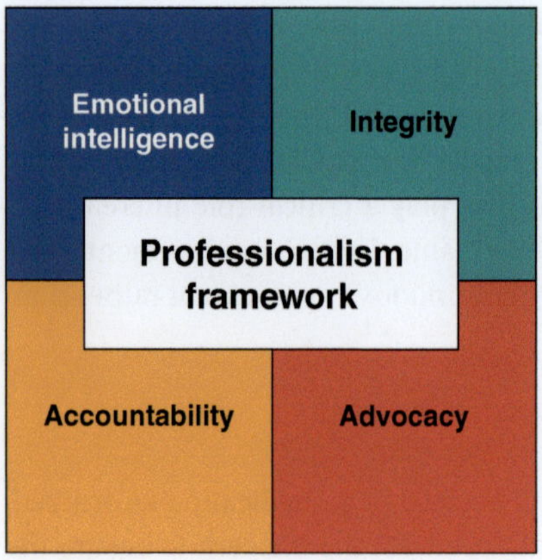

Figure 12.1 A three-level framework for supporting well-being in veterinary practice: individual, team, and organizational factors.

At the foundation of professionalism is integrity. Integrity refers to adherence to moral and ethical principles, even when it is inconvenient or challenging. A professional veterinary technician acts with honesty in every interaction, whether it involves delivering difficult news to a client, admitting a mistake to a supervisor, or advocating for a patient whose needs may be overlooked. Integrity also means aligning actions with ethical standards even when no one is watching. It is not the absence of mistakes that defines integrity but the willingness to take responsibility for them and make them right.

Accountability is intricately linked to integrity and is one of the most defining characteristics of a true professional. Veterinary technicians who consistently take ownership of their actions, whether those actions result in positive outcomes or errors, demonstrate accountability. This includes recognizing personal limitations and seeking guidance when necessary rather than proceeding with uncertainty that could compromise patient care. Professionals understand that admitting what they do not know is not a weakness but a critical step toward maintaining high standards of care.

Emotional intelligence is another hallmark of professionalism. In a high-stress, emotionally charged field like veterinary medicine, professionals must navigate not only their own emotions but also the emotional states of clients and colleagues. Emotional intelligence involves the ability to recognize, understand, and manage one's own emotions while also responding appropriately to the emotions of others. A professional veterinary technician remains calm under pressure, communicates with empathy, and practices active listening during client interactions. Emotional intelligence also fosters healthier workplace relationships, reducing interpersonal conflict and supporting effective collaboration within the veterinary team (Goleman 1995).

Reliability and consistency are essential traits that contribute to professional identity. Professionals do what they say they will do, meet deadlines, and deliver high-quality work regardless of external stressors. Clients and colleagues alike develop trust in veterinary technicians who consistently demonstrate reliability. This trust is critical in the fast-paced clinical environment where teamwork and efficiency directly impact patient outcomes.

Commitment to lifelong learning is a distinguishing characteristic of professionalism. Veterinary medicine is a dynamic field with constant advancements in treatments, technologies, and patient care protocols. Professionals recognize that their education does not end with formal training. Instead, they actively seek opportunities for continued growth through conferences, workshops, certification programs, and independent study. By staying informed about the latest developments in the field, veterinary technicians ensure that they remain competent and provide the best possible care for their patients.

Self-regulation is another critical factor. Professionals are capable of managing their emotional responses, even during demanding situations. They do not allow personal frustrations or external stress to negatively impact their interactions with clients or the quality of care they provide. Instead, they rely on healthy coping strategies to navigate workplace challenges and maintain a high standard of professionalism even under pressure.

Advocacy is a defining feature of what makes a professional. Veterinary technicians serve as advocates not only for their patients but also for their profession. They promote ethical treatment of animals, support the professional development of their colleagues, and actively participate in initiatives that advance the role of veterinary technicians within the broader veterinary healthcare system. Advocacy also extends to workplace culture; professionals foster environments where respect, integrity, and emotional well-being are valued and protected.

Professionalism in veterinary nursing is a multifaceted concept built on a foundation of integrity, accountability, emotional intelligence, reliability, and a dedication to continuous improvement. These qualities elevate the role of the veterinary technician beyond technical skill, shaping individuals who are not only highly competent but also deeply respected within their teams and by the clients they serve. True professionals understand that their actions and attitudes have a lasting impact on patients, on colleagues, and on the advancement of the veterinary nursing profession (Goleman 1995).

How to Gain Professionalism

Professionalism is not an inherent quality one is simply born with; it is a cultivated set of behaviors, attitudes, and skills that develop over time through intentional effort and self-reflection. For veterinary technicians, gaining professionalism involves a continuous journey of personal growth, ethical development, and mastery of both technical and interpersonal skills. It is a process rooted in conscious decision-making, learning from experience, and a commitment to embodying the values and standards of the veterinary nursing profession.

The first step in gaining professionalism is developing a keen sense of self-awareness. Self-awareness allows individuals to recognize their strengths, weaknesses, and emotional triggers. Veterinary technicians working to enhance their professionalism must engage in honest self-reflection, asking themselves whether their actions align with the core values of integrity, compassion, and accountability. This reflective practice can be fostered through journaling, mentorship conversations, and regular feedback from supervisors and colleagues. By identifying areas for growth, individuals can set clear goals to improve their professional conduct.

Establishing a solid ethical foundation is equally critical in the pursuit of professionalism. Veterinary technicians must familiarize themselves with the ethical guidelines established by organizations such as the NAVTA and the AVMA. However, gaining professionalism requires more than just knowing these codes, it involves internalizing them and applying them consistently in daily practice. When faced with ethical dilemmas, veterinary technicians should practice moral reasoning by carefully considering patient welfare, client needs, and institutional policies before making decisions. Seeking mentorship from experienced professionals can also provide valuable insight into navigating complex ethical scenarios with integrity.

Another key component of professionalism is mastering emotional intelligence. Veterinary technicians often operate in emotionally charged environments where client grief, patient suffering, and team stress can create tension and conflict. Gaining professionalism means developing the ability to manage personal emotions while responding empathetically to the emotions of others. This skill is cultivated through active listening, practicing patience, and remaining composed under pressure. Emotional intelligence also helps veterinary technicians engage in difficult conversations with clients and colleagues in a constructive and compassionate manner, ultimately fostering healthier relationships and better patient outcomes (Goleman 1995).

Veterinary technicians seeking to gain professionalism must also demonstrate a commitment to continuous learning. Medicine is a rapidly evolving field, and staying current with the latest research, techniques, and best practices is a hallmark of professionalism. Pursuing continuing education opportunities, attending conferences, seeking specialty certifications, and staying engaged with professional organizations are tangible ways to demonstrate a dedication to growth. Professionals who actively seek new knowledge not only improve their clinical competence but also become valuable resources for their colleagues, enhancing the overall quality of care provided by their teams.

Developing effective communication skills is another critical step toward professionalism. Veterinary technicians play a leading role in educating clients, relaying patient updates to the healthcare team, and ensuring continuity of care. Clear, respectful, and compassionate communication builds trust and strengthens professional relationships. Gaining professionalism means learning how to deliver information accurately and confidently, while also knowing when to listen without judgment. Participating in communication workshops and role-playing scenarios can help veterinary technicians refine their communication strategies, particularly in emotionally sensitive situations.

Time management and organization also contribute to the development of professionalism. Veterinary nursing is a demanding profession that requires the ability to juggle multiple responsibilities, prioritize tasks effectively, and work efficiently under pressure. By cultivating strong organizational habits, such as maintaining accurate patient records, preparing thoroughly for procedures, and meeting documentation deadlines, veterinary technicians demonstrate reliability and dedication to their professional role.

Perhaps one of the most challenging aspects of gaining professionalism is learning to set and maintain healthy boundaries. Compassion and empathy are essential qualities for veterinary technicians, but overextending oneself emotionally can lead to burnout and impaired judgment. Professionals understand the importance of caring deeply while maintaining the objectivity necessary to make sound clinical decisions. This balance is achieved through regular self-care, emotional resilience training, and the ability to recognize when additional support or time away from work is needed to maintain mental health.

Mentorship plays a significant role in fostering professionalism. Aspiring professionals benefit greatly from observing and learning from respected colleagues who model exemplary professional behavior. Engaging in mentorship relationships allows veterinary technicians to gain insight into how experienced professionals handle complex situations with grace, integrity, and confidence. These role models provide not only guidance but also encouragement, helping less experienced technicians navigate the challenges of their evolving careers.

Finally, professionalism is strengthened through a commitment to service and advocacy. Veterinary technicians who seek to advance their profession actively participate in professional organizations, support efforts to improve workplace culture, and advocate for patient welfare and the recognition of veterinary nursing as a critical component of veterinary healthcare.

This outward focus on contributing to the profession as a whole demonstrates a mature understanding of professionalism that transcends individual career advancement.

Gaining professionalism is an ongoing process that requires deliberate effort, self-reflection, and a willingness to grow. By developing self-awareness, building a strong ethical foundation, mastering emotional intelligence, committing to lifelong learning, and fostering healthy communication and boundaries, veterinary technicians elevate themselves and their profession. Professionalism is not a destination but a journey, one that enhances patient care, enriches professional relationships, and ultimately leads to a more fulfilling and impactful career (Goleman 1995).

Developing a Personal Professional Identity

Professionalism is often taught as a set of standards and behaviors, being punctual, communicating respectfully, and wearing clean scrubs, but true professionalism goes deeper. It is also about cultivating a personal professional identity, the internal compass that guides how a veterinary technician chooses to show up in their role every day.

While early-career technicians may begin by mimicking the behavior of respected mentors or instructors, long-term growth comes from actively shaping one's own values, communication style, and ethical principles. This identity evolves with experience, mentorship, self-reflection, and exposure to both success and adversity. A technician who once struggled to speak up during rounds may later become the person who advocates most fiercely for their patients. A team member who once avoided conflict may learn to navigate hard conversations with clarity and compassion. These shifts reflect not just clinical skill but professional maturity.

Developing a professional identity also means aligning personal values with workplace expectations. A technician may value advocacy, autonomy, or continual learning. When these values are honored and expressed through daily actions, such as speaking up about patient pain, seeking new knowledge, or modeling calm under pressure, they become part of the technician's professional brand. This alignment leads to greater job satisfaction, integrity, and resilience (Figure 12.2).

Mentorship and feedback are also powerful tools. Honest conversations with trusted colleagues can clarify blind spots and reinforce strengths. Journaling, coaching, and attending CE focused on leadership or ethics can further deepen this sense of self.

When technicians take ownership of their professional identity, they are more grounded in their actions, more resilient in the face of conflict, and better able to lead by example, no matter their title. In this way, professionalism becomes not just a checklist, but a personal and purposeful expression of who they are within the veterinary team.

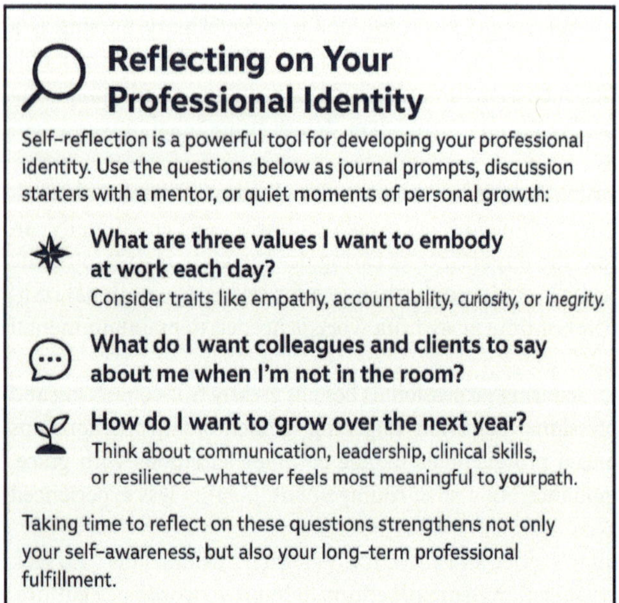

Figure 12.2 Time-bound debrief structure for reflective team discussions following stressful clinical events.

Professionalism in Client Interactions

Professionalism in client interactions is one of the most visible and impactful demonstrations of a veterinary technician's role. While technical skills are critical to patient care, the way a technician communicates with and supports clients can have a lasting effect on the client's perception of the veterinary team and the care their pet receives. In emotionally charged situations, such as delivering shocking news, discussing financial limitations, or guiding clients through end-of-life decisions, the professionalism of the veterinary technician becomes a source of stability and trust.

At the core of professionalism in client interactions is emotional intelligence. Veterinary technicians must recognize that clients often experience elevated levels of stress, anxiety, and grief when seeking medical care for their pets. These emotions can manifest in a range of behaviors, from sadness and confusion to frustration and anger. A professional veterinary technician approaches each client encounter with empathy, understanding that emotional responses are a natural part of the human–animal bond. By practicing active listening and responding with calm, measured language, technicians help de-escalate emotional situations and foster trust (Goleman 1995).

Communication clarity is also essential to professionalism in client interactions. Clients rely on veterinary technicians to explain complex medical information in a way that is easy to understand without being condescending. This requires the ability to translate medical terminology into layperson language, provide clear explanations of treatment options, and ensure that clients fully comprehend the care plans being presented. Professionalism dictates that technicians remain patient and respectful when clients ask repeated questions or struggle to process difficult information.

Boundary setting is another critical aspect of professional client interactions. While veterinary technicians should express empathy and compassion, it is important to avoid becoming overly involved in the personal lives of clients or blurring the lines between professional and personal relationships. Maintaining appropriate emotional distance helps preserve the technician's objectivity and emotional well-being while still providing effective support. For example, while it is appropriate to acknowledge a client's grief during euthanasia, it is not professionally appropriate to share deeply personal stories or overly immerse oneself in the client's emotional experience.

Handling difficult clients is one of the most challenging aspects of maintaining professionalism. Clients may express anger, frustration, or dissatisfaction, often in moments of high emotional stress. A professional veterinary technician remains composed and respectful, even in the face of inappropriate behavior. Rather than responding defensively, professionals use de-escalation techniques such as lowering their voice, maintaining open body language, and calmly acknowledging the client's concerns. Statements like, "I understand this situation is very stressful, and I want to help find the best solution for you and your pet," help redirect the conversation toward problem-solving rather than conflict.

Additionally, professionalism requires transparency in client interactions. Veterinary technicians must be honest about patient conditions, treatment limitations, and financial considerations. While it may be tempting to sugarcoat difficult news to avoid upsetting a client, true professionalism involves providing accurate, timely information while offering compassionate support. Clients appreciate honesty and are more likely to trust the veterinary team when they feel fully informed, even during challenging situations.

Cultural sensitivity also plays a significant role in professional client interactions. Veterinary technicians must be aware of and respectful toward diverse cultural beliefs and values that influence how clients approach pet ownership, healthcare decisions, and end-of-life considerations. Professionalism involves approaching these differences without judgment, asking respectful questions to understand client perspectives, and adapting communication styles to meet individual client needs.

Professionalism in client interactions means recognizing and respecting the emotional significance of the human–animal bond. Veterinary technicians should never minimize a client's grief or emotional response, regardless of the situation. Whether discussing the loss of a long-time companion or the treatment plan for a newly adopted pet, a professional acknowledges the depth of the client's attachment and treats each situation with compassion and dignity.

Professionalism in client interactions is about more than just delivering information, it is about building trust, providing emotional support, and ensuring that clients feel respected, heard, and cared for throughout their veterinary experience. Through empathy, clarity, respectful boundaries, and cultural sensitivity, veterinary technicians strengthen client relationships and uphold the highest standards of their profession.

Case Study: Navigating a Difficult Euthanasia Appointment

A veterinary technician was present during a euthanasia for a beloved family dog. When the client became overwhelmed with emotion and began lashing out at the team, the technician maintained a calm tone, validated the client's distress, and provided quiet reassurance. Her ability to remain professional and compassionate de-escalated the moment and allowed the appointment to proceed with dignity for both the pet and family.

Professionalism in Team Dynamics and Leadership

Professionalism in team dynamics and leadership is fundamental to creating a healthy, collaborative, and efficient workplace environment. Veterinary nursing is inherently team-based, requiring close collaboration among veterinary technicians, veterinarians, assistants, and administrative staff. In this interconnected environment, professionalism ensures that communication remains clear, conflicts are resolved constructively, and the shared goal of delivering high-quality patient care is consistently upheld.

One of the most important aspects of professionalism in team dynamics is respect for colleagues. This involves acknowledging the skills and contributions of each team member, regardless of their role within the hospital hierarchy. Professional veterinary technicians understand that every team member plays a vital role in patient care and that success is achieved through collaboration rather than competition. Respectful interactions foster an environment where ideas can be shared openly, and team members feel valued for their contributions. This sense of mutual respect promotes job satisfaction and enhances the overall effectiveness of the veterinary team.

Effective communication is also central to professionalism within team dynamics. Veterinary technicians must be able to clearly articulate patient updates, relay treatment plans, and provide constructive feedback to colleagues. This communication should be concise, respectful, and free from personal judgment. In high-stress environments, where emotions can run high, maintaining professionalism means managing one's tone and language carefully, avoiding gossip, and addressing concerns directly rather than through passive-aggressive behavior or indirect complaints.

Professionalism also plays a critical role in conflict resolution. Workplace disagreements are inevitable, particularly in fast-paced and emotionally demanding clinical settings. Professional veterinary technicians approach conflict with a problem-solving mindset, focusing on finding solutions rather than assigning blame. They address issues promptly and privately, using respectful dialogue to understand differing perspectives and work toward mutually acceptable outcomes. Conflict resolution strategies such as the LEARN model (Listen, Explain, Acknowledge, Recommend, Negotiate) can be effective tools for navigating workplace disagreements in a professional and constructive manner (Berlin and Fowkes 1983).

Leadership within the veterinary nursing profession is not limited to those in formal supervisory positions. Any veterinary technician can demonstrate leadership through their actions, professionalism, and willingness to support and mentor others. Leadership involves setting a positive example for colleagues by consistently demonstrating integrity, accountability, and a commitment to exceptional patient care. Professionals who lead by example inspire others to adopt similar behaviors, contributing to a workplace culture that values collaboration, respect, and continuous improvement.

Mentorship is another vital aspect of professional leadership. Experienced veterinary technicians are paramount in guiding newer colleagues, sharing their knowledge, and helping them navigate the challenges of the profession. Professional mentors provide constructive feedback, model appropriate behavior, and encourage the professional development of those they mentor. By investing time and effort in mentoring others, veterinary technicians strengthen their teams and contribute to the advancement of their profession.

Professionalism in leadership also involves advocating for positive workplace changes. This includes identifying systemic issues that impact staff well-being and patient care and working collaboratively with management to develop solutions. Professional leaders do not simply point out problems; they take initiative to propose and implement improvements that benefit both the team and the organization. Whether advocating for better scheduling practices, additional training opportunities, or improved communication protocols, these actions demonstrate a commitment to creating a healthier and more effective work environment.

Accountability is another critical component of professionalism in leadership and team dynamics. Professional veterinary technicians hold themselves accountable for their actions and encourage the same level of accountability among their colleagues. They address mistakes openly and constructively, focusing on learning from errors rather than placing blame. This fosters a culture of trust and psychological safety, where team members feel comfortable acknowledging mistakes and working collaboratively to prevent them in the future.

Recognizing and celebrating the successes of colleagues is an often-overlooked aspect of professionalism. Positive reinforcement builds morale and encourages continued high performance. Professional veterinary technicians make a point of acknowledging the contributions and achievements of their team members, fostering a supportive and motivating environment where everyone feels valued and appreciated.

Professionalism in team dynamics and leadership ultimately enhances the quality of care provided to patients and improves client satisfaction. When teams operate within a professional, respectful, and collaborative framework, patient outcomes improve, workplace stress is reduced, and job satisfaction increases across all roles. Veterinary technicians who consistently demonstrate professionalism in their interactions and leadership contribute to the long-term success and sustainability of both their teams and their profession.

Crisis Professionalism: Staying Grounded in High-Stress Moments

Veterinary medicine is inherently high-pressure. Emergencies, critical cases, emotionally distraught clients, and unpredictable outcomes test not only clinical skill, but also a technician's ability to maintain professionalism under stress. This ability to remain composed, compassionate, and effective during a crisis is what we might call crisis professionalism.

Crisis professionalism is not about denying emotion or detaching from difficult circumstances. Rather, it is about staying centered enough to fulfill one's role and communicate clearly, even when tension or chaos is mounting. A technician who can regulate their tone of voice, maintain situational awareness, and support the team during a code or euthanasia appointment demonstrates a level of leadership that extends beyond job title.

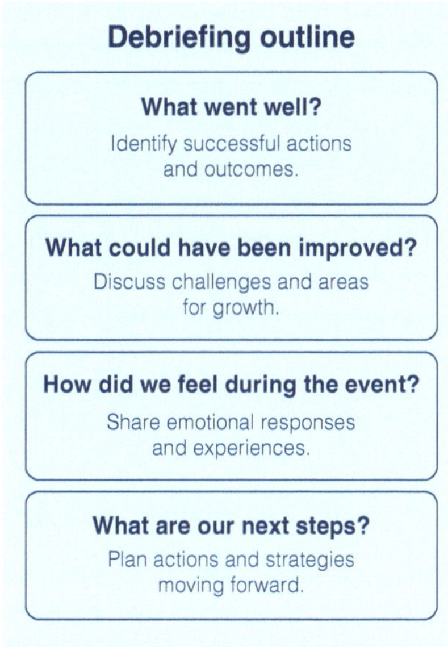

Figure 12.3 Boundary language examples and short-term tracking tool to reinforce respectful, time-bound communication.

Several strategies can help veterinary technicians strengthen the skill of crisis professionalism. One of the most effective is to pause and take a deep breath before responding in a high-stress situation. This brief moment of stillness can prevent impulsive reactions and allow the technician to reset, shifting from reactivity to intentional action. Internal self-talk is another powerful technique. Repeating grounding phrases such as "stay calm," "you've done this before," or "focus on what's in front of you" can help bring clarity when the mind feels overwhelmed. It is also important to maintain a steady, professional tone even when emotions are running high. Speaking slowly and deliberately, especially when a client is upset, can serve as a calming influence and reinforce trust. Finally, crisis professionalism does not end when the event is over. Debriefing afterward with colleagues, sharing emotions, and reflecting on what went well or what could be improved helps build resilience and foster a more connected, prepared team.

Debriefing is a vital part of crisis professionalism. It provides a structured opportunity for veterinary teams to process emotionally intense events, identify what went well, and discuss areas for improvement. Whether after a medical emergency, difficult euthanasia, or emotionally charged client interaction, debriefing strengthens resilience, fosters teamwork, and promotes continuous learning. Use the following outline to guide your post-event discussions and support a healthier, more connected workplace culture (Figure 12.3).

Case Example: Using the Debriefing Outline

Scenario:

A young Labrador Retriever was rushed into the clinic after being hit by a car. The emergency team performed CPR, but the dog could not be revived. The owner became distraught and shouted at the staff, blaming them for not saving the pet. The situation was emotionally charged and left the entire team shaken.

Post-Event Debrief (Using the Outline):

1) **What happened?**
   The team gathered in a quiet room after the shift. The lead technician recapped the timeline of events from intake to CPR and final outcome, allowing everyone to confirm or clarify details.
2) **What went well?**
   The team noted that triage and communication during the code were clear and efficient. One technician highlighted how the doctor calmly relayed updates to the client during the effort, maintaining professionalism despite high tension.

3) **What was difficult or stressful?**
   Several team members mentioned feeling helpless during CPR and emotionally affected by the owner's outburst. One CSR expressed that she froze during the client confrontation and felt unsure how to respond.
4) **What can we learn from this event?**
   The team recognized the need to better prepare for client grief reactions. They decided to develop a "code protocol" for CSRs to help manage the lobby during resuscitations, including designating a support staff member to be with the client.
5) **What support do team members need moving forward?**
   A technician who had bonded with the patient asked for time to step away from appointments to process. The team agreed to check in on each other the following week and planned a peer support huddle at their next staff meeting.

By practicing crisis professionalism, veterinary technicians not only safeguard the well-being of patients and clients but also lead by example. In moments of chaos, their calm presence becomes a stabilizing force for the entire team.

Inclusive Professionalism and Microaggressions in the Veterinary Workplace

Professionalism is not only about how a veterinary technician behaves individually, but also how they contribute to a safe and respectful environment for others. In modern veterinary settings, professionalism must include a commitment to inclusivity ensuring that all clients, team members, and students are treated with dignity, regardless of their background, identity, or beliefs.

Microaggressions are subtle, often unintentional comments or behaviors that communicate bias or exclusion toward individuals from marginalized groups. These might include offhand jokes about gender, assumptions about a person's ethnicity or language abilities, or dismissive comments toward someone's LGBTQ+ identity. Though they may appear minor in isolation, their cumulative impact can significantly harm psychological safety and contribute to workplace burnout or attrition.

Veterinary technicians play a key role in shaping workplace culture. Inclusive professionalism involves actively working to prevent microaggressions by avoiding them and by speaking up when they occur. For example, a technician who notices a colleague consistently misgendering a team member might gently intervene by modeling the correct pronoun use or checking in privately to offer support. These actions reinforce a culture of respect and accountability.

Inclusive professionalism also involves self-awareness. Reflecting on one's own biases, assumptions, or language habits helps technicians grow and ensure that their professionalism uplifts others rather than causes harm. This does not mean perfection, but it does require humility, a willingness to learn, and the courage to prioritize equity even when it's uncomfortable. By expanding the definition of professionalism to include inclusivity and cultural competence, veterinary teams build environments where all staff can thrive and where every client feels seen, respected, and safe.

Digital Professionalism and Social Media Conduct

In the digital age, professionalism extends far beyond in-person interactions. Veterinary technicians must also uphold professional standards in online spaces, including social media platforms, professional networking sites, and digital communications such as email and text messaging. How a veterinary technician conducts themselves online directly affects their personal reputation, the public image of their workplace, and the broader perception of the veterinary nursing profession. Digital professionalism is a critical, and often overlooked, component of maintaining credibility, trust, and ethical integrity in modern veterinary practice (Cain and Romanelli 2009).

One of the most fundamental aspects of digital professionalism is recognizing that online activity is rarely private. Even personal social media accounts can become accessible to clients, colleagues, and employers through shared connections or public-facing posts. Veterinary technicians must assume that anything they post, comment on, or share could ultimately be seen by professional contacts or clients. This awareness should guide their behavior online, prompting careful consideration before engaging in discussions, sharing content, or making public statements (Cain and Romanelli 2009).

Professional conduct in digital spaces requires always maintaining respectful and appropriate language. Engaging in online arguments, using inflammatory language, or making disparaging remarks about clients, colleagues, or employers violates the ethical standards of the profession and can have serious professional consequences. Even posts that are not directly related to the veterinary field can reflect poorly on a technician's professionalism if they demonstrate poor judgment or offensive behavior. Digital footprints are long-lasting, and content shared impulsively can resurface years later, potentially affecting career opportunities and professional relationships.

Confidentiality is a critical concern in online conduct. Veterinary technicians must never share patient information, client details, or sensitive workplace incidents on social media, even in closed or private groups. The Health Insurance Portability and Accountability Act (HIPAA) governs confidentiality in human healthcare, and while veterinary medicine is not subject to the same legal regulations, ethical standards regarding client and patient privacy are equally important. Sharing case details, even without using names, can inadvertently reveal client identities and is considered a breach of professional trust (Cain and Romanelli 2009).

In addition to social media activity, digital professionalism encompasses professional communication via email and other electronic platforms. Veterinary technicians should use clear, respectful language in all written communications, ensuring that messages are free of slang, abbreviations, and emoticons that may be perceived as unprofessional. Emails should be thoughtfully composed, using appropriate salutations and signatures, and checked carefully for spelling and grammatical errors before sending them. In professional settings, digital communication represents not only the individual but also the organization, making professionalism in written correspondence essential (Cain and Romanelli 2009).

Digital professionalism also involves managing one's online presence strategically. Veterinary technicians should periodically review their personal and professional social media accounts to ensure that content aligns with their desired professional image. This may include updating privacy settings, removal of inappropriate content, and curating a digital presence that reflects their values and professionalism. Creating or maintaining a professional online profile on platforms like LinkedIn allows veterinary technicians to highlight their qualifications, certifications, and ongoing professional development, demonstrating their commitment to growth and advancement within the field (Cain and Romanelli 2009).

One area where digital professionalism has become increasingly important is in online interactions with clients. Many clients may attempt to connect with veterinary staff on personal social media accounts or reach out for advice through unofficial communication channels such as direct messages. While this may seem harmless, it blurs professional boundaries and can create liability risks. Veterinary technicians should politely decline such requests and direct clients to appropriate professional communication channels for medical advice or patient care discussions. Establishing and maintaining these boundaries reinforces professionalism and protects both the technician and the organization from potential legal and ethical complications (Cain and Romanelli 2009).

Employers also play a role in promoting digital professionalism by providing clear guidelines and policies on social media use and digital communication. Veterinary practices should offer training on appropriate online behavior, confidentiality standards, and the potential professional consequences of inappropriate digital activity. By establishing clear expectations and fostering open discussions about digital professionalism, organizations help their staff navigate the complex landscape of online conduct more effectively (Cain and Romanelli 2009).

In the modern professional landscape, a veterinary technician's online presence is often an extension of their professional identity. Upholding professionalism in digital spaces reinforces trust with clients, enhances workplace relationships, and supports the advancement of the veterinary nursing profession. Through thoughtful, ethical, and respectful online behavior, veterinary technicians can maintain their personal and professional integrity while navigating the evolving digital world.

Case Study: A Misstep on Social Media

A technician posted a humorous meme about "difficult clients" on a private Facebook group, not realizing a client had access. The post was screenshot and shared publicly, resulting in a disciplinary conversation with hospital leadership. The technician later reflected on how a single online comment could undermine years of professionalism.

Navigating Professional Challenges and Ethical Dilemmas

Professional challenges and ethical dilemmas are an inevitable part of veterinary nursing. The complex nature of clinical environments, financial constraints of clients, and emotional intensity of animal care create situations where personal values, professional obligations, and workplace realities can come into conflict. Navigating these moments with professionalism requires a strong ethical foundation, critical thinking, and the ability to manage emotional responses while staying focused on patient welfare and professional integrity.

One of the most common professional challenges faced by veterinary technicians is working under leadership that does not always model professionalism or ethical behavior. In such situations, technicians may feel torn between following directives and advocating for what they believe is right for the patient or workplace environment. When confronted with questionable practices, such as cutting corners in patient care, ignoring safety protocols, or engaging in unprofessional conduct, technicians must rely on their ethical training and personal integrity to guide their actions. While it may not always be possible to change the behavior of leadership directly, veterinary technicians can maintain their own professional standards by modeling ethical behavior, documenting concerns appropriately, and seeking support through official reporting channels when necessary.

Another frequent dilemma involves financial limitations impacting patient care. Veterinary technicians often find themselves in emotionally challenging situations where clients are unable or unwilling to pursue recommended treatments due to cost. While the desire to provide the best possible care is strong, professionals must respect the financial boundaries and decisions of clients. Navigating these situations professionally means clearly presenting all treatment options, including lower-cost alternatives when appropriate, and ensuring clients have the information needed to make informed decisions. It also involves managing personal emotions, such as frustration or helplessness, and maintaining empathy for clients facing difficult financial choices.

Ethical dilemmas also arise when dealing with differing opinions within the healthcare team. Veterinary technicians may encounter situations where they disagree with a veterinarian's recommended treatment plan or a colleague's approach to patient care. While it is important to respect the authority and expertise of supervising veterinarians, professionals have a responsibility to advocate for their patients when they believe a different course of action would better serve the patient's welfare. Approaching these situations respectfully and constructively is critical. Using structured communication models, such as SBAR (Situation, Background, Assessment, Recommendation), allows veterinary technicians to present their concerns clearly and professionally without undermining their colleagues. For additional guidance on applying SBAR in clinical settings, refer to Chapter 10.

When faced with serious ethical concerns, such as suspected animal abuse, neglect, or workplace violations of legal and professional standards, veterinary technicians must know how to take appropriate action. Professionalism demands that technicians prioritize patient welfare and act in accordance with legal and ethical obligations, even when doing so may be personally or professionally uncomfortable. This may involve reporting suspected abuse to the appropriate authorities or escalating workplace concerns through management or external regulatory bodies. Knowing the reporting protocols and resources available within the practice and the broader profession empowers veterinary technicians to respond appropriately when serious issues arise.

In emotionally charged situations, maintaining professionalism also means recognizing when to step back and seek support before reacting impulsively. Ethical dilemmas often provoke strong emotions, and it is important to manage those emotions effectively to prevent escalation or unprofessional behavior. Practicing mindfulness, debriefing with trusted colleagues, or seeking mentorship support can help veterinary technicians process their feelings and approach difficult situations with greater clarity and composure.

It is also important for veterinary technicians to recognize that not every challenge will have a perfect or satisfying resolution. In some cases, compromises must be made, and the best available option may still fall short of ideal care or personal expectations. Professionalism involves accepting these realities without becoming cynical or disengaged. Instead, professionals focus on what is within their control, continuing to provide compassionate, ethical care to the best of their abilities while advocating for systemic improvements where possible.

Ultimately, navigating professional challenges and ethical dilemmas requires a balance of courage, humility, and emotional intelligence. Veterinary technicians who approach these situations with integrity, clear communication, and commitment to patient advocacy demonstrate the highest level of professionalism. By staying true to their ethical principles and seeking constructive solutions, veterinary technicians can manage even the most challenging situations with grace and professionalism (Goleman 1995).

The Role of Professional Organizations and Credentialing

Professional organizations and credentialing bodies play a vital role in shaping the identity, standards, and advancement of the veterinary nursing profession. These organizations provide structure to the field by establishing codes of ethics, developing educational standards, offering continuing education opportunities, and advocating for the recognition and expansion of the veterinary nursing role. For individual veterinary technicians, engagement with professional organizations and the pursuit of advanced credentials are powerful ways to strengthen professional identity, demonstrate commitment to the field, and elevate the quality of patient care.

One of the primary functions of professional organizations is to establish and uphold ethical and professional standards. Organizations such as the NAVTA and state veterinary technician associations provide guidelines that define appropriate professional behavior, patient advocacy responsibilities, and workplace conduct. These standards serve as a foundation for veterinary technicians to navigate complex clinical environments, ensuring that their actions consistently reflect the values of compassion, integrity, and competence.

Credentialing is another critical component of professional development. Earning and maintaining credentials demonstrates a technician's commitment to clinical excellence and ongoing professional growth. Credentialing processes typically require completion of accredited education programs, successful passage of certification exams such as the Veterinary Technician National Examination (VTNE), and compliance with state or provincial licensing regulations. These credentials not only validate a technician's technical knowledge and skills but also signify their adherence to the professional standards established by the field.

Beyond initial credentialing, the pursuit of specialty certifications further distinguishes veterinary technicians who wish to deepen their expertise in specific areas of practice. Organizations such as the Academy of Veterinary Emergency and Critical Care Technicians (AVECCT) and the Academy of Veterinary Technicians in Anesthesia and Analgesia (AVTAA) offer advanced certifications for veterinary technicians seeking to specialize. Earning these credentials requires significant clinical experience, mastery of advanced competencies, and successful completion of rigorous examinations. Specialized credentials enhance professional credibility, open new career opportunities, and position veterinary technicians as leaders within their chosen fields.

Professional organizations also play an essential role in providing access to continuing education, which is a cornerstone of professionalism. As veterinary medicine continues to evolve, staying current with emerging treatments, technologies, and best practices is critical to maintaining clinical competence. Through conferences, webinars, journals, and workshops, professional organizations offer veterinary technicians ongoing opportunities to expand their knowledge and refine their skills. Participation in these educational activities not only strengthens clinical abilities but also demonstrates a commitment to lifelong learning and professional growth.

In addition to education, professional organizations advocate for the advancement of the veterinary nursing profession at both the state and national levels. These organizations work to secure legislative recognition, expand the scope of practice, improve working conditions, and increase public awareness of the critical role that veterinary technicians play in animal healthcare. By joining and actively participating in professional associations, veterinary technicians contribute to these advocacy efforts, helping to shape the future of their profession and ensure that their voices are represented in policy discussions.

Networking is another valuable benefit of professional organization membership. Connecting with peers, mentors, and industry leaders creates opportunities for collaboration, professional development, and career advancement. Professional conferences and events offer veterinary technicians the chance to share ideas, learn from experts, and explore new career pathways. These connections often lead to mentorship relationships that support personal growth and help technicians navigate the challenges and opportunities of their careers more effectively.

Engagement with professional organizations also reinforces the value of professional service and community involvement. Many associations encourage members to participate in volunteer initiatives, serve on committees, or contribute to outreach programs that promote animal welfare and public education. These activities enhance professional fulfillment, build leadership skills, and strengthen the veterinary nursing profession's reputation within the broader community.

For veterinary technicians committed to professionalism, active participation in professional organizations and the pursuit of credentialing represent powerful affirmations of their dedication to the field. These efforts demonstrate a commitment to excellence, a willingness to lead by example, and a desire to continually elevate the standards of patient care. By investing in their own professional development and contributing to the advancement of their profession, veterinary technicians not only enrich their careers but also play a pivotal role in shaping the future of veterinary medicine.

A Global Perspective on Professionalism in Veterinary Nursing

Professionalism in veterinary nursing is not confined to a single national standard, it is a dynamic and evolving concept shaped by cultural values, regulatory frameworks, and the healthcare infrastructure of each country. Exploring how professionalism is defined and practiced across global contexts broadens understanding and highlights both the diversity and shared goals of the veterinary nursing community worldwide.

In the United Kingdom, veterinary technicians are registered through the Royal College of Veterinary Surgeons (RCVS), which enforces a mandatory Code of Professional Conduct. This code outlines specific expectations regarding clinical competence, ethical behavior, client communication, and lifelong learning (RCVS 2021). Unlike in the United States, where title protection and credentialing vary by state, the United Kingdom has a centralized register and legal recognition of the term "veterinary nurse," helping to elevate professional identity and accountability. Registration also entails the ability to be removed from practice for breaches of conduct, reinforcing the seriousness of professional responsibility.

Australia also recognizes veterinary technicians, though regulation differs between regions. In states like Western Australia, nurses are required to register and adhere to professional standards, while in others, credentialing is voluntary. Nonetheless, professional associations such as the Veterinary Nurses Council of Australia (VNCA) have established national guidelines promoting ethical behavior, continuing education, and advocacy for full professional recognition (VNCA 2023). The VNCA's code closely mirrors principles found in NAVTA's Code of Ethics in the United States, including a focus on animal welfare, competence, and respect for colleagues and clients (NAVTA 2016).

In Canada, the credentialed veterinary technician or technologist role is governed by provincial regulatory bodies. For example, Ontario's Ontario Association of Veterinary Technicians (OAVT) requires certification and adherence to a professional code that includes duties related to continuing competence, honesty, and collaboration with veterinary teams (OAVT 2024). Many Canadian provinces also require mandatory continuing education, aligning with global trends emphasizing lifelong learning as a core component of professionalism.

These international perspectives reveal shared foundations in ethical practice, patient advocacy, and ongoing education, yet also highlight structural differences in how professionalism is implemented and enforced. Countries with centralized regulatory systems and protected professional titles often enjoy clearer public understanding and greater autonomy for veterinary nurses. Conversely, in more fragmented systems, like in many parts of the United States, ongoing efforts are required to solidify recognition and standardize expectations.

Understanding global models allows veterinary technicians to reflect on their own professional identity, advocate for systemic improvements, and appreciate the broader impact of their role in animal healthcare. As veterinary nursing becomes more globalized through conferences, international credentialing programs, and online education, the ability to engage with diverse professional standards enhances collaboration and fosters a more unified global profession.

Conclusion

Professionalism is the cornerstone of success and fulfillment in veterinary nursing. It shapes not only the quality of patient care but also the integrity of workplace environments, the strength of professional relationships, and the public's perception of the veterinary nursing profession. By embracing the core values of integrity, accountability, emotional intelligence, and continuous learning, veterinary technicians elevate their roles from technical support staff to essential members of the healthcare team. Professionalism is not a singular achievement but a lifelong commitment to growth, reflection, and excellence (Goleman 1995).

Throughout this chapter, professionalism has been explored from multiple perspectives: in client interactions, where trust and empathy guide conversations; in team dynamics and leadership, where collaboration and respectful communication foster strong, supportive workplaces; and in digital environments, where online behavior reflects personal and professional integrity. Navigating professional challenges and ethical dilemmas with confidence further demonstrates maturity and commitment to patient advocacy, while active participation in professional organizations and pursuit of credentialing reinforces dedication to the highest standards of practice.

Ultimately, veterinary technicians who commit to professionalism not only enhance their own careers but also contribute to the advancement and recognition of the veterinary nursing profession as a whole. Through their actions, attitudes, and leadership, they help shape a future where veterinary technicians are respected as highly skilled healthcare professionals who play a vital role in improving the lives of animals and the people who care for them.

References

Berlin, E.A. and Fowkes, W.C. (1983). A teaching framework for cross-cultural health care: Application in family practice. *Western Journal of Medicine* 139 (6): 934–938.

Cain, J. and Romanelli, F. (2009). E-professionalism: A new paradigm for a digital age. *Currents in Pharmacy Teaching and Learning* 1 (2): 66–70. https://doi.org/10.1016/j.cptl.2009.10.001.

Goleman, D. (1995). *Emotional Intelligence: Why It Can Matter More Than IQ*. Bantam Books.

National Association of Veterinary Technicians in America. (2016). Code of ethics. https://www.navta.net/page/code-of-ethics

Ontario Association of Veterinary Technicians (2024). *OAVT professional practice standards.* https://www.oavt.org

Royal College of Veterinary Surgeons. (2021). *Code of professional conduct for veterinary technicians.* https://www.rcvs.org.uk/standards/code-of-professional-conduct-for-veterinary-technicians/

Veterinary Technicians Council of Australia (2023). *Code of professional conduct.* https://www.vnca.asn.au/veterinary-technicians/professional-standards

Part V

The Future of Veterinary Nursing

13

Innovations in Veterinary Nursing

Veterinary nursing is evolving at a remarkable pace. As companion animals, exotic species, and production animals continue to benefit from advances in veterinary medicine, the role of veterinary technicians has similarly expanded. Innovations in technology, clinical techniques, educational pathways, and scope of practice are not only redefining what veterinary technicians can do—but also reshaping what they must do to meet the demands of an increasingly complex, multidisciplinary profession. From cutting-edge diagnostics and remote patient monitoring to veterinary technician specialization and national advocacy efforts, the landscape of veterinary nursing is rapidly progressing toward a future defined by precision, specialization, and professional autonomy.

Emerging Technologies and Advancements in Practice

The integration of technology into veterinary nursing practice is no longer optional, it is essential. One of the most transformative advancements in recent years is the advent of point-of-care diagnostics. Handheld analyzers now allow for real-time measurement of lactate, glucose, electrolytes, and blood gases within minutes. These tools, once confined to tertiary care settings, are now commonplace in general practice and emergency departments alike. The rapidity of results supports early detection of critical conditions such as hypoperfusion, diabetic crises, and electrolyte disturbances, allowing technicians to initiate nursing interventions without delay.

Similarly, advancements in multimodal monitoring technologies have changed the way veterinary technicians manage anesthetic and critically ill patients. Capnography, invasive and noninvasive blood pressure monitoring, plethysmography, and continuous ECG telemetry are now expected standards of care in many facilities. Moreover, wearable biosensors capable of tracking real-time temperature, respiratory rate, heart rate, and activity levels are expanding postoperative monitoring outside the clinical setting. These wearable devices interface with cloud-based platforms, allowing veterinary technicians to remotely monitor patients and alert clinicians to concerning trends before they become emergencies.

Telemedicine, once viewed as a convenience, is now a vital component of client communication and triage. Veterinary technicians play an increasingly active role in virtual consultations, triage protocols, and remote recheck evaluations, enhancing continuity of care and client compliance. As artificial intelligence and machine learning algorithms continue to evolve, there is a growing presence of AI-assisted radiology, cytology interpretation, and predictive analytics for disease risk. Technicians are expected to interface with these systems, interpret results within a clinical context, and relay implications to the veterinary team.

Innovative Techniques and Expanding Competency

While technological advancements are remarkable, innovation in veterinary nursing is equally rooted in clinical skill. Advanced nursing techniques have moved far beyond traditional expectations. Veterinary technicians are now routinely performing nasoesophageal and nasogastric tube placements, placing peripherally inserted central catheters (PICC lines), managing blood product administration, and executing regional and local anesthetic blocks under the direction of a DVM. In emergency and critical care settings, technicians are actively engaged in mechanical ventilation, high-flow nasal oxygen therapy, closed chest drainage systems, and advanced wound care including vacuum-assisted closure.

The application of evidence-based nursing models, such as the Veterinary Nursing Process, ensures that patient care plans are not merely a collection of tasks but a dynamic and individualized process (Prittie 2010). This model allows for the delivery of individualized nursing care that integrates pathophysiology, pharmacology, behavioral needs, and environmental modification, reinforcing the intellectual and clinical autonomy of veterinary technicians.

Nutritional intervention, particularly for critically ill or cachectic patients, has become a central domain for advanced veterinary nursing care. Calculation of resting energy requirements (RER), consideration of metabolic modifiers, and implementation of assisted feeding plans (e.g., enteral tube nutrition, parenteral nutrition when applicable) require in-depth knowledge and interdisciplinary communication. Veterinary technicians who specialize in this domain are expected to understand nutrient-sparing pathways, immunonutrition, and refeeding syndrome mitigation.

The Veterinary Technician Specialist (VTS) Movement

In parallel to the evolution of clinical skills and technology, the emergence of recognized Veterinary Technician Specialist (VTS) credentials has redefined professional growth for credentialed veterinary technicians. The National Association of Veterinary Technicians in America (NAVTA) oversees the Committee on Veterinary Technician Specialties (CVTS), which governs the recognition of specialty academies. As of this writing, there are currently 16 NAVTA-recognized academies, each requiring rigorous demonstration of advanced knowledge, skills, and case experience in a defined area of practice (Committee on Veterinary Technician Specialties 2025).

These specialties include anesthesia and analgesia, emergency and critical care, internal medicine, behavior, dentistry, zoological medicine, equine nursing, nutrition, dermatology, clinical pathology, diagnostic imaging, laboratory animal medicine, physical rehabilitation, ophthalmology, surgery, and education. Each academy requires applicants to have been credentialed veterinary technicians for a minimum of three to five years, possess documented hours of specialty experience, submit detailed case logs and reports, and successfully pass a board examination. Many academies also require peer-reviewed publications or presentations as a demonstration of professional contribution to the field.

Attaining a VTS is not simply an academic achievement—it is a professional declaration of mastery. It demands years of clinical commitment, ongoing education, mentorship, and academic rigor. Veterinary technician specialists often serve as department leads, educators, clinical trainers, authors, and research assistants, helping to raise the standard of care across all sectors of veterinary medicine. The presence of a VTS in a hospital elevates patient outcomes, improves team confidence, and enhances client communication through specialized knowledge.

The Veterinary Nurse Initiative (VNI): National Unification and Title Clarity

In recognition of the variability and confusion surrounding the term "veterinary technician." The Veterinary Nurse Initiative (VNI) was developed as a national advocacy campaign aimed at standardizing credentialing, terminology, and scope of practice across the United States (NAVTA 2025). Spearheaded by NAVTA, the VNI seeks to legally adopt the title "Registered Veterinary Nurse (RVN)" across all states in the United States, aligning the profession with international standards found in countries such as the United Kingdom and Australia.

The initiative is based on the principle that title consistency, educational standardization, and public understanding are fundamental to professional recognition. In the current system, the titles "licensed," "certified," and "registered" veterinary technician vary by state and often carry different legal definitions and implications. This lack of clarity confuses clients, underrepresents the profession's contribution, and dilutes advocacy efforts. By unifying the title under the designation "veterinary nurse," the VNI aims to elevate public perception, reinforce professional identity, and promote reciprocity between states.

Critically, the VNI does not seek to devalue existing credentialing but instead to elevate the title to reflect the complexity of the work. Veterinary technicians are not assistants. They are trained professionals capable of advanced procedures, critical thinking, and independent patient assessment under veterinary supervision. Title protection and clarity serve as the scaffolding on which utilization, compensation, and respect can be constructed.

The Veterinary Professional Associate (VPA) Movement: Advanced Practice and Mid-Level Providers

While the VNI addresses standardization at the entry-level credentialing stage, the Veterinary Professional Associate (VPA) movement represents an even more progressive paradigm shift. The VPA is envisioned as a mid-level provider model, analogous to nurse practitioners (NPs) or physician associates (PAs) in human medicine. This role would be occupied by advanced credentialed veterinary technicians with graduate-level education and clinical residency experience, allowing for increased autonomy in patient care under a defined scope of indirect veterinary supervision.

The ideology behind the VPA is grounded in the increasing demand for veterinary services, the workforce shortage, and the need for accessible, affordable care. The VPA would serve in roles such as managing chronic disease, prescribing limited classes of medications, performing minor procedures, and leading client education and follow-up—particularly in underserved or rural areas where veterinary access is limited.

Educational pathways to the Veterinary Professional Associate (VPA) role are currently being forged through the evolving framework of graduate-level education in veterinary clinical care. The most appropriate academic foundation for this mid-level provider model is the Master of Veterinary Clinical Care (MVCC) degree, which is designed to equip credentialed veterinary technicians with advanced theoretical knowledge, clinical reasoning, and applied professional skills that mirror the graduate-level expectations of nurse practitioners and physician associates in human medicine.

As of the writing of this textbook, Colorado State University (CSU) is the only academic institution actively developing and offering the MVCC degree specifically for the purpose of advancing the VPA concept (Colorado State University 2025). In addition to CSU, Lincoln Memorial University (LMU) also offers a Master of Veterinary Clinical Care program, though the structure and emphasis of their curriculum differ (Lincoln Memorial University 2025). Their curriculum is designed not only to elevate clinical proficiency but also to prepare graduates for the professional, legal, and ethical challenges inherent in providing care under indirect veterinary supervision. The CSU MVCC program integrates coursework in clinical pharmacology, advanced physiology, diagnostic imaging interpretation, internal medicine, emergency, and critical care principles, nursing leadership, professional communication, evidence-based practice, and bioethics. A capstone project or clinical thesis is typically required, demonstrating the student's ability to critically assess, apply, and communicate scholarly research within a clinical framework. In addition to CSU, Lincoln Memorial University (LMU) also offers a Master of Veterinary Clinical Care program, though they differ in structure and emphasis. LMU's program emphasizes clinical mentorship, professional development, and advanced nursing intervention. Required coursework includes advanced pathophysiology, anesthetic pharmacology, emergency stabilization, critical care nursing, professional ethics, research methods, and curriculum design.

Across these programs, core competencies include advanced patient assessment, differential diagnosis, intervention planning, outcome evaluation, and interprofessional collaboration. Coursework is typically delivered in a hybrid or fully online format to accommodate working professionals, with synchronous components to support clinical discussion and mentorship.

Following completion of an MVCC degree, candidates pursuing the VPA designation would likely be expected to complete a clinical internship or residency in a designated area of focus such as internal medicine, emergency and critical care, or general practice. Credentialing for the VPA role—once formalized—would include a standardized examination, formal licensure, and mandated continuing education, aligning with the principles of professional accountability, clinical autonomy, and patient safety.

While legislative infrastructure to support the VPA role is still under development, the academic foundation now exists. These programs reflect a significant shift in how veterinary nursing is conceptualized—not merely as a technical support function, but as a clinical science requiring academic rigor, critical thinking, and clinical leadership. The promise of the VPA model is not only in expanding access to veterinary care but in redefining the trajectory of the veterinary nursing profession as a whole.

Future Landscape: Innovation, Advocacy, and Academic Expansion

The future of veterinary nursing lies at the intersection of innovation, advocacy, and education. As the demand for specialized care grows, so too will the expectations placed upon veterinary technicians. Artificial intelligence, robotics-assisted surgery, 3D printing for prosthetics and orthopedic implants, and gene editing for hereditary diseases will demand that veterinary technicians possess not only technical competence but also scientific literacy and ethical reasoning.

Academic institutions are beginning to respond. Graduate programs in veterinary nursing and clinical care are gaining traction, offering master's-level education in advanced nursing science, pathophysiology, research methodology, leadership, and education. These programs serve to advance the clinical voice of the veterinary technician, placing them at the center of translational medicine, policy advocacy, and interprofessional collaboration.

Leadership roles for veterinary technicians will continue to emerge—not only within hospitals, but also in regulatory boards, accreditation councils, nonprofit sectors, disaster response, and international development. Technicians will be integral to One Health initiatives, zoonotic disease control, antimicrobial stewardship, and climate-related animal welfare challenges.

Legislative Action and Association Advocacy: The Backbone of Veterinary Nursing's Future

As the veterinary nursing profession accelerates toward clinical specialization, mid-level provider models, and advanced educational opportunities, it becomes increasingly clear that sustainable progress hinges on strategic legislative engagement. While educational innovation lays the foundation for clinical advancement, only legislative and regulatory reform can cement these advancements into formalized practice. In this regard, state veterinary technician associations and national professional organizations are not peripheral to progress—they are the very infrastructure upon which the future of veterinary nursing must be built.

Historically, the scope of practice for veterinary technicians has been defined and constrained by individual state practice acts. These documents, often decades old, were not written with modern veterinary nursing in mind and frequently contain vague or inconsistent language around permissible duties, supervision categories, and title protection. Without active legislative advocacy, even the most skilled and well-educated veterinary technicians remain legally underutilized. As a result, patient outcomes, professional satisfaction, and retention are negatively impacted.

State associations serve as the critical liaison between credentialed veterinary technicians and their respective veterinary medical boards, state legislatures, and departments of professional licensing. Their role extends far beyond member benefits or continuing education—they act as the collective voice of the profession, championing statutory revisions, promoting workforce expansion, and ensuring that veterinary technicians are represented in policy decisions that directly affect clinical practice. When associations lack a robust governmental relations strategy, the profession risks stagnation or, worse, regression in the face of growing industry demands.

The Veterinary Nurse Initiative, for example, cannot achieve national title unification or scope protection without state-by-state legislative wins. Likewise, the future viability of the Veterinary Professional Associate model will depend on the establishment of a licensure pathway through legislative statutes. No matter how academically prepared a VPA graduate may be, their authority to diagnose, prescribe, or perform procedures under indirect supervision must be granted and protected by law. That law begins at the state level.

Several states have demonstrated what is possible when associations mobilize effectively. Legislative successes in states like Oregon, Tennessee, and Indiana have included title protection for credentialed veterinary technicians, recognition of specialty roles, and expanded procedural authority under appropriate supervision. These advancements were not accidental; they were the result of years of relationship building, public testimony, lobbying, and collaboration between veterinary technician associations, state VMAs, and supportive lawmakers. Associations that invest in professional lobbying services, regulatory committees, and policy education for their members are more likely to see meaningful progress.

Additionally, as veterinary technicians increasingly seek parity with human healthcare models, the strategic alliances they form with public health entities, human nursing boards, and advocacy groups become even more important. Issues such as opioid handling, zoonotic disease control, antimicrobial stewardship, and telehealth all involve state or federal legislation. Without a seat at the table, veterinary technicians may find their roles restricted or overlooked in emerging healthcare models.

The importance of governmental relations is further underscored by the growing need for reciprocity and licensure portability. As the veterinary workforce becomes more mobile and national organizations seek unification of credentials, state boards must collaborate to harmonize requirements. Advocacy through associations is essential in facilitating these conversations and ensuring that veterinary technicians are not penalized by outdated or inconsistent regulations.

Ultimately, the future of veterinary nursing will be shaped not only in lecture halls and surgery suites but in committee rooms and legislative chambers. If veterinary technicians are to realize their full potential—as educators, specialists, mid-level providers, and leaders—they must invest in the political infrastructure that supports these aspirations. This requires membership, engagement, and active participation in the associations that represent them.

Advocacy is not optional. It is a professional obligation. Through organized legislative action, veterinary technicians can secure authority, recognition, and respect that their education, skill, and dedication so clearly warrant. The blueprint for progress is already being written—one statute, one state, one association at a time.

Conclusion: A Profession in Evolution

Veterinary nursing is no longer a support role; it is a profession in its own right—one that demands intellectual rigor, technical expertise, and emotional intelligence. As innovations in technology, education, and legislative advocacy continue to unfold, veterinary technicians will be called upon not only to master new tools and techniques, but also to shape the policies and paradigms that govern their use.

The future of veterinary nursing will be one of purpose, power, and potential. The profession stands at the precipice of extraordinary opportunity—one where the veterinary technician is no longer behind the scenes, but rather at the heart of every patient's journey. The challenge now is to rise to meet it.

References

Colorado State University (CSU) (2025). *Master of Veterinary Clinical Care (MVCC) program.* College of Veterinary Medicine and Biomedical Sciences. [online] https://vetmedbiosci.colostate.edu (accessed 27 June 2025).

Committee on Veterinary Technician Specialties (CVTS) (2025). *Recognized veterinary technician specialty academies.* National Association of Veterinary Technicians in America. [online] https://www.navta.net/page/specialties (accessed 27 June 2025).

Lincoln Memorial University (LMU) (2025). *Master of Veterinary Clinical Care (MVCC).* [online] https://www.lmunet.edu (accessed 27 June 2025).

National Association of Veterinary Technicians in America (NAVTA) (2025). *Veterinary Nurse Initiative (VNI).* [online] https://www.navta.net/page/VNI (accessed 27 June 2025).

Prittie, J., 2010. Veterinary nursing process: A framework for care. *Veterinary Clinics of North America: Small Animal Practice,* 40(3), pp.461–470. doi:https://doi.org/10.1016/j.cvsm.2010.02.002.

14

Continuing Education and Professional Development

Introduction

Continuing education and` professional development are essential elements of a fulfilling and sustainable career in veterinary nursing. In a profession driven by innovation, advancing medical knowledge, and evolving patient care practices, the veterinary technician's role is continually expanding. To remain effective and confident in their clinical responsibilities, veterinary technicians must embrace a lifelong commitment to learning. This commitment goes beyond fulfilling required continuing education credits, and it reflects a deep dedication to personal growth, patient advocacy, and the advancement of the veterinary nursing profession.

The rapidly changing landscape of veterinary medicine presents both challenges and opportunities. New diagnostic technologies, advanced treatment protocols, and emerging specialties require veterinary technicians to remain informed and adaptable. As the profession continues to advocate for greater recognition and expanded roles for veterinary technicians, ongoing education becomes the foundation for building professional credibility and enhancing patient outcomes. Continuing education and professional development not only improve technical competencies but also contribute to personal satisfaction and long-term career success.

This chapter explores the importance of lifelong learning, the diverse opportunities available for advanced training and specialization, and the strategies veterinary technicians can use to develop personalized learning plans that support their career goals. By actively engaging in continuing education and seeking new professional challenges, veterinary technicians can remain at the forefront of their field, delivering the highest standard of care while achieving personal and professional fulfillment.

Self-Reflection and Professional Identity Development

Professional development begins with self-awareness. Before a veterinary technician can chart a path forward, they must first understand who they are, what motivates them, and how they define themselves within the profession. This process of self-reflection is not only a precursor to effective goal setting, but it is the foundation of professional identity. In a field as emotionally demanding and intellectually complex as veterinary medicine, a strong sense of self is essential for resilience, purpose, and long-term fulfillment.

Professional identity refers to how an individual sees themselves within their role. It includes the values they hold, the responsibilities they embrace, and the contributions they aspire to make. For veterinary technicians, this identity is shaped by a blend of clinical experience, educational background, ethical beliefs, and personal passion for animal care. However, it is not static. Like all meaningful identities, it evolves over time—molded by both triumphs and challenges. Continuing education plays a central role in this evolution, not only by enhancing clinical skills but by expanding one's sense of capability, responsibility, and vision.

Self-reflection invites veterinary technicians to pause and ask important questions about who they are and where they are headed. They might consider what kind of technician they want to be, which moments in practice have been the most meaningful, or what aspects of their role continue to challenge them. They may reflect on how their personal values influence patient care or ponder how their career goals align with their current experiences. These questions aren't easily answered in a single sitting. They require ongoing reflection, ideally supported by journaling, peer conversations, mentorship, or dedicated time during performance reviews. Veterinary technicians who engage in reflective practice are better prepared to make purposeful decisions about their continuing education, rather than simply reacting to external requirements or trends. Their learning becomes intentional, personal, and aligned with who they are becoming.

This type of reflection also supports emotional processing and mental wellness, which are the critical components of holistic veterinary care. Veterinary medicine is full of emotionally charged moments: euthanasia, financial limitations, patient suffering, and client conflict. Without reflection, these moments can accumulate, leading to burnout or disengagement. But when veterinary technicians create space to think about what they've experienced, how it aligns with their values, and what they've learned from it, they begin to transform stress into insight. Continuing education then becomes not just a way to gain knowledge, but a tool to refine judgment, build emotional intelligence, and strengthen professional confidence.

Clinical storytelling, writing, or speaking about real cases, is another effective tool for identity development. By recounting a difficult anesthesia, a challenging client interaction, or a successful recovery, veterinary technicians not only process their experience but also clarify what kind of technician they were in that moment and what kind they wish to become. These stories help form a narrative of growth and resilience that is essential for sustaining motivation and direction.

Professional identity is also reinforced by recognition and validation. Participating in CE events, contributing to case discussions, publishing articles, or earning credentials all affirm that a veterinary technician is not only a member of the profession, but a contributor to it. This sense of belonging and impact is vital to long-term engagement and satisfaction.

In holistic veterinary practice, the individual technician is seen not just as a task performer but as a thoughtful, value-driven clinician whose mindset shapes patient care. Cultivating professional identity through self-reflection ensures that the technical aspects of development are balanced by emotional and ethical grounding. When veterinary technicians know who they are and what they stand for, they can approach learning with clarity, confidence, and purpose.

Importance of Lifelong Learning

Lifelong learning is the continuous pursuit of knowledge and skill development throughout one's career. For veterinary technicians, this concept is not merely an ideal but a professional necessity. The veterinary field evolves rapidly, with new research findings, medical advancements, and technologies emerging at a pace that requires practitioners to remain informed and adaptable. Without a commitment to ongoing education, veterinary technicians risk falling behind in both their clinical skills and their understanding of best practices in patient care.

The importance of lifelong learning in veterinary nursing extends beyond staying current with medical knowledge. It is directly linked to patient outcomes and the technician's ability to advocate effectively for their patients. Veterinary technicians who engage in ongoing education are better equipped to recognize subtle changes in patient condition, understand advanced treatment options, and provide informed recommendations to both clients and the veterinary healthcare team. This depth of knowledge enhances critical thinking and clinical decision-making, leading to improved patient care and stronger outcomes.

Engaging in lifelong learning also contributes to greater job satisfaction and personal fulfillment. As veterinary technicians acquire new skills and expand their knowledge base, they experience increased confidence in their clinical abilities and a renewed sense of purpose in their work. This growth helps combat the feelings of stagnation and burnout that can arise from repetitive daily tasks. By continually challenging themselves to learn and improve, veterinary technicians keep their careers dynamic and personally rewarding.

Lifelong learning also strengthens the veterinary nursing profession as a whole. As more veterinary technicians pursue advanced education and develop specialized skills, the role of the technician becomes increasingly valuable within the veterinary healthcare team. This collective growth supports the ongoing effort to achieve greater professional recognition, expanded scopes of practice, and improved working conditions for veterinary technicians.

The holistic nursing model further reinforces the importance of lifelong learning. In this model, veterinary technicians are encouraged to view patient care from a comprehensive perspective that considers the physical, emotional, and environmental factors affecting health. Ongoing education in areas such as pain management, nutrition, behavior, and alternative therapies allows veterinary technicians to develop a more well-rounded understanding of patient needs, enabling them to provide holistic, individualized care that addresses the whole patient rather than isolated symptoms.

Moreover, the veterinary nursing profession faces an ever-growing need for leaders and mentors who can guide the next generation of professionals. Lifelong learning positions veterinary technicians to take on these leadership roles, whether through formal positions within their organizations or through informal mentorship relationships. Sharing knowledge and fostering the professional growth of colleagues not only elevates the individual technician's career but also strengthens the profession as a whole.

In embracing lifelong learning, veterinary technicians demonstrate a commitment to excellence that transcends individual achievement. They contribute to better patient outcomes, stronger healthcare teams, and a more respected and empowered professional community. Lifelong learning is not just a professional obligation—it is a pathway to personal and collective advancement that defines the highest standards of veterinary nursing.

Overcoming Barriers to Continuing Education

While the value of continuing education in veterinary nursing is widely recognized, many veterinary technicians face significant barriers that can hinder their ability to engage in lifelong learning. These obstacles—ranging from financial constraints to time limitations, emotional fatigue, and lack of institutional support—can make the pursuit of professional development feel out of reach. Understanding these common challenges and developing strategies to overcome them is essential for veterinary technicians who want to remain engaged, competent, and fulfilled in their roles.

One of the most prevalent barriers is financial limitations. Many veterinary technicians work in practices that offer limited or no reimbursement for continuing education courses, conferences, or certifications. The cost of travel, registration fees, and required materials can add up quickly, particularly for those pursuing advanced training or specialty credentials. However, several resources are available to help offset these costs. Many state and national veterinary technician associations offer scholarships and travel grants specifically for continuing education. Employers may be willing to contribute to CE expenses if the veterinary technician can demonstrate how the training will directly benefit the hospital—such as by enabling the technician to take on new responsibilities or train other team members. Additionally, a growing number of high-quality online CE opportunities are available at low or no cost, including webinars, podcasts, and digital workshops offered by universities, professional associations, and industry partners.

Time constraints are another major hurdle. Veterinary technicians often work long hours in emotionally demanding environments, leaving little time or energy for additional learning. Those with caregiving responsibilities, second jobs, or inconsistent schedules may find it especially difficult to attend live courses or travel for in-person events. To address this, it is essential to embrace flexible learning formats. Asynchronous online courses, self-paced certification programs, and recorded lectures allow veterinary technicians to learn on their own schedule. Breaking education into manageable segments—such as watching a 15-minute module during a lunch break or dedicating one evening per week to study—makes continuing education more accessible and sustainable. Employers who value professional development can also support learning by building CE time into work schedules or offering rotating shift coverage to allow team members to attend training events.

In some cases, emotional and psychological barriers may be even more limiting than financial or logistical ones. Veterinary technicians experiencing burnout or compassion fatigue may lack the motivation or mental bandwidth to pursue learning, even if resources are available. Others may struggle with imposter syndrome, feeling that they are not "smart enough" or "qualified enough" to pursue advanced education. In these moments, it is crucial to reconnect with the deeper reasons for choosing this profession: a love for animals, a desire to help, and a passion for clinical excellence. Starting small—with a single course or conversation with a mentor—can reignite a sense of curiosity and capability. Peer support also plays a vital role in overcoming these emotional obstacles. Talking with colleagues who have successfully pursued CE can demystify the process and offer encouragement through shared experiences.

Another significant barrier is lack of support or recognition from the workplace. In some veterinary hospitals, continuing education may not be prioritized, and veterinary technicians may not be given the time, funding, or encouragement to pursue learning opportunities. This can lead to stagnation and dissatisfaction, particularly for those who are eager to grow. In these settings, veterinary technicians may need to advocate for their own development. This includes initiating conversations with supervisors about CE goals, outlining how learning will benefit the practice, and requesting dedicated time or resources. Keeping a professional portfolio of completed CE activities and competencies gained can also help demonstrate value to the employer and open the door to future support.

Geographic isolation can also impact access to continuing education. Veterinary technicians in rural or underserved areas may have limited opportunities to attend in-person workshops or network with peers. In such cases, building a digital learning network is critical. Online discussion forums, social media groups for veterinary professionals, and virtual conferences can provide the sense of community and shared learning that is often missing in remote locations. Additionally, many national organizations offer recorded versions of their CE events, ensuring that content is accessible regardless of location.

Overcoming these barriers often requires creativity, persistence, and self-advocacy. Veterinary technicians who approach continuing education as an essential part of their professional identity—not an optional extra—are more likely to seek out solutions and remain committed to their growth. By recognizing and addressing the obstacles to learning, veterinary technicians take ownership of their careers and ensure that they remain resilient, knowledgeable, and empowered members of the veterinary healthcare team. This commitment also reinforces the principles of holistic nursing by acknowledging the real-life challenges veterinary technicians face and promoting compassionate, sustainable strategies for growth. In this way, overcoming barriers to continuing education is not only about gaining knowledge, but also about creating the conditions for a balanced, fulfilling, and long-lasting career in veterinary nursing.

Integrating Learning into Daily Practice

Continuing education does not have to be confined to conferences, formal coursework, or credentialing pathways. In fact, some of the most impactful professional development happens organically through everyday clinical experiences. Integrating learning into daily practice ensures that education is ongoing, dynamic, and immediately relevant. For veterinary technicians working in busy hospitals, this approach to development is both practical and empowering—it transforms routine work into meaningful opportunities for growth.

One of the most effective strategies for daily learning is microlearning: the practice of acquiring knowledge in small, digestible segments throughout the day. This might involve taking five minutes between appointments to read a clinical article, watching a short video on a new anesthetic protocol, or reviewing a case summary posted in the treatment area. Microlearning fits into even the most demanding schedules and helps reinforce information incrementally, making it easier to retain and apply in practice. When veterinary technicians approach each shift with curiosity and openness, even brief moments of downtime can become productive educational experiences.

Case-based learning is another powerful tool for integrating education into the clinical environment. Every patient encounter presents a chance to ask questions, reflect on outcomes, and build clinical reasoning. After completing a complex case, veterinary technicians can participate in informal case reviews with colleagues, discussing what went well, what could have been improved, and what they learned. This practice not only reinforces clinical knowledge but also strengthens communication and collaboration within the team. Encouraging these debriefs as a regular part of hospital culture fosters a shared commitment to growth and learning.

Daily rounds also present a rich opportunity for on-the-job education. Veterinary technicians can elevate their participation by preparing thoughtful questions about cases, sharing recent evidence-based practices, or requesting clarification on unfamiliar procedures. Asking a veterinarian to explain the rationale behind a particular treatment or to walk through an ultrasound interpretation transforms passive observation into active engagement. Over time, these interactions build confidence and deepen understanding, especially when technicians feel empowered to contribute observations and suggestions rooted in their own clinical knowledge.

To support this culture of continuous learning, many hospitals implement skills boards, clinical tip sheets, or "topic of the week" features in common areas. These simple tools provide quick access to relevant information and can be rotated regularly to reflect seasonal diseases, frequently asked client questions, or changes in hospital protocols. Having visual reminders and reference materials readily available supports memory retention and encourages all staff to stay informed. Some practices even dedicate a few minutes at each staff meeting to clinical mini-presentations, giving team members the opportunity to share a new technique or summarize a CE course they recently attended.

Mentorship and peer-to-peer learning are particularly valuable in reinforcing learning within daily practice. Experienced veterinary technicians can take newer team members under their wing and provide real-time teaching moments throughout the shift. Whether it's reviewing venipuncture technique, walking through a discharge conversation, or demonstrating catheter placement, hands-on instruction in the moment is one of the most effective ways to build technical and communication skills. These interactions also strengthen team dynamics, as they foster mutual respect, shared responsibility, and collaboration.

Integrating learning into daily practice also aligns with the principles of holistic nursing, which emphasize mindful presence, intentional action, and treating each patient interaction as a unique opportunity to apply knowledge with compassion. When veterinary technicians consciously reflect on their clinical decisions, engage with colleagues about patient care, and seek out small moments of growth throughout the day, they embody the values of holistic practice. This approach supports not only better patient outcomes, but also personal fulfillment and emotional resilience.

Technology can further support continuous learning in the workplace. Mobile apps, hospital intranets, and digital knowledge banks allow veterinary technicians to look up drug dosages, anatomy diagrams, or best practices in real time. Creating digital bookmarks or quick-access folders on hospital tablets or shared computers makes information retrieval more efficient and encourages the habit of consulting reliable, evidence-based sources during clinical decision-making.

Even administrative tasks can present learning opportunities. Reviewing vaccine protocols, double-checking controlled drug logs, or auditing patient discharge instructions can spark questions and lead to small but meaningful improvements in clinical accuracy. By viewing every aspect of the job through the lens of learning, veterinary technicians stay engaged and elevate the overall quality of care they deliver.

Ultimately, integrating learning into daily practice transforms professional development from a task on a checklist into a mindset—one that celebrates curiosity, embraces challenges, and seeks growth in every shift. This philosophy not only enriches the veterinary technician's career but also fosters a collaborative, progressive, and supportive workplace culture. In this way, learning becomes not something separate from practice, but an essential part of it (Figure 14.1).

Daily Learning Tip Sheet

- Watch a 5-minute clinical video during lunch
- Review a journal article between appointments
- Ask a teammate to walk you through a new protocol
- Take turns sharing one new thing learned during rounds
- Post a 'clinical tip of the week' on the treatment board
- Reflect on a case after your shift: What went well? What would you do differently?

Figure 14.1 Practical, time-efficient learning activities for integration into the clinical workday. M. Jennings, 2025.

The Role of Technology in Learning and Professional Development

In an increasingly digital world, technology has become an indispensable ally in the pursuit of continuing education and professional development for veterinary technicians. The rapid growth of online platforms, mobile applications, and virtual communities has reshaped how veterinary professionals access information, collaborate, and build expertise. For veterinary technicians who are balancing demanding work schedules, financial limitations, or geographic isolation, technology provides flexible, affordable, and effective avenues for learning. When used intentionally, it can enrich clinical practice, support credentialing goals, and foster a sense of belonging within the broader veterinary community.

One of the most significant advantages of technology in professional development is the accessibility of online continuing education. A wide variety of organizations, including veterinary schools, industry partners, state associations, and credentialing bodies, now offer high-quality webinars, asynchronous courses, and on-demand video libraries. These resources allow veterinary technicians to learn on their own time and at their own pace, removing the logistical barriers associated with traditional in-person events. Many platforms offer certificates of completion or provide CE credits that count toward state licensure requirements, making them both convenient and professionally relevant.

In addition to formal courses, podcasts and video content offer informal but powerful ways to stay engaged with clinical topics and emerging trends. Veterinary-focused podcasts often feature case discussions, interviews with specialists, and practical advice on communication and leadership. YouTube channels and social media accounts managed by credentialed professionals provide visual demonstrations of procedures, tutorials on equipment use, and bite-sized clinical updates. Veterinary technicians can incorporate these tools into their daily routines, listening to a podcast during a commute or watching a quick procedure video before a shift—to reinforce knowledge and stay inspired.

Mobile apps have also become valuable tools for veterinary technicians seeking real-time access to clinical information. Drug reference apps, dosage calculators, anatomy atlases, and diagnostic guidelines are now available at the touch of a button. These resources support clinical decision-making and improve confidence during high-pressure scenarios. Some hospitals adopt shared devices, like tablets or workstations with bookmarked resources, while others encourage veterinary technicians to personalize their own learning app libraries. The ability to instantly verify information promotes both accuracy and autonomy in the clinical setting.

Beyond content consumption, technology facilitates interactive and social learning. Online discussion forums, veterinary technician Facebook groups, and professional listservs create opportunities for peer-to-peer support, mentorship, and case sharing. These digital communities help veterinary technicians connect across geographical and institutional boundaries, fostering a sense of solidarity and collaboration. They also create space for dialogue around difficult cases, ethical dilemmas, and career advancement questions. Participating in these forums builds communication skills, promotes reflective practice, and introduces diverse perspectives that enhance clinical reasoning.

Technology also supports career visibility and documentation of growth. Maintaining a digital portfolio—through platforms like LinkedIn, Google Drive, or professional CE tracking software—allows veterinary technicians to organize certificates, case logs, mentorship records, and learning reflections. This portfolio not only serves as a motivational record of progress but is also useful when applying for jobs, specialty certification, or speaking opportunities. An active online presence can also increase professional visibility, attracting invitations to contribute to publications, present at conferences, or mentor others in the field.

Additionally, virtual simulation tools and online skills assessments are beginning to reshape clinical learning. While still emerging in veterinary nursing education, these tools allow users to interact with case scenarios, practice decision-making, and receive instant feedback. As these technologies become more sophisticated and accessible, they will offer new ways for veterinary technicians to hone critical thinking and prepare for real-world challenges (Table 14.1).

To use technology effectively, however, veterinary technicians must practice discernment and digital literacy. Not all online content is evidence-based or relevant to best practices. It is essential to evaluate the credibility of sources, favoring content from licensed professionals, academic institutions, or established organizations. Critical thinking is key when navigating online spaces—especially when advice is anecdotal, sensationalized, or disconnected from current standards of care. Participating in well-moderated forums and engaging with credentialed educators helps ensure that technology enhances, rather than undermines, clinical judgment.

The use of technology also aligns with the holistic model of veterinary nursing, which emphasizes adaptability, proactive learning, and emotional well-being. Technology reduces isolation by connecting veterinary technicians with peers and mentors; it supports autonomy by offering on-demand learning; and it promotes balance by allowing users to engage with content in ways that respect their time and energy. When thoughtfully integrated into daily practice, digital tools empower veterinary technicians to remain current, confident, and connected throughout their careers.

As technology continues to evolve, it will offer even more innovative ways to support veterinary technician education—from virtual reality training simulations to AI-assisted learning platforms. Embracing these tools not only positions veterinary technicians at the forefront of clinical excellence but also reaffirms their commitment to a growth mindset and to the compassionate, evidence-based care at the heart of their profession.

Building and Sustaining Motivation for Lifelong Learning

The decision to pursue continuing education is not a one-time event. It is a commitment to ongoing personal and professional evolution. While many veterinary technicians begin their careers with a strong desire to grow, sustaining that motivation over time can be difficult. Workplace fatigue, emotional burnout, personal obligations, or a sense of stagnation can

Table 14.1 Top 5 tools for Tech-Savvy veterinary technicians.

Tool	Description	How to Leverage
Veterinary Apps	Mobile apps that provide instant access to drug dosages, anatomical references, and clinical calculators.	Download and organize apps like Plumb's, VetPDA, or Merck Vet Manual. Use daily for quick referencing on the floor.
Online Learning Platforms	Websites and platforms offering CE courses, webinars, and certification programs tailored to veterinary medicine.	Subscribe to platforms like VSPN, VetFolio, or NAVTA's learning hub. Block time weekly for professional learning.
Web-Based Practice Management Software	Cloud-based software that manages appointments, patient records, billing, and inventory in real time.	Use integrated tools to streamline workflow, reduce duplication, and track technician-driven metrics.
Digital Imaging Systems	Technology used to capture, store, and interpret radiographic, ultrasound, or CT images efficiently.	Improve diagnostic accuracy and speed. Collaborate with veterinarians to enhance patient imaging protocols.
Portable Devices	Tablets, laptops, or mobile phones that provide flexibility for documentation, communication, and mobile learning.	Create digital notebooks, bookmark key websites, and stay updated with medical news via push notifications.

dull even the most passionate learners. Understanding how to cultivate and maintain motivation is therefore essential for ensuring that learning remains a vibrant and rewarding part of a veterinary technician's career.

One of the most powerful motivators is connecting learning to purpose. Veterinary technicians are often driven by a deep desire to make a difference in the lives of animals and their caregivers. When continuing education is viewed through the lens of patient advocacy, the value of learning becomes more immediate and personal. For example, learning a new pain management technique isn't just about expanding clinical skills; it's about relieving suffering and improving comfort. Acquiring knowledge about behavior or nutrition becomes a way to help clients better support their pets. When learning is rooted in compassion, motivation becomes intrinsic and sustainable.

Another strategy for maintaining motivation is to set meaningful, personal goals. Rather than pursuing CE simply to meet licensing requirements, veterinary technicians should reflect on what they want to achieve in their careers and lives. This might include becoming a specialist, mentoring others, increasing clinical confidence, or transitioning into a leadership role. When learning goals are tied to these larger aspirations, they become more compelling. Writing down these goals and revisiting them regularly can serve as a personal contract reminder of what inspired the journey and where it is headed.

Celebrating milestones—even small ones—is crucial to sustaining enthusiasm. Finishing a CE course, participating in a successful case discussion, or getting positive feedback from a mentor all represent progress. These moments deserve acknowledgment. Veterinary technicians should consider maintaining a professional journal, blog, or digital portfolio to track their achievements, reflect on lessons learned, and document personal growth. Looking back on these records during moments of self-doubt can rekindle pride and momentum.

Accountability partnerships can also help maintain learning momentum. Whether it's a mentor, colleague, or friend, having someone to check in with about educational goals creates external reinforcement. Study groups, CE "buddies," or team-based learning challenges in the workplace foster shared commitment and mutual support. These social learning relationships also make the process more enjoyable and help counter feelings of isolation.

At times, motivation may dip not due to lack of desire but because of emotional exhaustion or mental overload. Veterinary technicians often give so much to others that they have little energy left to invest in themselves. In these cases, motivation must begin with self-compassion. It is okay to step back, rest, and return to learning when emotional reserves have been restored. Reframing education as an act of self-care, one that nurtures professional identity and personal fulfillment, can help veterinary technicians reconnect with their intrinsic drive. Sometimes, the most powerful motivator is not ambition, but the need for renewal and clarity.

Visualization techniques can also support motivation. Creating a vision board—whether physical or digital—with images or phrases that represent future goals can serve as a daily visual reminder of what continued growth can lead to. This practice transforms abstract intentions into something tangible and inspiring. Others may benefit from writing a future bio or imagining a job interview where they talk about the skills they want to develop. These exercises help turn long-term aspirations into short-term actions.

Changing learning formats can also refresh motivation. If lectures have grown stale, switching to interactive webinars, podcasts, or hands-on labs may reignite curiosity. If clinical cases feel repetitive, seeking out a new area of focus—such as hospice care, exotic animals, or rehabilitation—can introduce novelty. Varying the types of educational experiences prevents burnout and keeps learning dynamic.

Lastly, veterinary technicians should give themselves permission to learn for the sake of learning. Not all continuing education needs to result in a certification or credential. Sometimes, reading a book about empathy in medicine or attending a wellness workshop can be just as transformative as mastering a clinical technique. Lifelong learning is as much about growing as a person as it is about expanding technical proficiency. Embracing this broader definition of education keeps motivation expansive and inclusive.

Sustaining motivation is not about staying in a constant state of inspiration—it's about building systems, habits, and support structures that make learning a natural part of life. It's about remembering the "why" behind the work, honoring progress, and remaining flexible in how growth is pursued. When veterinary technicians approach learning with curiosity, intention, and self-awareness, they ensure that their careers remain alive with purpose—and that their impact on patients, clients, and colleagues continues to deepen with every year of practice (Figure 14.2).

Opportunities for Advanced Training and Specialization

The veterinary nursing profession offers a diverse range of opportunities for advanced training and specialization, allowing technicians to deepen their expertise, expand their clinical roles, and pursue areas of personal and professional interest.

Specialization not only enhances the quality of patient care but also contributes to career advancement, increased job satisfaction, and greater recognition within the veterinary healthcare team. As the field continues to evolve, veterinary technicians who pursue specialized knowledge position themselves at the forefront of patient advocacy and clinical excellence.

One of the most well-established avenues for specialization is through obtaining a Veterinary Technician Specialist (VTS) certification. Administered by academies recognized by the National Association of Veterinary Technicians in America (NAVTA), VTS credentials are available in several disciplines, including emergency and critical care, anesthesia and analgesia, internal medicine, dentistry, behavior, nutrition, and zoological medicine, among others. Earning a VTS designation requires rigorous clinical experience, demonstrated mastery of advanced competencies, and successful completion of comprehensive examinations. This credential not only validates specialized knowledge but also opens doors to leadership roles, teaching opportunities, and positions in referral and specialty practices (National Association of Veterinary Technicians in America [NAVTA] n.d.).

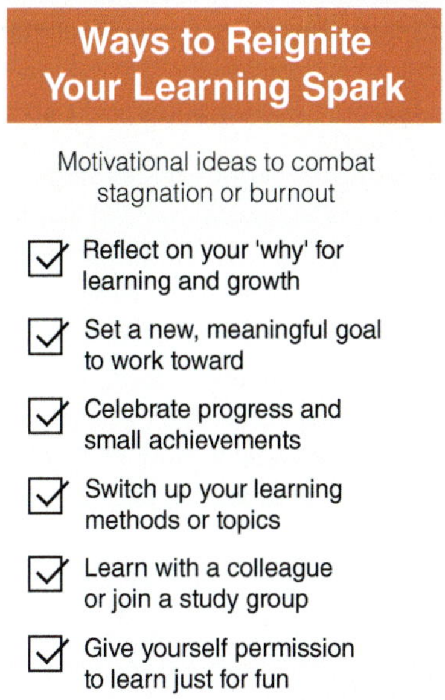
Ways to Reignite Your Learning Spark
Motivational ideas to combat stagnation or burnout
Reflect on your 'why' for learning and growth
Set a new, meaningful goal to work toward
Celebrate progress and small achievements
Switch up your learning methods or topics
Learn with a colleague or join a study group
Give yourself permission to learn just for fun

Figure 14.2 Strategies for rekindling motivation and engagement in professional learning. M Jennings, 2025.

Advanced training is not limited to formal credentialing programs. Veterinary technicians can also pursue focused continuing education in specific areas of interest, such as pain management, rehabilitation therapy, fear-free handling, and integrative medicine. These specialized skill sets allow technicians to offer advanced services within their current practice or transition into roles in specialty hospitals, research facilities, or academic institutions. For example, a veterinary technician trained in rehabilitation therapy may work closely with postoperative orthopedic patients to develop and implement recovery plans that improve mobility and reduce pain, directly enhancing patient outcomes.

The rise of telemedicine and remote patient monitoring technologies has also created new specialization opportunities for veterinary technicians. Technicians with advanced training in digital health tools and remote client communication are becoming increasingly valuable in practices that offer virtual consultations and follow-up care. This emerging area of specialization reflects the broader shifts in healthcare delivery and positions veterinary technicians to play key roles in expanding access to veterinary services (American Animal Hospital Association & American Veterinary Medical Association 2021).

Specialization can also extend beyond direct patient care. Veterinary technicians interested in practice management, education, and research may pursue advanced degrees or certifications in these areas. Programs in veterinary practice management prepare technicians to take on administrative and leadership roles, overseeing hospital operations, managing staff development, and improving business performance. Those passionate about education may pursue teaching opportunities within veterinary technology programs or contribute to professional conferences and continuing education platforms as subject matter experts. Technicians involved in research contribute to advancing veterinary medicine by participating in clinical trials, developing new protocols, and publishing in scientific journals.

Advanced training and specialization also play a critical role in supporting holistic nursing approaches. Veterinary technicians who pursue education in areas such as acupuncture, therapeutic massage, herbal medicine, and nutritional counseling can integrate these modalities into their patient care strategies. This holistic perspective addresses the full spectrum of patient needs, promoting physical, emotional, and environmental well-being. As pet owners increasingly seek integrative and alternative therapies for their animals, veterinary technicians trained in these areas provide valuable expertise that enhances client satisfaction and patient outcomes. In addition to formal programs, professional organizations and specialty academies frequently offer workshops, hands-on labs, and certification courses that support skill development in specialized areas. Attending these events not only strengthens clinical skills but also provides opportunities to connect with leaders in the field and explore emerging trends in veterinary medicine.

Pursuing advanced training and specialization requires dedication, time, and often financial investment, but the professional and personal rewards are significant. Veterinary technicians who commit to specialization experience greater confidence in their abilities, increased respect from colleagues and clients, and a more fulfilling career path. They become key contributors to their healthcare teams, playing specialized roles that directly impact patient care and the overall success of the practice. By seeking out opportunities for advanced training and specialization, veterinary technicians embrace a proactive approach to career development and patient advocacy. In doing so, they ensure that they remain not only relevant but indispensable in an ever-evolving field of veterinary medicine.

Navigating Credentialing and Certification Pathways

Navigating the various credentialing and certification pathways available to veterinary technicians is a critical step in advancing clinical expertise, professional recognition, and career satisfaction. While initial credentialing lays the foundation for clinical practice, the pursuit of specialized certifications and advanced academic degrees reflects a deep commitment to excellence and a desire to contribute at the highest levels of patient care and professional leadership.

The first milestone for most veterinary technicians is earning their initial credential through completion of an accredited veterinary technology program and successful passage of the Veterinary Technician National Examination (VTNE) (American Association of Veterinary State Boards [AAVSB] n.d.). This foundational credential allows veterinary technicians to meet state or provincial licensure or registration requirements, enabling them to legally practice and demonstrate competency in fundamental nursing skills. However, true professional growth often requires going beyond these minimum qualifications.

One of the most respected and rigorous forms of advanced credentialing is the VTS designation. Managed by academies recognized by the National Association of Veterinary Technicians in America (NAVTA), the VTS designation is available in several highly specialized areas. Each specialty academy sets strict requirements for eligibility, including a minimum number of years of clinical experience in the specialty area, a detailed skills log documenting advanced competency, comprehensive case reports, and successful completion of a specialty board examination (National Association of Veterinary Technicians in America [NAVTA] n.d.).

The most recognized VTS specialties include:

- **Emergency and Critical Care (VTS-ECC):** This specialty focuses on advanced knowledge and skills in the management of critically ill and emergent patients. Veterinary technicians working toward this certification gain expertise in life-saving interventions, advanced monitoring techniques, and critical care pharmacology.
- **Anesthesia and Analgesia (VTS-AA):** Technicians specializing in anesthesia and analgesia become highly skilled in anesthesia protocols, advanced monitoring, pain management strategies, and perioperative patient care, often working closely with board-certified veterinary anesthesiologists.
- **Internal Medicine (VTS-IM):** This specialty emphasizes advanced knowledge in complex disease processes across areas such as cardiology, nephrology, endocrinology, and gastroenterology, preparing technicians to support diagnostic and treatment plans for chronic and challenging medical conditions.
- **Dentistry (VTS-Dentistry):** Technicians specializing in dentistry focus on advanced dental procedures, oral surgery assistance, radiographic interpretation, and patient education regarding oral health.
- **Behavior (VTS-Behavior):** This specialty addresses advanced behavior modification techniques and management strategies for patients with behavioral disorders, including fear, aggression, and anxiety, integrating both medical and environmental solutions.
- **Nutrition (VTS-Nutrition):** Veterinary technicians in this specialty develop expertise in formulating nutritional plans for patients with specific medical conditions, including critical care nutrition, weight management, and therapeutic diets.
- **Zoological Medicine (VTS-ZM):** This highly specialized certification focuses on the care of exotic, zoo, and wildlife species, covering unique handling techniques, husbandry, and species-specific medical considerations.
- **Clinical Practice (VTS-CP):** This specialty allows veterinary technicians to demonstrate advanced competency in general clinical practice, often with a focus on one of three subcategories: canine/feline, production animal, or exotic companion animal.
- **Clinical Pathology (VTS-Clinical Pathology):** Technicians in this area specialize in laboratory diagnostics, including advanced hematology, cytology, urinalysis, and microbiology, playing a critical role in diagnostic interpretation and laboratory quality control.
- **Rehabilitation (VTS-Rehabilitation):** This emerging specialty focuses on physical therapy and rehabilitation for recovering patients, including postoperative orthopedic care, neurologic rehabilitation, and pain management through therapeutic exercise and modalities such as laser therapy and hydrotherapy.

In addition to the VTS credentials, many veterinary technicians are exploring academic pathways through advanced degree programs, including emerging master's degree opportunities. Traditionally, advanced academic pursuits for veterinary technicians were limited to bachelor's degrees; however, recent developments have created opportunities for master's-level education specifically tailored to veterinary nursing and technology.

Master's degree programs in Veterinary Nursing or Advanced Veterinary Practice provide a more comprehensive understanding of complex clinical concepts, leadership strategies, research methodology, and healthcare education. These programs often cater to veterinary professionals seeking roles in academia, clinical leadership, or advanced patient care management. Some universities offer Master of Science (MS) degrees in Veterinary Nursing, while others offer specialized tracks focusing on areas such as animal welfare, veterinary education, or hospital administration.

An example of this trend is the growing interest in combining advanced clinical certifications with formal academic credentials. A veterinary technician may pursue a VTS in Emergency and Critical Care while simultaneously earning a master's degree focused on leadership or healthcare education, preparing them for roles in hospital management, teaching, or research. These academic pathways support the ongoing evolution of veterinary nursing as a profession that demands both advanced clinical expertise and leadership capability.

For those interested in non-clinical advancement, there are also credentialing opportunities in areas such as practice management and education. The Certified Veterinary Practice Manager (CVPM) designation, for example, is a respected credential for veterinary professionals pursuing leadership and administrative roles. Earning the CVPM requires extensive experience in practice management, continuing education, and successful completion of a rigorous examination focused on business operations, human resources, and financial management within veterinary practices (Veterinary Hospital Managers Association [VHMA] n.d.).

Pursuing these advanced certifications and academic degrees requires significant time, financial investment, and dedication. However, the long-term benefits are substantial. Veterinary technicians with advanced credentials enjoy expanded career opportunities, increased earning potential, and greater professional recognition. They often become sought-after contributors to specialty hospitals, research institutions, veterinary schools, and leadership positions within their organizations.

By thoughtfully navigating credentialing and academic pathways, veterinary technicians not only elevate their own careers but also contribute to the growth and professionalization of veterinary nursing as a whole. Through specialization and advanced education, they help define the future of the profession, ensuring that veterinary nursing continues to evolve as a respected, highly skilled, and essential component of modern veterinary medicine.

Global and Interdisciplinary Perspectives on Continuing Education

Veterinary nursing is a dynamic and evolving profession that exists within a global healthcare ecosystem. While continuing education is a core professional value in many regions, its structure, accessibility, and recognition can vary widely across the world. By examining global and interdisciplinary perspectives, veterinary technicians can gain a broader understanding of what lifelong learning looks like beyond their immediate environment and discover fresh inspiration from other professions and cultures. This global awareness not only enhances personal growth but also strengthens the collective identity of veterinary technicians as essential healthcare providers in a rapidly changing world.

Across different countries, the expectations and models for continuing education in veterinary nursing reflect diverse regulatory systems and cultural values. In the United States, most states require a set number of CE hours for license renewal, often with guidelines around approved content or providers. In contrast, countries like the United Kingdom and Australia often include CE requirements within formal career development frameworks, such as the Royal College of Veterinary Surgeons' (RCVS) Continuing Professional Development (CPD) scheme or Australia's Veterinary Technicians Council CPD program. These systems emphasize reflection, goal-setting, and documentation—not just credit hours—encouraging veterinary technicians to engage in intentional and self-directed learning (Royal College of Veterinary Surgeons [RCVS] n.d.; Veterinary Nurses Council of Australia [VNCA] 2025).

Some countries have well-established credentialing systems for veterinary technicians and nurses, while others are still developing pathways toward national recognition. In regions where formal licensure does not yet exist, continuing education becomes even more critical for ensuring consistent standards of care and for building professional credibility. International veterinary nursing and technician organizations, such as the International Veterinary Technicians and Technicians Association (IVNTA), play an important role in supporting global learning efforts and sharing resources across borders. Engaging with these organizations can provide veterinary technicians with access to international webinars, virtual conferences, and networking opportunities that transcend geographical boundaries (International Veterinary Nurses and Technicians Association [IVNTA] n.d.).

Learning from human healthcare professions can also provide valuable insights into the future of continuing education in veterinary nursing. In human nursing, for example, professional development often includes competencies in leadership, research literacy, evidence-based practice, and ethics—areas that are increasingly relevant to veterinary medicine. Many human nursing programs use portfolios, mentorship frameworks, and reflective journaling as core components of CE, highlighting the importance of personal insight and professional identity formation alongside technical knowledge. By adopting similar strategies, veterinary technicians can create more holistic and individualized learning experiences.

Additionally, interdisciplinary collaboration offers rich opportunities for growth. Veterinary technicians who attend CE events with colleagues from fields like animal behavior, social work, rehabilitation, or shelter medicine gain exposure to different philosophies, communication styles, and problem-solving approaches. These cross-disciplinary experiences can broaden clinical insight and improve the ability to work within complex, team-based environments. For example, attending a workshop on grief counseling led by a licensed therapist may enhance a veterinary technician's ability to support clients during euthanasia appointments. Engaging with a physiotherapist during a pain management course may inspire a deeper understanding of rehabilitation techniques. Learning does not always have to remain within the veterinary bubble—in fact, it becomes more impactful when it transcends it.

Technology has further blurred geographical and disciplinary lines, making it easier than ever to engage in cross-cultural and cross-professional learning. Veterinary technicians can now join global online communities, attend international conferences virtually, and participate in educational exchanges with professionals around the world. These opportunities not only provide exposure to different clinical protocols but also promote cultural sensitivity, respect for diversity, and a sense of global solidarity in the pursuit of animal welfare.

Veterinary technicians working in multicultural communities also benefit from understanding how cultural norms and belief systems influence client decision-making, treatment adherence, and perceptions of veterinary care. Continuing education that includes cultural competence, global ethics, and communication across cultural barriers enhances a technician's ability to provide compassionate, inclusive care. For example, learning how different cultures view end-of-life decisions, animal ownership, or pain expression allows veterinary technicians to approach clients with greater empathy and clarity.

By embracing global and interdisciplinary perspectives, veterinary technicians expand their professional horizons and discover new possibilities for growth, collaboration, and innovation. This broader view fosters humility, adaptability, and curiosity—key traits in both holistic nursing and lifelong learning. Whether exploring international CE offerings, attending interprofessional seminars, or engaging in cross-cultural mentorship, veterinary technicians position themselves at the forefront of an interconnected, progressive, and deeply compassionate profession (Table 14.2).

Developing a Personal Learning Plan

A personal learning plan is a structured approach to professional growth that allows veterinary technicians to assess their current skills, identify areas for improvement, set realistic goals, and track progress over time. In a fast-paced field like veterinary medicine, where new technologies, treatments, and best practices are constantly emerging, having a clear and organized learning plan ensures that professional development remains intentional and aligned with long-term career aspirations. Without this level of structure, continuing education efforts can become reactive and fragmented, leading to missed opportunities for meaningful growth.

The first step in developing a personal learning plan is conducting an honest self-assessment. This involves reflecting on both strengths and weaknesses across a wide range of competencies, including technical skills, clinical knowledge, communication abilities, leadership qualities, and emotional resilience. Veterinary technicians should ask themselves what

Table 14.2 Global CE comparison table.

Country	CE Required?	System or Organization	Unique Feature
The United States	Yes (varies by state)	State Boards/AVMA/AAVSB RACE	Focus on CE hours and state renewal
The United Kingdom	Yes	Royal College of Veterinary Surgeons (RCVS)	Portfolio-based CPD with reflective documentation
Australia	Yes	Veterinary Technicians Council of Australia (VNCA)	CPD logbook required for credentialed technicians
Canada	Yes (in most provinces)	Provincial Veterinary Technician Associations	Peer-reviewed CE often required for renewal

aspects of their daily work bring confidence and satisfaction, and where they experience uncertainty or discomfort. Seeking feedback from supervisors, colleagues, and mentors can provide valuable outside perspectives that reveal skill gaps or developmental opportunities that might not be immediately apparent.

Once areas for growth have been identified, the next step is to establish clear, measurable goals. These goals should be specific and actionable, rather than vague aspirations. For example, rather than setting a general goal like "improve anesthesia skills," a more effective objective would be "complete an advanced anesthesia monitoring workshop within the next six months and apply learned techniques in daily practice." Setting timelines and defining success criteria helps maintain focus and accountability, ensuring that goals remain a priority even amidst the demands of daily clinical work.

Personal learning plans should also include a variety of educational modalities to support different learning styles and maximize engagement. Formal continuing education courses, hands-on workshops, professional conferences, and specialty certification programs provide structured opportunities for in-depth learning. Informal learning activities, such as reading veterinary journals, participating in case discussions, and watching instructional videos, complement these experiences and help reinforce new knowledge. Engaging in mentorship relationships, both as a mentee and mentor, further supports skill development and fosters professional growth through shared experiences.

Personal Learning Plan Template

Name:
Role:
Date Started:
Review Date:

1. Self-Assessment

Describe your current role and primary responsibilities.
What are your strengths as a veterinary technician?
What challenges or areas for improvement have you identified?

2. Learning Goals

List 2–3 specific, measurable learning goals.
Include a mix of technical, soft skills, and professional development goals.

Goal	Why it Matters	Timeline	How You'll Achieve It

An important component of any learning plan is ongoing self-evaluation and progress tracking. Veterinary technicians should regularly review their learning goals, assess their progress, and make adjustments as needed. Career development is a dynamic process, and as new opportunities arise or career interests evolve, learning plans should be updated to reflect these changes. Keeping a professional portfolio that documents completed courses, certifications, case studies, and personal reflections is a valuable tool for tracking achievements and identifying new learning.

Veterinary technicians should also consider how their personal learning plans align with their long-term career goals. Those interested in pursuing leadership roles may include training in management, mentorship, or conflict resolution. Technicians focused on clinical excellence may prioritize advanced technical skills and specialty certifications. By aligning short-term learning goals with broader career aspirations, veterinary technicians create a roadmap for long-term success and satisfaction.

Developing a personal learning plan also supports emotional well-being and job satisfaction. When veterinary technicians have a clear path toward professional growth, they experience a greater sense of purpose and direction. This proactive approach reduces the likelihood of career stagnation and burnout, common challenges in a demanding profession where emotional labor is high and recognition is sometimes limited. A well-structured learning plan provides a sense of control and progress, even during challenging times.

Incorporating the principles of holistic nursing into a personal learning plan ensures that professional development efforts address not only technical competencies but also the emotional and relational aspects of patient care. Including goals related to improving client communication, learning about animal behavior and welfare, and developing stress management techniques enhances the technician's ability to provide comprehensive, compassionate care that supports the well-being of both patients and their human caregivers.

Ultimately, a personal learning plan is a powerful tool for veterinary technicians who are committed to lifelong learning and professional excellence. By taking ownership of their growth and intentionally seeking opportunities for development, veterinary technicians ensure that they remain engaged, competent, and fulfilled throughout their careers. This structured approach to learning not only benefits the individual but also contributes to the advancement of the veterinary nursing profession as a whole.

Personal Learning Plan: Sophia—Emergency/Critical Care Technician

Sophia, a veterinary technician working in an emergency and critical care facility, realized during a particularly difficult overnight shift that she struggled to manage ventilator-dependent patients confidently. After reviewing her experiences and discussing them with her clinical manager, she identified advanced respiratory management as an area for growth. Her personal learning plan included attending a critical care ventilation workshop, completing online continuing education courses in advanced respiratory support, and shadowing a VTS-certified technician during ventilator cases for additional hands-on experience. Within six months, Sophia had developed a new level of comfort with ventilator management, and her supervisors noticed a significant improvement in her confidence and effectiveness during critical cases.

A comprehensive learning plan should also include a balance of formal and informal learning opportunities. Formal education may include attending conferences, enrolling in advanced certification programs, or participating in hands-on workshops. Informal learning can involve activities like reading clinical journals, joining case discussions, or participating in hospital-based learning rounds. Diversifying the types of learning experiences not only accommodates different learning styles but also ensures that knowledge is reinforced through multiple modalities.

Veterinary technicians should also consider how their personal learning plans support long-term career aspirations. For instance, if a technician aspires to specialize in oncology, their plan may include shadowing an oncologist, attending a conference focused on cancer therapies, and beginning to prepare for the VTS certification in oncology when available. If leadership is the desired path, the plan may focus on developing soft skills, such as conflict resolution, mentorship, and practice management education.

Name: Sophia
Role: Emergency/Critical Care Technician
Date Started: January 10, 2025
Review Date: July 10, 2025

1. Self-Assessment

I work in an overnight ER setting. My strengths include patient triage and catheter placement. I struggle with confidence when managing patients on ventilators. I also want to improve my client communication, especially during discharge.

2. Learning Goals

Goal	Why it Matters	Timeline	How You'll Achieve It
Learn ventilator management protocols	Improve confidence and patient outcomes in critical cases	Within six months	Attend CE, shadow VTS-EC, complete three hands-on shifts
Strengthen communication during discharge	Enhance client trust and reduce callback errors	Within three months	Role-play with mentor, study written scripts, get feedback
Begin preparing for VTS-ECC certification	Long-term career development goal	Ongoing	Download handbook, join online study group

Personal Learning Plan: James—Transitioning into Management

James, a veterinary technician with five years of general practice experience, aspired to move into a practice management role. His learning plan included completing a leadership course through a veterinary management organization, enrolling in a business communication class at his local community college, and attending his state veterinary technician association's annual leadership workshop. Over the next year, he actively pursued mentorship from his hospital manager and began participating in hiring interviews and team meetings. His proactive approach positioned him to be promoted to lead technician within his practice, setting the stage for a future transition into management.

Tracking progress is a vital component of any personal learning plan. Veterinary technicians should maintain a professional portfolio that includes completed courses, certifications earned, case studies or presentations developed, and personal reflections on lessons learned. This portfolio serves not only as a record of achievement but also as a motivational tool, providing tangible evidence of growth and development over time. In addition, incorporating holistic nursing principles into a personal learning plan ensures that professional growth addresses more than just technical skills. For example, a technician might set a goal to improve patient handling techniques that reduce stress and fear, becoming certified in fear-free or low-stress handling practices. Another goal might focus on improving client communication during emotionally challenging situations, particularly surrounding end-of-life care. These goals enhance the technician's ability to provide well-rounded, compassionate care that supports the physical and emotional well-being of both patients and clients.

Name: James
Role: Veterinary Technician, General Practice
Date Started: February 1, 2025
Review Date: August 1, 2025

1. Self-Assessment

I have five years of experience in general practice and am interested in moving into a management role. I enjoy mentoring new technicians and participating in hospital operations, but I lack formal leadership training and business communication skills. I'd like to build confidence in leading team discussions and handling staff concerns professionally.

2. Learning Goals

Goal	Why it Matters	Timeline	How You'll Achieve It
Complete leadership training	Prepare for practice management responsibilities	Within six months	Enroll in a veterinary management leadership course
Improve communication skills	Support team leadership and client interaction	Within three months	Take a business communication course at local community college
Gain mentorship and leadership exposure	Build real-world leadership experience	Over one year	Shadow hospital manager, participate in interviews and staff meetings

Personal Learning Plan: Maria—Emotional Resilience in Shelter Medicine

Maria, a veterinary technician working in a busy shelter environment, found that she was emotionally drained by the constant exposure to euthanasia cases and the stress of managing high case volumes. Her personal learning plan included attending a compassion fatigue workshop, integrating mindfulness practices into her daily routine, and leading monthly emotional debriefing sessions for her team. Over time, she experienced improved emotional resilience and became a peer leader in helping colleagues manage workplace stress.

By building a structured, realistic, and actionable personal learning plan, veterinary technicians can remain proactive about their growth and well-being. This deliberate approach fosters a greater sense of purpose and satisfaction, keeps skills sharp and relevant, and positions veterinary technicians to take advantage of emerging opportunities throughout their careers. In doing so, they not only advance their own professional journey but also contribute to the continuous elevation of the veterinary nursing profession.

Name: Maria
Role: Veterinary Technician, Shelter Medicine
Date Started: March 15, 2025
Review Date: September 15, 2025

1. Self-Assessment

Working in a high-volume shelter has taken an emotional toll on me, especially with frequent euthanasias and limited resources. I feel myself becoming emotionally exhausted and less present with patients. I want to improve my emotional resilience and become a supportive presence for my team.

2. Learning Goals

Goal	Why it Matters	Timeline	How You'll Achieve It
Address compassion fatigue	Improve emotional resilience and prevent burnout	Within three months	Attend a compassion fatigue workshop
Integrate self-care practices	Support mental health and sustainable performance	Immediate and Ongoing	Adopt mindfulness into daily routine
Support team wellness	Foster a culture of emotional well-being within the workplace	Monthly	Lead emotional debriefing sessions for shelter team

The Role of Mentorship in Professional Development

Mentorship plays a pivotal role in the professional development of veterinary technicians, providing a bridge between foundational knowledge and advanced clinical expertise. While formal education and continuing education programs offer critical theoretical and technical instruction, mentorship brings those lessons to life through real-world application and personal guidance. Engaging in both sides of the mentorship relationship, as a mentee and eventually as a mentor, supports lifelong learning, strengthens professional identity, and fosters a culture of collaboration and growth within the veterinary profession.

For veterinary technicians in the early stages of their careers, having a mentor provides a trusted source of support and guidance as they navigate the complexities of clinical practice. The transition from the academic environment to a fast-paced clinical setting can be overwhelming, and new veterinary technicians often face challenges in building confidence, mastering advanced technical skills, and learning how to handle emotionally charged client interactions. A skilled mentor helps ease this transition by sharing practical knowledge, demonstrating critical thinking during patient care, and offering constructive feedback that builds competence without diminishing confidence.

Mentorship is particularly valuable in helping veterinary technicians develop the soft skills that are essential to professional success but are not always covered comprehensively in formal education. These skills include effective communication with clients and colleagues, conflict resolution, stress management, and leadership development. Observing how a mentor handles complex situations—such as delivering difficult news to a client or managing disagreements within the veterinary team—provides mentees with practical models of professionalism in action. Through regular check-ins and reflective discussions, mentors help mentees process their experiences, recognize their progress, and identify areas for continued growth.

Mentorship also facilitates access to professional networks and career advancement opportunities. Experienced mentors can introduce their mentees to influential professionals, recommend valuable continuing education programs, and provide guidance on navigating credentialing pathways. This exposure broadens the mentee's understanding of the diverse career opportunities available within veterinary nursing, from clinical specialization to roles in education, research, and practice management.

As veterinary technicians gain experience and confidence, stepping into the role of mentor becomes a natural progression in their professional development. Serving as a mentor not only reinforces the mentor's own knowledge but also fosters leadership skills and deepens their commitment to the profession. By guiding less experienced colleagues, mentors contribute to the ongoing improvement of patient care standards and help build a supportive, collaborative workplace culture. This reciprocal relationship between mentor and mentee benefits both parties, enhancing job satisfaction and promoting professional resilience.

The impact of mentorship extends beyond individual relationships; it shapes the culture of veterinary practices and the profession as a whole. Organizations that cultivate structured mentorship programs often experience lower staff turnover, higher job satisfaction, and stronger teamwork. When mentorship is prioritized, new employees feel welcomed and supported, experienced staff are empowered to lead, and the entire team benefits from a shared commitment to continuous improvement.

From a holistic nursing perspective, mentorship also supports the emotional well-being of veterinary technicians. The demands of the profession can lead to burnout and compassion fatigue, particularly when technicians feel isolated or unsupported in their roles. Having a mentor to provide guidance, encouragement, and emotional support helps veterinary technicians navigate difficult situations with greater resilience. Mentorship relationships create safe spaces for discussing professional challenges, processing emotional experiences, and developing healthy coping strategies.

To fully benefit from mentorship, both mentees and mentors must approach the relationship with intention and openness. Mentees should be proactive in seeking feedback, asking questions, and reflecting on their experiences. Mentors should provide honest, constructive guidance while fostering a supportive and nonjudgmental learning environment. Setting clear expectations and goals for the mentorship relationship ensures that both parties remain engaged and focused on professional growth.

Mentorship is a cornerstone of professional development in veterinary nursing. It accelerates skill acquisition, builds confidence, and creates lasting professional relationships that support career advancement and personal well-being. Through mentorship, veterinary technicians contribute to a culture of excellence that elevates their profession and ensures the delivery of compassionate, high-quality care to the patients and clients they serve.

Interview at a High Level

Interviewing at a high level is not only a valuable skill for career advancement but also a critical component of a veterinary technician's broader professional development journey. Each interview is an opportunity to assess how well a prospective role aligns with personal growth goals and to demonstrate the competencies and mindset that have been intentionally cultivated through continuing education and skill development. Viewing interviews as part of a strategic professional development plan transforms them from stressful events into purposeful conversations about career progression and the pursuit of excellence.

A key element of high-level interviewing is demonstrating how past professional development efforts have prepared you for advanced responsibilities. Veterinary technicians who have invested time in continuing education courses, pursued specialty certifications, or participated in mentorship programs should be prepared to articulate how these experiences have shaped their clinical expertise and professional identity. Employers seeking high-caliber candidates want to understand not just what skills you have acquired, but how you have applied them to improve patient outcomes, mentor colleagues, or contribute to workplace initiatives.

For example, a veterinary technician who recently completed a leadership development program might share how they successfully led a project to improve discharge instructions for postoperative patients, resulting in better client compliance and reduced complications. This kind of real-world application demonstrates that the candidate is not only committed to learning but also capable of translating that learning into meaningful workplace improvements.

High-level interviews also provide a platform to outline future development goals. A candidate who is actively working toward a VTS certification or planning to pursue an advanced degree in veterinary nursing demonstrates ambition and a forward-thinking approach to career growth. Framing these future goals within the context of how they will benefit the hospital or team shows interviewers that you are invested in mutual success, not just personal advancement.

In this way, interviews become an extension of a veterinary technician's personal learning plan. Preparing for a high-level interview should include a review of this plan, allowing candidates to confidently discuss both past achievements and how the prospective role fits into their broader vision for growth. This reinforces the idea that career advancement is a continuous process, driven by intentional learning and self-reflection.

Employers seeking highly qualified veterinary technicians are not only interested in clinical proficiency but also in the leadership qualities and emotional intelligence that contribute to a positive and productive workplace culture. Candidates who can articulate how their professional development efforts have enhanced their soft skills—such as conflict resolution, team collaboration, and effective client communication—position themselves as well-rounded professionals who bring both technical expertise and emotional maturity to their roles.

Finally, high-level interviews are an opportunity for candidates to evaluate how well a prospective employer supports professional development. Asking thoughtful questions about mentorship opportunities, access to continuing education, and support for advanced certifications ensures that the next career move aligns with long-term growth objectives. By approaching interviews through this lens, veterinary technicians actively participate in shaping a career path that fosters ongoing learning, personal fulfillment, and professional excellence.

Finding a Workplace that Prioritizes Continued Development

Choosing the right workplace is one of the most critical decisions a veterinary technician can make to support their long-term professional development. While salary, location, and job duties are important considerations, the true measure of a fulfilling and sustainable career often lies in the opportunities a workplace provides for growth, education, and advancement. Veterinary technicians who align themselves with organizations that actively support continuing education and professional development set the stage for a career marked by ongoing learning, increased job satisfaction, and expanded opportunities for advancement.

Identifying a workplace that prioritizes development begins with careful evaluation of the organization's culture. Practices that value professional growth often make their commitment visible through structured mentorship programs, regular continuing education events, and financial support for certifications and advanced training. During the interview process, candidates should inquire about how the hospital supports the professional development of its nursing team. A practice that proudly describes its mentorship initiatives, education stipends, or in-house training opportunities is more likely to foster a growth-oriented environment.

One of the clearest indicators of a development-focused workplace is the presence of formal mentorship programs. In these environments, new hires are paired with experienced veterinary technicians or supervisors who provide guidance, feedback, and hands-on training during the onboarding process and beyond. Structured mentorship not only helps new staff members acclimate to the hospital's protocols and expectations but also demonstrates that the organization values its employees' long-term success and growth.

Another key factor to assess is the practice's willingness to support and fund continuing education. High-quality veterinary hospitals often provide paid time off for attending conferences, reimburse tuition for relevant courses, or host in-house educational workshops. Some organizations even maintain formal partnerships with credentialing bodies and actively encourage their veterinary technicians to pursue advanced certifications such as the VTS designation. When a workplace invests financially in its employees' development, it signals a genuine commitment to fostering professional excellence.

Real-world Example: At a progressive specialty hospital, the leadership team implemented a continuing education allowance of $1,500 per technician annually, in addition to covering travel expenses for national conferences. The hospital also hosted quarterly skills labs and brought in specialists to conduct workshops on advanced anesthesia techniques and emergency critical care protocols. As a result, the nursing team not only developed advanced clinical skills but also experienced higher job satisfaction and lower turnover rates. Many of the technicians successfully obtained VTS certifications and moved into senior leadership roles within the hospital.

In addition to formal education support, a development-focused workplace encourages cross-training and exposure to specialized areas of veterinary medicine. Veterinary technicians are provided opportunities to rotate through different departments, learn from specialists, and develop competencies in areas such as surgery, internal medicine, critical care, and rehabilitation. This exposure not only builds clinical expertise but also allows veterinary technicians to discover areas of interest that may shape their future career paths.

Workplaces that prioritize continued development also emphasize leadership and career advancement opportunities. Rather than viewing veterinary technicians as static roles within the organization, these hospitals create clear pathways for growth into leadership positions, such as lead technician, department supervisor, or practice manager. Veterinary technicians interested in teaching or mentorship may be offered opportunities to develop and lead training programs or become involved in onboarding new staff. This culture of advancement ensures that motivated professionals have opportunities to contribute at higher levels, fostering long-term engagement and satisfaction.

Another important consideration is the hospital's approach to emotional and mental well-being. Development-focused workplaces understand that supporting their teams extends beyond clinical education. They offer resources for managing compassion fatigue and burnout, encourage healthy work-life balance, and promote open communication about workplace challenges. A holistic approach to development recognizes that personal well-being and professional growth are interconnected and equally important.

When evaluating a potential employer, candidates should ask specific questions to determine whether the workplace supports professional development:

- "What opportunities are available for continuing education and advanced certification?"
- "Does the hospital offer financial support or paid time off for attending conferences or workshops?"
- "Are there mentorship programs or structured onboarding processes for new team members?"
- "How does the hospital support veterinary technicians interested in pursuing leadership roles or specialization?"

Veterinary technicians who intentionally seek out workplaces that invest in their growth not only advance their careers but also ensure that they work in environments where their contributions are valued and their futures are supported. This proactive approach to workplace selection fosters a career defined by continued learning, personal satisfaction, and professional excellence.

Conclusion

Continuing education and professional development are not optional luxuries in veterinary nursing—they are essential components of a thriving, sustainable, and fulfilling career. In a profession that evolves rapidly with new medical advancements, patient care techniques, and growing expectations for the veterinary technician's role, those who remain committed to lifelong learning ensure that their skills remain sharp, their knowledge current, and their contributions impactful.

Throughout this chapter, we have explored how veterinary technicians can intentionally shape their careers through personal learning plans, strategic credentialing pathways, mentorship, and the pursuit of advanced training and specialization. These efforts not only elevate individual competence and confidence but also advance the profession as a whole. As veterinary technicians achieve higher levels of clinical expertise, leadership capability, and professional recognition, they play a critical role in shaping the future of patient care and advocating for their profession's rightful place within the healthcare team. Finding workplaces that support continued development and mastering the art of high-level interviewing empower veterinary technicians to align their career paths with environments that foster growth, collaboration, and excellence. By prioritizing professional development, veterinary technicians create opportunities for themselves to lead, mentor, and inspire others while delivering the highest quality of care to their patients. The journey of professional development is a lifelong commitment to becoming not only a more skilled veterinary technician but also a more fulfilled and resilient professional. Through this commitment, veterinary technicians ensure that their careers remain dynamic, their personal growth continuous, and their impact on the lives of patients, clients, and colleagues immeasurable.

References

American Animal Hospital Association, & American Veterinary Medical Association. (2021). 2021 AAHA/AVMA telehealth guidelines for small-animal practice. https://www.aaha.org/wp-content/uploads/globalassets/02-guidelines/telehealth/2021-aaha-avma-telehealth-guidelines.pdf

American Association of Veterinary State Boards. (n.d.). Veterinary Technician National Exam (VTNE). https://www.aavsb.org/students-exams/veterinary-technician-national-exam/

International Veterinary Nurses and Technicians Association. (n.d.). IVNTA. https://www.ivnta.org/

National Association of Veterinary Technicians in America. (n.d.). List of approved academies (VTS). https://navta.net/veterinary-technician-specialties/list-of-approved-academies/

Royal College of Veterinary Surgeons. (n.d.). Continuing professional development (CPD). https://www.rcvs.org.uk/lifelong-learning/continuing-professional-development-cpd/

Veterinary Hospital Managers Association (n.d.). About certification: Certified Veterinary Practice Manager (CVPM). https://www.vhma.org/certificatesandcertification/cvpmroadmap/cvpmaboutcertification

Veterinary Nurses Council of Australia. (2025). AVNAT Registration Scheme. https://www.vnca.asn.au/avnat/

Index

d

i

m

n

t

u